THIRD EDITION

Tunable Laser Applications

OPTICAL SCIENCE AND ENGINEERING

Founding Editor
Brian J. Thompson
University of Rochester
Rochester, New York

RECENTLY PUBLISHED

Tunable Laser Applications, Third Edition, *edited by F. J. Duarte*
Laser Safety: Tools and Training, Second Edition, *edited by Ken Barat*
Optical Materials and Applications, *edited by Moriaki Wakaki*
Lightwave Engineering, *Yasuo Kokubun*
Handbook of Optical and Laser Scanning, Second Edition, *Gerald F. Marshall
    and Glenn E. Stutz*
Computational Methods for Electromagnetic and Optical Systems, Second Edition,
    John M. Jarem and Partha P. Banerjee
Optical Methods of Measurement: Wholefield Techniques, Second Edition, *Rajpal S. Sirohi*
Optoelectronics: Infrared-Visible-Ultraviolet Devices and Applications, Second Edition,
    edited by Dave Birtalan and William Nunley
Photoacoustic Imaging and Spectroscopy, *edited by Lihong V. Wang*
Polarimetric Radar Imaging: From Basics to Applications, *Jong-Sen Lee and Eric Pottier*
Near-Earth Laser Communications, *edited by Hamid Hemmati*
Slow Light: Science and Applications, *edited by Jacob B. Khurgin and Rodney S. Tucker*
Dynamic Laser Speckle and Applications, *edited by Hector J. Rabal and Roberto A. Braga Jr.*
Biochemical Applications of Nonlinear Optical Spectroscopy, *edited by Vladislav Yakovlev*
Optical and Photonic MEMS Devices: Design, Fabrication and Control, *edited by Ai-Qun Liu*
The Nature of Light: What Is a Photon?, *edited by Chandrasekhar Roychoudhuri,
    A. F. Kracklauer, and Katherine Creath*
Introduction to Nonimaging Optics, *Julio Chaves*
Introduction to Organic Electronic and Optoelectronic Materials and Devices,
    edited by Sam-Shajing Sun and Larry R. Dalton
Fiber Optic Sensors, Second Edition, *edited by Shizhuo Yin, Paul B. Ruffin, and Francis T. S. Yu*
Terahertz Spectroscopy: Principles and Applications, *edited by Susan L. Dexheimer*
Photonic Signal Processing: Techniques and Applications, *Le Nguyen Binh*
Smart CMOS Image Sensors and Applications, *Jun Ohta*
Organic Field-Effect Transistors, *Zhenan Bao and Jason Locklin*
Coarse Wavelength Division Multiplexing: Technologies and Applications,
    edited by Hans Joerg Thiele and Marcus Nebeling

*Please visit our website **www.crcpress.com** for a full list of titles*

THIRD EDITION

Tunable Laser Applications

EDITED BY

F.J. DUARTE

Interferometric Optics
Rochester, New York, USA

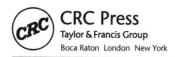

CRC Press
Taylor & Francis Group
Boca Raton London New York

CRC Press is an imprint of the
Taylor & Francis Group, an **informa** business

MATLAB® is a trademark of The MathWorks, Inc. and is used with permission. The MathWorks does not warrant the accuracy of the text or exercises in this book. This book's use or discussion of MATLAB® software or related products does not constitute endorsement or sponsorship by The MathWorks of a particular pedagogical approach or particular use of the MATLAB® software.

CRC Press
Taylor & Francis Group
6000 Broken Sound Parkway NW, Suite 300
Boca Raton, FL 33487-2742

First issued in paperback 2019

ISBN-13: 978-1-4822-6106-6 (hbk)
ISBN-13: 978-0-367-87102-4 (pbk)

Visit the Taylor & Francis Web site at
http://www.taylorandfrancis.com

and the CRC Press Web site at
http://www.crcpress.com

Dedication

In memory of our dear friends, colleagues, and coauthors:
Roberto Sastre (1944–2010) and Robert Owens James (1944–2015).

Contents

Preface

Broadly tunable lasers continue to have a tremendous impact in many and diverse fields of science and technology. From a renaissance in laser spectroscopy, to Bose–Einstein condensation, the one nexus is … *the tunable laser*. In this regard, numerous applications, from physics, to isotope separation, and all the way to medicine, depend on the tunable laser. This third edition includes 14 chapters. In this collection of chapters, two chapters are new, and all the other chapters have been updated and extended in their coverage. The subject matter ranges from the physics of tunable coherent sources and coherent microscopic instrumentation to exciting applications such as astronomy, defense, medicine, laser isotope separation, microscopy, and spectroscopy.

It is indeed a pleasure to offer to the scientific community this updated and enlarged third edition of *Tunable Laser Applications*. As editor, I remain indebted to all the contributing authors.

F. J. Duarte
Rochester, New York

MATLAB® is a registered trademark of The MathWorks, Inc. For product information, please contact:

The MathWorks, Inc.
3 Apple Hill Drive
Natick, MA 01760-2098 USA
Tel: 508 647 7000
Fax: 508-647-7001
E-mail: info@mathworks.com
Web: www.mathworks.com

Editor

F. J. Duarte is a research physicist with Interferometric Optics, Rochester, New York, and adjunct professor at Electrical and Computer Engineering, University of New Mexico. He graduated with first-class honors in physics from the School of Mathematics and Physics at Macquarie University (Sydney, Australia), where he was also awarded a PhD in physics for his research on optically pumped molecular lasers. At Macquarie, he was a student of the well-known quantum physicist J. C. Ward. Duarte's research has taken place at a number of institutions in academia, industry, and the defense establishment. Dr. Duarte is the author of the generalized multiple-prism dispersion theory and has made various unique contributions to the physics and architecture of tunable laser oscillators. He has also pioneered the use of Dirac's quantum notation in interferometry, oscillator physics, and classical optics. These contributions have found applications in the design of laser resonators, laser pulse compression, imaging, microscopy, medicine, optics communications, the nuclear industry, and quantum entanglement. He is the lead author of numerous refereed papers and several U.S. patents. Dr. Duarte is author and editor of *Dye Laser Principles* (Academic 1990), *High-Power Dye Lasers* (Springer 1991), *Selected Papers on Dye Lasers* (SPIE 1992), *Tunable Lasers Handbook* (Academic 1995), *Tunable Laser Applications* (1st edn, Marcel Dekker 1995; 2nd edn, CRC Press 2009; 3rd edn, CRC Press 2016), *Coherence and Ultrashort Pulsed Laser Emission* (InTech 2010), and *Laser Pulse Phenomena and Applications* (InTech 2010). He is also the sole author of *Tunable Laser Optics* (1st edn, Elsevier-Academic 2003; 2nd edn, CRC Press 2015) and *Quantum Optics for Engineers* (CRC Press 2014). Dr. Duarte is a fellow of the Australian Institute of Physics and a fellow of the Optical Society, and received the Engineering Excellence Award from the Optical Society of America.

Contributors

A. Costela
Instituto de Química Física
   "Rocasolano", C.S.I.C.
Madrid, Spain

F. J. Duarte
Interferometric Optics
Rochester, New York

and

Electrical and Computer Engineering
University of New Mexico
Albuquerque, New Mexico

I. García-Moreno
Instituto de Química Física
   "Rocasolano", C.S.I.C.
Madrid, Spain

C. Gómez
Instituto de Química Física
   "Rocasolano", C.S.I.C.
Madrid, Spain

J. G. Haub
Laser Technologies Group
Cyber & Electronic Warfare Division
Defence Science and Technology Group
Edinburgh, South Australia, Australia

Y. He
National Measurement Institute

and

MQ Photonics Research Centre
Department of Physics and Astronomy
Macquarie University
Sydney, New South Wales, Australia

R. O. James
Interferometric Optics
Rochester, New York

B. J. Orr
MQ Photonics Research Centre
Department of Physics and
   Astronomy
Macquarie University
Sydney, New South Wales, Australia

S. Popov
Royal Institute of Technology
Stockholm, Sweden

R. Sastre
Instituto de Ciencia y Tecnología de
   Polímeros, C.S.I.C.
Madrid, Spain

T. M. Shay
Shay Electro-Optical Engineering
Saint George, Utah

R. T. White
Institute for Photonics and Advanced
   Sensing and School of Physical
   Sciences
The University of Adelaide
Adelaide, South Australia, Australia

1 Introduction

F. J. Duarte

CONTENTS

1.1 INTRODUCTION

The ability to yield tunable coherent radiation enhances the applicability of a given laser substantially. Indeed, tunable lasers are among the most studied and successful lasers known today. For instance, the first broadly tunable laser, *the organic dye laser*, introduced circa 1966 [1–4], has enjoyed a significant amount of attention directed toward the study of its inherent physical properties and technology [5–12]. At the same time, these organic lasers have had a profound impact on a plethora of fields, including physics, spectroscopy, laser isotope separation, medicine, and astronomy [6,13–16].

Today, the field of broadly tunable lasers includes an array of different lasers, which have markedly extended the applicability domain of lasers. In addition to the broadly tunable organic dye lasers, there are broadly tunable semiconductor lasers, optical parametric oscillators (OPOs), tunable fiber lasers, tunable quantum cascade lasers, and free electron lasers (FELs). Also, at this stage, it should be realized that in addition to the class of broadly tunable lasers, there is an additional group of discretely tunable or line-tunable lasers. This latter class of laser, besides being able to shift emission frequency from transition to transition, can also be fine-tuned within the emission spectrum of a given transition.

In Tables 1.1 through 1.5, basic tuning ranges and energetic properties of tunable sources of coherent radiation are provided to facilitate rapid familiarity with the emission characteristics offered by these sources.

Table 1.1 lists the wavelength coverage published for various broadly tunable pulsed sources of coherent radiation, including the OPO and the FEL. Table 1.2 lists reported short pulse durations demonstrated in several types of broadly tunable lasers, while Table 1.3 includes the energetic and power characteristics capabilities for tunable pulsed lasers.

Table 1.4 lists the emission characteristics from broadly tunable lasers in the continuous-wave (CW) regime, including wavelength range and reported

1

TABLE 1.1
Wavelength Range of Broadly Tunable Coherent Sources in the Pulsed Regime

Tunable Source	Spectral Range
Dye laser	$320 \leq \lambda \leq 1200$ nm[a] [17]
$Ti^{3+}:Al_2O_3$ laser	$660 \leq \lambda \leq 986$ nm [18]
$Cr^{3+}:BeAl_2O_4$ laser	$701 \leq \lambda \leq 818$ nm [19]
Fiber laser[b]	$980 \leq \lambda \leq 1070$ nm [20]
OPO (BBO)[c]	$0.3 \leq \lambda \leq 3.0$ µm [21]
OPO (KTP)[c]	$0.7 \leq \lambda \leq 4.0$ µm [21]
FEL	$0.9 \leq \lambda \leq 10$ µm[d] [22]
	$830 \leq \lambda \leq 940$ nm[e] [23]
	$31 \leq \lambda \leq 32$ nm [24]

[a] Tuning range resulting from the use of several dyes.
[b] Yb-doped fiber.
[c] BBO, β-barium borate; KTP, potassium titanyl phosphate.
[d] The combined tuning range from various FEL facilities extends into the millimeter range.
[e] Large bandwidth.

TABLE 1.2
Short Pulse Emission Characteristics of Broadly Tunable Coherent Sources

Tunable Source	Δt
Dye laser	6 fs[a] [25]
$Ti^{3+}:Al_2O_3$ laser	5 fs[b] [26]
ECS[c] laser (AlGaAs)	200 fs[a] [27]
Fiber laser	24 fs [28]
OPO (BBO)	4 fs [29]
FEL	25 fs [30]

[a] Using prismatic intracavity pulse compression.
[b] Using extracavity in addition to intracavity pulse compression.
[c] Semiconductor.

laser power. It should be noted that although some types of lasers have been reported with higher power figures at a single emission wavelength, these are not included, given the emphasis on broad wavelength tunability. The extension of the tuning ranges cited in these tables can be established via nonlinear optical techniques [6,11].

TABLE 1.3

Energetic Characteristics of Broadly Tunable Coherent Sources in the Pulsed Regime[a]

Tunable Source	Pulse Energy	Average Power
Dye laser	400 J[b] [31]	2.5 kW[c] [16]
$Ti^{3+}:Al_2O_3$ laser	6.5 J[d] [32]	5.5 W[e] [33]
$Cr^{3+}:BeAl_2O_4$ laser	100 J[f] [34]	—
Fiber laser[f]	31 nJ [35]	3 W [35]
OPO (BBO)	>100 mJ [36]	5.4 W [37]
FEL	—	100 W[g] [22]

[a] Energy and average power figures are from unrelated experiments.

[b] From a flashlamp-pumped dye laser.

[c] CVL-pumped dye laser operating at a prf of 13.2 kHz.

[d] Under flashlamp excitation.

[e] Under CVL excitation at a prf of 6.5 kHz.

[f] Oscillator amplifier configuration using a Tm-doped amplifier. System is tunable in the 1900–2040 nm region [35].

[g] Under broadly tunable conditions at the FEL of the Thomas Jefferson National Accelerator Facility. The average power can increase to over 10 kW at selected individual wavelengths [22].

Spectral information on discretely tunable pulsed lasers is given in Table 1.5; line-tunable CW lasers such as Ar+, Kr+, He–Ne, and He–Cd are listed in Table 10.1 (Chapter 10). An interesting laser listed in Table 1.5 is XeF. It can be classified as discretely tunable, given the characteristics of its $B \rightarrow X$ transitions. However, the wide tunability of its $C \rightarrow A$ transition qualifies it as a broadly tunable laser. At this stage, it should be mentioned that a distinct feature of the gas lasers listed in Table 1.5 is their ability to yield high pulse energies and, in some cases, very high average powers [16].

1.2   TUNABLE LASER COMPLEMENTARITY

The information conveyed in Tables 1.1 through 1.5 suggests that the field offers a wide variety of sources of tunable coherent radiation that have distinct optimal modes of operation. Hence, a useful generalized approach to the field should be from a perspective of complementarity. This principle of *tunable laser complementarity* [64,65] offers a dual advantage, which encourages the use of the most efficient and apt type of laser for a given application, and the integration of different lasers into a single system if necessary. This latter approach has been fairly well demonstrated in hybrid laser systems using one class of laser at the oscillator stage and a different type of laser at the amplifier stage. Examples of these systems involve the use of a dye laser oscillator and an XeF laser amplifier [54], a semiconductor laser oscillator

TABLE 1.4

Emission Characteristics Available from Broadly Tunable Sources of Coherent Radiation in the CW Regime

Tunable Source	Spectral Range	CW Power
Dye laser	$365 \leq \lambda \leq 1000$ nm[a] [38]	43 W[b] [39]
$Ti^{3+}:Al_2O_3$ laser	$710 \leq \lambda \leq 870$ nm[c] [40]	43 W[b,d] [41]
$Cr^{3+}:BeAl_2O_4$ laser	$744 \leq \lambda \leq 788$ nm	6.5 W [42]
ECS laser (InGaAsP/InP)	$1255 \leq \lambda \leq 1335$ nm[e]	≥ 1 mW [43]
ECS laser (GaAlAs)	$815 \leq \lambda \leq 825$ nm	5 mW [44]
ECS laser array	$750 \leq \lambda \leq 758$ nm	13.5 W [45]
EC QCL[f]	$8.2 \leq \lambda \leq 10.4$ μm	15 mW [46]
EC QCL[f]	$7.6 \leq \lambda \leq 11.4$ μm[g]	65 μW [47]
OPO (PPLN[j])	$3.3 \leq \lambda \leq 3.9$ μm	>1 W [48]
Fiber laser	$1032 \leq \lambda \leq 1124$ nm[h]	10 W [49]
Fiber laser	$1532 \leq \lambda \leq 1568$ nm[i]	>100 W [50]

[a] Tuning range resulting from the use of several dyes.
[b] Under Ar^+ laser excitation.
[c] Tuning range of single-longitudinal-mode emission.
[d] Uses liquid-nitrogen cooling.
[e] Measured laser linewidth is $\Delta v \leq 100$ kHz [43].
[f] QCL, quantum cascade laser.
[g] Measured laser linewidth is $\Delta v \approx 2.5$ GHz [47].
[h] Measured laser linewidth is $\Delta v \approx 3.6$ GHz [49].
[i] Measured laser linewidth is $\lambda \approx 1$ nm [50].
[j] PPLN, periodically poled lithium niobate.

in conjunction with a dye laser amplifier [66], and a solid-state dye laser oscillator [67] with an OPO as amplifier [68]. A better-known example of complementarity is the excitation of one class of laser by a different type of laser. Recent versions of this synergy include the fiber laser excitation of an optical parametric amplifier (OPA) [69] and the fiber laser excitation of tunable mid-infrared (IR) solid-state lasers [70]. Albeit arguably more attractive examples than those listed might be available, the principal message is that different types of lasers can be integrated in a system to provide an optimum solution.

However, more fundamental than the skillful integration of hybrid systems is the appropriate, and most efficient, use of a laser system for a given application. For instance, if an application requires high average powers, in the $580 \leq \lambda \leq 590$ nm region, the choice should still be a copper-vapor laser (CVL)–pumped dye laser. If large pulsed energies, tens or hundreds of joules per pulse, were necessary in the same spectral region, then a flashlamp-pumped dye laser would have to be considered. On the other hand, for an application requiring very narrow-linewidth CW emission in the near IR, an external-cavity semiconductor (ECS) laser should be the preference. Further, for spectroscopic applications demanding considerable

TABLE 1.5

Spectral Emission Characteristics of Discretely Tunable High-Power Pulsed Lasers

Laser	Transition	Bandwidth (GHz)	Wavelength (nm)
ArF	—	~17,000[a] [51]	193
KrF	$B^2\Sigma^+_{1/2} - X^2\Sigma^+_{1/2}$	~10,500[a] [51]	248
XeCl	$B^2\Sigma^+_{1/2} - X^2\Sigma^+_{1/2}$	374 [52]	308
	—	397 [52]	308.2
XeF	B–X	187 [53]	351
	—	330 [53]	353
	C–A	—	466–514[a] [54]
N_2	$C^3\Pi_u - B^3\Pi_g$	203 [55]	337.1
HgBr	—	918 [56]	502
	—	1,012 [56]	504
Ca^{2+}	$5^2S_{1/2}-4^2P_{3/2}$	—	373.7
Sr^{2+}	$6^2S_{1/2}-5^2P_{3/2}$	2–12[b] [57]	430.5
Cd^{2+}	$4^2F_{5/2}-5^2D_{3/2}$	—	533.7
Cu	$^2P_{3/2}-^2D_{5/2}$	7 [58]	510.5
	$^2P_{1/2}-^2D_{3/2}$	11 [58]	578.2
Au	$^2P_{1/2}-^2D_{3/2}$	1.5 [59]	627.8
Nd:YAG	$^4F_{3/2}-^4I_{11/2}$	15–32	1,064
CO_2	P14(00°1–10°0)[c]	—	10,532.09
	P16(00°1–10°0)	—	10,551.40
	P18(00°1–10°0)	—	10,571.05
	P20(00°1–10°0)	3–4[d] [60]	10,591.04

[a] Tuning range.

[b] Variable-linewidth range.

[c] Emission transitions obtained in a hybrid CO_2 laser [61]. For a comprehensive listing of CO_2 laser transitions, see [62].

[d] Observed bandwidth in a transversely excited atmospheric pressure CO_2 laser in the absence of intracavity linewidth-narrowing optics or injection from a CW CO_2 laser. Tunable narrow-linewidth emission, at $\Delta\nu \approx 107$ MHz, has been reported for this transition [63].

wavelength agility throughout the visible, an OPO system would be a most attractive option. In this context, at present, tunable fiber lasers appear best suited for applications requiring high-CW powers in the near IR. This perspective of complementarity is compatible with the rationale that, under ideal conditions, *it should be the application that determines the use of a particular laser* [71,72]. Note that under this utilitarian rationale, complementarity does not marginalize competition.

The logic to determine the usefulness of a given laser for an application of interest should follow the criteria of providing tunable coherent radiation, at a given spectral region, within specified emission parameters, using the simplest and most efficient means. However, in practice, this approach can be complicated by extraneous issues, such as existing managerial guidelines or cost constraints.

In the absence of extraneous constraints, parameters that should determine the suitability of a laser to a given application include the required spectral region of emission, tuning range, output power or energy, emission linewidth, and amplified spontaneous emission (ASE) level. In the case of pulsed lasers, pulse duration and pulse repetition frequency (prf) can often be considered important parameters.

At this juncture, it should be mentioned that although the word *laser* has been used throughout this chapter, an important source of coherent tunable radiation, the OPO, does not involve the process of population inversion. Nevertheless, what is important is that this source emits tunable coherent radiation that is indistinguishable from laser radiation. Hence, the title of the book and the ample use of the word laser are justified.

1.3 TUNABLE LASER APPLICATIONS

Applications for tunable lasers are extraordinarily widespread and varied, so that only some limited highlights can be mentioned in this introduction. For instance, the dye laser alone has been applied to physics [73–75], astronomy [16], spectroscopy [15,76–79], laser isotope separation [16,80–95], material diagnostics [96], material processing [96,97], remote sensing [96,98,99], defense [17,87,100], and medicine [101].

Tunable solid-state coherent sources have found numerous applications, including spectroscopy [21,102,103], and remote sensing [104]. A remarkable application of short-pulse solid-state lasers has been their use in the generation of frequency combs for *optical clockworks* [105,106], which has led to a revolution in high-precision optical measurements.

Tunable semiconductor lasers are particularly well suited for application to atomic physics [107–109] and spectroscopy [110,111]. These sources are also useful in application to metrology, interferometry, and imaging. Furthermore, simple and compact external-cavity tunable semiconductor lasers have made essential contributions to studies in laser cooling [108,110] and Bose–Einstein condensation [112]. They have also been applied to laser isotope separation [113] and have become a central component in the field of optical communications [114].

1.4 TUNABLE LASER APPLICATIONS: 1ST EDITION

The first edition of *Tunable Laser Applications* [115], published in 1995, included the following chapters:

1. Introduction, by F. J. Duarte
2. Spectroscopic Applications of Pulsed Tunable Optical Parametric Oscillators, by B. J. Orr, M. J. Johnson, and J. G. Haub
3. Dispersive External Cavity Semiconductor Lasers, by F. J. Duarte

4. Applications of Ultrashort Pulses, by X. M. Zhao, S. Diddams, and J. C. Diels
5. Interferometric Imaging, by F. J. Duarte
6. Medical Applications of the Free Electron Laser, by F. E. Carroll and C. A. Brau
7. Lidar for Atmospheric and Hydrospheric Studies, by W. B. Grant

1.5 TUNABLE LASER APPLICATIONS: 2ND EDITION

The second edition of *Tunable Laser Applications* [116], published in 2009, included the following chapters:

1. Introduction, by F. J. Duarte
2. Spectroscopic Applications of Tunable Optical Parametric Oscillators, by B. J. Orr, Y. He, and R. T. White
3. Solid State Dye Lasers, by A. Costela, I. García-Moreno, and R. Sastre
4. Tunable Lasers Based on Dye-Doped Polymer Gain Media Incorporating Homogeneous Distributions of Functional Nanoparticles, by F. J. Duarte and R. O. James
5. Broadly Tunable External-Cavity Semiconductor Lasers, by F. J. Duarte
6. Tunable Fiber Lasers, by T. M. Shay and F. J. Duarte
7. Fiber Laser Overview and Medical Applications, by S. Popov
8. Medical Applications of Dye Lasers, by A. Costela, I. García-Moreno, and R. Sastre
9. Biological Microscopy with Ultrashort Laser Pulses, by J. L. Thomas and W. Rudolph
10. Pulsed, Tunable, Monochromatic X-Rays: Medical and Nonmedical Applications, by F. E. Carroll
11. Lithium Spectroscopy Using Tunable Diode Lasers, by I. E. Olivares
12. Interferometric Imaging, by F. J. Duarte
13. Multiple-Prism Arrays and Multiple-Prism Beam Expanders: Laser Optics and Scientific Applications, by F. J. Duarte
14. Coherent Electrically Excited Organic Semiconductors, by F. J. Duarte
15. Appendix on Optical Quantities and Conversion Units, by F. J. Duarte

In fairness to readers, in this new edition, it was decided not to reproduce a chapter unless it had been updated by at least one of the original authors. Thus, Chapters 1 through 8 and Chapters 12 through 15 are included in this third edition of *Tunable Laser Applications* [117] in an expanded and updated format. In addition, two new chapters extend the scope and coverage of this third edition, which is introduced and explained in the next section.

1.6 FOCUS OF THIS BOOK

The purpose of this book is to focus on topics that highlight the utilitarian ethos of tunable lasers. In this regard, the emphasis in this book is to highlight the synergy between tunable laser development and *tunable laser applications*. The topics selected focus on applications judged to be of broad interest, historical significance, and sustained value: spectroscopy, laser isotope separation, selective laser excitation, biology, medicine, imaging, and interferometry. Among these, one of the most prevalent themes of interest in this third edition of *Tunable Laser Applications* continues to be medicine and biomedical applications.

Although there is no predetermined order of presentation, and each chapter can be read independently, Chapters 2 through 5 deal with issues of gain media, device physics, and technology. Chapter 2, written by B. J. Orr, J. G. Haub, Y. He, and R. T. White, is entitled "Spectroscopic Applications of Pulsed Tunable Optical Parametric Oscillators" and is the leading chapter, given the wider spectral coverage of these sources of coherent radiation and its extensive and detailed discussion on spectroscopy. In this new edition, this chapter has been substantially updated and enlarged, thus providing perhaps the most complete and authoritative treatise on the application of optical parametric oscillators available in the contemporary literature. The applications sections include biomedical, defense, and microscopy applications.

Chapter 3, authored by A. Costela, I. García-Moreno, and R. Sastre, is entitled "Solid-State Organic Dye Lasers," and focuses on solid-state dye lasers, with a thorough emphasis on organic and organic–inorganic gain media. Chapter 4, by F. J. Duarte and R. O. James, entitled "Organic Dye-Doped Polymer-Nanoparticle Tunable Lasers," provides an updated performance survey of tunable narrow-linewidth solid-state dye lasers and describes the characteristics of new dye-doped polymer gain media incorporating homogeneous nanoparticle distributions. Chapter 5, by F. J. Duarte, entitled "Broadly Tunable Dispersive External-Cavity Semiconductor Lasers," focuses on the performance of dispersive external-cavity semiconductor lasers and describes intracavity optics and tuning methods that are also relevant to other tunable sources of coherent radiation discussed in this book. Both Chapters 4 and 5 include a brief survey of biomedical applications. Chapter 6, written by T. M. Shay and F. J. Duarte, is entitled "Tunable Fiber Lasers" and focuses on the main approaches currently used to achieve tunability in these lasers. This is followed by Chapter 7, by S. Y. Popov, which is entitled "Fiber Laser Overview and Medical Applications." This chapter provides a survey of fiber laser gain media and introduces the reader to the medical applications of these lasers. This chapter signals a shift in emphasis in the book toward applications.

The emphasis on medical and biomedical applications becomes a central theme in Chapter 8. This chapter is authored by A. Costela, I. García-Moreno, and C. Gómez and is entitled "Medical Applications of Organic Dye Lasers." This work provides an updated and extensive survey of the applications of tunable dye lasers to medicine, including subjects such as dermatology, photodynamic therapy, and lithotripsy. Chapter 9, written by F. J. Duarte, is entitled "Tunable Laser Microscopy" and provides a survey of various coherent techniques used in the fields of microscopy and nanoscopy. Biomedical applications are also considered in Chapter 10, written by F. J. Duarte, which is on "Interferometric Imaging." This chapter also considers applications of *N*-slit interferometric techniques in optical metrology and optical free-space communications.

The following chapter focuses on selective laser excitation. Chapter 11, by F. J. Duarte, is entitled "Tunable Laser Atomic Vapor Laser Isotope Separation" and provides an overview of this field, mainly from the perspective of high-power tunable lasers.

The remaining two chapters focus on multiple-prism optics and its applications, plus coherent emission from organic semiconductors. Chapter 12, by F. J. Duarte, focuses on a description of experiments on electrically excited pulsed organic semiconductors and is entitled "Coherent Electrically Excited Organic Semiconductors." Chapter 13, by F. J. Duarte, is entitled "Multiple-Prism Arrays and Multiple-Prism Beam Expanders: Laser Optics and Scientific Applications," and provides a brief referenced survey of numerous fields of applications that use multiple-prism arrays either directly, deployed within a narrow-linewidth tunable laser, or deployed within an ultrashort pulse laser. The book concludes with Chapter 14, by F. J. Duarte, listing useful optical quantities and explaining the linewidth equivalence, which is entitled "Optical Quantities and Conversion Units."

Tunable Laser Applications includes the applications of tunable coherent sources, in various degrees of detail, to the following fields:

Astronomy
Atomic spectroscopy
Biomedicine
Coherent Raman microscopy
Communications
Characterization of textiles
Defense
Densitometry
Dentistry
Dermatology
Digital imaging
Digital microscopy
Environmental monitoring
Infrared countermeasures
Interferometric communications
Interferometric imaging
Interferometric microscopy
Interferometry
Laser cooling
Laser guide star
Laser isotope separation
Laser printing
Laser pulse compression
Light sheet microscopy
Medical applications of dye lasers
Medical applications of fiber lasers
Microdensitometry
Molecular spectroscopy

Nanoparticle transparency
Optical coherence tomography (OCT)
Optical metrology
Photodynamic therapy
Surgery
Ultrashort pulse microscopy

ACKNOWLEDGMENTS

This third edition of *Tunable Laser Applications* has been made possible by the support of Interferometric Optics and the integrated effort of the contributing authors. In addition to discussions of laser physics and technology, they have provided an up-to-date and vibrant description of an enormous variety of applications of tunable sources of coherent radiation. The encouragement and cooperation of Ashley Gasque at CRC Press is also acknowledged.

REFERENCES

1. Sorokin, P. P. and J. R. Lankard, Stimulated emission observed from an organic dye, chloroaluminum phthalocyanine, *IBM J. Res. Dev.* 10: 162–163, 1966.
2. Schäfer, F. P., W. Schmidt, and J. Volze, Organic dye solution laser, *Appl. Phys. Lett.* 9: 306–309, 1966.
3. Soffer, B. H. and B. B. McFarland, Continuously tunable narrow-band organic dye lasers, *Appl. Phys. Lett.* 10: 266–267, 1967.
4. Stepanov, B. I., A. N. Rubinov, and V. A. Mostovnikov, Optic generation in solutions of complex molecules, *JETP Lett.* 5: 117–119, 1967.
5. Schäfer, F. P. (Ed.), *Dye Lasers*, Springer, Berlin, 1990.
6. Duarte, F. J. and L. W. Hillman (Eds), *Dye Laser Principles*, Academic, New York, 1990.
7. Duarte, F. J. (Ed.), *High Power Dye Lasers*, Springer, Berlin, 1991.
8. Stuke, M. (Ed.), *Dye Lasers: 25 Years*, Springer, Berlin, 1992.
9. Duarte, F. J. (Ed.), *Selected Papers on Dye Lasers*, SPIE Optical Engineering, Bellingham, WA, 1992.
10. Duarte, F. J. (Ed.), *Tunable Lasers Handbook*, Academic, New York, 1995.
11. Duarte, F. J., *Tunable Laser Optics*, Academic, New York, 2003.
12. Maeda, M., *Laser Dyes*, Academic, New York, 1984.
13. Radziemski, L. J., R. W. Solarz, and J. A. Paisner (Eds), *Laser Spectroscopy and Its Applications*, Marcel Dekker, New York, 1987.
14. Duarte, F. J., J. A. Paisner, and A. Penzkofer, Dye lasers: Introduction by the feature editors, *Appl. Opt.* 31: 6977–6878, 1992.
15. Demtröder, W., *Laser Spectroscopy*, 3rd edn, Springer, Berlin, 2003.
16. Bass, I. L., R. E. Bonanno, R. P. Hackel, and P. R. Hammond, High-average-power dye laser at Lawrence Livermore National Laboratory, *Appl. Opt.* 31: 6993–7006, 1992.
17. Duarte, F. J. and L. W. Hillman, Introduction. In F. J. Duarte and L. W. Hillman (Eds), *Dye Laser Principles*, Chapter 1, Academic, New York, 1990.
18. Moulton, P. F., Spectroscopic and laser characteristics of Ti:Al$_2$O$_3$, *J. Opt. Soc. Am. B* 3: 125–132, 1986.
19. Walling, J. C., O. G. Peterson, H. P. Jenssen, R. C. Morris, and E. W. O'Dell, Tunable alexandrite lasers, *IEEE J. Quantum Elect.* QE–16: 1302–1315, 1980.

20. Okhonikov, O. G., L. Gomes, N. Xiang, T. Jouhti, and A. B. Grudinin, Mode-locked ytterbium fiber laser tunable in the 980–1070 nm spectral range, *Opt. Lett.* 28: 1522–1524, 2003.

21. Orr, B. J., M. J. Johnson, and J. B. Haub, Spectroscopic applications of pulsed tunable optical parametric oscillators. In F. J. Duarte (Ed.), *Tunable Laser Applications*, 1st edn, Chapter 2, Marcel-Dekker, New York, 1995.

22. Benson, S. V., Private communication, 2007.

23. Andonian, G., A. Murokh, J. B. Rosenzweig, R. Agustsson, M. Babzien, I. Ben-Zvi, P. Frigola, et al., Observations of anomalously large spectral bandwidth in a high-gain self- amplified spontaneous emission free electron laser, *Phys. Rev. Lett.* 95: 054801, 2005.

24. Düsterer, S., P. Radcliffe, G. Geloni, U. Jastrow, M. Kuhlmann, E. Plönjes, K. Tiedke, P., et al., Spectroscopic characterization of vacuum ultraviolet free electron laser pulses, *Opt Lett.* 31: 1150–1152, 2006.

25. Fork, R. L., C. H. Brito-Cruz, P. C. Becker, and C. V. Shank, Compression of optical pulses to six femtoseconds by using cubic phase compensation, *Opt. Lett.* 12: 483–485, 1987.

26. Ell, R., U. Morgner, F. X. Kärtner, J. G. Fujimoto, E. P. Ippen, V. Scheuer, G. Angelow, et al., Generation of 5-fs pulses and octave-spanning spectra directly from a Ti:sapphire laser, *Opt. Lett.* 26: 373–375, 2001.

27. Delfyett, P. J., L. Florez, N. Stoffel, T. Gmitter, N. Andreadakis, G. Alphonse, and W. Ceislik, 200 fs optical pulse generation and intracavity pulse evolution in a hybrid mode-locked semiconductor diode-laser/amplifier system, *Opt. Lett.* 17: 670–672, 1992.

28. Tauser, F., F. Adler, and A. Leitenstorfer, Widely tunable sub-30-fs pulses from a compact erbium-doped fiber source, *Opt. Lett.* 29: 516–518, 2004.

29. Baltuska, A., T. Fuji, and T. Kobayashi, Visible pulse compression to 4 fs by optical parametric amplification and programmable dispersion control, *Opt. Lett.* 27: 306–308, 2002.

30. Chalupsky, J., L. Juha, J. Kuba, J. Cihelka, V. Hájková, S. Koptyaev, J. Krása, et al., Characteristics of focused soft X-ray free-electron laser beam determined by ablation of organic molecular solids, *Opt. Express* 15: 6036–6043, 2007.

31. Baltakov, F. N., B. A. Garikhin, and L. V. Sukhanov, 400-J pulsed laser using a solution of rhodamine 6 G in ethanol, *JETP Lett.* 19: 174–175, 1974.

32. Brown, A. J. W. and C. H. Fisher, A 6.5-J flashlamp-pumped Ti:Al$_2$O$_3$ laser, *IEEE J Quantum Elect.* 29: 2513–2518, 1993.

33. Knowles, M. R. H. and C. E. Webb, Efficient high-power copper-vapor-laser-pumped Ti:Al$_2$O$_3$ laser, *Opt. Lett.* 18: 607–609, 1993.

34. Walling, J. C., High energy pulsed alexandrite lasers. In *Technical Digest International Conference on Lasers '90*, paper MH.3, San Diego, CA, 1990.

35. Imeshev, G. and M. E. Fermann, 230 kW peak power femtosecond pulses from a high-power tunable source based from amplification in Tm-doped fiber, *Opt. Express* 13: 7424–7231, 2005.

36. Fix, A., T. Schröder, R. Wallenstein, J. G. Haub, M. J. Johnson, and B. J. Orr, Tunable β-barium borate optical parametric oscillator: Operating characteristics with and without injection seeding, *J. Opt. Soc. Am. B* 10: 1744–1750, 1993.

37. Maruyama, Y., 0.5-kHz, 5-W optical parametric oscillator pumped by the second harmonic of a Nd:YAG laser, *Opt. Eng.* 44: 094202, 2005.

38. Hollberg, L., CW dye lasers. In F. J. Duarte and L. W. Hillman (Eds), *Dye Laser Principles*, Chapter 5, Academic, New York, 1990.

39. Baving, H. J., H. Muuss, and W. Skolaut, CW dye laser operation at 200 W pump power, *Appl. Phys. B* 29: 19–21, 1982.

40. Adams, C. S. and A. I. Ferguson, Frequency doubling of a single frequency Ti:Al$_2$O$_3$ laser using an external enhancement cavity, *Opt. Commun.* 79: 219–223, 1990.

41. Erbert, G., I. Bass, R. Hackel, S. Jenkins, K. Kanz, and J. Paisner, 43-W, CW Ti:sapphire laser, in *Conference on Lasers and Electro-Optics*, pp. 390–393, Optical Society of America, Washington, DC, 1991.

42. Walling, J. C., O. G. Peterson, and R. C. Morris, Tunable CW alexandrite laser, *IEEE J. Quantum Elect.* QE-16: 120–121, 1980.

43. Zorabedian, P., Characteristics of a grating-external-cavity semiconductor laser containing intracavity prism beam expanders, *J. Lightwave Technol.* 10: 330–335, 1992.

44. Fleming, M. W. and A. Moorodian, Spectral characteristics of external-cavity controlled semiconductor lasers, *IEEE J. Quantum Elect.* QE-17: 44–59, 1981.

45. Meng, L. S., B. Nizamov, P. Nadasami, J. K. Brasseur, T. Henshaw, and D. K. Newmann, High-power 7-GHz bandwidth external-cavity diode laser array and its use in optically pumping singlet delta oxygen, *Opt. Express* 14: 10469–10474, 2006.

46. Maulini, R., A. Mohan, M. Giovannini, J. Faist, and E. Gini, External cavity quantum-cascade laser tunable from 8.2 to 10.4 µm using a gain element with a heterogeneous cascade. *Appl. Phys. Lett.* 88: 201113, 2006.

47. Hugi, A., R. Terazzi, Y. Bonetti, A. Wittmann, M. Fischer, M. Beck, J. Faist, and E. Gini, External cavity quantum cascade laser tunable from 7.6 to 11.4 µm, *Appl. Phys. Lett.* 95: 061103, 2009.

48. Bosenberg, W. R., A. Drobshoff, J. I. Alexander, L. E. Myers, and R. L. Byer, 93% pump depletion, 3.5 W continuous-wave, singly resonant optical parametric oscillator, *Opt. Lett.* 21: 1336–1338, 1996.

49. Auerbach, M., P. Adel, D. Wandt, C. Fallnich, S. Unger, S. Jetschke, and H-R. Müller, 10 W widely tunable narrow linewidth double-clad fiber ring laser, *Opt. Express* 10: 139–144, 2002.

50. Shen, D. Y., J. K., Sahu, and W. A. Clarkson, Highly efficient Er, Yb-doped fiber laser with 188 W free running and >100 W tunable output power, *Opt. Express* 13: 4916–4921, 2005.

51. Loree, T. R., K. B. Butterfield, and D. L. Barker, Spectral tuning of ArF and KrF discharge lasers, *Appl. Phys. Lett.* 32: 171–173, 1978.

52. Lyutskanov, V. L., K. G. Khristov, and I. V. Tomov, Tuning the emission frequency of a gas-discharge XeCl laser, *Sov. J. Quantum Electron.* 10: 1456–1457, 1980.

53. Yang, T. T., D. H. Burde, G. A. Merry, D. G. Harris, L. A. Pugh, J. H. Tillotson, C. E. Turner, and D. A. Copeland, Spectra of electron beam pumped XeF laser, *Appl. Opt.* 27: 49–57, 1988.

54. Hofmann, T. and F. K. Tittel, Wideband-tunable high-power radiation by SRS of a XeF($C{\rightarrow}A$) excimer laser, *IEEE J. Quantum Elect.* 29: 970–974, 1993.

55. Woodward, B. W., V. J. Ehlers, and W. C. Lineberger, A reliable repetitively pulsed, high-power nitrogen laser, *Rev. Sci. Instrum.* 44: 882–887, 1973.

56. Shay, T. M., F. E. Hanson, D. Gookin, and E. J. Schimitscheck, Line narrowing and enhanced efficiency of an HgBr laser by injection locking, *Appl. Phys. Lett.* 39: 783–785, 1981.

57. Bukshpun, L. M., V. V. Zhukov, E. L. Latush, and M. F. Sem, Frequency tuning and mode self locking in He-Sr recombination laser, *Sov. J. Quantum Electron.* 11: 804–805, 1981.

58. Tenenbaum, J., I. Smilanski, S. Gabay, L. A. Levin, G. Erez, and S. Lavi, Structure of 510.6 and 578.2 nm copper laser lines, *Opt. Commun.* 32: 473–477, 1980.

59. Wang, Y., B. Lin, and Y. Qian, Spectral structure of the 627.8 nm gold vapor laser line. *Appl. Phys. B* 49: 149–153, 1989.

60. Duarte, F. J., Variable linewidth high-power TEA CO$_2$ laser, *Appl. Opt.* 24: 34–37, 1985.

61. Mehendale, S. C., D. J. Biswas, and R. G. Harrison, Single mode multiline emission from a hybrid CO_2 laser, *Opt. Commun.* 55: 427–429, 1985.

62. Chang, T. Y., Vibrational transition lasers. In M. J. Weber (Ed.), *Handbook of Laser Science and Technology*, Chapter 3.3.2, CRC, Boca Raton, FL, 1991.

63. Duarte, F. J., Multiple-prism Littrow and grazing-incidence pulsed CO_2 lasers, *Appl. Opt.* 24: 1244–1245, 1985.

64. Duarte, F. J., Introduction. In F. J. Duarte (Ed.), *Tunable Laser Applications*, 1st edn, Chapter 1, Marcel-Dekker, New York, 1995.

65. Duarte, F. J., Introduction. In F. J. Duarte (Ed.), *Tunable Lasers Handbook*, Chapter 1, Academic, New York, 1995.

66. Farkas, A. M. and J. G. Eden, Pulsed dye amplification and frequency doubling of single longitudinal mode semiconductor, *IEEE J. Quantum Elect.* 29: 2923–2927, 1993.

67. Duarte, F. J., Solid-state multiple-prism grating dye-laser oscillators, *Appl. Opt.* 33: 3857–3860, 1994.

68. Orr, B. J., Private communication, 1995.

69. Andersen, T. V., O. Schmidt, C. Bruchmann, J. Limpert, C. Aguergaray, E. Cormier, and A. Tünnermann, High repetition rate tunable femtosecond pulses and broadband amplification from fiber laser pumped parametric amplifier, *Opt. Express* 14: 4765–4773, 2006.

70. Eichhorn, M., Development of a high-pulse-energy Q-switched Tm-doped doubled-clad fluoride fiber laser and its application to the pumping of mid-IR lasers, *Opt. Lett.* 32: 1056–1058, 2007.

71. Duarte, F. J., Letter, *Laser Focus World* 27(5): 25, 1991.

72. Duarte, F. J., Letter, *Lasers Optron.* 10(5): 8, 1991.

73. Drell, P. S. and E. D. Commins, Parity nonconservation in atomic thallium, *Phys. Rev. A* 32: 2196–2210, 1985.

74. Gould, P. L., G. A. Ruff, and D. E. Pritchard, Diffraction of atoms by light: The near-resonant Kapitza-Dirac effect, *Phys. Rev. Lett.* 56: 827–830, 1986.

75. Letokhov, V. S., Atomic optics with tunable dye lasers. In M. Stuke (Ed.), *Dye Lasers: 25 Years*, Chapter 11, Springer, Berlin, 1992.

76. Hall, R. J. and A. C. Eckbreth, Coherent anti-Stokes Raman spectroscopy, CARS: Application to combustion diagnostics. In J. F. Ready and R. K. Erf (Eds), *Laser Applications*, Volume 5, Chapter 4, Academic, New York, 1984.

77. Majewski, W. A., J. F. Pfanstiel, D. F. Plusquellic, and W. D. Pratt, High resolution optical spectroscopy in the ultraviolet. In A. B. Myers and T. R. Rizzo (Eds), *Laser Techniques in Chemistry*, Chapter 4, Wiley, New York, 1995.

78. Sneddon, J., T. L. Thiem, and Y-I. Lee (Eds), *Lasers in Analytical Atomic Spectroscopy*, Wiley-VCH, New York, 1996.

79. Demtröder, W., *Laserspektroscopie: Grundlagen und Techniken*, Springer, Berlin, 2007.

80. Pease, A. A. and W. M. Pearson, Axial-mode structure of a copper vapor pumped dye laser, *Appl. Opt.* 16: 57–60, 1977.

81. Hargrove, R. S. and T. Kan, High power efficient dye amplifier pumped by copper vapor lasers, *IEEE J. Quantum Elect.* 16: 1108–1113, 1980.

82. Duarte, F. J. and J. A. Piper, Comparison of prism-expander and grazing-incidence grating cavities for copper laser pumped dye lasers, *Appl. Opt.* 21: 2782–2786, 1982.

83. Duarte, F. J. and J. A. Piper, Narrow-linewidth, high-prf copper laser-pumped dye-laser oscillators, *Appl. Opt.* 23: 1391–1394, 1984.

84. Broyer, M. and J. Chevaleyre, CVL-pumped dye laser for spectroscopic applications, *Appl. Phys. B* 35: 31–36, 1984.

85. Paisner, J. A. and R. W. Solarz, Resonance photoionization spectroscopy. In L. J. Radziemski, R. W. Solarz, and J. A. Paisner (Eds), *Laser Spectroscopy and Its Applications*, Chapter 3, Marcel Dekker, New York, 1987.

86. Paisner, J. A., Atomic vapor laser isotope separation, *Appl. Phys. B* 46: 253–260, 1988.

87. Duarte, F. J., H. R. Aldag, R. W. Conrad, P. N. Everett, J. A. Paisner, T. G. Pavlopoulos, and C. R. Tallman, High power dye laser technology. In R. C. Sze and F. J. Duarte (Eds), *Proceedings of the International Conference on Lasers '88*, pp. 773–790. STS, McLean, VA, 1989.

88. Akerman, M. A., Dye-laser isotope separation. In F. J. Duarte and L. W. Hillman (Eds), *Dye Laser Principles*, Chapter 9, Academic, New York, 1990.

89. Duarte, F. J., Dispersive dye lasers. In F. J. Duarte (Ed.), *High Power Dye Lasers*, Chapter 9, Springer, Berlin, 1991.

90. Tallman, C. and R. Tennant, Large-scale excimer-laser-pumped dye lasers. In F. J. Duarte (Ed.), *High Power Dye Lasers*, Chapter 4, Springer, Berlin, 1991.

91. Webb, C. E., High-power dye lasers pumped by copper-vapor lasers. In F. J. Duarte (Ed.), *High Power Dye Lasers*, Chapter 5, Springer, Berlin, 1991.

92. Singh, S., K. Dasgupta, S. Kumar, K. G. Manohar, L. G. Nair, and U. K. Chatterjee, High-power high-repetition-rate copper-vapor-pumped dye laser, *Opt. Eng.* 33: 1894–1904, 1994.

93. Sugiyama, A., T. Nakayama, M. Kato, Y. Maruyama, and T. Arisawa, Characteristics of a pressure-tuned single-mode dye laser oscillator pumped by a copper vapor laser, *Opt. Eng.* 35: 1093–1097, 1996.

94. Ready, J. F., *Industrial Laser Applications*, Academic, New York, 1997.

95. Bokhan, P. A., V. V. Buchanov, N. V. Fateev, M. M. Kalugin, M. A. Kazaryan, A. M. Prokhorov, and D. E. Kakrevskii, *Laser Isotope Separation in Atomic Vapor*, Wiley-VCH, Weinheim, 2006.

96. Klick, D., Industrial applications of dye lasers. In F. J. Duarte and L. W. Hillman (Eds), *Dye Laser Principles*, Chapter 8, Academic, New York, 1990.

97. Hargrove, R. S., Industrial applications of high power lasers. In *Technical Digest International Conference on Lasers '91*, paper THA.2, San Diego, CA, 1991.

98. Browell, E. V., Ozone and aerosol measurements with an airborne lidar system, *Opt. Photonics News* 2(10): 8–11, 1991.

99. Grant, W. B., Lidar for atmospheric and hydrospheric studies. In F. J. Duarte (Ed.), *Tunable Laser Applications*, 1st edn, pp. 213–305, Marcel-Dekker, New York, 1995.

100. Duarte, F. J., Organic dye lasers: Brief history and recent developments, *Opt. Photonics News* 14(10): 20–25, 2003.

101. Goldman, L., Dye lasers in medicine. In F. J. Duarte and L. W. Hillman (Eds), *Dye Laser Principles*, Chapter 10, Academic, New York, 1990.

102. Vassen, W., C. Zimmermann, R. Kallenbach, and T. W. Hänsch, A frequency-stabilized titanium sapphire laser for high-resolution spectroscopy, *Opt. Commun.* 75: 435–440, 1990.

103. Gilmore, D. A., P. V. Cvijin, and G. H. Atkinson, Intracavity absorption spectroscopy with a titanium:sapphire laser, *Opt. Commun.* 77: 385–389, 1990.

104. Bruneau, D., T. Arnaud des Lions, P. Quaglia, and J. Pelon, Injection-seeded pulsed alexandrite laser for differential absorption Lidar application, *Appl. Opt.* 33: 3941–3950, 1994.

105. Diddams, S. A., D. J. Jones, J. Ye, S. T. Cundiff, J. L. Hall, J. K. Ranka, R. S. Windeler, et al., Direct link between microwave and optical frequencies with 300 THz femtosecond laser comb, *Phys. Rev. Lett.* 84: 5102–5105, 2000.

106. Holzwarth, R., Th. Udem, T. W. Hänsch, J. C. Knight, W. J. Wadsworth, and P. S. J. Russell, Optical frequency synthesizer for precision spectroscopy, *Phys. Rev. Lett.* 85: 2264–2267, 2000.

107. Camparo, J. C., The diode laser in atomic physics, *Contemp. Phys.* 26: 443–477, 1985.

108. Wieman, C. E. and L. Hollberg, Using diode lasers in atomic physics, *Rev. Sci. Instrum.* 62: 1–20, 1991.

109. Camparo, J., The rubidium atomic clock and basic research, *Phys. Today* 60(11): 33–39, 2007.
110. Weidemüller, M., C. Gabbanini, J. Hare, M. Gross, and S. Haroche, A beam of laser-cooled lithium Rydberg atoms for precision microwave spectroscopy, *Opt. Commun.* 101: 342–346, 1993.
111. Atutov, S. N., E. Mariotti, M. Meuchi, C. Marinelli, and L. Moi, 670 nm external-cavity single mode diode laser continuously tunable over 18 GHz range, *Opt. Commun.* 107: 83–87, 1994.
112. Myatt, C. J., N. R. Newbury, R. W. Ghrist, S. Loutzenhizer, and C. E. Wieman, Multiply loaded magneto-optical trap, *Opt. Lett.* 21: 290–292, 1996.
113. Olivares, I. E., A. E. Duarte, E. A. Saravia, and F. J. Duarte, Lithium isotope separation with tunable diode lasers, *Appl. Opt.* 41: 2973–2977, 2002.
114. Berger, J. D. and D. Anthon, Tunable MEMS devices for optical networks, *Opt. Photonics News* 14(3): 43–49, 2003.
115. Duarte, F. J. (Ed.), *Tunable Laser Applications*, 1st edn, Marcel-Dekker, New York, 1995.
116. Duarte, F. J. (Ed.), *Tunable Laser Applications*, 2nd edn, CRC Press, New York, 2009.
117. Duarte, F. J. (Ed.), *Tunable Laser Applications*, 3rd edn, CRC Press, New York, 2015.

2 Spectroscopic Applications of Tunable Optical Parametric Oscillators

Brian J. Orr, John G. Haub, Yabai He, and Richard T. White

CONTENTS

2.1   INTRODUCTION

2.1.1   "Good-bye to Ti: and Dye"?

The corresponding chapter in the first edition of this book [1] was written in the mid-1990s, at a time when a prominent scientific laser manufacturer had advertised its latest optical parametric oscillator (OPO) with the motto "Good-bye to Ti: and Dye," signaling the possible demise of tunable dye lasers that had served laser spectroscopists and others well for at least 20 years [2,3]. At that time, a book review speculated that solid-state tunable lasers "might relegate the dye laser to the pages of the history book," counterpoised by a view that "the dye laser in its many incarnations looks set to be with us for quite some time yet" [4]. Approximately 15 years later, the corresponding chapter in the second edition of this book [5] recorded that Ti:sapphire and dye lasers continued to occupy a significant place in the tunable laser market alongside many others (such as diode and quantum cascade lasers), but that solid-state nonlinear optical (NLO) devices, such as OPOs, were by then preferred as tunable coherent light sources for many spectroscopic purposes in the ultraviolet (UV), visible, near-infrared (IR), and mid-IR [6,7]. The same is true at the time of preparation of this updated chapter (~20 and ~5 years, respectively, after our contributions to the first [1] and second [5] editions of this book), although the spectroscopic dye laser market continues to contract substantially.

This chapter focuses on developments in the design, operation, and spectroscopic applications of tunable OPOs, as well as in the closely related optical parametric generator (OPG) and optical parametric amplifier (OPA) devices. Such optical parametric devices have now been available for more than 40 years [8,9], but it is only in the last 25 years that the spectroscopic community at large has found tunable OPOs to be sufficiently reliable for routine, trouble-free operation. Pulsed OPO devices operating in the nanosecond (ns) regime had long been recognized as potentially useful sources of broadly tunable, coherent radiation for spectroscopy, typically yielding high peak and average powers [8–12]. Their solid-state character and high efficiency offer substantial advantages in some respects over the previously ubiquitous dye laser. Moreover, the wide range of wavelengths over which many OPOs can be tuned has opened up prospects for laser spectroscopy in otherwise inaccessible spectral regions, such as the near- and mid-IR, on which much of this chapter will concentrate [6,7].

The first precursor of this chapter [1] displayed an IR absorption spectrum of the 2–0 first-overtone band of carbon monoxide (CO) gas in the near IR at ~2.35 µm; that spectrum was remarkably fine by the standards that prevailed when it was recorded in 1972 (over 40 years ago), using idler radiation from an ns-pulsed, singly resonant LiNbO₃ OPO [10,13]. The spectrum displayed in Figure 2.1 shows the P ($\Delta J=-1$) and R ($\Delta J=+1$) branches of that rovibrational band, spanning a 180 cm⁻¹ (5.4 THz) range with an instrument-limited linewidth of ~0.5 cm⁻¹ (~15 GHz) at a CO sample pressure (P) of 3 atm in a 4 cm cell. It was accompanied by a (subsequently fulfilled) prophecy that "the use of parametric oscillator sources for molecular spectroscopy should increase rapidly as the frequency range is extended further into the IR and the bandwidth is reduced" [10].

Within 2 years, Stanford University's OPO technology had further advanced: pulsed LiNbO₃ OPO idler radiation, continuously tunable with an optical bandwidth of 0.35 cm⁻¹ (10.5 GHz), enabled better-resolved reference spectra of the same 2.35 µm 2–0 band of CO gas to be recorded [14]. These were used in the context of an OPO-based transmitter–receiver system that was able to detect CO in air at a range of 107 m against a topographical backscattering target, providing an early

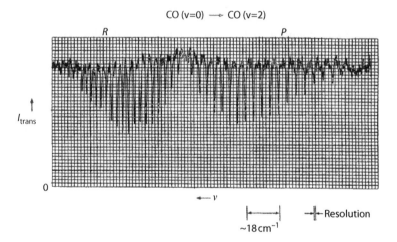

FIGURE 2.1 Continuously scanned IR absorption spectrum of the 2.35 µm 2–0 rovibrational absorption band of carbon monoxide (CO) gas, recorded in a 4 cm cell at a pressure of 3 atm using an ns-pulsed, singly resonant LiNbO₃ OPO: an early demonstration of the spectroscopic potential of tunable OPO technology [10,13]. (Reproduced with permission from R. L. Byer, Optical parametric oscillators. In H. Rabin and C. L. Tang (Eds), *Quantum Electronics: A Treatise*, Volume I, Part B, Chapter 9, pp. 578–702, Academic, New York, 1975; Sackett, P. (US Air Force Cambridge Research Laboratory), cited in [10] as a private communication to R. L. Byer (1972).

indication of the utility of OPO-based IR spectroscopy for stand off detection and density measurement of pollutant gases [15].

However, despite some significant early progress, the spectroscopic potential of pulsed OPOs was not readily realized [9–12,14,16]. Many research laboratories had dark recesses to which their original pulsed OPO systems had been relegated, either optically damaged or used occasionally as "one-wavelength-at-a-time" instruments, rather than the continuously scannable spectroscopic workhorses that they were originally intended to be (and have now become). This shortcoming was attributable to several critical factors:

- The low optical damage limits and high oscillation thresholds in available OPO gain materials.
- The relative complexity of early pulsed OPO cavity designs (including phase-matching schemes and line-narrowing strategies) necessary to achieve narrowband, continuously tunable operation [6,9,10,17–23].
- The need for intense, pulsed lasers with adequate temporal and spatial coherence to serve as OPO pump sources.

Within the last 25 years, these problems have diminished appreciably with the availability of new OPO materials [24,26] and high-quality pump lasers [27]. As a variety of pulsed tunable OPO systems became commercially available, the spectroscopic community, sections of which had in earlier days been disappointed by the difficulty of implementing OPO technology, were attracted to the cost-effectiveness and practical utility of such systems.

Since the first edition of this book [1], tunable OPOs, their applications, and relevant aspects of nonlinear optics have matured considerably. There have been numerous review articles, both by our research group at Macquarie University, Sydney [28–33] and by others [34–59], as well as relevant feature issues of topical journals on OPOs [60–67] and related spectroscopic techniques [68–70]. In this chapter, therefore, we do not intend to provide a comprehensive coverage of the field, but, rather, to indicate some of its foundations and address a number of issues concerning the design and operation of tunable OPOs for various spectroscopic applications. This overview will include continuous wave (CW) and ultrafast pulsed systems, as well as the ns-pulsed devices on which our earlier versions of this chapter [1,5] and our own ongoing research have focused. Our approach here is essentially that of a selective series of case studies sampling representative examples of progress in this area.

2.1.2 OPO-Based Spectroscopy Has Come a Long Way …

OPO-based spectroscopy has come a long way since 1972, when Figure 2.1 was recorded. To illustrate how far this field has progressed, we retain CO molecular studies as a benchmark and examine several more recent OPO-spectroscopic accomplishments (but without many technological details at this introductory stage of the chapter).

For instance, a diode-pumped CW OPO with an optical linewidth of <60 MHz was used in 1999 to measure higher-resolution spectra of CO ($P = 4$ Torr) in a single pass of a 60 cm gas cell; the 2.3337 μm $R(6)$ rovibrational line of CO (in the same 2–0 band as in Figure 2.1) was recorded with a Doppler- and pressure-broadened linewidth of 0.013 cm^{-1} (390 MHz) [71]. Around the same time, an advanced, commercially available, computer-controlled tunable OPO/OPA system (based on the ns-pulsed design of Bosenberg and Guyer [20,21]) was used for IR planar laser-induced fluorescence (LIF) imaging of fluid dynamics in CO gas flows and of CO combustion diagnostics [72–74]. Figure 2.2 shows a single-shot planar LIF image of a vortex in a CO/Ar gas jet [72].

Our ultimate illustration of the extensive recent progress in this field, still in the context of molecular spectroscopy of CO(g), is provided by recent work of Vodopyanov and colleagues [75,76]. They have developed state-of-the-art broadband OPOs operating in the spectral range 2.5–5 μm for intracavity spectroscopy with sub-parts per million by volume (ppmv) detection limits for various gases, including CO, for which a mid-IR spectrum is shown in Figure 2.3. The black trace is an absorption spectrum measured within 2 min for 50 parts ppmv of CO in He at $P = 1$ atm. In the calculated spectrum (gray; offset and inverted), the effective path length is taken to be seven times the physical length (48 cm) of the intracavity gas cell.

Figure 2.4 illustrates the layout of the degenerate broadband OPO that was used. The pump source is a femtosecond (fs) fiber laser, either Er doped operating at 1.56 μm or Tm doped operating at 2.05 μm. The corresponding NLO material is either periodically poled lithium niobate (PPLN) or orientation-patterned gallium arsenide (OP GaAs); wedge pairs composed of either ZnSe or CaF$_2$ are used for dispersion compensation and beam out-coupling.

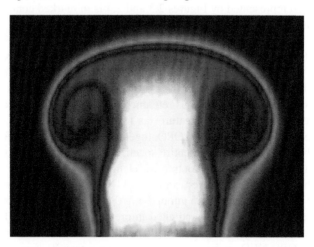

FIGURE 2.2 Single-shot IR planar laser-induced fluorescence image of a vortex in a CO/Ar gas jet, formed by releasing a 50:50 mixture of CO and Ar through a 6 mm tube into air [72]. A computer-controlled tunable OPO/OPA system operating at ~2.35 μm was used to excite CO molecules via their near IR 2–0 overtone absorption band (the same as in Figure 2.1), and then 2–1 and 1–0 fundamental-band mid-IR emission was detected at ~4.7 μm. (With kind permission from Professor R. K. Hanson and Springer Science+Business Media: B. J. Kirby and R. K. Hanson, Planar laser-induced fluorescence imaging of carbon monoxide using vibrational (infrared) transitions, *Appl. Phys. B* 69: 505–507, 1999.)

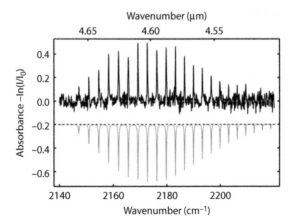

FIGURE 2.3 Comparison of measured (black) and calculated (gray) mid-IR rovibrational absorption spectra at ~4.6 μm for 50 ppmv CO in He at 1 atm pressure. The spectra correspond to the R branch of the 1–0 fundamental band of CO gas at ~4.6 μm, observed by means of an fs-pumped broadband frequency comb OPO incorporating an intracavity gas cell, as depicted in Figure 2.4 [75]. (From M. W. Haakestad, T. P. Lamour, N. Leindecker, A. Marandi, and K. L. Vodopyanov, Intra-cavity trace molecular detection with a broadband mid-IR frequency comb source, *J. Opt. Soc. Am. B* 30: 631–640, 2013. With permission from Professor K. L. Vodopyanov and Optical Society of America.)

The approach represented by Figures 2.3 and 2.4 is in marked contrast to that of more traditional OPO-spectroscopic techniques, in several respects [75,76]:

- Many traditional OPO-spectroscopic studies use a narrow-bandwidth source, of which the tunable output wavelength (signal or idler) is either scanned through the spectrum of interest (as in Figure 2.1 [10,13] and in other examples cited in previous references [14,15,71]) or tuned to a single characteristic spectroscopic feature (as in Figure 2.2 [72–74]). However, here the fs-pumped broadband OPO, together with Fourier-transform (FT) methods, is able to record an entire spectrum without needing to continuously tune or select the OPO output wavelength.
- All of the previously considered examples of OPO spectroscopy have focused on near IR absorption at ~2.35 μm in the 2–0 first-overtone absorption band of CO gas (as in Figure 2.1 and cited in previous references [10,13–15,71–74]), due to the limited long-wavelength range of idler radiation from readily available OPO NLO media and ns-pulsed pump lasers. By contrast, the use of an OP GaAs OPO fs-pumped by a 2.05 μm Tm-doped fiber laser provides broadband spectroscopic access to the much stronger 1–0 fundamental band of CO gas at ~4.6 μm; the rovibrational R branch of that spectrum is displayed in Figure 2.3. Innovative aspects of OP GaAs as a relatively new NLO medium are further considered later in this chapter (e.g., in Section 2.2.3).
- The instrument shown in Figure 2.4 comprises a doubly resonant, degenerate OPO that is synchronously pumped [75,76]. The spectrum of its fs-pump

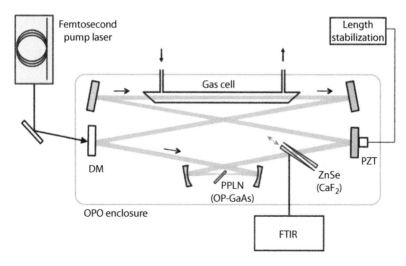

FIGURE 2.4 Schematic layout of the degenerate broadband OPO used to measure the mid-IR 1–0 fundamental-band absorption spectrum (as in Figure 2.3) of CO gas contained in an intracavity cell [75]. In that application, the pump beam from an fs-pulsed Tm-doped fiber laser (operating at 2.05 µm) was introduced through an in-coupling dielectric mirror DM; the other five mirrors were gold coated. A pair of CaF$_2$ wedges (for dispersion compensation and mid-IR beam out-coupling) were used, and the nonlinear optical crystal was OP-GaAs (placed at Brewster's angle) to generate a broadband frequency comb output spectrum centered at ~4.1 µm. Alternative shorter-wavelength applications (with an output spectrum centered at ~3.4 µm) have employed a 1.56 µm Er-doped fiber laser, a ZnSe wedge pair, and an AR-coated PPLN nonlinear optical crystal. (From M. W. Haakestad, T. P. Lamour, N. Leindecker, A. Marandi, and K. L. Vodopyanov, Intra-cavity trace molecular detection with a broadband mid-IR frequency comb source, *J. Opt. Soc. Am. B* 30: 631–640, 2013. With permission from Professor K. L. Vodopyanov and Optical Society of America.)

frequency comb is downconverted with high fidelity, thereby generating mid-IR frequency combs with large parametric gain bandwidth. Extensive mixing of comb components results in an extremely large instantaneous mid-IR bandwidth that spans more than one octave and is suitable for molecular spectroscopy at wavelengths out to ~6 µm.

- The spectroscopic sensitivity of this broadband mid-IR source is enhanced for trace gas detection by coupling the frequency comb into a high-finesse Fabry–Perot cavity to attain long effective optical path lengths and conveniently short measurement times. This has been realized for the following six trace gases (with reported detection limits, all diluted at 1 atm pressure, at chosen operating wavelengths): methane (CH$_4$, 1.7 parts per billion by volume [ppbv] at ~3.3 µm), formaldehyde (H$_2$CO, 0.31 ppmv at ~3.5 µm), acetylene (C$_2$H$_2$, 0.11 ppmv at ~3.0 µm), ethylene (C$_2$H$_4$, 0.32 ppmv at ~3.3 µm), CO (0.27 ppmv at ~4.8 µm), and isotopic carbon dioxide (^{13}CO$_2$, 2.4 ppbv at ~4.4 µm) [75,76]. The two longer-wavelength intracavity measurements (of CO in He and of ^{13}CO$_2$ in ambient air) employed the OP GaAs OPO system with a Tm-doped fiber laser pump, while the other four (at

shorter wavelengths, in N_2) employed the PPLN OPO system pumped by an Er-doped fiber laser, as in Figure 2.4.
- In these OPO-spectroscopic measurements, the line shapes are found to have dispersive features (e.g., as for CO in the upper trace of Figure 2.3), which can be adequately described by a model that takes into account intra-cavity passive loss and round-trip group delay dispersion across the broad OPO frequency band.

The foregoing five bullet points, together with Figures 2.3 and 2.4, provide a representative demonstration of the significant scale of technological and scientific advances that continue to be made in the area of OPO-based spectroscopy [75,76].

2.2 OPTICAL PARAMETRIC DEVICES: HOW THEY OPERATE

2.2.1 OPTICAL PARAMETRIC PROCESSES

Optical parametric devices are useful sources of coherent, laser-like radiation that are typically intense and tunable over a wide range of wavelengths. They invariably arise via nonlinear optics, most frequently through a three-wave mixing process mediated by the NLO susceptibility tensor $\chi^{(2)}$ in a noncentrosymmetric crystalline medium [77–80]. Three forms of optical parametric device are illustrated in Figure 2.5: (a) OPG, (b) OPA, and (c) OPO. Also illustrated is a closely related (but distinct) NLO device: (d) the difference-frequency generator (DFG). Coherent light waves are represented by arrows, with their associated optical angular frequency ω_j and wave vector $\mathbf{k}_j$ (as defined later in this section). In Figure 2.5, input and output waves are shown as arrows on the left and right, respectively, with their breadth indicating typical relative intensities.

An OPG is the simplest form of optical parametric device. As depicted in Figure 2.5a, it entails a single input wave (pump P, at frequency ω_P) and two output waves: signal S (at ω_S) and idler I (at ω_I), where $\omega_S \geq \omega_I$. The NLO process itself is initiated by spontaneous parametric processes that comprise naturally occurring emission/noise/fluorescence at low intensity, effectively "splitting" a pump photon into two new photons [81]. There is considerable interest in *spontaneous parametric downconversion* at the single-photon level, in view of its relevance to quantum optics, quantum entanglement, and quantum computing [82,83]. However, for relatively high-power optical parametric generation as considered here, a semiclassical description can be retained without quantum-optical subtleties [81].

Once a signal or idler wave has been generated, it can be coherently amplified by passing it through an OPA together with input pump radiation, as depicted in Figure 2.5b. A further order of sophistication is reached in an OPO, as depicted in Figure 2.5c, in which the functions of an OPG and an OPA are combined by multi-passing one or more of the optical waves involved inside a resonant optical cavity, formed by two or more appropriately aligned reflectors (M_1, M_2).

A DFG, as depicted in Figure 2.5d, is *not* an optical parametric device, although the DFG source term is central to the NLO mechanism of OPGs, OPAs, and OPOs. In a DFG, two intense input waves (with frequencies ω_1 and ω_2) interact coherently to generate a third output wave (with frequency ω_{diff}) at the difference frequency

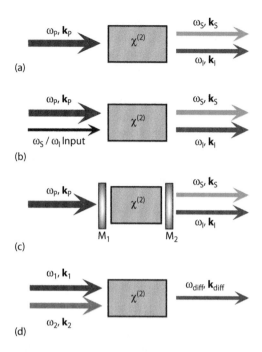

FIGURE 2.5 Schematic diagrams of three forms of optical parametric device. (a) Optical parametric generator (OPG). (b) Optical parametric amplifier (OPA). (c) Optical parametric oscillator (OPO). Note that, by convention, optical frequencies of the signal (S) and idler (I) output waves are defined such that $\omega_S \geq \omega_I$. Also shown is a fourth closely related device: (d) Difference-frequency generator (DFG). Nonlinear optical (NLO) media are denoted by their susceptibility tensor $\chi^{(2)}$. Arrows represent input and output waves, together with their optical frequencies ω_j and wave vectors $\mathbf{k}_j$. An OPO requires an optical resonator, comprising at least two aligned reflectors (M_1, M_2).

of the two input waves [11,84]. There are now two relatively high-power driving waves (rather than one), and the frequencies of these waves are subtracted from each other (rather than effectively splitting a single incident frequency in two, as in an optical parametric process). Nevertheless, the outcome and utility of a DFG can be similar to those of an optical parametric device. For instance, if coherent radiation is required at a particular IR wavelength, it can be generated either as the idler wave of an optical parametric device, with frequency $\omega_I = (\omega_P - \omega_S)$, or as the output wave of a DFG, with frequency $\omega_{diff} = |\omega_1 - \omega_2|$. Moreover, the NLO source term for a DFG entails a form of susceptibility tensor $\chi^{(2)}$ that is very similar to that for an OPG, OPA, or OPO. Furthermore, the mechanistic description of a DFG, as in Figure 2.5d, converges on that of an OPA, as in Figure 2.5b, when the field strength of the signal or idler input wave in the OPA case is increased to approach that of its pump wave.

Many desirable attributes of optical parametric devices in general, and tunable OPOs in particular, arise from the fact that any such instrument is derived from non-linear optics [77–80] and is therefore distinctively different from a laser. This yields flexible, versatile design features, such as modes of temporal and wavelength control to which lasers are not amenable. Lasers generally depend on population inversion of an optical gain medium, with associated optical lifetime and saturation limitations. On the other hand, optical parametric gain, oscillation, and amplification facilitate modular system design because they entail NLO coefficients and phase-matching conditions, as explained in this section.

In nonlinear optics, a number (σ, >2) of optical waves interact in a medium with NLO susceptibility tensor $\chi^{(\sigma-1)}$. For inelastic optical processes, these waves (with angular frequencies ω_1, ω_2,..., ω_σ) obey two *conservation conditions*. One is for energy (or frequency):

$$\omega_1 + \omega_2 + \cdots + \omega_\sigma = 0 \qquad (2.1)$$

The other conservation condition is effectively for momentum; this is expressed in terms of wave vectors $\mathbf{k}_j$ (with $j = 1, 2,..., \sigma$) that have magnitudes $k_j = n_j\omega_j/c = 2\pi n_j/\lambda_j$, where n_j is the refractive index at vacuum wavelength λ_j, and c is the speed of light:

$$\mathbf{k}_1 + \mathbf{k}_2 + \cdots + \mathbf{k}_\sigma + \Delta\mathbf{k} = 0 \qquad (2.2)$$

where $\Delta\mathbf{k}$ is the phase-mismatch vector between the σ interacting waves. Each frequency component ω_j and wave vector $\mathbf{k}_j$ is ascribed a positive or a negative sign, according to its phase relationships. Equation 2.2 defines a phase-matching condition, in which $\Delta\mathbf{k}$ must be minimized to optimize the efficiency of the NLO process of interest.

Two specific three-wave NLO processes that are relevant to this chapter are those for either an optical parametric device (i.e., OPG, OPA, or OPO) or a DFG. Each of these is mediated by the second-order NLO susceptibility tensor $\chi^{(2)}$, which is non-zero in a crystalline medium only if it is noncentrosymmetric. Many such crystals are available [24,25]. For example, lithium niobate ($LiNbO_3$) has been popular since the early days of pulsed tunable OPOs. Subsequent interest and activity in optical parametric device technology have been stimulated by the availability of NLO materials such as BBO (β-barium borate, BaB_2O_4) and KTP (potassium titanyl phosphate, $KTiOPO_4$). Much impetus has come from quasi-phase-matched (QPM) NLO media, such as periodically poled (PP) materials PPLN and PPKTP, tailored for specific wavelengths by the periodic structuring of ferroelectric domains. QPM media offer compact, efficient, low-threshold alternatives to conventional birefringently phase-matched (BPM) media. The characteristics of many BPM and QPM NLO crystalline media are accessible, both in books [24,25] and via the versatile SNLO software package [26].

For a three-wave optical parametric device, which is of principal interest in this chapter, the energy and momentum conservation conditions of Equations 2.1 and 2.2 become

$$\omega_P - \omega_S - \omega_I = 0; \quad \mathbf{k}_P - \mathbf{k}_S - \mathbf{k}_I - \Delta\mathbf{k} = 0 \qquad (2.3)$$

where a laser input wave ("pump," frequency ω_P, wave vector $\mathbf{k}_P$) yields two coherent output waves ("signal," ω_S, $\mathbf{k}_S$; "idler," ω_I, $\mathbf{k}_I$), such that $\omega_P > \omega_S \geq \omega_I$. Note that the idler frequency ω_I equals the difference $(\omega_P - \omega_S)$ between pump and signal frequencies. Equation 2.3 should be viewed in the context of parts (a–c) of Figure 2.5.

Equation 2.2 and the second half of Equation 2.3 apply strictly only to the conventional case of BPM media. In such media, the phase-matching condition $\Delta \mathbf{k} \approx 0$ is attained by adjusting its ordinary- and extraordinary-ray refractive indices via the angle and temperature of a birefringent NLO crystal. Such adjustments are used to optimize parametric conversion efficiency for a particular set of frequencies $(\omega_P, \omega_S, \omega_I)$ and thereby control the output signal and idler wavelengths, λ_S and λ_I. If it is assumed that the three waves are collinear and $\Delta \mathbf{k}$ is exactly zero, then the signal frequency/wavelength is given simply in terms of the pump frequency/wavelength and the refractive indices n_j $(j = P, S, I)$ as

$$\omega_S = \omega_P \frac{(n_P - n_I)}{(n_S - n_I)}; \quad \lambda_S = \lambda_P \frac{(n_S - n_I)}{(n_P - n_I)} \tag{2.4}$$

Various angle-dependent index-matching schemes are applicable in the case of OPOs based on BPM crystals: for example, Type I (eeo/ooe) and Type II (oeo/eoe) in positive/negative uniaxial birefringent crystals, where "o" and "e" denote the ordinary and extraordinary waves listed in the order "I S P" [24,84]. Many BPM optical parametric devices (especially those in the ns-pulsed regime) employ so-called critical phase matching (CPM, which may be either collinear or noncollinear), which depends on the orientation of the optical-wave propagation directions relative to the optic axis of the NLO crystal [10,11,24,43,47,48,84].

An alternative approach is so-called noncritical phase matching (NCPM, also known as 90° phase matching), in which the propagation direction is normal to the optic axis of the NLO crystal, and the ordinary- and extraordinary-wave refractive indices n_o and n_e have a zero first-order dependence on the orientation of the crystal [10,11,24,43,47,48,84]. NCPM enables the phase-matched interaction to be along a principal optical axis of the NLO material with no spatial walk-off. This also has the advantage that the effective interaction length is determined by the length of the crystal and is not reduced by spatial walk-off. For a fixed pump wavelength, the output signal and idler wavelengths of an NCPM OPO can then be tuned by varying the temperature (and hence the refractive indices) of the crystal at a fixed (90°) orientation. Alternatively, NCPM OPO output can be tuned by varying the pump wavelength (e.g., from a tunable dye or Ti:sapphire laser—so much for "Good-bye to Ti: and Dye," as proclaimed in Section 2.1.1 [1,5]), while maintaining the fixed crystal temperature and orientation. Such a NCPM approach was popular in the early days of OPO spectroscopy [10,11,16,17] and has since seen a resurgence, particularly for CW OPOs or for ultrafast OPOs, in which the absence of beam walk-off facilitates tight focusing of the (relatively low-power) CW or ultrafast pump beam to exceed the threshold of the OPO (as discussed in Sections 2.3.2 and 2.3.3).

The QPM approach was first recognized by pioneers of nonlinear optics in 1962 as an alternative to birefringent phase matching [85–87]. However, this QPM approach was not realized practically until ~30 years later, via NLO media such as PPLN [49,50,88–92]. For a QPM device, grating contributions, arising from the engineered microscale structure of the crystal, need to be included in phase-matching conditions. For instance, the z-component Δk of the wave-vector mismatch $\Delta \mathbf{k}$ in the second half of Equation 2.3 needs to be replaced by $\Delta k = [\Delta k_{QPM} + (2\pi \, m/\Lambda)]$, where m is the QPM order (usually an odd-numbered integer), Λ is the QPM grating period, and a collinear interaction along the z-axis is assumed.

In the corresponding case of a DFG (which, we repeat, is *not* an optical parametric device), two coherent input waves (frequencies ω_1, ω_2; wave vectors $\mathbf{k}_1$, $\mathbf{k}_2$) yield a single coherent output wave at the difference frequency $\omega_{diff} = |\omega_1 - \omega_2|$ (with wave vector $\mathbf{k}_{diff}$). The energy and momentum conservation conditions of Equations 2.1 and 2.2 then become

$$|\omega_1 - \omega_2| - \omega_{diff} = 0; \quad \mathbf{k}_1 - \mathbf{k}_2 - \mathbf{k}_{diff} - \Delta \mathbf{k} = 0 \tag{2.5}$$

as depicted in Figure 2.5d. As in Equations 2.2 and 2.3, phase matching is achieved when $\Delta \mathbf{k} \approx 0$ for BPM media. In the case of QPM media, there is an additional grating contribution in the second half of Equation 2.5, in which the z-component Δk of the vector $\Delta \mathbf{k}$ in the second half of Equation 2.3 needs to be replaced by $\Delta k = [\Delta k_{QPM} + (2\pi \, m/\Lambda)]$.

In a general sense (which is incidental to this chapter), other important forms of coherent wavelength conversion arise from four-wave mixing processes that are mediated by the third-order NLO susceptibility tensor $\chi^{(3)}$, which can be nonzero even in isotropic or centrosymmetric media such as gases, liquids, optical fibers, and all classes of crystal. Optical parametric processes of this type contribute to stimulated Raman scattering (SRS), involving an optical medium with Raman-active resonance frequencies, ω_R, that coincide with the difference between two optical frequencies. This can yield a relatively straightforward source of coherent radiation, Raman-shifted at discrete intervals from the frequency ω_L of an input pump laser (either tunable or fixed wavelength). These Raman-shift intervals, both added to (anti-Stokes) and subtracted from (Stokes) the laser frequency ω_L, are integer multiples of ω_R. Other NLO Raman parametric processes give rise to various forms of nonlinear Raman spectroscopy, such as coherent anti-Stokes Raman scattering (CARS), and to Raman fiber-optical amplifiers, used in optical telecommunications. Another developing area of optical parametric device technology entails OPGs, OPAs, and OPOs based on $\chi^{(3)}$ nonlinearities in highly NLO fibers, with either pulsed or CW pump lasers. Such processes typically use two pump waves (P) to generate tunable signal (S) and idler (I) output waves, so that $\omega_I = 2\omega_P - \omega_S$.

2.2.2 $\chi^{(2)}$-BASED OPTICAL PARAMETRIC GAIN AND AMPLIFICATION

The central theme of this chapter concerns $\chi^{(2)}$-based OPGs, OPAs, and OPOs, for which we can consider the intrinsic NLO process semiclassically in terms of three complex plane-wave radiation fields and the corresponding polarizations in the medium of interest:

$$\mathbf{E}_j(t) = \tfrac{1}{2} \mathbf{E}_j \exp\left[i\left(\mathbf{k}_j . \mathbf{r} - \omega_j t\right)\right] + \tfrac{1}{2} \mathbf{E}_j^* \exp\left[-i\left(\mathbf{k}_j . \mathbf{r} - \omega_j t\right)\right] \tag{2.6}$$

$$\mathbf{P}_j(t) = \tfrac{1}{2}\mathbf{P}_j \exp\left[i\left(\mathbf{k}_j.\mathbf{r} - \omega_j t\right)\right] + \tfrac{1}{2}\mathbf{P}_j^* \exp\left[-i\left(\mathbf{k}_j.\mathbf{r} - \omega_j t\right)\right] \qquad (2.7)$$

where the suffix $j = $ P, S, or I. Interaction with the NLO susceptibility tensor $\chi^{(2)}$ of a noncentrosymmetric medium then causes these to be interrelated as follows:

$$\mathbf{P}_S^{(2)} = \varepsilon_0\chi^{(2)}\mathbf{E}_P\mathbf{E}_I^*; \quad \mathbf{P}_I^{(2)} = \varepsilon_0\chi^{(2)}\mathbf{E}_P\mathbf{E}_S^*; \quad \mathbf{P}_P^{(2)} = \varepsilon_0\chi^{(2)}\mathbf{E}_S\mathbf{E}_I \qquad (2.8)$$

where ε_0 is the vacuum permittivity (8.854×10^{-12} C^2/(J m)). Here, only the second-order polarizations $\mathbf{P}_j^{(2)}$ need be considered, and, in the interest of simplicity, the functional dependence of $\chi^{(2)}$ on the optical frequencies ω_S, ω_I, ω_P has been suppressed.

It is significant that the polarizations $\mathbf{P}_j^{(2)}(t)$ for the coherent NLO processes, such as those represented in Equation 2.8, depend functionally on phase-dependent radiation fields $\mathbf{E}_j(t)$ as in Equation 2.6, rather than on phase-independent optical power or intensity. This phase dependence gives rise to phase-matching conditions—such as those in Equations 2.2, 2.3, and 2.5—in which the amplitude of $\mathbf{P}_j^{(2)}(t)$ is optimized (and hence the NLO output) when pump, signal, and idler waves are in phase for a maximum distance in the NLO medium.

Incidentally, use of the word *parametric* here is sometimes the cause of ambiguity. Parametric conversion processes were first recognized in the microwave context and were later carried over into the NLO domain. One highly regarded author suggests that all "elastic" NLO processes (in which initial and final material quantum states are identical and no real population is created elsewhere during the NLO process, which depends on a real susceptibility tensor $\chi^{(2)}$) can be regarded as "parametric" [80]. This is in contrast to so-called nonparametric NLO processes, which are "inelastic" (with nonidentical initial and final material quantum states, and the photon energy is not conserved, because energy is transferred between the radiation field and the material); such nonparametric processes are independent of phase matching and depend on a complex susceptibility, for example, as in the $\chi^{(1)}$ description of SRS [79,80]. All of the former "elastic" types of NLO process can, indeed, be treated by applying a parametric approximation, for example, to Equation 2.8, in the limit of low-strength signal and idler fields. However, the more widespread use [7–11,77–79] is for NLO parametric conversion to be a description that is confined to include processes such as those in OPGs, OPAs, and OPOs, but not those, for instance, in second harmonic, sum frequency, and DFGs (although these are "parametric processes" in the sense of [80]).

Continuing from Equations 2.6 through 2.8, we introduce a suitably defined, effective NLO coefficient d_{eff} (units: m V^{-1} or, more typically, pm V^{-1}) to yield [1,5]

$$P_S^{(2)} = 2\varepsilon_0 d_{\text{eff}} E_P E_I^*; \quad P_I^{(2)} = 2\varepsilon_0 d_{\text{eff}} E_P E_S^*; \quad P_P^{(2)} = 2\,\varepsilon_0 d_{\text{eff}} E_S E_I \qquad (2.9)$$

where d_{eff} is a linear combination of elements of the NLO susceptibility tensor $\chi^{(2)}$ for the medium of interest. For a particular BPM crystal, d_{eff} depends on its (noncentrosymmetric) crystal class and its cut and orientation relative to the propagation and polarization directions of the incident light waves. The vector/tensor notation used in Equation 2.8 is not needed in Equation 2.9 for a specific experimental configuration.

By combining Equations 2.6, 2.7, and 2.9 with Maxwell's equations, our algebraic treatment of optical parametric amplification yields a set of relevant coupled wave equations for plane waves propagating in the z direction. These are common to various forms of three-wave NLO process, but are specified here for OPGs, OPAs, and OPOs [1,5]:

$$\left(\frac{dE_S}{dz}\right)+\alpha_S E_S = i\left(\frac{k_S}{n_S^2}\right)d_{eff}E_P E_I^* \exp\left(i\Delta k z\right) \tag{2.10}$$

$$\left(\frac{dE_I}{dz}\right)+\alpha_I E_I = i\left(\frac{k_I}{n_I^2}\right)d_{eff}E_P E_S^* \exp\left(i\Delta k z\right) \tag{2.11}$$

$$\left(\frac{dE_P}{dz}\right) = i\left(\frac{k_P}{n_P^2}\right)d_{eff}E_S E_I \exp\left(-i\Delta k z\right) \tag{2.12}$$

where α_j (j=S, I, P) are loss factors and the wave-vector mismatch Δk is the z-component of $\Delta \mathbf{k}$.

Equation 2.12 corresponds to the customary limit of negligible pump-field losses ($\alpha_P = 0$). In addition, the pump wave may be treated as undepleted ($dE_P/dz = 0$) when it is much more intense than the other two waves, leaving only two coupled differential equations.

In parametric generation, the pump field, E_P, is assumed to be relatively strong, whereas the signal and idler fields, E_S and E_I, grow from a low level. In the zero-loss limit (with all $\alpha_j = 0$), Equations 2.10 through 2.12 yield what is effectively a photon conservation condition:

$$\omega_S^{-1}\left(\frac{dI_S}{dz}\right)=\omega_I^{-1}\left(\frac{dI_I}{dz}\right)=-\omega_P^{-1}\left(\frac{dI_P}{dz}\right);\ \lambda_S\left(\frac{dI_S}{dz}\right)=\lambda_I\left(\frac{dI_I}{dz}\right)=-\lambda_P\left(\frac{dI_P}{dz}\right) \tag{2.13}$$

where $I_j = \frac{1}{2} c \varepsilon_0 n_j |E_j|^2$ (with j=S, I, or P) is the optical intensity or flux (units: W m^{-1}). The conversion of each photon from the pump field (P) is then seen to generate two photons, one in the signal field (S) and the other in the idler field (I).

A situation that is more realistic than this zero-loss limit is that with finite but equal signal and idler losses ($\alpha_S = \alpha_I = \alpha$). This yields a tractable general solution describing the evolution of the signal and idler fields. In the case where a single-frequency idler field, $E_I(z)$, is incident on a pumped medium of length L, it experiences a single-pass power gain of the form:

$$G_I(L)=\left[\frac{|E_I(z=L)|^2}{|E_I(z=0)|^2}\right]-1=\Gamma^2 L^2 (gL)^{-2}\sinh^2(gL) \tag{2.14}$$

where g and Γ are the total and parametric gain coefficients, respectively, defined by

$$\Gamma = \left(k_S k_I\right)^{1/2} |d_{\text{eff}}| \frac{|E_P^0|}{n_S n_I} \tag{2.15}$$

$$g = \left[\left|\Gamma^2 - \left(\frac{\Delta k}{2}\right)^2\right|\right]^{1/2} \tag{2.16}$$

where, in the limit of zero pump depletion, $E_p^0 \equiv E_p(z=0)$ is taken to be constant over the range $0 \leq z \leq L$ and the incident signal field $E_S(z=0)$ is zero. The relatively simple functional form of Equations 2.14 through 2.16 applies only to the case of an effectively monochromatic incident idler wave. If more than one frequency is present, then the solutions become critically dependent on the phases of those incident waves relative to that of the pump radiation field.

In the high-gain limit, where $\Gamma^2 \gg (\Delta k/2)^2$, the single-pass power gain corresponds to the extreme case of superfluorescent parametric emission:

$$G_I(L) = \tfrac{1}{4}\exp(2\Gamma L) \tag{2.17}$$

where zero loss has again been assumed. This situation arises when the medium is pumped by a high-intensity pulsed laser source, as in pulsed OPGs and OPOs.

Alternatively, pumping by a CW or low/moderate-peak-power pulsed laser corresponds to the low-gain limit of parametric generation, with $\Gamma L < 1$ or $\Gamma^2 < (\Delta k/2)^2$:

$$G_I(L) = \Gamma^2 L^2 \text{sinc}^2 \left\{\left[\left|\left(\frac{\Delta k}{2}\right)^2 - \Gamma^2\right|\right]^{1/2} L\right\} \tag{2.18}$$

where sinc $x = (\sin x)/x$. When $\Gamma^2 \ll (\Delta k/2)^2$, the argument of the sinc^2 function is $(\Delta k\, L/2)$, with the phase mismatch Δk exerting a dominant influence on the single-pass gain. Near phase matching $\Delta k \approx 0$ and $\Gamma L \ll 1$, the single-pass power gain $G_I(L) \approx \Gamma^2 L^2$.

An alternative form of Equation 2.15 can be derived in terms of the intensity or flux $I_p^0 \equiv I_p(z=0)$ of the incident pump radiation, yielding the square of the total gain coefficient Γ:

$$\Gamma^2 = \left[\frac{8\pi^2 d_{\text{eff}}^2}{(c\varepsilon_0 n_p n_S n_I \lambda_S \lambda_I)}\right] I_p^0 = \left[\frac{2d_{\text{eff}}^2 \omega_S \omega_I}{(c^3 \varepsilon_0 n_p n_S n_I)}\right] I_p^0 \tag{2.19}$$

where pump depletion is assumed to be zero.

Another useful transformation [8,43,47] is to use a parameter $\delta = [2(\omega_S/\omega_P) - 1] = [2(\lambda_P/\lambda_S) - 1]$, such that $\omega_S = \frac{1}{2}\omega_P(1 + \delta)$ and $\omega_I = \frac{1}{2}\omega_P(1 - \delta)$ and Equations 2.15 and 2.19 become

$$\Gamma = k_0 n_0^{-2}\left|d_{\mathrm{eff}}\right|\left|E_P^0\right|\left(1 - \delta^2\right)^{1/2} \tag{2.20}$$

$$\Gamma^2 = \left[\frac{8\pi^2 d_{\mathrm{eff}}^2}{\left(c\varepsilon_0 n_P n_0^2 \lambda_0^2\right)}\right]\left(1 - \delta^2\right)I_P^0 = \left[\frac{2d_{\mathrm{eff}}^2 \omega_0^2}{\left(c^3\varepsilon_0 n_P n_0^2\right)}\right]\left(1 - \delta^2\right)I_P^0 \tag{2.21}$$

where zero subscripts (i.e., on k_0, n_0, λ_0, and ω_0) denote the degeneracy point such that $\omega_0 = \frac{1}{2}\omega_P$, $\lambda_0 = 2\lambda_P$, and $n_0 \approx n_S \approx n_I$. The so-called degeneracy factor $(1 - \delta^2)^{1/2}$ measures the reduction in parametric gain as ω_S and ω_I (or λ_S and λ_I) move away from the degeneracy point ω_0 (or λ_0).

In view of the functional forms of Γ and Γ^2 in Equations 2.15 and 2.19 through 2.21, it is useful to a define a NLO figure of merit (FOM) as follows:

$$\mathrm{FOM} = \frac{d_{\mathrm{eff}}^2}{n_P n_S n_I} = d_{\mathrm{eff}}^2 n_{\mathrm{eff}}^{-3} \tag{2.22}$$

where $n_{\mathrm{eff}} = (n_P n_S n_I)^{1/3}$ is a geometric mean of refractive indexes. This arbitrary definition is consistent with that of Vodopyanov [46], although other (equally arbitrary) definitions of the FOM are in current usage [47,84]. Whatever definition is chosen for the FOM, it incorporates NLO properties that are critical in determining the optical parametric gain and hence the relative efficiencies of OPGs, OPAs, and OPOs based on different NLO media and operating regimes.

The FOM has an intrinsic wavelength dependence, not only from the dispersion of n_{eff} but also from the dispersion of $\chi^{(2)}$ and hence d_{eff}, which, using Miller's rule [93], can be predicted empirically to vary as $(n_{\mathrm{eff}}^2 - 1)^3$; the net effect is that the FOM as defined in Equation 2.22 is expected to be approximately proportional to n_{eff}^9 [47]. An outcome of this is that, for a given pump intensity I_P^0 and crystal length L, normal dispersion causes the optical parametric gain to decline markedly as one moves from the visible and near IR regions to longer wavelengths in the mid-IR ($\lambda > \sim 4\ \mu m$) and far-IR ($\lambda > \sim 20\ \mu m$) regions; this is aggravated by the dependence of Γ^2 on $(\lambda_S \lambda_I)^{-1}$, as in Equations 2.19 and 2.21. Optical parametric devices operating at longer wavelengths (e.g., in the mid-IR and far-IR regions) therefore posed early instrumental challenges.

2.2.3 CHOICE OF OPTICAL PARAMETRIC GAIN MEDIUM

The choice of NLO crystal for optical parametric devices depends on various well-established factors [8–11,22–26,35,46,47,84]. In the traditional BPM case, these include

- The symmetry class of the crystal, as only noncentrosymmetric crystals (also capable of piezoelectric response) can have nonzero $\chi^{(2)}$ tensor components (or values of d_{eff}).

- The magnitude of $\chi^{(2)}$ (or d_{eff}) to ensure sufficient optical nonlinearity.
- The form of phase matching (e.g., Type I or Type II, CPM or NCPM) to be used.
- The capability of growing large crystals of high optical quality, to maximize path length in a wide-aperture, blemish-free NLO medium.
- The transparency of the material at all three wavelengths (λ_S, λ_I, and λ_p) to enable the device to operate over as wide a tuning range as possible.
- The optical damage threshold, particularly at the nominated pump wavelength, but also at signal and idler wavelengths in high-gain devices.
- The ease of handling of the crystal (e.g., hygroscopic properties, durability, and hardness).
- The refractive indices, dispersion, and birefringent properties of the crystal, which need to be suitable for phase matching to be established.
- The thermal coefficients of the refractive index, either to enhance temperature tuning or to minimize temperature sensitivity.

The choice of a particular NLO material is also influenced by the affordability and ready availability of suitable crystals. In the corresponding chapter in the first edition of this book [1], it was feasible to tabulate on two facing pages the key properties of most of the BPM crystals that were in common use. Such a task is now impractical, in view of the improved availability and quality of BPM crystals, together with the advent of QPM media, which are in high demand for OPG, OPA, and OPO applications over a wide range in the IR and UV regions.

Table 2.1 lists a representative selection of uniaxial (*ua*) and biaxial (*ba*) NLO crystals that are used in near IR and mid-IR optical parametric devices; their relevant characteristics include FOM values. Also crucial, but not listed in Table 2.1, are estimates of optical damage thresholds, which limit the pump laser intensity, fluence, pulse duration, and repetition rate that can reliably be used for a given NLO material [24,25]. A diversity of NLO materials is available for use in optical parametric devices, but surveying them comprehensively is beyond the scope of this chapter [24,25], as is balancing the many design considerations [24] that arise when selecting such a material.

The QPM materials listed in the lower half of Table 2.1 are seen to have relatively high FOMs, primarily because it is then possible to take advantage of the largest NLO tensor element (e.g., d_{33} in various PP materials) rather than smaller d_{ij} values (with $i \neq j$) for BPM devices. For instance, the widely used QPM medium PPLN with all waves z-polarized offers an NLO gain enhancement of $(2d_{33}/\pi d_{31})^2 \approx 16$, relative to its BPM counterpart, bulk LiNbO$_3$ [46]. The ready availability of PPLN and other QPM materials has revolutionized the design of optical parametric wavelength-conversion techniques (such as OPG, OPA, and OPO), as well as DFG. However, applications such as high-power NLO devices and the generation of coherent mid-IR radiation continue to rely on bulk crystalline BPM materials [46,47,84,94].

As indicated in Table 2.1, OP GaAs has a remarkable FOM advantage due to its enormous d_{eff} value of $(2d_{14}/\pi) = 60$ pm/V, approximately five times that of PPLN [46,95]. However, GaAs is a cubic crystal with a zincblende structure, so that it is neither birefringent (i.e., a BPM device is not feasible) nor ferroelectric (i.e., it

TABLE 2.1
Characteristics of Selected NLO Crystals Commonly Used in Near IR and Mid-IR Optical Parametric Devices[a]

NLO Crystal (Biaxial, ba/uniaxial, ua)	Transparency Range (µm)	$\|d_{eff}\|$ (pm/V)	$n_{eff} = (n_P n_S n_I)^{1/3}$	FOM, $d_{eff}^2 n_{eff}^{-3}$ (pm²/V⁻²)
BPM Materials				
AgGaS₂ (ua)	0.47–13	12	2.40	10.4
AgGaSe₂[b] (ua)	0.71–19	33	2.65	2.8
β-BaB₂O₄ (BBO)[c] (ua)	0.20–2.6	2.2	1.7	1.0
KTiOAsO₄ (KTA) (ba)	0.35–5.3	4	1.8	1.4
KTiOPO₄ (KTP) (ba)	0.35–4.3	4	1.8	1.4
LiB₃O₅ (LBO)[c] (ba)	0.16–2.6	0.9	1.6	0.2
LiNbO₃ (LN) (ua)	0.33–5.5	5	2.13	2.6
RbTiOAsO₄ (RTA) (ba)	0.35–5.3	4	1.8	2.7
ZnGeP₂ (ZGP)[b] (ua)	0.74–12	75	3.13	8.8
QPM Materials[d]				
PP KTiOAsO₄ (PPKTA) (ba)	0.35–5.3	10.3	1.8	18
PP KTiOPO₄ (PPKTP) (ba)	0.35–4.3	10.8	1.8	20
PP LiNbO₃ (PPLN) (ua)	0.40–5.5	14.2	2.13	20.9
PP RbTiOAsO₄ (PPRTA) (ba)	0.35–5.3	10.1	1.8	17.5
OP GaAs (orientation-patterned)[a]	0.9–17	60	3.3	100

Source: Derived and adapted from: Tables 1–3 of Vodopyanov, K. L., *Solid-State Mid-Infrared Sources*, Springer, Berlin, 2003 [46]; table 2 of Ebrahim-Zadeh, M., *Solid-State Mid-Infrared Sources*, Springer, Berlin, 2003 [47], and table 2 of Fischer, C., and M. W. Sigrist, *Solid-State Mid-Infrared Sources*, Springer, Berlin, 2003 [84]; Dmitriev, V. G., G. G. Gurzayan, and D. N. Nikogosyan, *Handbook of Nonlinear Optical Crystals*, 3rd edn, Springer, New York, 1999 [24]; and Smith, A. V., *SNLO Nonlinear Optics Code*, freeware from http://www.as-photonics.com/snlo [26].

[a] Typical operating conditions are $\lambda_P = 1.06$ µm, $\lambda_S \approx 1.6$ µm, $\lambda_I \approx 3.2$ µm.

[b] Because of transparency and phase matching, it is not feasible to have $\lambda_P < \sim 2$ µm.

[c] Because of low IR transparency, typical operating conditions are taken to be $\lambda_P = 0.35$ µm, $\lambda_S \approx 0.46$ µm, $\lambda_I \approx 1.5$ µm.

[d] Values of $|d_{eff}|$ for QPM materials correspond to $2 |d_{33}|/\pi$. Ferroelectric media, such as KTA, KTP, LN, and RTA, can be periodically poled (PP), but GaAs, which is cubic and therefore not birefringent, must be used as an orientation-patterned NLO medium [46].

cannot be periodically poled). OP GaAs is an extremely promising medium for NLO wavelength conversion, given its large NLO coefficient [46,49,50,95]; its dispersion relationships, which influence phase matching [96]; its low absorption and high transparency over a wide IR wavelength range (0.9–17 µm); its high laser-damage threshold; and its high thermal conductivity. Moreover, GaAs is a widely used semiconductor with well-tried material technology. The availability of OP GaAs is still limited, due to the complicated fabrication processes (e.g., epitaxial growth [49,50,94,97–100]) that are needed to produce it. Early NLO wavelength-conversion applications of OP

GaAs included second-harmonic generation (SHG) [95], DFG-based spectroscopy at ~7–9 μm [101–103], pulsed tunable OPO operation at ~2–9 μm [104], a mid-IR continuum OPG spanning ~5–10 μm [105], and the generation of terahertz (THz) waves in the range ~0.9–3 THz (~0.3–0.1 mm) [106,107]. Aspects of more recent OP GaAs applications in an fs-pumped degenerate broadband OPO, used for frequency comb mid-IR absorption spectroscopy [75,76], have already been introduced in Section 2.1.2. OP GaAs OPOs also have potential for IR-countermeasure defense applications, as discussed in Section 2.5.5.

2.2.4   Operating Regimes for Optical Parametric Processes

Typical operating regimes for different classes (A–D) of single-pass optical parametric gain processes are examined in Table 2.2 under phase-matched conditions ($\Delta k = 0$) and near-degenerate operation with $\lambda_S \approx \lambda_I \approx 2$ μm, as previously reported by Majid Ebrahim-Zadeh [47]. In terms of Equations 2.14 through 2.21, the parametric gain factor ΓL (which equals gL when $\Delta k = 0$) is calculated and yields the single-pass power gain $G_I(L)$, which equals $\sinh^2 \Gamma L$. Typical NLO material parameters (e.g., $|d_{eff}| \approx 3$ pm/V and $n_{eff} \approx 1.5$, FOM ≈ 2.7) are assumed, and the four operating regimes are distinguished by the choice of pump power, focal geometry, crystal

TABLE 2.2

Typical Operating Regimes for Different Classes (Labeled A–D) of Single-Pass Optical Parametric Gain Process[a]

Class of Single-Pass Optical Parametric Gain	Class A Continuous-Wave (CW)	Class B ns-Pulsed	Class C ps/fs-Pulsed	Class D ps/fs-Pulsed and Amplified
Pump pulse energy	—	10 mJ	15 nJ	10 μJ
Pump pulse duration	—	10 ns	100 fs	200 fs
Peak pump power	5 W	1 MW	150 kW	50 MW
Focused waist radius (w_0)	20 μm	1 mm	15 μm	15 μm
Peak pump intensity I_p	0.4 MW/cm²	30 MW/cm²	20 GW/cm²	7 TW/cm²
Crystal length:	10 mm	10 mm	1 mm	1 mm
ΓL ($\equiv g L$ if $\Delta k = 0$)	0.09	0.77	1.99	37
$G_I(L)$, as in Equation 2.14	0.008	0.72	13	3.4×10^{31}
Relevant optical parametric device(s)[b]	OPO	OPO	OPO	OPO, OPG, OPA

Source: Adapted from Table 1 of Ebrahim-Zadeh, M., *Solid-State Mid-Infrared Sources*, Springer, Berlin, 2003 [47].

[a]   The table is based on typical experimental values for pump laser and NLO material parameters (e.g., $|d_{eff}| \approx 3$ pm/V and $n_{eff} \approx 1.5$, so that FOM = 2.7) in each operating regime. The parametric gain factor ΓL [$\equiv g L$, assuming phase-matched interaction ($\Delta k = 0$)], as in Equations 2.15 and 2.19 through 2.21, and single-pass power gain $G_I(L)$ [$\equiv \sinh^2 \Gamma L$], as in Equation 2.14, are calculated on the basis of near-degenerate operation with $\lambda_S \approx \lambda_I \approx 2$ μm.

[b]   Operational option(s) if output power must build up from spontaneous parametric emission.

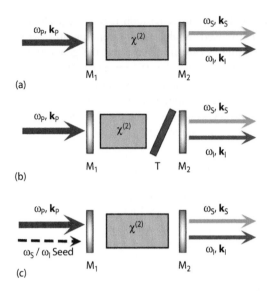

FIGURE 2.6 Schematic diagrams of three forms of optical parametric oscillator (OPO) [32]. (a) Free-running OPO (with no active wavelength control), similar to Figure 2.5c. (b) OPO with an intracavity tuning element (T). (c) Injection-seeded OPO.

length L, and (for pulsed cases B–D) pump pulse duration. The resulting values of $G_1(L)$ range over 33 orders of magnitude, from low-power CW operation (A) to high-energy ultrafast pulsed operation (D).

Usually, the signal and idler output power from an optical parametric device must build up from spontaneous parametric emission, so that only the high-energy ultra-fast pulsed case (D) has sufficiently high single-pass power gain $G_1(L)$ to enable practical operation as an OPG or an OPA, as in Figure 2.5a and b, respectively. In such a situation, the parametric gain in the other three operating regimes (CW, Q switched, and ps/fs-pulsed; cases A, B, and C, respectively) is typically too small to build up to a significant output power from spontaneous parametric emission. It is then necessary to adopt the OPO strategy, as in Figure 2.5c, with the NLO medium enclosed in an optical cavity to provide resonant optical feedback at the signal and/or idler wavelengths. On the other hand, if a sufficiently intense second input wave at the signal or idler frequency can be injected into the NLO medium together with the pump, then these three lower-power regimes (A–C) are still amenable to OPA or DFG operation, as in Figure 2.6b and d, respectively.

2.3 ELEMENTS OF OPTICAL PARAMETRIC OSCILLATOR DESIGN

As already explained in Section 2.1.1, we are primarily concerned in this chapter with tunable OPOs as coherent light sources for spectroscopic applications. Moreover, because such devices correspond inevitably to the downconversion of input pump radiation (and are particularly well suited to that task), much interest is concentrated on the spectroscopic applications of tunable OPOs generating coherent light in the near IR and mid-IR regions [46,47]. Most of the arbitrarily chosen examples that are considered in later sections of this chapter are therefore more relevant to the IR region than to the visible and UV regions, as are the selected NLO materials surveyed in Table 2.1. Meanwhile, we consider a few specific examples of tunable OPO designs, many based on the ubiquitous QPM NLO material, PPLN.

There are many ways to design an OPO, depending on whether it is CW, ns pulsed, or ps/fs pulsed (i.e., corresponding to Class A, B, or C, respectively) and what its end use is intended to be [7,41–48]. A key objective is invariably to ensure that the OPO has sufficiently high gain to overcome parasitic losses in the cavity. Two of the primary considerations concern the extent to which the OPO's optical cavity is resonant with one or both of the signal and idler output waves and with the pump wave, and whether the OPO itself is inside the cavity of the pump laser. Assorted OPO design strategies have been reviewed elsewhere; for instance, figure 2 of [41], figure 3 of [43], figure 1 of [45], and figure 3 of [46] each provide a useful pictorial compilation. Likewise, as discussed in Sections 2.4 and 2.5, control of the OPO output wavelengths (and their optical bandwidth) is critical to many spectroscopic applications. This generally depends on the tuning of the OPO cavity itself (e.g., by varying the cavity length or by incorporating a suitable intracavity wavelength-selective element), by tuning the pump laser wavelength, or (in the case of Class B OPOs) by injection seeding of control radiation from an independent tunable low-power source (which often requires control of OPO cavity length).

Another means of using an OPO as a spectroscopic source is to take advantage of the intrinsically broad bandwidth of a free-running OPO and to use its signal or idler output for multiplex spectroscopy, with the collection of the dispersed radiation by an optical-array detector. This approach has been demonstrated in various forms of OPO-based multiplex spectroscopy. The multiplex option (as discussed in Section 2.4) is able to use an extremely simple OPO cavity design, with much of the instrumental complexity transferred to the optical multichannel detection electronics. It is therefore attractive for various industrial laser-based monitoring applications, where coherent light sources (e.g., OPOs) need to be as rugged, compact, and simple to control as possible. Another application of broadband free-running OPOs is in defense, where thermal emissions from aircraft can be simulated by IR countermeasure systems that are able to repel and divert hostile heat-seeking missiles, as discussed in Section 2.5.5.

As already indicated in Section 2.1.2 [75,76], there has been much recent interest in using synchronously pumped, fs-pulsed OPOs to generate frequency combs with large parametric gain bandwidth for spectroscopic purposes. Such developments will be considered in more detail in Sections 2.3.3 through 2.3.5.

The amenability of pulsed OPO radiation to NLO processes also enables it to be used in various NLO wavelength-extension schemes, such as SFG, DFG, SHG, and SRS. These have been investigated as ways to extend the fundamental tuning range of pulsed OPOs further into the UV and IR regions [1,5,29,30].

2.3.1 NANOSECOND-PULSED OPTICAL PARAMETRIC OSCILLATORS

The initially reported PPLN-based OPO of Myers et al. [91] provides a useful example of typical operating conditions for an ns-pulsed OPO, as follows. A PPLN crystal

($L = 5$ mm, 0.5 mm thick) with a 31 μm QPM grating period was pumped at 1.064 μm by a pulsed, diode-pumped Nd:YAG laser (repetition rate, 100 Hz; pulse duration, 7 ns) with a focal spot diameter of 177 μm. A linear OPO cavity was formed by two carefully aligned reflectors (one 6.7 cm radius of curvature, the other flat) separated by 2.2 cm, each reflective (99% and 70% in this preliminary study [91]), and therefore resonant at the signal wavelength and transmissive at the pump and idler wavelengths. By varying the temperature of the PPLN crystal between room temperature and 180°C, this OPO was continuously tunable from 1.66 to 2.95 μm. At 145°C and $\lambda_S = 1.83$ μm, it was measured to have a pump threshold of 135 μJ, enabling damage-free pumping of the OPO as much as 10 times above threshold.

Subsequently, Myers et al. demonstrated an extended tuning range of 1.36–4.83 μm by implementing a multigrating PPLN chip (26 mm long, 0.5 mm thick), accommodating 25 gratings (each 0.5 mm wide) with QPM grating periods ranging from 26 to 32 μm in 0.25 μm steps [108]. With this longer multigrating PPLN crystal and with a higher-quality OPO cavity, an oscillation threshold of only 6 μJ was achieved, using a 7 ns pump pulse with a fluence of 0.09 J/cm². The average output power at an idler wavelength of 4 μm was 6 mW (with an average pump power of 100 mW at a repetition rate of 1 kHz).

The foregoing examples [91,108] represent a relatively straightforward approach to ns-pulsed OPO operation, namely, in the form of a singly resonant oscillator (SRO), with either the signal wave or the idler wave (but not both) resonated in the cavity. Some other OPO designs incorporate a nonresonant oscillator (NRO) stage, which comprises an OPA-type medium in an optical cavity that is resonant at neither ω_S nor ω_I [20,21]. Many additional examples of wavelength-control strategies for ns-pulsed OPOs will be presented in Section 2.4 of this chapter. Meanwhile, we briefly consider CW and ultrafast (ps/fs-pulsed) OPOs.

2.3.2 CONTINUOUS-WAVE OPTICAL PARAMETRIC OSCILLATORS

While the SRO approach is often used in ns-pulsed (Class B) OPO designs, the realization of CW OPOs (i.e., Class A) has presented much greater challenges [41,43,47,64]. A doubly resonant oscillator (DRO), in which both signal and idler waves are resonated in the cavity, is intrinsically more complicated than an SRO, but yields a lower oscillation threshold and has therefore been favored in many CW OPO designs [41,43,47]. Various multiparameter tuning approaches [43,109,110] have been devised to overcome mode- and cluster-hopping effects that complicate the continuously tunable, single-longitudinal-mode (SLM) operation of CW DROs. In one early example, a CW KTP DRO with a 40 mW oscillation threshold was pumped at ~1.047 μm near the signal/idler degeneracy point by a continuously tunable Nd:YLF laser, while maintaining resonance for a signal/idler pair at a discrete cavity length (stabilized to <0.4 nm) and tuning the OPO output frequencies over a range of ~4.5 GHz by tuning the pump laser frequency over a range of ~9 GHz [110]. In another example, a CW KTP DRO with an oscillation threshold of <50 mW was pumped at ~0.769 μm by a single-stripe GaAlAs diode laser [110]. Furthermore, by making the OPO cavity triply resonant (with the pump wave as well as the signal and idler waves), a pump-enhanced DRO attained an oscillation threshold as low as

~6 mW and yielded a 1.1 μm signal output power of ~10 mW with a diode-laser pump power of ~80 mW [111]. A CW PPLN DRO pumped at 0.810 μm by a 100 mW single-mode laser diode realized oscillation thresholds down to 16 mW, with quasi-continuous signal and idler tuning ranges of 1.15–1.25 and 2.31–2.66 μm, respectively, by variation of the crystal temperature, pump wavelength, and grating period [112].

Singly resonant CW OPO operation can also be attained by pump enhancement, with the OPO cavity resonant to the pump wave as well as signal or idler [41,43,47,113]. In an early (but complicated) 1993 example of a CW pump-enhanced SRO [114], a KTP OPO was pumped at 532 nm by frequency-doubling an injection-locked single-frequency Nd:YAG laser and operating at approximately two times above threshold by double passing both idler and pump waves and maintaining optimal phase relationships between all three waves in the standing-wave OPO cavity; with an oscillation threshold of 1.4 W, a CW pump power of 3.2 W yielded 1.07 W, 1.09 μm idler output. Schiller and coworkers have reported CW pump-enhanced SROs based on PPLN [115] and MgO-doped LiNbO$_3$ (MgO:LiNbO$_3$) [116], with theoretical analysis [113].

Another way to achieve singly resonant CW OPO operation is to locate the NLO medium inside the cavity of the pump laser itself, comprising an intracavity SRO [41,43,47,117–119]. For example, an early CW intracavity SRO comprising a KTP OPO located inside the cavity of a Ti:sapphire laser yielded idler output tunable from 2.53 to 2.87 μm with a maximum output power of ~0.4 W [120]. Corresponding Ti:sapphire-pumped intracavity SROs based on QPM NLO media such as PPLN (with signal and idler tuning ranges of 1.07–1.28 and 2.30–3.33 μm) [121] and PPKTP (with signal and idler tuning ranges of 1.14–1.27 and 2.23–2.73 μm) [119] have also been developed. A compact PPLN SRO sharing a dual cavity with a 1.064 μm Nd:YVO$_4$ mini-laser, pumped at 0.810 μm by a 1 W diode laser, yielded a diode-pump threshold of 310 mW; its quasi-continuous signal and idler tuning ranges were 1.45–1.60 and 3.16–4.02 μm, respectively [119,122].

The availability of QPM NLO materials such as PPLN has greatly enhanced the feasibility of CW SROs, which are much more readily tunable than CW DROs [41]. This was first shown by Bosenberg et al. using either standing-wave [123,124] or ring [124] cavities. The ring OPO operated on an SLM when pumped at 1.064 μm by a 13.5 W diode-pumped multiple-axial-mode CW Nd:YAG laser; by using a multi-grating PPLN chip, combined with an intracavity étalon and temperature tuning, the idler output could be tuned quasi-continuously from 3.95 to 3.25 μm with an optical bandwidth Δν < 6 GHz and 3.6 W maximum power.

This PPLN SRO approach was extended by replacing the multigrating PPLN chip with a "fan-out" grating on a 5 cm long, 2 cm wide PPLN crystal across which the QPM period changed continuously from 29.3 to 30.1 μm; single-frequency tuning of signal and idler outputs was achieved coarsely by translating the fan-out grating laterally, with finer tuning by rotating an intracavity étalon and varying the OPO cavity length at constant temperature [125].

Subsequent advances in PPLN-based CW SRO technology include a singly resonant OPO ring cavity pumped at 0.925 μm by a 2.5 W diode laser (generating up to 0.48 W of idler output with a tuning range of 2.0–2.3 μm) [126]; a CW PPLN SRO pumped at 1.03–1.10 μm by a tunable 8 W Yb-doped CW fiber laser (generating up to 1.9 W of idler output with a tuning range of 3.0–3.7 μm) [127]; extended mode-hop-free tuning of a dual-cavity, pump-enhanced CW PPLN SRO (with idler tuning ranges of 2.71–3.26 μm and 4.07–5.26 μm) [128]; a pump-enhanced CW PPLN SRO pumped at ~0.81 μm by a tunable extended-cavity diode laser (generating up to 4 mW of idler output with a tuning range of 2.58–3.44 μm) [129]; a CW PPLN OPO, pumped at 1.064 μm by a CW Nd:YAG laser, for near IR spectroscopic sensing by cavity-ringdown [130] and photoacoustic (PA) absorption [131] techniques; and a critical comparison of the performance of CW QPM OPOs based on PPLN and PPRTA [132].

2.3.3 Ultrafast Optical Parametric Oscillators

We now turn from CW OPOs to ultrafast OPOs (Classes C and D of Table 2.2). Despite the relatively high peak power of very short (subnanosecond) pulses of coherent laser light, it was at first nontrivial to use such light to pump the NLO medium of an OPO and to exceed its oscillation threshold [41–43,47]. This is because an ultrafast light pulse, on the timescale of picoseconds (10^{-12} s) or femtoseconds (10^{-15} s), does not have a sufficiently wide temporal window to enable a coherent parametric wave to build up coherent signal and idler waves in the NLO medium. Light travels only ~0.3 mm in 1 ps, which does not allow it to make multiple traversals of the NLO medium. Moreover, in contrast to the storage of population inversion in a laser, the NLO polarization in an OPO depends on the instantaneous optical field strength.

This significant problem is overcome by synchronous pumping (also used in some ultrafast lasers), in which a train of many consecutive ultrafast pulses from a pump laser interacts sequentially with a single signal or idler pulse circulating within the OPO cavity. The mode-locking interval of the pump laser (essentially the round-trip transit time in the laser cavity) must therefore equal the round-trip time of the down-converted (signal or idler) pulse in the OPO cavity. The situation is aggravated when subpicosecond (e.g., ~100 fs) pump pulses are used, because the pump and signal (or idler) waves have sufficiently different group velocities that they undergo "temporal walk-off," becoming separated in space after traversing a relatively short distance (typically 1–10 mm for 100 fs pulses) in the NLO medium.

Practical ultrafast OPOs were introduced around 1990, and their utility grew as improved pump lasers, NLO materials (e.g., KTP, PPLN), and OPO cavity designs became available [41–43,47,48,61–65]. Research on ps- and fs-pulsed OPOs remains extremely active, and numerous broadly tunable commercial ultrafast optical parametric systems (not only OPOs, but also OPGs and OPAs) are now on the market. This is driven, at least in part, by the key role that ultrafast OPG/OPA/OPO-based spectroscopy and imaging play in applications to biology and medicine, in which many key processes occur on picosecond and femtosecond timescales.

It is customary to classify synchronously pumped optical parametric systems as either CW ultrafast OPOs (i.e., pumped by a continuous train of ultrashort pulses) or quasi-CW/pulsed ultrafast OPOs (i.e., pumped by a burst of ultrashort pulses, contained in a nanosecond or microsecond envelope) [43,47]. Because the former are effectively steady-state devices, the output is a genuinely continuous train of identical pulses, whereas output from the latter comprises groups of ultrashort pulses in which the duration and amplitude of any pulse can vary across the pulse envelope.

Nevertheless, quasi-CW/pulsed ultrafast OPOs tend to yield significantly higher peak powers than their more stable CW ultrafast counterparts, and have in the past, therefore, been more readily realized. More recently, the advent of CW ultrafast OPOs has been promoted by the availability of high-power CW mode-locked lasers and improved NLO materials, which enable CW ultrafast OPOs to be operated in the (highly desirable) SRO format.

Specific operational aspects are discussed for fs-pulsed OPOs with regard to frequency comb spectroscopy (in Section 2.3.5) and for some ps-pulsed tunable OPOs in the context of nonlinear Raman microscopy (in Sections 2.5.3 and 2.5.4). The additional technical intricacies of ultrafast optical parametric devices (corresponding to Classes C and D of Table 2.2) are beyond the scope of this chapter. The reader is directed to relevant review articles [41–43,47,48,61–65,133–135] (particularly those concerning near- or mid-IR OPOs) and to various examples of tunable OPOs operating on picosecond and femtosecond timescales [75,76,133–194], as well as work on ultrafast travelling-wave OPGs and OPAs [195–198].

2.3.4 Optical Parametric Devices for Spectroscopic Applications

Spectroscopic measurement is an area of laser-based science and technology in which optical parametric devices such as OPOs play a significant role as versatile NLO sources of tunable coherent light. Some traditional elements of the spectroscopic applications of tunable OPOs, on which this chapter focuses, are listed in Table 2.3. Aspects of Table 2.3 are also relevant to Section 2.4, which considers in more detail the ways to control and enhance the optical bandwidth and tunability of ns-pulsed OPOs.

Practical laser-spectroscopic measurements usually require a source of coherent light (e.g., a tunable OPO) that is narrowband, continuously tunable (without mode-hops or other discontinuities), and sufficiently stable and powerful to yield high signal-to-noise ratios in recorded spectra. In the case of NLO spectroscopic measurements, the intensity of coherent radiation is a key factor. Many developments of tunable OPOs and other optical parametric devices for spectroscopic purposes (as reviewed in Sections 2.3.1 through 2.3.3 and Section 2.4) aim to meet such performance criteria. Moreover, particular applications (e.g., field-based spectroscopic sensing or military IR countermeasures) impose additional constraints concerning system cost, compactness, ruggedness, portability, and ease of operation.

The optical bandwidth of tunable OPO radiation will often limit the attainable spectroscopic resolution. The full width half-maximum (FWHM) linewidth arising in a particular spectroscopic application will usually define the optimal optical bandwidth of OPO output light: typically a few cm^{-1} (1 cm^{-1} = 30 GHz) for condensed phases or complicated biomolecular species, ~0.2 cm^{-1} (~6 GHz) for pressure-broadened gas-phase samples, and less than ~0.02 cm^{-1} (~0.6 GHz) for sub-Doppler spectra of atoms and molecules (e.g., with mass ~30 g/mol detected at 300 K and an absorption wavelength of 1 μm). High-resolution laser spectroscopy therefore requires narrowband radiation, preferably on an SLM basis.

Traditionally, the fineness of spectroscopic resolution is inherently limited in the case of pulsed light. A single coherent light pulse with a FWHM duration, Δt, can

TABLE 2.3

Operational Strategies for Tunable OPOs Applied to Spectroscopy

Objectives	Operational Strategies	Comments on Instrument/Technique
Wavelength range: what spectra are to be measured?	• UV/visible (0.2–0.7 μm) • Near infrared (0.7–4.0 μm) • Longwave IR (>4.0 μm)	Many nonlinear optical OPO materials are available, but are less well developed for the longwave IR. The UV/visible region is not considered thoroughly here.
Phase matching: BPM or QPM?	• BPM, angle- or T-tuned • QPM in periodic NLO materials	BPM is well established and preferred for high-power operation, also mid-IR. Low-threshold QPM media are available for both pulsed and CW OPOs.
Temporal: pulsed or continuous-wave (CW)?	• Pulsed for power and timing • CW for narrowest bandwidth	Mode-locked pulse trains from ultrafast (ps, fs) OPOs enable high-resolution frequency comb spectroscopy—see Sections 2.1.2, 2.3.3, and 2.3.4.
Optical bandwidth: narrowband or broadband?	• Broadband (e.g., free-running) • Single-longitudinal-mode (SLM)	The Fourier-transform limit is 44 MHz (0.0015 cm^{-1}) for an ideal 10 ns pulse. CW OPOs enable even lower $\Delta\nu$.
Mode of recording spectra: multiplex or continuously tunable?	• Scan narrowband signal/idler OPO output wavelength • Free-running OPOs operate broadband in multiplex cases	Wavelength control gives continuously tuned narrowband spectra. Multiplex spectroscopy with dispersed detection or multiwavelength tailored.
Output wavelength control: via cavity length or intracavity tuning elements or a variation of pump wavelength or injection seeding?	• Cavity length control + intracavity grating or étalon • Tuned pump with fixed cavity • Injection seeding of signal or idler by a tunable low-power coherent light source	Intracavity-element designs yield broad tunability but can be complicated. Pump tuning is particularly useful for CW OPOs. Injection seeding enables narrowband, mode-hop-free spectroscopy and tailored multiwavelength studies.

The operational strategies offer ways to use OPOs for spectroscopic applications, such as:

- Linear absorption (e.g., with multipass cell)
- Cavity ringdown (CRD) absorption spectra
- High-resolution spectra ($\Delta\nu \approx$ MHz/kHz/Hz)
- Nonlinear optical (e.g., coherent Raman)
- Atmospheric remote sensing (e.g., DIAL)
- Fast (μs, ns) and ultrafast (ps, fs) processes

Source: Adapted from He, Y., et al., *Opt. Photon. News*, 13(5) 56–60, 76, 2002 [30]; Orr, B. J., *Encyclopedia of Modern Optics*, Elsevier, Oxford, 2004 [31].

have a FWHM optical bandwidth, Δv, no finer than the associated Fourier-transform (FT) limit. For example (as explained on p. 334 of Siegman's textbook [199]), a transform-limited light pulse with pure Gaussian temporal and power-spectrum profiles is defined by the time–bandwidth product:

$$\Delta v \cdot \Delta t = \left(\frac{2 \ln 2}{\pi} \right) = 0.441 \qquad (2.23)$$

An illustrative consequence of this relationship is that a Gaussian light pulse with $\Delta t = 10$ ns has an FT-limited optical bandwidth $\Delta v = 44$ MHz (i.e., 0.0015 cm^{-1}), while the corresponding FT limits for shorter Gaussian pulses with $\Delta t = 10$ ps and 10 fs are $\Delta v = 44$ GHz and 44 THz (i.e., 1.5 and 1500 cm^{-1}), respectively. It is apparent that CW (or at least long-pulse) coherent light sources are more directly amenable to traditional forms of high-resolution spectroscopy.

However, such traditional FT limits to the effective spectroscopic bandwidth of pulsed coherent radiation can be greatly diminished in a coherent mode-locked train of short-duration light pulses. The phase relationship between successive short-Δt coherent optical pulses then forms a frequency comb structure, with effective spectroscopic resolution Δv much narrower than that suggested by the time–bandwidth product of Equation 2.23. Experimental indications of this effect can be seen [200] in early two-photon Ramsey-fringe spectroscopy [201,202]. Another instance of this effect is the case of mode-locked laser pulse trains (e.g., as discussed in Chapter 27 of Siegman's textbook [199]); extension to the context of optical frequency combs needs to take account of the additional effect of carrier-envelope phase shifts [203].

For instance, Diddams [204] has considered an octave-spanning mode-locked laser with repetition rate (mode spacing) f_r or pulse interval f_r^{-1}, carrier-envelope-offset (CEO) frequency f_0, and its nth comb frequency at $v_n = (n f_r + f_0)$; to stabilize the comb frequencies, both f_r and f_0 must be stabilized. Stabilization of f_0 is usually achieved by a $(f - 2f)$ interferometric technique [205], in which a portion of the long-wavelength end of the comb is frequency doubled and compared (via an optical heterodyne [OH] measurement) with the corresponding short-wavelength end of the comb spectrum; the resulting beat frequency is f_0. The mode spacing f_r can be stabilized directly, either by comparison with a radio-frequency (RF) standard (such as a Cs beam clock) or in the optical domain by heterodyning comb mode N with an external CW laser at frequency v_{opt}. In the latter case, active feedback can phase-lock the comb mode N (and hence all modes of the mode-locked laser) to the CW laser such that $f_r = (v_{opt} - f_0)/N$, assuming that there is no frequency offset in the lock. This mechanism is shown pictorially in figure 2 of Diddams's paper [204], and the outcome is that "each of the ~10^6 modes of the frequency comb can be thought of as a frequency-stabilized CW laser available for precision spectroscopy."

Residual errors in the phase lock of a frequency comb to a reference laser can be <1 mHz [206], which allows the impressive stability of ultrastable CW lasers (e.g., locked to external reference cavities) to be transferred to combs. For example, the frequency stability of a laser locked to a stabilized silicon cavity was recently measured by comparing it, via a frequency comb, to a strontium lattice clock [207]. The fractional frequency instability was found to be <2×10^{-16} (86 mHz) for averaging times of 10^2–10^3 s—14 orders of magnitude less than the FT bandwidth limit of a single 100 fs pulse, as derived from Equation 2.23.

2.3.5 SPECTROSCOPY WITH ULTRAFAST OPOs AND FREQUENCY COMBS

Before returning in Section 2.4 to our central theme of spectroscopic applications of ns-pulsed OPOs, it is topical to survey significant recent advances involving fs-pulsed OPOs and frequency combs. Section 2.1.2 includes an introductory example [75,76] in the case of OPO-based spectroscopy of CO(g)—see Figures 2.3 and 2.4. Likewise, additional technical aspects of synchronously pumped fs-pulsed OPOs, generating frequency combs for spectroscopic purposes, have been cited in Section 2.3.3 [164–167,169–194]. For the purposes of this chapter, we merely highlight ongoing progress by several of the leading research groups in this area.

Konstantin Vodopyanov—together with Ginzton Laboratory colleagues at Stanford, such as Stephen Harris, Robert Byer, and Martin Fejer—has made fundamental contributions to ns-pulsed and CW OPOs and their spectroscopic applications [6,8–12,40,45,46,49,67]. Vodopyanov's recent initiatives in the area of ultrafast synchronously pumped PPLN and OP GaAs OPOs and their frequency comb applications have already been surveyed in Sections 2.1.2 [75,76] and 2.3.3 [177,178,182–184,191–193]. Apart from our introductory example of OPO applications to CO(g) IR spectra (at ~4.8 μm with a detection limit of 0.27 ppmv in He), we note again that Vodopyanov et al. have also used their cavity-enhanced broadband-OPO frequency comb techniques for IR-spectroscopic measurements of the following trace gases: CH_4 (1.7 ppbv at ~3.3 μm), H_2CO (0.31 ppmv at ~3.5 μm), C_2H_2 (0.11 ppmv at ~3.0 μm), C_2H_4 (0.32 ppmv at ~3.3 μm), and $^{13}CO_2$ (2.4 ppbv at ~4.4 μm) [75,76].

Derryck Reid and coworkers from the Scottish laser physics community have long been prominent in the science, technology, and applications of fs-pulsed OPOs [133–135]. Their early (pre-2005) work was on ultrafast tunable OPOs based on $RbTiOAsO_4$, $LiNbO_3$, and their QPM variants [141,147–151,153–155], on tandem OPOs using consecutive PPLN gratings [161,163], and on chirped-pulse frequency conversion in PPKTP [162]. They have since used fs-pulsed OPOs to record Fourier-transform IR (FTIR) spectra of CH_4 in a 10 cm gas cell, spanning 3.25–3.85 μm (i.e., ~14 THz) with ~60 GHz (~2 cm^{-1}) linewidth [164–166]. An fs-OPO FTIR system has also been used to measure spectra of CH_4(g) inside a photonic crystal fiber (PCF) over a range of 3.15–3.35 μm with ~90 GHz (~3 cm^{-1}) linewidth [167,169]. More recently, development of an MgO:PPLN OPO source pumped by a pair of asynchronous amplified Yb:KYW-laser ultrafast pulse trains [181] has enabled higher-quality dual-comb IR spectra of CH_4(g) to be recorded with ~5 GHz (~0.2 cm^{-1}) linewidth at 3.25–3.45 μm [188]. A broadband fs OPO spanning 3.1–3.7 μm has also been used for active FTIR-based stand-off detection (e.g., of thiodiglycol, a chemical warfare agent) [194]. Reid and coworkers have made substantial progress in controlling carrier-envelope phases in synchronously pumped fs OPOs [170,173–175, 186]. In particular, the CEO frequency of an fs-pulsed OPO (with a Ti:sapphire laser pumping an MgO:PPLN ring cavity) has been locked by using a simplified approach that entails coherent sum-frequency mixing of pump-laser and OPO-signal frequencies to avoid the complexities of (f – 2f) self-referencing. They have also recently introduced various measures to optimize the power-scaling and tuning range of ultrafast OPOs [172,179,180,187,189].

Jun Ye and colleagues at JILA, National Institute of Standards and Technology (NIST), and University of Colorado have pioneered many applications of broadband frequency combs to near IR molecular spectroscopy [200,208,209], using a variety of ultrafast broadband laser sources [171,176,190,208–219]. Highly sensitive IR-spectroscopic measurements have been reported for the following gas-phase molecules: CH_4, C_2H_2 (including its ^{13}C isotopomer), C_2H_4, C_2H_6, C_5H_8 (isoprene), CO_2 (including its ^{13}C and ^{18}O isotopomers), H_2CO, CH_3OH, H_2O, H_2O_2, O_2, NH_3, N_2O, NO_2, H_2S, and AsH_3 [176,190,200,208–218]. Specific applications include diagnostic breath analysis [190,208,210,213,214], the detection of H_2O as an impurity in AsH_3 semiconductor process gas [200,210,216], tomography of cold molecules in supersonic jets [208,210,214,215], and plasma-effluent monitoring [210]. Recently, ~25 µs time-resolved frequency comb spectra of transient *trans*-DOCO (deuterated hydroxyformyl) free radicals in a photolytic flow reactor have been measured at 3.70–3.75 µm [219]. All these frequency comb spectroscopic investigations have relied on broadband coherent excitation by an fs-pulse train from a mode-locked laser (e.g., a Yb-fiber similariton laser with a chirped-pulse fiber amplifier [220]), with an OPO frequency comb stage (e.g., based on a fan-out MgO:PPLN NLO element) added to shift the spectral range out to 2.8–4.8 µm when necessary [171,176,190,210,214,218,219].

Additional investigations of OPO-based frequency comb spectroscopy are as follows:

- Sub-Doppler spectroscopy of the 895 nm D1 line of cesium (Cs) [221], by Hajime Inaba et al. in Japan, using a CW optical frequency synthesizer based on a monolithic CW MgO:LiNbO₃ OPO and an optical frequency comb phase-locked to an atomic clock [222].
- Cavity-enhanced FTIR multipass absorption spectroscopy of C_2H_2 at 1.50–1.55 µm with linewidths down to 0.005 cm⁻¹ (0.15 GHz), both in a gas cell and in a supersonic expansion, using an fs-pulsed OPO source, by Michel Herman's group in Brussels [223].
- Sub-Doppler saturated absorption spectroscopy of iodomethane (CH_3I) in a 50 cm cell at ~88.8 THz (~2.96 µm), using a frequency comb-referenced PPLN OPO, by the INO-CNR/LENS group of Paolo De Natale in Florence [185].
- Absorption and dispersion dual-comb spectroscopy of $C_2H_2(g)$ at 3.0–3.1 µm and $CH_4(g)$ at 3.1–3.45 µm, using an fs-pulsed OPO system containing two MgO:PPLN crystals in a single resonant ring cavity, by Frans Harren and coworkers in Nijmegen [224].

2.4 OPTICAL BANDWIDTH CONTROL IN NANOSECOND-PULSED OPOS

In this section, we consider pulsed tunable OPOs that operate on nanosecond (10^{-9} s) timescales, and design features that make them fit for spectroscopy—one of the principal areas of application for optical parametric devices. Some design and wavelength-control features used in ns-pulsed OPOs are depicted schematically in Figure 2.6.

Our research group at Macquarie University has made some substantial contributions to this area of instrumental development. The first edition of this book [1] reviewed much of our foundation work on injection-seeded, ns-pulsed tunable OPOs based on the popular NLO medium β-BaB$_2$O$_4$ (BBO), pumped at 355 nm, operating in the visible and near IR regions (~0.4–2.7 µm) [225–233] and upconverted by NLO techniques to the near UV [29,227]. Since then (and before publication of the second edition of this book [5]), our interest shifted to injection-seeded, ns-pulsed tunable OPOs based on LiNbO$_3$ and its QPM counterpart PPLN [29,30,32,234–238] and, more recently, on PPKTP [32,239–246] and on photorefractive phase-conjugate reflectors [248,249]. The outcomes of our research on injection-seeded tunable ns-pulsed OPOs are surveyed in Section 2.4.2, preceded in Section 2.4.1 by a discussion of other methods of tunable OPO wavelength control.

2.4.1 FACTORS INFLUENCING OPTICAL BANDWIDTH AND TUNABILITY

The first OPO, demonstrated by Giordmaine and Miller in 1965 [250], was ns pulsed; it was based on LiNbO$_3$, tunable over the range ~0.96–1.16 µm, spanning a signal and idler wavelength range of approximately ±0.1 µm on either side of the degeneracy point defined by the 529 nm pump radiation (from a frequency-doubled, Q-switched Nd:CaWO$_4$ laser). This advance occurred soon after lasers were discovered and the potential of nonlinear optics had been realized through harmonic-generation processes such as frequency doubling [85,86]. As already outlined in Section 2.1.1, ns-pulsed OPOs were soon established as practical sources of tunable coherent light for significant applications such as spectroscopic sensing of chemical processes, in industrial or environmental diagnostics, and in basic science. However, it was far from trivial to be able to control the optical bandwidth and tunability of OPO output sufficiently finely for OPOs to become a convenient form of spectroscopic instrumentation.

In a typical ns-pulsed OPO, the pump laser delivers sufficient power for parametric gain to build up from noise during the pump pulse, thereby exceeding the threshold for oscillation. To maximize gain, the parametric (signal and idler) waves are amplified by multipassing them during the pump pulse in an optical resonator, as depicted in Figures 2.5c and 2.6. Light travels ~3 m during a 10 ns pump pulse, so that the parametric waves can then make approximately 15 round trips of a 10 cm linear OPO cavity. Multiple passes in the OPO cavity also tend to reduce the optical bandwidth of light emerging from a simple free-running pulsed OPO [12]. Such a free-running OPO, comprising simply an optical cavity with input and output mirrors M$_1$ and M$_2$ but with no wavelength-selective elements, is depicted in Figures 2.5c and 2.6a.

It is reasonably straightforward to predict the single-pass gain bandwidth of an idealized OPO in the low-gain, plane-wave limit [9–12,251], as is shown in Equations 2.14 through 2.21 and borne out by some early experimental demonstrations [9,10]. However, this idealized gain bandwidth does not necessarily correspond at all closely to the actual spectroscopic bandwidth of the OPO output radiation under operating conditions well above the oscillation threshold and in a multipass optical resonator [230,231,251]. In fact, it is the spectroscopic bandwidth, rather than the single-pass gain bandwidth, that is required to assess the practical utility of a free-running ns-pulsed OPO in a given spectroscopic application.

The spectroscopic bandwidth of output radiation from a free-running, ns-pulsed OPO is influenced by many factors, such as dispersion and absorption of the OPO medium; wavelengths λ_P, λ_S, and λ_I; type of phase matching (BPM or QPM, CPM or NCPM, whether collinear or not); crystal dimensions and orientation; characteristics of the optical resonator, such as the cavity reflectivity and the effective number of passes of the resonated wave; beam quality, optical bandwidth, divergence, pulse duration, and pulse energy of the pump radiation; the OPO's oscillation threshold and NLO conversion efficiency [1,5,9–12,22,23,29,32,35,230,231]. For instance, the collective outcome of most of these effects can be modeled by means of the versatile SNLO software package [26].

For example, our measurements of a free-running, ns-pulsed BBO OPO [230,231] agreed well with model predictions [10,251] of optical bandwidth as a function of OPO signal wavelength λ_S and indicated accompanying spatio-spectral characteristics. Moreover, our later measurements of a free-running, ns-pulsed PPLN OPO have shown that the spectral profiles of successive single signal output shots vary quasi-chaotically, due to random cavity-mode competition, but that these variations are smoothed out by multishot averaging [237].

As noted in Section 2.3.4, additional constraints, such as simplicity and ease of operation, are imposed on the design of an OPO system for certain applications (e.g., field-based spectroscopic sensing and IR countermeasures). In such cases, a free-running ns-pulsed OPO therefore represents an ideal solution. Moreover, there is scope for control of the various factors discussed in this section to provide limited tailoring of the output bandwidth of free-running OPOs. At one extreme, it is possible to devise simple, free-running, ns-pulsed OPO devices with output bandwidths adequate for certain spectroscopic applications requiring moderate resolution (~1 cm^{-1}, say). Typical free-running OPOs display optical bandwidths an order of magnitude greater, which makes them suitable for multiplex spectroscopy [230]. At another extreme, ns-pulsed OPOs for IR countermeasure applications routinely generate optical bandwidths of several hundred reciprocal centimeters in each of the signal and idler outputs.

As already indicated in Section 2.3.1 [91,108], there has been much interest in ns-pulsed tunable OPOs based on QPM NLO media, such as PPLN, PPKTP, PPKTA, and PPRTA. Operation of ns-pulsed QPM OPOs has been realized with much lower pump pulse energies than for ns-pulsed BPM OPOs, in view of the higher FOM of QPM media (see Table 2.1) as well as their NCPM amenability and long interaction lengths. Q-switched laser pump sources with relatively low peak powers can therefore be used to drive efficient ns-pulsed OPOs based on PPLN [252,253] and PPKTP [254]. Moreover, there were early reports of intracavity ns-pulsed OPOs based on PPLN [255–258] and MgO:PPLN [258]. We note also a cascaded PPLN OPO [259], in which the signal field of a primary OPO internally pumps a secondary OPO, with multiple output wavelengths controlled by temperature tuning and a dual fan-out grating structure. In this context, an early free-running tandem BPM

OPO system [260,261] was based on a CdSe OPO pumped by a KTA OPO, with 1.5–10 μm output wavelength range. Another early longer-wavelength ns-pulsed tandem OPO [262] comprised a $ZnGeP_2$ (ZGP) OPO, pumped by the 2.55 μm idler output of a $LiNbO_3$ OPO, itself pumped at 1.064 μm by a Q-switched Nd:YAG laser. These were precursors of tandem PPKTP and ZGP OPO systems for mid-IR generation [263–267] and a cascaded BPM system comprising KTP and ZGP OPOs followed by a ZGP OPA [264], generating mid-IR output for optical countermeasure defense applications, which will be discussed in Section 2.5.5.

There are numerous additional representative early examples of free-running ns-pulsed QPM OPOs [268–280]. Free-running ns-pulsed OPOs represent one extreme of operational simplicity, yielding relatively broadband output radiation suitable for low-resolution or multiplex spectroscopy. Additional OPO wavelength-control measures are usually necessary for higher-resolution spectroscopic applications.

At the other extreme of operational complexity, intracavity wavelength-selective elements, such as gratings or étalons, provide a traditional way to control the output wavelength of an ns-pulsed OPO and to attain a narrow optical bandwidth. One such approach is depicted schematically in Figure 2.6b, where a tuning element T (in this case, a tilted étalon or filter; in other designs, an intracavity diffraction grating replacing the output cavity mirror M_2) is inserted in the cavity. Such approaches were used in early ns-pulsed $LiNbO_3$ OPOs that were continuously tunable in the near IR with an optical bandwidth of ~0.1 cm^{-1} (~3 GHz) [1,5,10–12,14,281–284]. However, these tended to be difficult to operate and to be damage prone (because intracavity losses from gratings and étalons cause the oscillation threshold to approach the damage threshold of OPO NLO materials such as $LiNbO_3$). Many of these problems had been addressed by the mid-1980s, and assorted designs now abound for grating tuned ns-pulsed OPOs, both BPM [17–19,29,30,285–287] and QPM [288–293]. Other novel tuning strategies for QPM OPOs include use of a photorefractive distributed-feedback grating written by UV light into the PPLN NLO element [294] and electro-optic tuning by means of a three-segment PPLN crystal [295]. Specialized cavity designs that are appropriate for CW and ultrafast tunable OPOs have been outlined in Sections 2.3.2 and 2.3.3, respectively.

As explained in Section 2.3.4, continuous narrowband (preferably SLM) tunability is a performance characteristic of ns-pulsed OPOs that makes them amenable to high-resolution spectroscopy. The pre-1980 initiatives of Brosnan and Byer laid the foundations for this objective [10]. As a commercially viable approach to this ideal, the advanced KTP OPO/NRO/OPA system of Bosenberg and Guyer was continuously tunable under computer control in the near IR (1.3–4 μm) with narrow optical bandwidth (~0.02 cm^{-1} or better) [20,21]. Rakestraw and colleagues [296,297] have used tunable SLM IR radiation from such an OPO system to record high-quality rovibrational cavity ringdown (CRD) spectra of molecules (e.g., in combustion media [297]). CRD spectroscopy uses the temporal decay of light traversing a high-finesse optical cavity to enhance resolution, sensitivity, and photometric precision [298,299].

Another grating tuned OPO, developed by Kung and coworkers [291–293], is an ns-pulsed PPLN OPO, tuned by a grazing-incidence intracavity grating (optical bandwidth ≈ 0.3 cm^{-1}). This has been used to record PA absorption spectra of CH_4 in nitrogen (N_2) gas with a trace-level sensitivity approaching 1 ppbv (one part in 10^9 by volume).

Vodopyanov [45,46] has reviewed various ns-pulsed mid-IR tunable OPOs, of which a few can generate output radiation that is sufficiently narrowband (with subreciprocal centimeter optical bandwidth) to enable rotationally resolved spectroscopic sensing of molecules in the gas phase.

Richman et al. [300] developed an ns-pulsed SLM-tunable OPO system, comprising a three-mirror signal-resonant ring cavity with a fan-out PPLN grating and an electronically tunable intracavity étalon (free spectral range = 420 GHz; finesse = 60; insertion loss = 30%); it was pumped at a 1 kHz repetition rate by 200 μJ pulses from an SLM Nd:YAG laser. Its signal and idler tuning ranges were 1.45–1.8 and 2.6–4 μm with maximum pulse energies of 18 and 15 μJ, respectively; continuous SLM tuning was feasible over ~10 cm^{-1} (~300 GHz) with ~0.005 cm^{-1} (~150 MHz) optical bandwidth. The output wavelengths and optical bandwidth of an earlier ns-pulsed tunable LiNbO$_3$ OPO, pumped at 930 nm by a Ti:sapphire laser, were controlled by an electronically tunable intracavity Fabry–Perot étalon [301].

In the previously mentioned long-wavelength ns-pulsed tandem OPO system, comprising a ZGP OPO pumped at 2.55 μm by an LiNbO$_3$ OPO, the signal-resonant ZGP OPO cavity incorporated a Littrow diffraction grating and a tiltable Si-plate étalon as tuning elements, yielding mid-IR output with 0.1 cm^{-1} (3 GHz) optical bandwidth [262].

A further development by Aniolek et al. comprised narrowband PPLN-based OPG/OPA tunable coherent light sources, in which broadband (~15 cm^{-1} FWHM) output from a PPLN OPG was spectrally filtered before being amplified by a PPLN OPA [302,303]. In the latter case [303], both OPG and OPA stages were pumped at 1.064 μm by a 120 Hz Nd:YAG microlaser incorporating a Cr^{4+}:YAG passive Q switch. After pre-OPA spectral filtering via a high-finesse air-spaced étalon, the idler output of the system was continuously tunable in 15 cm^{-1} (450 GHz) segments and had an optical bandwidth of ~0.05 cm^{-1} (~1.5 GHz) FWHM.

A closely related development comprises an injection-seeded ns-pulsed OPG/OPA system, based on diode laser–pumped BBO (β-barium borate, BaB$_2$O$_4$), which combines relatively low thresholds with good conversion efficiencies [304]. Because there is no need for active control of the optical properties of an OPO cavity, so that it matches the injected radiation field, external seeding over wide ranges by CW SLM lasers is straightforward. The signal (~0.628 μm) and idler (~0.815 μm) outputs of this OPG/OPA system had an optical bandwidth of ~0.07 cm^{-1} (~2.1 GHz) FWHM and were continuously tunable over a range of 20–30 cm^{-1} (600–900 THz).

The associated subject of injection-seeded, ns-pulsed tunable OPOs will be dealt with in greater detail in Sections 2.4.2 and 2.4.3.

2.4.2 Injection-Seeded Nanosecond-Pulsed OPOs: Early Days

Injection seeding, by a low-power tunable coherent source such as a tunable diode laser (TDL), as depicted in Figure 2.6c, is another means of OPO wavelength control. In practice, a ring cavity can avoid feedback from the OPO to the seed laser. A significant advantage of injection seeding is that OPO construction is simplified by putting the wavelength-control function into a module that is effectively separate from the optical generation and amplification functions.

2.4.2.1 Historical Overview

Injection seeding of an OPO was first demonstrated and qualitatively explained by Bjorkholm and Danielmeyer, who used ns-pulsed, single-mode ruby and Nd:YAG lasers as pump and seed, respectively, for an $LiNbO_3$ OPO [305]. This was reported in 1969—a short while before Kreuzer first used an intracavity étalon to achieve single-mode operation of an OPO [306]. An early rate-equation model was developed by Cassedy and Jain to provide a realistic qualitative model of such an injection-seeded ns-pulsed OPO [307]. Subsequent studies of ns-pulsed OPOs have used a variety of sources for injection seeding, as reviewed elsewhere [1,5,29–32].

Many of the early (pre-1995) studies of injection-seeded OPOs were performed with a fixed seed-laser wavelength and therefore appear to have focused primarily on attaining lower OPO oscillation threshold, higher efficiency, and narrower linewidth, rather than on continuous tunability [1,5,22,305,308]. Later research, at Macquarie University [225–249] and elsewhere [304,309–356], has aimed to transfer the continuous tunability of a low-power seed laser to the signal and idler outputs of a higher-power ns-pulsed tunable OPO. Even so, actual reports [29,30,235–237,304,313,316,321–323,327,328,330,334,336–341,343,349,352,355,356] of the use of injection-seeded ns-pulsed OPO systems for high-resolution spectroscopy were relatively slow to emerge. Such applications generally require that the OPO radiation (and hence its seed source) should have a narrow optical bandwidth (close to the FT limit of the OPO pulse), high spatial beam quality, and continuously tunable SLM operation.

Our own early work in this area (initiated in collaboration with Richard Wallenstein, Andreas Fix et al. at Universität Kaiserslautern [225–228]) showed that a singly resonant BBO OPO, injection seeded at the signal wavelength by narrowband radiation from a low-intensity tunable dye laser, could be continuously tuned in a spectroscopically useful fashion. This OPO yielded narrowband (~0.1 cm^{-1}) signal and idler outputs, continuously tunable over a wide range (>100 cm^{-1}) and with sufficient intensity and spatial coherence to enable applications to coherent Raman spectroscopy, as further discussed in Section 2.5 of this chapter.

2.4.2.2 Mechanism of Injection-Seeded OPOs

The mechanism of ns-pulsed OPO wavelength control by injection seeding was well explained in qualitative terms from the outset [305]. It is understood that when a singly resonant OPO is switched on by a pulse of pump radiation exceeding the oscillation threshold, the various resonant cavity modes falling within its gain bandwidth build up exponentially from noise at different rates, which depend on the extent of their phase mismatch Δk. When the pump intensity is very close to the oscillation threshold, the output of an ideal OPO is expected to build up to a steady state in which only the cavity mode with $\Delta k \approx 0$ is oscillating. In reality, however, an OPO pumped at any practical margin above oscillation threshold tends to oscillate on more than one cavity mode, so that the output of a free-running ns-pulsed OPO is intrinsically multimode (MM) and broadband. This can be overcome by injecting narrowband radiation coinciding with the frequency of one (or more) of the OPO cavity modes: if this injected radiation is significantly more intense than the noise level, the OPO will tend to oscillate predominantly on the injection-seeded resonant OPO cavity mode(s), which need not correspond to $\Delta k \approx 0$. It has been verified that the exact OPO resonant output frequency is determined by the optical cavity length, but not the seed frequency [236,237]. If the duration of pumping is sustained, noise-generated oscillations will eventually build up and compete with the seeded mode(s) (e.g., as in CW OPOs, which do not respond markedly to injection seeding). However, this does not occur if the pump pulse is sufficiently short (or is terminated by pump depletion in the OPO gain process).

The theory of Cassedy and Jain [307] is consistent with this injection-seeding mechanism for an ns-pulsed OPO. Moreover, this mechanism is borne out by the experiments of Fix and coworkers with a ns-pulsed BBO OPO operating close to its oscillation threshold; these reveal a halving of threshold pump energy as the seed radiation (from a pulsed dye laser) is increased in intensity 1000-fold (ranging from a pump threshold of 14 mJ per pulse with seed energies around 0.1 nJ per pulse to a 7 mJ threshold with 100 nJ seeding) [312,320,325].

If the seed radiation is sufficiently narrowband (as in several early instances of injection-seeded OPOs [22,226,305,308–312]), then it is possible to match the seed frequency to that of a single cavity resonance and thereby to attain SLM OPO wavelength control. Continuous tuning of the resonant OPO output without mode-hopping is then feasible by varying the OPO cavity length synchronously with the seed-frequency scan. For scans over moderate frequency ranges, in the case of a BPM OPO, the angular setting of the NLO gain medium must also be varied to keep the seeded mode near the $\Delta k \approx 0$ peak of the gain profile. Further work by Fix and Wallenstein, on an injection-seeded ns-pulsed BBO OPO with a very short (3.5 mm) optical cavity, was able to resolve discrete longitudinal mode structure and to examine its SLM dependence and fluctuations in output power on pump pulse energy and times above threshold [320].

2.4.2.3   Passively Seeded OPO Cavities

Passive OPO cavity control is a distinctive approach to injection-seeded tuning of ns-pulsed OPOs for spectroscopic purposes [1,5,28–32,225–227,232,234]. This has been used at Macquarie University in the context of BPM media such as BBO and LiNbO$_3$. Our initial work [225–227] sought continuous tuning with moderate spectral bandwidth, rather than SLM operation. The tunable source used for injection seeding at the signal wavelength of our BBO OPO was a MM dye laser, which is still sufficiently narrowband to generate rotationally resolved molecular spectra with linewidths approaching Doppler- and pressure-broadened limits. By continuously scanning the seed wavelength (and, on occasions, detuning the OPO cavity), it was possible for the signal output wavelength of the OPO to be scanned smoothly over several reciprocal centimeters, without adjusting the phase-matching angle of the BBO crystal.

This approach was similar in some respects to a report by Abdullin et al. in 1984 [357], in which a MM Nd:YAG laser pumped two ns-pulsed SROs, one an étalon-narrowed OPO based on Ba$_2$NaNb$_5$O$_{15}$ (popularly known as "banana") used to seed the other, an LiNbO$_3$ OPO. It was reported [357] that the output of the latter OPO could be tuned over a range of ~10 cm^{-1} (~300 GHz) by varying only the injection-seeding wavelength from the former. However, it is not clear that the output wavelengths from this injection-seeded OPO system could actually be continuously scanned (e.g., as usually required to record spectra).

At that stage, approximately 30 years ago, it was evident [1] that injection seeding could play a key role in OPO technology, as a way to control and continuously tune signal and idler outputs of an ns-pulsed, tunable OPO (instead of intracavity gratings and étalons), and that it was becoming increasingly well understood. By transferring wavelength-control complexities from the OPO cavity to the tunable seed source, it is possible for an injection-seeded OPO to be extremely small and simple: just two mirrors and a NLO crystal, all on appropriate optical mounts that do not need to be adjusted during moderate wavelength scans over several reciprocal centimeters.

In our distinctive approach to passive OPO cavity control, one or more of the cavity reflectors is slightly misaligned to facilitate continuous tuning of the injection-seeded OPO signal and idler outputs. This measure decreases the effective finesse of the OPO cavity, so that it is not necessary to lock the OPO cavity length to the seed wavelength, and effectively dispenses with active control of the OPO cavity, and is therefore simpler both optically and electronically. The method depends on the OPO cavity having a high Fresnel number, so that a series of high-order transverse modes can smooth out the sharp, widely separated resonances that occur when the OPO cavity is well aligned; a resulting disadvantage is that the multiple transverse modes tend to cause some degradation of output beam quality. Nevertheless, this approach has proved useful for many applications of tunable OPOs, with seeding by either pulsed dye lasers or CW TDLs [1,5,28–32,232,234].

2.4.2.4 Multiplex and Multiwavelength-Seeded OPOs

The preceding passive, misaligned-cavity approach to injection seeding of ns-pulsed BPM OPOs is well suited for multiline spectroscopic applications requiring a coherent light source that simultaneously generates two or more adjustable output wavelengths. This has previously been verified by OPO CARS experiments in our laboratory [232]. Dual-wavelength, ns-pulsed OPO signal output at ~607 nm was generated by a passive-cavity BBO OPO, pumped at 355 nm by a pulsed, SLM Nd:YAG laser and injection seeded at two separate 855 nm idler wavelengths by a pair of SLM TDLs. The 607 nm signal output served as the Raman Stokes beams in an NLO CARS process, with monochromatic 532 nm radiation (from the same SLM Nd:YAG laser) serving as the Raman pump beam. In this way, single-shot coherent Raman thermometric spectra were recorded for N$_2$ in furnace air by tuning the two signal/Stokes wavelengths to different rotational-state features in the Q branch of the Raman spectrum [232]. This is an example of the so-called spectroscopic tailoring of OPO output radiation to match the spectral features of interest. By turning the injection seeding off, multiplex broadband OPO CARS measurements were also made of a portion of the same Raman spectrum, but these were less sensitive than the dual-line Raman spectra recorded with the dual-wavelength injection-seeded OPO [232].

In closely related dual-pump CARS experiments, Robert Lucht and coworkers have employed two distinct coherent pump wavelengths, separated by the interval between the characteristic Raman-shift frequencies of two molecular species of interest (e.g., N_2 and CO_2), so that the two beams of anti-Stokes light emerge at a common wavelength [353,354]. These pump wavelengths are typically generated by a frequency-doubled Nd:YAG laser and the appropriately tuned output from an injection-seeded OPO.

Incidentally, the above dual-wavelength approach to injection seeding of an ns-pulsed OPO [232] had a useful mechanistic outcome in the context of NLO backconversion effects in the OPO itself [233]. By injection seeding an ns-pulsed passive-cavity BBO OPO at two distinct idler wavelengths (separated by a frequency interval Δ falling within the 350 GHz free-running OPO bandwidth), above-threshold operation was found to yield sidebands at multiples of Δ in the signal output spectrum and extending well beyond the regular free-running OPO gain profile [233]. The sideband spacing varied smoothly as Δ was tuned, and corresponding sidebands were observed on the transmitted pump radiation. This provides direct evidence of the backconversion of signal and idler waves in the ns-pulsed OPO, consistent with temporal observations and other aspects of OPO performance, such as the phase-matching conditions for the various OPO pump and idler (seed) frequencies that are involved.

Dual-wavelength injection seeding of ns-pulsed OPOs is relevant to atmospheric remote sensing techniques such as differential absorption lidar (DIAL) [28]. This has been borne out in several OPO-based IR DIAL demonstrations [323,327,328,342] to be reviewed in Section 2.5.2.2, as well as multiwavelength spectroscopic tailoring schemes for OPOs by injection seeding of either BPM [5,28,30,31,232] or QPM NLO media [290,358,359].

2.4.3   INJECTION-SEEDED NANOSECOND-PULSED OPOs: SUBSEQUENT PROGRESS

2.4.3.1   Actively Seeded OPO cavities

As already explained in Sections 2.3.1, 2.3.4, and 2.4.1, narrowband operation (preferably SLM, with mode-hop-free continuous tunability) of an ns-pulsed OPO is traditionally achieved by means of wavelength-selective elements, such as intracavity gratings or étalons, as sketched in Figure 2.6b. Within the last approximately 25 years, accompanying the revival in OPO technology, it has been recognized that injection seeding (by means of narrowband, tunable radiation from a low-power external light source) is an especially efficient way to control the output wavelengths and optical bandwidth of ns-pulsed OPOs intended for spectroscopic applications, as sketched in Figure 2.6c [1,5,29–32]. Early progress in this regard has been surveyed in Section 2.4.2. In the current section, subsequent progress on injection-seeded ns-pulsed OPOs is examined, with an emphasis on high-performance instruments of this type that are closely associated with our own research at Macquarie University.

Injection seeding simplifies the design of an ns-pulsed OPO by separating its wavelength-control function from that of power amplification. In this context, we have exploited an SLM TDL for continuously tunable, mode-hop-free injection seeding of ns-pulsed near IR OPOs based on $LiNbO_3$ in either its bulk [234] or QPM (PPLN) [235–238] forms, pumped at 1.064 μm by a high-performance Q-switched SLM Nd:YAG laser. This yields optical bandwidths that have been spectroscopically verified to be ~0.005 cm⁻¹ (~150 MHz) or better, approaching the FT limit of the single coherent light pulses as defined in Equation 2.23 [199].

Applications of injection-seeded ns-pulsed OPO systems to high-resolution spectroscopy require narrow optical bandwidth (close to the FT limit), high spatial beam quality, and continuously tunable SLM operation. Traditionally, the performance criteria of such a spectroscopic OPO system therefore included the following three design features:

- An ns-pulsed pump laser, typically a 1.064 µm flashlamp-pumped, Q-switched Nd:YAG oscillator/amplifier system, usually with an injection seeder for SLM operation [27].
- A tunable low-power CW laser (usually an SLM TDL) to be injection seeder for the OPO.
- Control of the injection-seeded OPO cavity length, usually achieved by actively varying the OPO cavity length synchronously with the wavelength scan of the seed source, employing some form of stabilization by optoelectronic feedback.

An early modular tunable OPO- spectroscopic system, relying on these design features, is illustrated photographically and schematically in Figures 2.7 and 2.8 [29,235–238]. This representative example is based on the QPM NLO medium PPLN, with a multigrating design [108] to provide a broad tuning range. There have been many subsequent technological developments, such as diode-pumped and fiber lasers.

2.4.3.2   Intensity-Dip OPO Cavity Control

The TDL-seeded, ns-pulsed PPLN OPO system uses an actively controlled ring cavity and depends on our distinctive intensity-dip feedback scheme, in which CW TDL

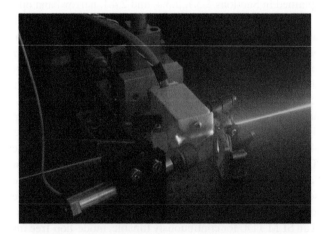

FIGURE 2.7   Photograph of an injection-seeded pulsed OPO ring cavity, with a green 532 nm laser beam simulating pump radiation and a red 633 nm laser beam simulating signal radiation [30,32]. The layout of such an OPO is shown in Figure 2.8.

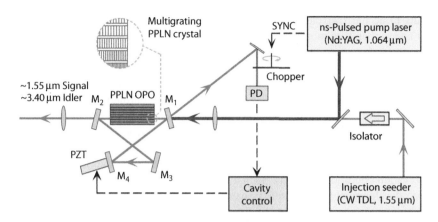

FIGURE 2.8 Layout of an injection-seeded tunable ns-pulsed OPO system, based on a multigrating PPLN chip with active intensity-dip cavity control [29–32,233–237]. The OPO comprises a four-mirror ring cavity that is pumped at 1.064 μm by an ns-pulsed Nd:YAG laser and seeded (typically at ~1.55 μm) by a CW tunable diode laser (TDL). The resulting signal and idler outputs at wavelengths λ_S and λ_I (typically ~1.55 μm and ~3.4 μm), respectively, are continuously tunable on an SLM. PD = photodetector; PZT = piezoelectric translator; M_{1-4} = cavity reflectors; SYNC, synchronization circuit. The inset shows the QPM multigrating structure of the PPLN nonlinear optical crystal.

seed light reflected off the four-mirror OPO ring cavity is monitored by a photodetector (PD) and used to optimize the cavity length by means of a piezoelectric translator (PZT) in the interval (typically 100 ms) between successive pulses from the ns-pulsed 1.064 μm Nd:YAG pump laser [235–237]. Typical signal and idler output wavelengths generated by this OPO system are $\lambda_S \approx 1.55$ μm (equal to the wavelength λ_{seed} of the CW TDL injection seeder) and $\lambda_I \approx 3.40$ μm. Using a pump pulse energy of ~1 mJ (delivered to the PPLN crystal with a beam waist of ~0.1 mm FWHM), the total output power is typically ~0.1 mJ (of which ~70% is signal radiation), but this OPO output can be pulse amplified to a total output pulse energy of ~2 mJ by using an additional OPA stage based on a bulk BPM LiNbO$_3$ crystal [29,235–237].

Such a high-performance narrowband tunable PPLN OPO system can be pumped at 1.064 μm and 10 Hz either by an elaborate injection-seeded SLM Nd:YAG laser [235,236] or by a more compact and economical MM Nd:YAG laser [237]. In the former (SLM-pumped) case, both signal and idler output beams are narrowband, with $\Delta\nu \approx 130$ MHz (~0.0045 cm^{-1}) FWHM, approaching the FT limit [235,236]. The latter (MM-pumped) version generates coherent near IR (~1.55 μm) signal radiation that is continuously tunable, comparably narrowband (sub-0.005 cm^{-1}), pulsed (~5 ns duration), and moderate energy (~0.1 mJ/pulse); the accompanying idler radiation is broader band (MM) [237].

The less elaborate MM-pumped PPLN OPO relies only on the second and third of the aforementioned design features [29,237,238]. It does not need an elaborate, costly SLM pump laser as in the first design feature, and is pumped instead by a compact, inexpensive MM Nd:YAG laser. An MM-pumped OPO system is advantageous and cost-effective for many OPO applications that do not require both signal and idler outputs to be narrowband. It is more readily transportable than an SLM-pumped OPO and is therefore more amenable to operation in field settings for industrial or environmental monitoring applications requiring coherent, tunable near IR pulses.

Resonance properties of the actively controlled, TDL-seeded PPLN OPO ring cavity are used in the MM-pumped OPO to constrain the resonated wave (here, the signal wave) to an SLM of the OPO cavity and to tune it continuously without mode-hops. The nonresonated wave (here, the idler) carries all the broadband character of the MM pump radiation. In this way, we are able to employ a *multimode* pump laser and still attain *single-mode* tunability of signal (or idler, if that is the resonated wave) output radiation. We note that this property is associated with the intrinsic energy-conservation condition of OPOs. Such a possibility was recognized from the outset of their development [8] but rarely implemented.

2.4.3.3 Self-Adaptive Tunable OPO

A novel advance in injection-seeded OPO wavelength control [248,249] is a self-adaptive tunable (SAT) OPO design for an ns-pulsed tunable OPO system that needs no active variation of the cavity length or other mechanical adjustment, as the wavelength λ_{seed} of the injection seeder is scanned. As depicted schematically in Figure 2.9, this SAT OPO employs a photorefractive crystal [360] to serve as a phase-conjugate cavity mirror (M_1). A phase-conjugate Bragg grating mirror is formed within a few seconds in an $Rh:BaTiO_3$ crystal by photorefractive interaction with the forward-propagating and retroreflected CW seed beams. Its reflectivity is centered at the wavelength λ_{seed} of the tunable CW seed laser, and it adapts automatically to remain wavelength selective as λ_{seed} is scanned.

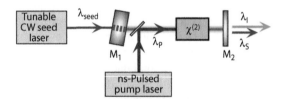

FIGURE 2.9 Schematic layout of a narrowband OPO, pumped by an ns-pulsed laser at wavelength λ_p and tuned by injection seeding a self-adaptive tunable (SAT) optical cavity. The SAT OPO cavity includes a photorefractive crystal M_1 (e.g., $Rh:BaTiO_3$), in which a phase-conjugate Bragg grating is written by interfering CW tunable seed laser light (at wavelength λ_{seed}) with its own backreflection from cavity mirror M_2. The central wavelength of the induced reflective grating tracks λ_{seed} as it is scanned, such that the injection-seeded OPO cavity stays resonant at λ_{seed} and is automatically controlled to yield continuously tunable SLM signal and idler output beams at wavelengths λ_S and λ_I, respectively. This novel SAT approach to narrowband, mechanical adjustment–free control of OPO output wavelength and optical bandwidth has been demonstrated in the form of a compact, rugged OPO system that is based on periodically poled $KTiOPO_4$ (PPKTP), injection seeded (typically in the range 820–850 nm) by a CW tunable diode laser, and pumped at 532 nm by an ns-pulsed Nd:YAG laser [32,248,249]. (From Y. He, and B. J. Orr, *Appl. Phys. B* 96: 545–560, 2009.)

This SAT approach has been realized with an OPO system pumped at 532 nm by a frequency-doubled SLM Nd:YAG laser (~8 ns pulse duration at 10 Hz), a PPKTP NLO medium, and a CW SLM TDL as an injection seeder (~5 mW CW at 820–855 nm). This injection-seeded, self-adaptive, ns-pulsed OPO cavity stays resonant at λ_{seed} and generates continuously tunable SLM output beams at signal and idler wavelengths λ_S and λ_I. Étalon measurements confirm that they are SLM, with the optical bandwidth close to the FT limit, and continuously tunable without mode-hopping. This adjustment-free SAT OPO approach [248,249] is potentially useful for high-resolution, time-resolved laser spectroscopy close to the FT limit. It is particularly promising for applications that require a stable, continuously tunable SLM source of coherent, narrowband, ns-pulsed near IR radiation without any active wavelength-selective feedback or mechanically adjustable elements in the OPO cavity.

This robust, simple design provides a remarkably simple way to achieve reliable narrowband (SLM) tuning of the OPO signal and idler output. It takes advantage of the high photorefractive efficiency of $Rh:BaTiO_3$ [360], which can be used with seed radiation at near IR wavelengths (0.6–1.1 μm). Other photorefractive materials may be suitable for SAT OPOs that are injection seeded at longer IR wavelengths, such as the 1.55 μm optical telecommunications band. For example, vanadium-doped cadmium telluride (V:CdTe) [361] has been used as an adaptive intracavity filter to facilitate SLM tuning of an external-cavity diode laser operating at ~1.55 μm [362]. We note that a photorefractive grating, permanently written in PPLN by UV light, has been used for the distributed-feedback operation of an ns-pulsed PPLN OPO [294]; a less dynamic and adaptable arrangement than in our SAT OPO [248,249].

Incidentally, in a related application that does not involve OPOs [363], we have developed a form of extended-cavity TDL that includes a self-pumped $Rh:BaTiO_3$ photorefractive phase-conjugate reflector for wavelength-adaptive narrowband feedback. A compact, high-finesse tunable intracavity ring filter provides SLM selectivity and control, enabling robust tunable single-frequency operation with submegahertz linewidth. The device's performance at a wavelength of ~830 nm has been verified with a Fabry–Perot laser diode and by sub-Doppler two-photon spectroscopy in atomic Cs [363].

As a precursor to the aforementioned research on SAT optical devices based on photorefractive phase-conjugate elements [248,249,363], we had developed a self-injection-seeded OPO concept employing a wavelength-selective tunable filter (WSTF) external to a PPKTP OPO ring cavity [364]. This entailed optical feedback from the WSTF (comprising either a spatially filtered Littman–Metcalf diffraction grating or a tunable étalon or a high-finesse ringdown cavity) instead of the customary TDL seed source. Our WSTF work preceded innovative research by Darrell Armstrong and Arlee Smith on a high-efficiency self-injection-seeded KTP OPO as a key component in an all-solid-state satellite-based ozone (O_3) UV DIAL sensing system [345,346].

2.4.3.4   Chirp-Controlled, Injection-Seeded OPOs

Ongoing collaboration between Macquarie University and the Australian National University is directed toward optical-heterodyne measurement and control of frequency chirp in the output of a high-performance ns-pulsed injection-seeded OPO system intended for advanced high-resolution atomic and molecular spectroscopic applications [239–247]. As shown in Figure 2.10, this chirp-controlled OPO system is based on PPKTP, pumped at 532 nm by the second harmonic of a long-pulse SLM Nd:YAG laser, and injection seeded by a CW SLM TDL at a signal wavelength, λ_{seed}, of ~842 nm. The Nd:YAG pump radiation employed in our most recent work [241–247] has a relatively long pulse duration of ~27 ns FWHM (3.5 times that used to pump a previously reported 8 ns pulsed OPO system [239,240]). According to Equation 2.23 [199], the corresponding FT-limited optical bandwidth of the resulting 842 nm OPO signal output pulses (duration ≈ 25 ns FWHM) is reduced to ~17.5 MHz (~0.0006 cm^{-1}) FWHM. The chirp-controlled OPO system generates SLM pulsed coherent signal and idler output radiation that is continuously tunable with a narrow optical bandwidth (<20 MHz) and low frequency chirp (<10 MHz).

The chirp-control module of the OPO system shown in Figure 2.10 is able to measure the optical phase properties of its ns-pulsed coherent output radiation by

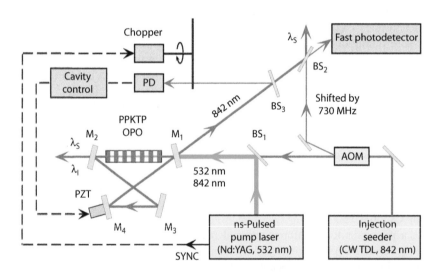

FIGURE 2.10 Injection-seeded, ns-pulsed tunable OPO with an optical-heterodyne (OH) detection system that is able to log the chirp and other instantaneous-frequency characteristics of each signal output pulse [32,239–245]. The OPO system comprises a four-mirror ring cavity based on periodically poled KTiOPO$_4$ (PPKTP), is controlled by intensity-dip feedback to a piezoelectric translator (PZT), is injection seeded (typically at ~842 nm) by a CW tunable diode laser (TDL), and is pumped at 532 nm by an ns-pulsed SLM Nd:YAG laser. The pulsed OPO signal output beam (typically at ~842 nm) is combined at BS$_2$ with frequency-shifted light from the CW seed source via an acousto-optic modulator (AOM; typically driven at ~730 MHz). The resulting beats are detected by a fast photodetector and analyzed by the OH method. M$_1$–M$_4$, OPO cavity mirrors; BS$_1$–BS$_3$, beam splitters; SYNC, synchronization circuit. (From R. T. White, et al., *Opt. Lett.* 28: 1248–1250, 2003; R. T. White, et al., *J. Opt. Soc. Am. B* 21, 1577–1585, 2004; R. T. White, et al., *J. Opt. Soc. Am. B* 21: 1586–1594, 2004; R. T. White, et al., *Opt. Express* 12: 5655–5660, 2004.)

means of OH techniques [365–368], in which OPO output pulses beat against CW TDL-seed radiation that is frequency shifted by an acousto-optic modulator (AOM). Of central importance in such considerations is the instantaneous-frequency profile, $f_{inst}(t)$, of the pulse, which is expressed [240,366] in terms of the time-derivative of the optical phase $\varphi(t)$:

$$f_{inst}(t) = (2\pi)^{-1}[d\varphi(t)/dt] \qquad (2.24)$$

where any phase perturbations during an optical pulse are assigned to $\varphi(t)$, and $f_{inst}(t)$ is defined relative to the time-independent central frequency ($\langle\omega\rangle/2\pi$) of the pulsed optical field. The phenomenon of frequency chirp can then be understood in terms of an approximately linear or monotonic change in $f_{inst}(t)$, which may include quadratic and other higher-order chirp terms.

A representative set of temporal and frequency profiles, extracted from typical observed output for a single pulse from the long-pulse OPO, is depicted in Figure 2.11. The successive FT analysis steps [240,366] needed to process such measurements are indicated by arrows. The beat waveform in panel (b) contains intrinsic information about the instantaneous frequency and the frequency chirp. An FT algorithm is used to extract from these beats the temporal profile of the narrowband OPO pulse amplitude—used to reconstruct the pulse intensity profile in panel (d) for comparison with the raw intensity profile in panel (a)—and to determine the associated instantaneous-frequency profile $f_{inst}(t)$ as in panel (e). A key step, as in panel (c), entails the isolation of one of the two OH sidebands (each displaced from the central peak in the power spectrum by the AOM frequency of ~730 MHz) by means of a suitable numerical filter prior to the second FT step. The vertical dashed lines in panels (d) and (e) denote 10%-intensity points of the OPO pulse's temporal profile, indicating the range of signal output amplitude over which frequency chirp can be conservatively estimated. In this particular example (in which the OPO operating conditions are chosen to ensure that phase mismatch $\Delta k \approx 0$), the frequency chirp is very small (less than 10 MHz) on the basis of either the spread of $f_{inst}(t)$ values or a straight-line fit slope of $f_{inst}(t)$ in panel (e) of Figure 2.11.

The chirp-controlled PPKTP OPO and the OH detection system used to measure the instantaneous-frequency characteristics of its signal output are depicted schematically in Figure 2.10. The essential features of this instrument [241,242] are as follows:

- A high-performance Q-switched, injection-seeded SLM Nd:YAG laser system [241,242], custom built to deliver spatially and temporally smooth 1064 nm pump pulses with relatively long durations (e.g., ~27 ns FWHM at 10 Hz pulse repetition rate) that minimize their FT-limited optical bandwidth.
- A four-mirror signal-resonant OPO ring cavity containing a temperature-controlled PPKTP crystal (e.g., with grating period $\Lambda = 9.35$ μm for free-running OPO signal wavelengths λ_{free} ranging from 815 to 877 nm at $T_{PPKTP} = 200°C$ and 20°C, respectively [239]).

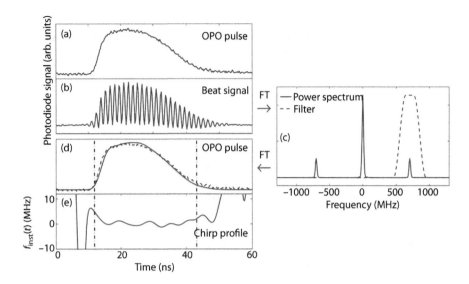

FIGURE 2.11 Fourier-transform (FT) chirp analysis method applied to signal output from a long-pulse injection-seeded PPKTP OPO [32,239–245]. Panels (a) and (b) depict the measured temporal profiles for amplitude and optical-heterodyne (OH) beat waveform, respectively, as measured for an actual OPO signal pulse. The FT algorithm converts panel (b) into the power spectrum in panel (c), where two OH sidebands are displaced from a central peak by the AOM frequency (~730 MHz), then one OH sideband is numerically filtered and FT analyzed to yield the temporal profiles of reconstructed OPO pulse amplitude and instantaneous frequency $f_{inst}(t)$ in panels (d) and (e), respectively. The pump-pulse energy (64 μJ) is twice the unseeded threshold level, and the PPKTP temperature is $T_{PPKTP} = 125.0°C$, so that the signal wavelength of the free-running PPKTP OPO is $\lambda_{free} = 841.75 \pm 0.02$ nm. The TDL-seeded signal wavelength λ_s (841.76 ± 0.01 nm) is virtually identical to λ_{free}; this minimizes phase mismatch and attains a frequency chirp of less than 10 MHz, as is evident from the f_{inst} profile in panel (e). (From R.T. White, et al., *Opt. Express* 12: 5655–5660, 2004.)

- A TDL injection seeder delivering continuously tunable CW SLM radiation at ~842 nm (e.g., with OPO signal seed wavelengths λ_{seed} that are tunable over 834–851 nm [239]) via an optical isolator and spatial filter or a single-mode optical fiber.
- A piezoelectrically controlled intensity-dip cavity locking system [235–237] that maintains the OPO cavity in resonance at a signal wavelength λ_S that coincides with the TDL injection-seeder wavelength λ_{seed}.
- An AOM (e.g., driven at ~730 MHz), with the undiffracted CW seed beam directed into the OPO cavity while the diffracted, frequency-shifted CW beam is combined with output from the OPO system to generate OH beats on a fast square-law PD (e.g., with 1 GHz bandwidth) [239–242].

Additional pulsed optical amplifier stages (either OPA [243–245] or Ti:sapphire [246,247]) can be added for higher-power applications. In early work, an OPA based on BPM LiNbO$_3$ was used for fourfold amplification of output at ~850 nm from our chirp-controlled OPO prior to NLO upconversion [243–245]. This was found to reduce the optical pulse duration from ~23 to ~15 ns FWHM, with corresponding degradation of the FT-limited optical bandwidth. Subsequently, an advanced two-stage Ti:sapphire laser amplifier was installed [246,247]; its booster and multipass stages (pumped at 532 nm by ~35 and ~200 mJ pulses from the long-pulse Nd:YAG laser) amplify the chirp-controlled SLM OPO signal output pulse energies from ≤5 to ~1 and ~40 mJ, respectively, with good spatial beam profile. The chirp from this Ti:sapphire amplifier is well below 10 MHz FWHM, but the amplified pulse duration is disappointingly short (≤6 ns FWHM, compared with ~25 ns for the OPO output pulse itself). The corresponding fourfold optical-bandwidth deterioration (which seems to arise from the extraction of most of the gain of the Ti:sapphire pulsed amplifier by the leading part of each OPO pulse) has imposed an unwelcome trade-off between high OPO output pulse energy and narrow spectroscopic bandwidth.

This chirp-controlled, injection-seeded PPKTP OPO system exhibits stable SLM operation, with frequency chirp that is minimal when the phase mismatch Δk is close to zero, which is attained by minimizing the wavelength difference $|\lambda_S-\lambda_{free}|$. The OH module of this OPO system allows us to monitor the frequency chirp and central-frequency fluctuations in the SLM signal output on a real-time, pulse-by-pulse capability basis. This capability to log instantaneous-frequency data for each OPO output pulse has resulted in a new form of sub-Doppler spectroscopy: coherent heterodyne-assisted pulsed spectroscopy (CHAPS) [243,244], as will be discussed in Sections 2.5.1 and 2.5.3.

Under certain conditions (excessive pump-pulse intensity or Δk), seeding is found [241,242] to fail partway through the output pulse, such that operation on multiple longitudinal modes ensues, as observed via irregularities in the temporal profiles of the injection-seeded long-pulse PPKTP OPO signal output at higher pump-laser energies (e.g., approximately three times the unseeded OPO threshold) and with phase mismatch $|\Delta k| \gg 0$ (e.g., at large values of $|\lambda_S-\lambda_{free}| \approx 0.2$ nm) [241,242,245]. The buildup of MM operation becomes a significant problem in OPOs when longer pump-pulse durations (e.g., ~27 ns [241,242]) are used to produce a narrower FT-limited optical bandwidth, particularly when pump-laser intensities are high. However, a reliable SLM operation is feasible throughout each pulse when the buildup time for free-running modes exceeds the pump-pulse duration; this holds if the phase mismatch $\Delta k \approx 0$ (i.e., if $|\lambda_S-\lambda_{free}| \approx 0$) for moderate pump-laser intensities, approaching the PPKTP damage threshold.

This versatile all-solid-state tunable NLO light source [241,242] produces tunable narrowband SLM pulses (with ~25 ns duration and ≤5 μJ energy) in the fundamental IR wavelength range of 820–850 nm. Its output can be amplified and upconverted to generate coherent tunable UV radiation for high-precision spectroscopy [239–247], for example, at the fourth-harmonic wavelength (λ_{UV}) of 205–213 nm. It is especially useful for applications in the vacuum UV (VUV), region where a high peak power and a narrow optical bandwidth are needed (e.g., in pulses of tens of nanoseconds) for NLO upconversion. This instrument has been used, together with our distinctive CHAPS technique, for sub-Doppler two-photon excitation (TPE) spectroscopy of gaseous atoms such as Cs at ~822.5 nm [243,244], krypton (Kr) at ~212.5 nm [246], and xenon (Xe) at 205–213 nm [247]. Our long-term objective has been to improve the accuracy of a previous determination [367] of the absolute frequency for the $1\,^1S \rightarrow 2\,^1S$ two-photon transition of helium (He), excited at a VUV wavelength of ~120 nm; this may provide a measure of the Lamb shift in ground-state He as a significant test of quantum-electrodynamic theory. Such OPO-spectroscopic applications will be further discussed in Section 2.5.2.1.

2.4.3.5 Dynamics of SLM Nanosecond-Pulsed OPO Operation

There has been much fundamental interest in the temporal, spatial, and spectral performance of ns-pulsed OPOs, both within our own research group [225,239–247] and elsewhere [314,315,331,347–349,351,369–374]. Effects such as frequency chirp, the breakdown of seeding during signal and idler pulse generation, reduced backconversion, spatial beam quality, and spectro-temporal dynamics have been measured and modeled under various operating conditions for both BPM and QPM NLO media [245,314,315,331,347–349,351,369–374]. Numerical simulation studies of such processes, in and beyond the range in which they are observed, has offered insight into mechanisms that are at work in injection-seeded ns-pulsed OPOs and thereby enabled their design and performance to be improved.

In particular, we have employed the SNLO code [26] to perform numerical simulations to reveal mechanisms of spectro-temporal dynamics and to model the performance characteristics of our injection-seeded chirp-controlled PPKTP OPO system [241,242]. These simulations [245] are in satisfactory agreement with our OH measurements of instantaneous-frequency profiles and frequency chirp in the narrowband signal output from this OPO.

Frequency chirp in narrowband signal output pulses from such an OPO system has been observed to depend on phase mismatch between the pump, signal, and idler waves, and also on the pump pulse energy. Our simulations accurately predict the observed dependence of the frequency chirp on phase mismatch between the pump, signal, and idler waves, and also on the pump pulse energy. They yield realistic estimates of the frequency chirp, optical bandwidth, and spectral purity of the signal output pulse as it evolves, including effects that are not readily observed directly. For instance, rapid walk-off oscillations, which are predicted [347,348,370] to be associated with a breakdown in backconversion and injection seeding due to group-velocity mismatch, are evident in our simulations [245]; these oscillations are too rapid to observe with the PDs regularly used in our OH detection system. The combination of our experiments [241,242] and simulations [245] provides a dynamic, time-resolved view of the partial failure of injection seeding and the transition from SLM to MM OPO operation.

Our simulations [245] explore instrumental conditions allowing continuously tunable SLM operation of the chirp-controlled, injection-seeded PPKTP OPO [241,242], with optical bandwidth as close as possible to the FT limit. The excellent agreement between the simulations and experiment confirms that this OPO system is a well-characterized, reliable source of tunable, narrowband, coherent radiation for high-resolution spectroscopy on a nanosecond timescale.

2.5 OPO-BASED SPECTROSCOPIC MEASUREMENTS

2.5.1 SPECTROSCOPIC VERIFICATION OF OPO PERFORMANCE

The operational strategies listed in Table 2.3 indicate that, in many of their applications, OPOs (particularly the ns-pulsed and CW varieties) are used as spectroscopic instruments. The utility of such OPOs in this regard depends on a variety of distinctive properties, including:

- Continuous tunability, particularly in spectroscopic regions that are inaccessible to other tunable coherent light sources
- Narrow optical bandwidth (narrowest in the case of CW OPOs, FT limited in the case of ns-pulsed OPOs) for high-resolution spectroscopy
- High optical intensity, enabling assorted forms of NLO spectroscopy and up- or downconversion to more remote regions of the spectrum (e.g., VUV, mid-IR, or far IR)
- Laser-like beam quality, comprising sufficiently high spatial coherence, collimation, and directionality to facilitate long-path absorption for high sensitivity, remote sensing of distant targets, fine focusing for microimaging, and so forth
- Pulsed capability (e.g., nanoseconds, picoseconds, or femtoseconds), enabling time-resolved spectroscopy
- Broadband capability, as an option that may be useful for multiplex spectroscopy

Within this spectroscopic context, the ultimate test of OPO performance characteristics may entail a spectroscopic measurement itself, rather than relying solely on optical diagnostic instruments such as étalons, spectrum analyzers, wavemeters, and spatial beam profilers. For instance, spectra recorded by tuning the signal or idler output wavelength of an OPO may reveal scanning irregularities or discontinuities (such as mode-hops) that are difficult to detect in practice simply by analyzing Fabry–Perot étalon fringes. Moreover, the finesse of such an étalon may be insufficient to resolve the optical bandwidth of a narrowband SLM-tunable OPO.

This approach, in which actual spectra are used to confirm spectroscopic performance, was evident in the early OPO literature, as exemplified by the OPO-recorded 2.35 μm 2–0 band of CO shown in Figure 2.1 [1,10,13] and by other early investigations [11,14,16,281–284]. Nevertheless, many early reports of "tunable" OPOs failed in practice to provide convincing demonstrations of continuously tunable operation suitable for convenient spectroscopic scanning. In many cases, OPO performance characteristics such as optical bandwidth have been reported at a single, fixed wavelength with little or no evidence that the OPO can be continuously tuned on an SLM basis, or at least reliably stepped from one longitudinal mode to another at which spectroscopic data can be collected.

The Bosenberg/Guyer KTP OPO/NRO/OPA system is an instance of spectroscopic verification of the narrow optical bandwidth, SLM character, and continuous tunability of output OPO radiation [20,21]. In a sub-Doppler degenerate four-wave mixing (DFWM) spectrum [21], continuously scanned over a 30 GHz (1 cm^{-1}) range at ~2963.5 cm^{-1} (~3.3745 μm), the $R(3)$ line in the 1–0 absorption band of H^{35}Cl has an FWHM width of 0.45 GHz (0.015 cm^{-1}), indicating that the OPO has an SLM optical bandwidth of ~0.42 GHz (~0.014 cm^{-1}).

A central theme of our own research on injection-seeded ns-pulsed OPOs [1,5,29–32,234–249] has been to confirm performance by using the generated OPO radiation in actual spectroscopic applications. In Tables 2.4 and 2.5, we present chronologically ordered summaries of these investigations, together with a noncomprehensive sampling of examples from other research groups. These highly selective tabular surveys are confined to the period 1972–2006, as presented in the second edition of this book [5]. Table 2.4 is devoted to gas-phase spectroscopic measurements with moderate resolution, in which linewidths are limited by inhomogeneous broadening due to the Doppler effect. Table 2.5 concerns higher-resolution spectroscopy, designated "sub-Doppler," in which inhomogeneous broadening is circumvented in various ways.

The survey in Tables 2.4 and 2.5 refers predominantly to ns-pulsed OPOs; the few instances of spectroscopically characterized CW OPOs are designated "CW." The distinctive spectroscopic characteristics of mode-locked pulse trains from ultrafast (picosecond, femtosecond) OPOs, as well as their manifestation in frequency comb applications, have been considered separately in Sections 2.1.2 and, 2.3.3 through 2.3.5. Likewise, the emphasis is primarily on near IR tunable OPO sources, with a few examples of UV [29], visible [227,228,230–234,316,383,385], and mid-IR ($\lambda > \sim 4$ μm) [258,378] sources. Tables 2.4 and 2.5 focus on continuous tunability and optical bandwidth, although other characteristics are implicated indirectly (e.g., optical intensity and beam quality in the case of NLO spectroscopic methods).

It is evident from Tables 2.4 and 2.5 that a diverse range of laser-spectroscopic techniques [51,387–388] is available for OPO performance characterization. These can be subdivided somewhat arbitrarily into "linear" optical absorption spectroscopy and NLO spectroscopy. The former include the following linear spectroscopic techniques:

- Simple absorption, in which direct transmission of an absorbing medium is measured [10,13,262,323,377]
- PA spectroscopy, in which optically absorbed energy is detected as sound waves generated by thermal relaxation [131,225,227,229,231,234,376, 378–382]
- LIF, entailing luminescence excited by optical absorption [29,229,231,243,244,385]
- CRD spectroscopy [298,299], in which temporal decay of light in an optical cavity is measured instead of transmitted intensity [130,237,238,248,249]

The latter include the following nonlinear spectroscopic techniques:

- CARS, a form of coherent Raman spectroscopy [389–392] depending on the third-order NLO susceptibility $\chi^{(3)}$, in which molecules are excited by two coherent waves (Raman pump and Stokes; frequencies

TABLE 2.4

Performance Characteristics of Various ns-Pulsed and CW Tunable Optical Parametric Systems Spectroscopically Measured under Doppler-Limited Conditions, 1972–2007

Type of OPO System[a] [Ref(s)]	Description of Spectrum and Doppler-Limited Technique[b]	$\Delta\nu_{spectrum}{}^{c}$ (cm^{-1})	$\Delta\nu_{OPO}{}^{d}$ (cm^{-1})
Grating/étalon-controlled BPM LiNbO$_3$ OPO (Byer et al., 1972–1975) [10,13]	Absorption of CO gas in a 3 cm cell at 3 atm; continuous 180 cm^{-1} scan over the 2.35 μm 2–0 band of CO; see Figure 2.1.	~0.5 (OPO limited)	~0.5 (~15 GHz)
Grating/étalon-controlled BPM LiNbO$_3$ OPO (Byer et al., 1975–1977) [11]	CARS spectrum of H$_2$ gas @ 325 Torr; 50 cm^{-1} scan in 0.25 cm^{-1} steps of the signal @ ~1.9 μm, with 1.064 μm Raman pump, in the Q branch, with 4155 cm^{-1} $J=1$ peak.	2 (grating only)	2 (grating only); 0.1 (with étalon)
Dye laser–seeded passive-cavity BBO OPO (Haub et al., 1991–1993) [225,226]	PA spectra of C$_2$H$_2$ gas @ 100 Torr; continuous scans of idler @ ~965 nm in the C$_2$H$_2$ ($\nu_1+2\nu_3+\nu_5$) band: A 8.5 cm^{-1} scan of the Q branch and four 1 cm^{-1} scans of the 10,382.3 cm^{-1} $R(7)$ line.	0.12 (pressure broadened)	~0.1 (~3 GHz)
LiNbO$_3$ OPO, injection seeded by SFG in LiTO$_3$ (Huisken et al., 1992) [310]	IR spectra of HCl vapor @ 19 Torr; continuous 60 cm^{-1} scan of idler @ ~2.7 μm over the $P(1)$, $P(2)$, and $P(3)$ lines in the HCl 1–0 band.	2.3 cm^{-1} H^{35}Cl/H^{37}Cl splittings resolved	~0.1 (seeded by narrowband dye laser)
Dye laser–seeded passive-cavity BBO OPO (Fix et al., 1993) [226]	PA spectrum of C$_2$H$_2$ gas @ 80 Torr; continuous 135 cm^{-1} scan of idler @ ~1.04 μm in the P and R branches of the C$_2$H$_2$ $3\nu_3$ band.	0.25 (~7.5 GHz)	<0.25 (<7.5 GHz)
Dye laser–seeded passive-cavity BBO OPO (Haub et al., 1993) [227,228]	CARS spectra of N$_2$ in air @ 1 atm; continuous 5 cm^{-1} signal scan @ ~607 nm with 532 nm Raman pump, in the 2330 cm^{-1} Q branch.	0.2 (pressure broadened)	~0.1 (~3 GHz)
TDL–seeded passive ring-cavity BBO OPO (Johnson et al., 1995) [227,231]	PA spectrum of C$_2$H$_2$ gas @ 14 Torr; continuous 1.1 cm^{-1} scan of idler @ ~865.5 nm covering part of the C$_2$H$_2$ ($\nu_2+3\nu_3$) band.	0.03 (Doppler broadened)	≤0.008 (≤250 MHz) from TPE
Aperture-selected free-running BBO OPO (Haub et al., 1995) [230,232]	DFWM spectrum of Na in an air–acetylene flame; continuous 17 cm^{-1} scan of signal over the 589.0 and 589.6 nm Na D-lines.	~4 (aperture-limited)	~4 (full beam: ~20 cm^{-1})

(Continued)

TABLE 2.4 (CONTINUED)

Performance Characteristics of Various ns-Pulsed and CW Tunable Optical Parametric Systems Spectroscopically Measured under Doppler-Limited Conditions, 1972–2007

Type of OPO System[a] [Ref(s)]	Description of Spectrum and Doppler-Limited Technique[b]	$\Delta\nu_{spectrum}$[c] (cm⁻¹)	$\Delta\nu_{OPO}$[d] (cm⁻¹)
TDL-seeded passive ring-cavity BBO OPO (Baxter et al., 1996) [232]	CARS spectra of N_2 gas @ 75 Torr; continuous 1.6 cm⁻¹ signal scan @ ~607 nm with 532 nm Raman pump, in 2330 cm⁻¹ Q branch of N_2.	0.018 (0.54 GHz)	~0.01 (~0.3 GHz)
Dual-wavelength passive ring-cavity LiNbO₃ OPO seeded by 2 TDLs (Baxter et al., 1996) [232]	Dual-wavelength CARS spectra of N_2 gas in furnace air @ 300–1200 K, enabling instantaneous single-shot OPO CARS thermometry.	0.4 (12 GHz), diode-array limited	~0.01 (~0.3 GHz) for each wavelength
Dual-wavelength passive ring-cavity LiNbO₃ OPO seeded by 2 TDLs (Baxter et al., 1997) [233]	Dual-wavelength signal output spectra display sidebands due to backconversion when OPO is operated above threshold.	0.4 (12 GHz), diode-array limited	~0.01 (~0.3 GHz) for each wavelength
TDL-seeded LiNbO₃ OPO (Milton et al., 1997) [323]	Absorption of 2% CH_4 in 1 atm of air; stepwise scan over a 1.2 cm⁻¹ range @ ~3.428 μm over several lines @ 2916.5–2918.0 cm⁻¹ v_3 band of CH_4.	0.02 (pressure broadened)	0.005 (135 MHz) estimated
TDL-seeded passive ring-cavity LiNbO₃ OPO (Baxter et al., 1998) [234]	PA and CARS spectra of CH_4 gas @ 10 Torr; continuous scans of idler and signal in 3019 cm⁻¹ v_3 and 2916.5 cm⁻¹ v_1 Q branches, respectively.	≤0.02 (≤0.6 GHz)	~0.01 (~0.3 GHz)
Single-frequency CW PPLN OPO system (Kühnemann et al., 1998) [376]	PA detection of C_2H_6 (83 ppm in N_2 @ 1 atm) at a single frequency @ ~3.3 μm of ^rQ subbranches in the 2985.4 cm⁻¹ C_2H_6 v_7 band.	~0.4 (multiline, pressure broadened)	Not specified (probably <1 MHz)
Grazing-incidence grating-tuned PPLN OPO system (Yu and Kung, 1999) [291]	PA spectra of CH_4 gas @ 16 Torr; continuous 40 and 60 cm⁻¹ scans of signal and idler @ ~1.645 and ~3.28 μm, in the v_3 and (v_1+v_3) bands of CH_4, respectively.	0.3 (signal) and 0.9 (idler)	0.3 (signal) and 0.9 (idler)
BPM-angle-scanned AgGaS₂ OPO with wide tuning range (4–11 μm) (Vodopyanov et al., 1999) [377]	Absorption spectrum of CO gas @ 630 Torr; continuous 200 cm⁻¹ scan of resonated signal over the ~4.65 μm 1–0 band of CO.	~1 (30 GHz)	~1 (30 GHz)

System	Application		
TDL-seeded passive-cavity BBO OPO/SFG system (Baxter et al., 2000) [29]	LIF-detected spectrum of NO gas @ 0.25 Torr; continuous 2.1 cm⁻¹ scan within the NO A $^2\Sigma+ \leftarrow$ X $^2\Pi$ 0–0 band @ ~226 nm.	0.115 (3.45 GHz)	0.06 (1.8 GHz)
TDL-seeded PPLN OPO with intensity-dip control, MM-pumped (He and Orr, 2001) [237]	CRD spectra of C_2H_2 gas @ 100 Torr; continuous 1 cm⁻¹ scan of 1.528 µm TDL-seeded signal over weak lines @ 6543.3–6544.0 cm⁻¹ near the $(\nu_1+\nu_3)$ P branch of C_2H_2.	0.016 (Doppler broadened)	<0.004 (<120 MHz)
TDL-seeded PPLN OPO, MM- and SLM-pumped with intensity-dip control (He and Orr, 2001) [237,238]	CRD spectra of CO_2 gas @ 1 atm; continuous 120 cm⁻¹ scans of TDL-seeded signal @ 1.54 µm over the 6503 cm⁻¹ CO_2 $(3\nu_1+\nu_3)$ band.	0.0065 (195 MHz)	<0.004 (<120 MHz)
Grating/étalon-controlled mid-IR $ZnGeP_2$ OPO (Ganikhanov et al., 2001) [262]	Absorption spectra of H_2O vapor @ 60°C; continuous 2 and 7 cm⁻¹ scans of resonated signal within the range 1615–1630 cm⁻¹.	0.3–0.4 (9–12 GHz)	0.1–0.15 (3–4.5 GHz) estimated
TDL-seeded PPKTP OPO, with photorefractive SAT control (He and Orr, 2001) [248]	CRD spectrum of CO_2 gas @ 20 Torr; continuous 0.15 cm⁻¹ scan of 1.44 µm idler over the 6948.76 cm⁻¹ CO_2 $3\nu_3$ P(24) line.	0.017 (507 MHz)	≤0.0033 (≤100 MHz)
Nd:YAG-laser-pumped CW fan-grating PPLN OPO (Bisson et al., 2001) [378]	PA spectroscopy of CH_4 @ 1 atm; a 9 cm⁻¹ idler mode-hop scan in the 3019 cm⁻¹ Q branch of the CH_4 ν_3 band.	~0.1 (pressure broadened)	Sub-MHz (mode-hop scanned)
Nd:YAG-laser-pumped CW fan-grating PPLN OPO (van Herpen et al., 2002) [379–381]	PA spectroscopy of C_2H_6 (0.4 ppb in N_2 @ 1 atm; a continuous 0.6 cm⁻¹ idler scan over the 2996.85 cm⁻¹ Q branch of the C_2H_6 ν_7 band.	~0.15 (pressure broadened)	Sub-MHz (pump-frequency scanned)
Nd:YAG-laser-pumped CW PPLN OPO system (Popp et al., 2002) [130]	CRD detection of C_2H_6 @ 77 Torr at a single frequency (2990.096 cm⁻¹) in the 3.34 µm $^rQ_1$ subbranch of the C_2H_6 ν_7 band, yielding 0.3 ppb detection limit.	~0.5 (multiline, pressure broadened)	Sub-MHz (fixed single frequency)

(Continued)

TABLE 2.4 (CONTINUED)

Performance Characteristics of Various ns-Pulsed and CW Tunable Optical Parametric Systems Spectroscopically Measured under Doppler-Limited Conditions, 1972–2007

Type of OPO System[a] [Ref(s)]	Description of Spectrum and Doppler-Limited Technique[b]	$\Delta\nu_{spectrum}$[c] (cm⁻¹)	$\Delta\nu_{OPO}$[d] (cm⁻¹)
Nd:YAG-laser-pumped CW dual-cavity PPLN OPO system (Müller et al., 2003) [131]	PA spectroscopy of C_2H_6 (1 ppm in N_2 @ 1 atm); a 1 cm⁻¹ idler mode-hop scan in 2983.4 cm⁻¹ $^\nu Q_1$ subbranch of the C_2H_6 ν_7 band, yielding 0.11 ppb detection limit.	~0.13 (multiline, pressure broadened)	Sub-MHz (±30 MHz stability in 45 min)
Diode laser–pumped CW PP MgO:LiNbO₃ OPO system (Ngai et al., 2007) [382]	Quartz-enhanced PA spectroscopy (QEPAS) of trace-level CH_4, C_2H_6, H_2O, … in 0.2 atm of laboratory air; continuous scan over 15 cm⁻¹ range @ ~3.35 μm.	0.03 (pressure broadened)	Sub-MHz

a   OPOs are ns pulsed unless otherwise specified (e.g., continuous-wave designated CW). Distinctive spectroscopic characteristics of mode-locked pulse trains from ultrafast (ps, fs) OPOs and frequency combs are considered separately in Sections 2.1.2, 2.3.3, and 2.3.4.

b   Acronyms for spectroscopic techniques (CARS, PA, DFWM, CRD) are defined in the text; ppbv = parts per billion (by volume).

c $\Delta\nu_{spectrum}$ is the FWHM spectroscopic linewidth (in units of reciprocal centimeter; also gigahertz or megahertz).

d $\Delta\nu_{OPO}$ is the FWHM optical bandwidth of the OPO output radiation, inferred from the spectrum (unless otherwise specified), allowing for Doppler or pressure broadening.

TABLE 2.5

Performance Characteristics of Various ns-Pulsed and CW Tunable Optical Parametric Systems Spectroscopically Measured under Sub-Doppler Conditions, 1993–2006

Type of OPO System[a] [Ref(s)]	Description of Spectrum and Sub-Doppler Technique[b]	$\Delta\nu_{spectrum}$[c] (cm^{-1})	$\Delta\nu_{OPO}$[d] (cm^{-1})
Grating/étalon-tuned KTP OPO/ NRO/OPA (Bosenberg and Guyer, 1993) [21]	DFWM, continuous 1 cm^{-1} scan @ ~3.374 µm of $R(3)$ line in 1–0 band of H^{35}Cl (pressure not specified).	0.015 (450 MHz)	~0.014 (~420 MHz)
TDL-seeded passive-cavity BBO OPO (Johnson et al., 1995) [229,231]	LIF-detected TPE of Rb vapor @ ~90°C; continuous scan of idler @ ~778.1 nm over the 25,703.5 cm^{-1} 5 s^2 $S\frac{1}{2} \to 5d\,^2 S\frac{1}{2}$ ^{85}Rb ($F=3$) line.	0.01 (315 MHz)	≤0.008 (≤250 MHz)
TDL-seeded BBO OPO system (Boon-Engering et al., 1995) [316]	Ionization-detected TPE in beam of Ba metastables; 0.8 cm^{-1} continuous scan @ ~620.6 nm over 16,112.864 cm^{-1} $5d\,7d\,^3D_2 \to 6s\,5d\,^3P_0$ Ba line.	0.02 (600 MHz)	0.012 (~400 MHz)
TDL-seeded passive ring-cavity LiNbO$_3$ OPO (Baxter et al., 1998) [234]	CARS of a CH$_4$ supersonic free jet with $T_{rot} = 10$–20 K; continuous 0.2 cm^{-1} scans of signal @ ~1.54 µm (with 1064 nm Raman pump) in 2330 cm^{-1} ν_1 Q branch.	0.008 (240 MHz)	0.007 (210 MHz)
TDL-seeded PPLN OPO with intensity-dip control (Baxter et al., 1998) [235]	CARS of a CH$_4$ supersonic free jet with $T_{rot} = 15$ K; continuous 0.15 cm^{-1} scan of signal @ ~1.54 µm (with 1064 nm Raman pump) in 2330 cm^{-1} ν_1 Q branch.	0.0065 (195 MHz)	~0.0045 (135 MHz)
TDL-seeded PPLN OPO with intensity-dip control, SLM- or MM-pumped (He and Orr, 1999) [237]	CRD spectra of a C$_2$H$_2$ supersonic free jet with $T_{rot} \approx 20$ K; continuous 0.03 cm^{-1} scans of 1.528 µm TDL-seeded signal over the $P(5)$ line @ 6544.442 cm^{-1} in the $\nu_1+\nu_3$ band of C$_2$H$_2$.	SLM pump: 0.0037 (110 MHz) MM pump: 0.0042 (125 MHz)	<0.004 (<120 MHz)

(Continued)

TABLE 2.5 (CONTINUED)

Performance Characteristics of Various ns-Pulsed and CW Tunable Optical Parametric Systems Spectroscopically Measured under Sub-Doppler Conditions, 1993–2006

Type of OPO System[a] [Ref(s)]	Description of Spectrum and Sub-Doppler Technique[b]	$\Delta\nu_{spectrum}$ [c] (cm⁻¹)	$\Delta\nu_{OPO}$ [d] (cm⁻¹)
Multistage Nd:YAG/SHG–pumped CW MgO:LiNbO₃ DRO system with SHG stage (Petelski et al., 2001) [383]	Hyperfine spectral hole-burning spectrum of $^5D_0 \rightarrow {}^7F_0$ transition in Eu^{3+}: Y_2SiO_5 @ 4 K; continuous 6.7 cm⁻¹ scan @ ~580 nm.	≤0.1 (≤3 GHz) inhomogeneous width	<3.3×10^{-5} (<1 MHz) ex hole-burning
Étalon- and pump-frequency-scanned CW SLM PPLN OPO system (Kovalchuk et al., 2001) [384]	High-resolution Doppler-free FM saturation spectroscopy in 6 mTorr of CH_4 @ 3.39 µm; 1.8 GHz (0.06 cm⁻¹) continuous tuning range.	1.7×10^{-5} (0.5 MHz), pressure broadened	0.1 MHz (with ~0.2–0.4 MHz jitter)
TDL-seeded BBO OPG/OPA system (Kulatilaka et al., 2005) [385]	LIF-detected TPE spectra of 0.3% NO in 2 Torr of N_2; continuous 0.5 cm⁻¹ scan within the NO A $^2\Sigma^+ \leftarrow X\,^2\Pi$ 0–0 band @ ~452 nm.	~0.01 (~300 MHz)	0.007 (220 MHz) ex spectrum analyzer
TDL-seeded PPKTP OPO with intensity dip and OH chirp control (Kono et al., 2005–6) [243,244]	LIF-detected TPE CHAPS of Cs vapor @ ~90°C; signal-pulse histogram sampled @ ~822.47 nm on a 2 MHz grid at the $^2S\frac{1}{2} \rightarrow 8s\ ^2S\frac{1}{2}$ ($F=4$) 2-photon transition of Cs.	0.0006 (18 MHz) from TPE histogram	0.0006 (18 MHz), with jitter suppressed by CHAPS

a OPOs are ns pulsed unless otherwise specified (e.g., continuous wave designated CW). Distinctive spectroscopic characteristics of mode-locked pulse trains from ultrafast (picosecond, femtosecond) OPOs and frequency combs are considered separately in Sections 2.1.2, 2.3.3, and 2.3.4.

b Acronyms for spectroscopic techniques (DFWM, LIF, TPE, CARS, CRD, CHAPS, FM) are defined in the text.

c $\Delta\nu_{spectrum}$ is the FWHM spectroscopic linewidth (in units of reciprocal centimeter; also gigahertz or megahertz).

d $\Delta\nu_{OPO}$ is the FWHM optical bandwidth of the OPO output radiation, inferred from the spectrum (unless otherwise specified), allowing for Doppler or pressure broadening.

ω_{pump} and ω_{Stokes}), and a third coherent anti-Stokes wave is generated (at $2\omega_{pump} - \omega_{Stokes}$) when ($\omega_{pump} - \omega_{Stokes}$) matches a Raman frequency of the molecules [11,227,228,232–235,353,354]

- DFWM spectroscopy [393], another $\chi^{(3)}$-dependent NLO technique in which three coherent input waves (all at frequency ω) generate a fourth coherent wave (also at ω) [21,230,231,393–396]
- TPE spectroscopy, detected by either ionization [246,247,316] or LIF [229,231,243,244,385]

Sub-Doppler spectroscopic measurements in the gas or vapor phase by techniques such as DFWM [21,230,231,393–396] and TPE (with counterpropagating beams) [229,231,243,244,246,247,385] have played a key role in verifying the performance of tunable injection-seeded OPOs. Sub-Doppler CARS [234,235] and CRD [237] spectra can be detected in supersonic molecular beams or jets, with the optical path(s) carefully aligned to be transverse to the direction of the beam or jet. Narrow homogeneously broadened spectral features can also be extracted from inhomogeneously broadened spectra by various forms of saturation or hole-burning spectroscopy [51,383,384]. Moreover, CARS spectroscopy (with copropagating beams) is able to provide some reduction, by a factor of at least ($\omega_{pump} - \omega_{Stokes}$)/$\omega_{Stokes}$, of the inhomogeneous line broadening in the case of gas-phase molecules, given that the relevant Doppler width is proportional to ($\omega_{pump} - \omega_{Stokes}$), rather than the tunable OPO frequency ω_{Stokes} itself; such reduction effects are evident in Table 2.4.

Another form of high-precision OPO-based spectroscopy with sub-Doppler resolution is CHAPS [243,244,246,247], which relies on our OH-based capability to make shot-to-shot instantaneous frequency measurements of the OPO output radiation [241,242]. This technique has been used [243] to verify the performance of our chirp-controlled, injection-seeded PPKTP OPO system, described in Section 2.4.3.4. The instrumental layout illustrated in Figure 2.12a has been used to characterize the fundamental OPO signal output at ~822.5 nm via the LIF-detected TPE 6S $\rightarrow$ 8S spectrum of Cs vapor, with counterpropagating coherent beams to attain sub-Doppler resolution. Figure 2.12b shows the spectroscopic scheme for LIF-detected TPE of $6s\ ^2S_{1/2} \rightarrow 8s\ ^2S_{1/2}$ transitions in Cs ($F=4$ at 822.49 nm and $F=3$ at 822.45 nm). In our original CHAPS approach [243], the reference frequency of the CW Ti:sapphire seed laser was held fixed, within ~1 MHz of a Cs TPE resonance peak. Using our OH method, it was then feasible to log the central frequency of each OPO pulse (pre- or postamplification) and thereby record a sub-Doppler histogram-style spectrum in which the OPO frequency jitter spanned the full sub-Doppler spectrum (18 MHz FWHM). As illustrated in Figure 2.12c, the TPE spectral lineshape has a ~27 MHz FWHM Lorentzian fit, approaching the FT limit [243].

2.5.2   OPO-Spectroscopic Sensing of Atoms and Molecules

Tables 2.4 and 2.5 provide ample evidence of a wide range of spectroscopic measurements to which tunable OPOs may be applied. However, most of the spectra involved are of little intrinsic spectroscopic interest or novelty, given that they are already well known and may be recorded routinely in less elaborate ways, such as FTIR,

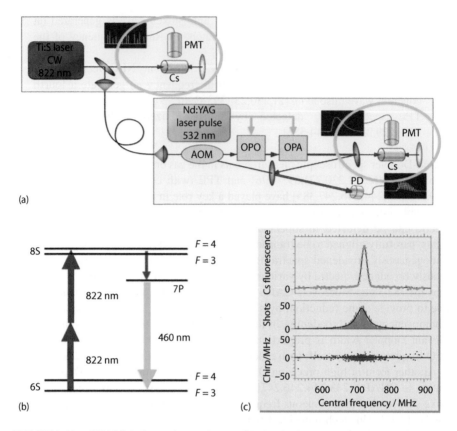

FIGURE 2.12 CHAPS (coherent heterodyne-assisted pulsed spectroscopy) approach to sub-Doppler spectroscopic measurements that are designed to verify the performance of a pulsed injection-seeded tunable OPO with a chirp-control system [32,243,244]. Here, the CHAPS method is used to characterize the fundamental OPO signal output at ~822.5 nm via the fluorescence-detected two-photon 6S → 8S spectrum of Cs vapor. (a) Layout of the CHAPS instrument used for these measurements. (b) The relevant LIF-detected TPE scheme for Cs (in which $\Delta F = 0$ selection rules apply). (c) Cs TPE LIF plotted as a function of OH-detected central frequency (top panel), together with a histogram of the number of OPO shots recorded (middle panel), and the corresponding distribution of linear frequency chirp (bottom panel). PMT, photomultiplier tube; Cs, optical cell containing Cs vapor; AOM, acousto-optic modulator; OPO, injection-seeded PPKTP OPO system as in Figure 2.10; OPA, LiNbO₃ optical parametric amplifier; PD, fast photodetector for optical-heterodyne diagnostics. (From Kono, M. et al., *Opt. Lett.* 30: 3413–3415, 2005; Kono, M. et al., *J. Opt. Soc. Am. B* 23: 1181–1189, 2006.)

linear Raman spectrometry, or conventional forms of sub-Doppler spectroscopy. In this section, we consider spectroscopic applications in which the spectra themselves provide not only a way to characterize OPO performance but also a fresh source of information about fundamental atomic and molecular processes, or highly sensitive analytical methodologies, or spectroscopic sensing strategies for atmospheric and other industrial, environmental, or biological media. Section 2.5.2 covers only a selective, representative sample of a wide range of the many spectroscopic applications of optical parametric devices.

2.5.2.1 Fundamental OPO Spectroscopy of Atoms, Molecules, and Ions

Sub-Doppler OPO spectroscopy, as outlined in Section 2.5.1 (including Table 2.5), is now established as a source of fundamental spectroscopic information. For instance, Kovalchuk et al. [384] reported a CW OPO system based on multigrating PPLN. This was SLM tuned by combined tilting of an intracavity étalon and scanning the frequency of the CW Nd:YAG pump laser; the OPO idler output had a continuous, mode-hop-free tuning range of 1.8 GHz (0.06 cm^{-1}) and an optical bandwidth of ~0.1 MHz (with 0.5 ms integration time and typical idler-frequency drift of 0.5 MHz/min), measured by beating the OPO idler at 3.39 μm against a CH_4-stabilized He–Ne laser. The sub-Doppler spectroscopic performance of this OPO system was demonstrated [384] by recording frequency-modulation (FM) saturation spectra of the classic 3.39 μm resonance in CH_4 gas, with counterpropagating saturating (10 mW) and probe (2 mW) beams in a 2 m long cell at pressures of 6–54 mTorr; the sub-Doppler linewidth at 6 Torr was observed to be ~0.5 MHz (1.7×10^{-5} cm^{-1}), which is attributable to a combination of pressure broadening (~0.2 MHz) and medium-term OPO frequency jitter (~0.2–0.4 MHz). OPOs have enabled various other lower-resolution measurements of $CH_4(g)$ absorption spectra [75,76,164–167,169,176,188,211,212,216,224,234,282,291–293,303,323,378,382,395,396].

Another relevant example (although not strictly "sub-Doppler") is that of Petelski et al. [383], who used a frequency-doubled CW MgO:LiNbO$_3$ tunable OPO system to measure hyperfine hole-burning spectra of the 580 nm $^5D_0 \rightarrow {}^7F_0$ transition in Eu^{3+}:Y$_2$SiO$_5$ at 4 K. The inhomogeneously broadened two-site spectrum of this low-temperature crystalline medium had a linewidth of ≤ 3 GHz (0.1 cm^{-1}) FWHM; after 40 min of spectral hole burning, its 580.070 nm peak was found to have a homogeneous linewidth of <1 MHz ($<3.3 \times 10^{-5}$ cm^{-1}) and a decay time of ~15 h.

As outlined at the end of Section 2.4.3, our OH chirp-controlled, injection-seeded PPKTP OPO/OPA system [241,242] has been designed as the primary stage of an all-solid-state narrowband SLM-tunable source of coherent VUV radiation for fundamental spectroscopic experiments in atomic and molecular physics. Our CHAPS spectroscopic technique [243,244], as mentioned in Section 2.5.1 and in Table 2.5, was a preliminary stage in this program, yielding sub-Doppler LIF-detected 6S → 8S TPE spectra of Cs vapor at ~822.5 nm, as illustrated in Figure 2.12.

We have subsequently developed a scanned-reference variant of CHAPS [246], in which the CW Ti:sapphire seed-laser frequency is slowly tuned (rather than having its frequency fixed, as in our previous CHAPS measurements of Cs at ~822.5 nm [243,244]) and monitored by a high-resolution wavemeter. This technique has been used to measure the ionization-detected sub-Doppler spectral profile of the two-photon resonance of Kr excited to its 5p[1/2]$_0$ state, with optical amplification and fourth-harmonic generation of fundamental PPKTP OPO signal radiation at ~850.2 nm yielding upconverted pulsed coherent TPE radiation at ~212.55 nm [246], thereby confirming the spectroscopic utility of this tunable SLM source of upconverted coherent pulsed UV radiation. The sub-Doppler TPE spectral profile of Kr was recorded by logging the central frequency for each amplified OPO pulse at

~850.2 nm, using our OH chirp-analysis software. Scanned-reference sub-Doppler CHAPS spectra were produced by controlled tuning of the CW laser over a frequency range exceeding that spanned by frequency jitter of the pulsed OPO. The sub-Doppler CHAPS lineshape indicated that the amplified, upconverted UV pulses at ~212.5 nm had an optical bandwidth of ~100 MHz, consistent with the FT limit of their amplifier-shortened duration (~4.5 ns FWHM).

More recently, a similar ionization-detected sub-Doppler TPE technique has been used for OPO-based spectroscopic studies of 33 Rydberg levels of Xe, UV excited at 205–213 nm [247]. The pulsed coherent UV beam was retroreflected through an ionization cell containing pure Xe (or Kr) gas at room temperature and ~0.1 Torr (~0.13 mbar), avoiding signal saturation and pressure broadening (as in our previous study of Kr [246]). This counterpropagating optical geometry yielded sub-Doppler TPE spectra of the Xe atoms, with the ionization signal recorded by means of a 36 V biased electrode and gated boxcar integrator. The outcome is a diverse set of spectra corresponding to excitation of the following five sets of high-energy Rydberg levels of Xe: $5p^5 np [1/2]_0$ $(n=9-13)$, $5p^5 np [3/2]_2$ $(n=9-13)$, $5p^5 np [5/2]_2$ $(n=9-17)$, $5p^5 nf [3/2]_2$ $(n=6-14)$, and $5p^5 nf [5/2]_2$ $(n=6-10)$. These levels lie at TPE energies in the range of $94,100-97,300 \text{cm}^{-1}$ $(11.67-12.06 \text{eV})$ above the $5p^6$ $^1 S_0$ electronic ground state of Xe. The sub-Doppler spectra display diverse isotope energy shifts and hyperfine-coupling effects, for which least-squares-fit spectroscopic parameters reflect the influence of angular momentum within the Xe atom. In ongoing research, we have adapted the atomic-beam apparatus employed previously in early TPE experiments on the He 1 ^{1}S → 2 ^{1}S transition [367]. This provides isotopic-mass selectivity to distinguish spectral contributions from individual Xe isotopes and thereby to resolve some of the heavily overlapped spectra that were previously recorded in natural isotopic abundance [247]. This approach is expected to help to reduce uncertainties in our previous results, particularly for the nf $[5/2]_2$ $(n=6-10)$ levels, for which remarkably small magnetic-dipole hyperfine coupling parameters A^{129} and A^{131} are found, and best-fit values of electric-quadrupole hyperfine coupling parameter B^{131} are ambiguous [247].

As already mentioned in Section 2.4.3.4, further development of the amplification and upconversion stages of our OH chirp-controlled, injection-seeded PPKTP OPO/OPA system (with wavelength conversion from ~842 to ~210 nm and, ultimately, to ~120 nm) should facilitate spectroscopic access to the quantum-electrodynamically significant 1 ^{1}S – 2 ^{1}S two-photon transition of He, excited at a VUV wavelength of ~120 nm [367]. That would enable us to emulate earlier measurements of the ground-state Lamb shift of He [367], but with an all-solid-state laser and NLO system. Such an experiment would complement relevant recent advances in high-precision VUV spectroscopy of He [397–402], based on frequency combs and high-order harmonic generation. We note a very early (1978) experiment [403] that used a VUV spontaneous anti-Stokes light source, pumped by an ns-pulsed $LiNbO_3$ OPO, to measure the 7.8 cm^{-1} isotope shift between the 2 ^{1}S levels of ^{4}He and ^{3}He, excited in a glow discharge in a mixture of He and Ne.

As mentioned in Section 2.4.1, Rakestraw and coworkers have used a commercial Bosenberg/Guyer-type KTP OPO/NRO/OPA system [20,21] to record high-resolution rovibrational DFWM spectra, realizing a spectroscopic bandwidth of ≤ 450 MHz (≤ 0.015 cm^{-1}) in the 3 µm region. High-quality spectra of this type have been published for the 3.37 µm 1–0 band of HCl (near the $R(3)$ line) [21], for the 3.30 µm v_3 band of CH$_4$ [395,396], and for the 3.05 µm $v_3/(v_2+v_4+v_5)^0$ Fermi-dyad bands of C$_2$H$_2$ [395,396].

Such a high-performance, computer-controlled SLM-tunable coherent IR source [20,21] has been used for various forms of laser spectroscopy (CRD, DFWM, long-path absorption, etc.), including investigations of chemically reactive media, combustion diagnostics, and studies of processes in molecular beams. For instance, Bieske and coworkers have used a similar OPO/NRO/OPA system to record mechanistically significant IR spectra of mass-selected complexes of a halide ion with various molecules, such as acetylene (C$_2$H$_2$), Cl$^-$–(C$_2$H$_2$)$_n$ ($n = 1-9$) [404], Br$^-$–(C$_2$H$_2$)$_n$ ($n = 1-8$) [405,406], and I$^-$–(C$_2$H$_2$)$_n$ ($n = 1-4$) [407]. Such gas-phase IR-spectroscopic studies [408] have explored the nature of hydrogen bonds between "solute" atomic or molecular anions and neutral "solvent" molecules.

The alternative injection-seeding approach to narrowband OPO tuning was used by Frieder Huisken and colleagues in Göttingen [310] in a 1.064 µm pumped BPM LiNbO$_3$ OPO seeded at its idler wavelength by a LiIO$_3$ DFG stage that mixes 532 nm Nd:YAG and tunable visible dye laser radiation; continuous tuning over ranges of at least 50 cm^{-1} was achieved by "look-up table" computer-based control of NLO phase-matching angles as the dye-laser diffraction grating was rotated. This DFG-seeded LiNbO$_3$ OPO system was used to record vibrational spectra of small water complexes embedded in large liquid He clusters [318] and to measure gas- and supersonic-jet-phase DFWM and resonance-enhanced SRS spectra of C$_2$H$_2$, CO$_2$, and nitrous oxide (N$_2$O) [324].

David Nesbitt and coworkers in Colorado have also developed a high-performance injection-seeded tunable OPO system with peak output energies ≥ 10 mJ and optical bandwidth (160 ± 20 MHz) close to the FT limit [321]. They applied it to high-resolution vibrational overtone studies of HOD and H$_2$O in the $3v_{OH}$ and $4v_{OH}$ regions, to high-resolution LIF Doppler spectroscopy of OH radicals, and to IR-UV multiple resonance spectroscopy of H–OH bond breaking in quantum-state-selected Ar–H$_2$O molecular clusters [322,330,334].

In another example of fundamental molecular spectroscopy, Michael Ashworth, Colin Western, and coworkers in Bristol used an injection-seeded narrowband ns-pulsed SLM-tunable OPO to record sub-Doppler LIF spectra displaying hyperfine structure in the A $^3\Pi$ electronic states of the molecular radicals PF [338,339] and PH [341] in a supersonic jet expansion.

At Macquarie University, an early objective of our OPO-related research was to devise convenient tunable, narrowband coherent sources of ns-pulsed IR and UV radiation for time-resolved, LIF-detected IR-UV (IR-UV DR) spectroscopy to probe energy-transfer dynamics of small gas-phase polyatomic molecules such as C$_2$H$_2$ [409]. At the outset, UV-scanned IR-UV DR spectra of the "$3v_{CH}$" manifold at ~9600 cm^{-1} in the electronic ground state $\tilde{X}$ of C$_2$H$_2$ were recorded using an injection-seeded passive-cavity BBO OPO as IR source (e.g., pumping the 9567.36 cm^{-1} $3v_3$ $R(7)$ rovibrational transition) to reveal interesting anomalies in the resulting collision-induced IR-UV DR spectra [1,29,227]. Our subsequent OPO-based IR-UV DR research has focused on the "$4v_{CH}$" manifold at ~12,700 cm^{-1} in the electronic ground state $\tilde{X}$ of C_2H_2, where discrete rovibrational structure is known [409–411] to be complicated by an underlying collision-induced quasi-continuous background (CIQCB). We therefore introduced two tunable OPO systems to attain higher spectroscopic resolution (relative to that of the tunable dye lasers regularly used for our IR-UV DR experiments [409–411]): as continuously tunable narrowband IR pump source, a Bosenberg/Guyer-type KTP OPO/NRO/OPA system [20,21]; as UV probe source, an injection-seeded passive-cavity BBO OPO with additional BBO SFG upconversion stage tuned to a characteristic rovibronic transition of C_2H_2 (e.g., by probing the $v_1 + 3v_3$, $J = 19$ rovibrational level). It was of particular interest in this later IR-UV DR study that the narrower optical bandwidths of these OPO-based IR pump and UV probe sources resulted in no fresh insight into IR-UV DR effects such as CIQCB [409–411].

2.5.2.2 OPO Applications to Atmospheric Sensing

There is extensive literature on the foundations of laser-based atmospheric sensing [15,28,412–422]. This field offers opportunities for OPOs in the IR region, where IR lidar (light detection and ranging—an optical analogue of radar) usually embraces techniques that monitor an optically defined column of the atmosphere, as well as true range-resolved lidar. IR lidar relies on two key factors: the strength of IR light scattering from aerosols and particulates (relative to that from molecules) and the amenability of most small molecules to being monitored via their IR absorption spectra. Such factors are vital in the range-resolved form of IR DIAL, which relies on elastic scattering from atmospheric aerosols (to act as a "distributed mirror") and on characteristic rovibrational absorption spectra as signatures of specific atmospheric molecules, such as H_2O, CH_4, O_3, and various pollutant species. The latter attribute also enables retroreflected long-path IR laser absorption, which entails a trade-off between range resolution and sensitivity. There are additional opportunities for atmospheric sensing by OPO-based sources in the visible and UV regions, where the optical processes involved arise predominantly from electronic properties of molecules: Rayleigh and Raman scattering, electronic absorption, and fluorescence.

The high output power, optical coherence, and narrowband tunability of ns-pulsed OPOs are all advantageous for remote sensing of the atmosphere. Moreover, OPO pulse durations of 2–10 ns are amenable to the range-resolution requirements of many lidar and DIAL applications. Narrowband ns-pulsed $LiNbO_3$ OPOs, with intracavity grating and étalon control, were realized before 1980 by Byer and coworkers [9–12] and successfully applied in a number of atmospheric remote-sensing demonstrations involving the following molecular species: CO (at 2.3 μm and a range of >100 m) [14,15], SO_2 (at 4.0 μm and 120 m range) [281,282], CH_4 (at 1.66 μm and over a 2.7 km column) [282], and H_2O (around 1.75 μm, both for a 2 km atmospheric column [283] and range resolved up to ~1 km [284]). There were relatively few OPO-based advances in IR lidar or DIAL during the next 15 years, after which OPOs appear to have regained acceptance as high-power pulsed tunable sources suitable for such applications. For example, a TDL-seeded $LiNbO_3$ OPO was used by Milton et al. [323] to demonstrate range-resolved 3.4 μm IR DIAL measurements of atmospheric CH_4 at ranges up to 0.5 km.

Gerhard Ehret, Andreas Fix, and coworkers at Germany's Deutsches Zentrum für Luft- und Raumfahrt (DLR) [327,328,340] have devised significant TDL-seeded OPO systems for airborne H_2O-vapor IR DIAL measurements: typically, they comprise a BBO or KTP ring-cavity OPO pumped at 532 nm and TDL seeded at signal wavelengths in the range of 920–950 nm with an average output power of 1.2 W and a spectral purity > 99%. This system was designed to monitor the second-overtone 3–0 absorption band ($3v_{OH}$) of H_2O, which offers higher sensitivity than the third-overtone 4–0 band ($4v_{OH}$) region at ~725 nm, which was accessed in earlier airborne dye-laser-based IR DIAL studies by the same group [423]. This form of OPO has been incorporated in an airborne all-solid-state DIAL system, and enabled, for the first time, daytime measurements of two-dimensional H_2O-vapor cross sections with high vertical (500–750 m) and horizontal (6–20 km) resolution in the tropopause region [340]. Subsequently, the DLR group has further developed airborne H_2O-vapor IR DIAL measurements [424–428] and extended the technique to spaceborne missions [429,430].

Multiwavelength or multiplex OPO operation (as briefly discussed in the final part of Section 2.4.2) is an essential feature of many DIAL instruments, so that (resonant) atmospheric signals of interest can be actively distinguished from the (nonresonant) background. This has been borne out in several OPO-based IR DIAL demonstrations [323,327,328,340,342]. In one case [323], narrowband TDL-seeded OPO output was switched between on- and off-resonance wavelengths on alternate ns-pulsed pump laser shots to make range-resolved measurements of atmospheric CH_4. In another case [342], a dual-injection-seeded OPO for IR DIAL measurements was realized by synchronously switching between two TDL seed sources for a KTP OPO pumped by a dual-pulse Nd:YAG laser. The third approach entailed a system designed for airborne H_2O-vapor DIAL [327,328,340], in which the ns-pulsed OPO output was switched rapidly from narrowband, TDL-seeded, on resonance to broadband, unseeded, (predominantly) off resonance. DLR has subsequently been engaged in further OPO-based IR DIAL measurements of CO_2, CH_4, and N_2O [429–433].

At Macquarie University, we have shown [232,233] that injection seeding facilitates multiwavelength or multiplex OPO operation for multiline spectroscopic sensing (e.g., by dual-wavelength CARS diagnostics of N_2 in furnace air [232]). A proposed novel spectroscopic tailoring scheme (e.g., for DIAL) provides a source of coherent, pulsed radiation simultaneously generating a set of discrete wavelengths, each selected (e.g., by injection seeding an ns-pulsed OPO via an array of TDLs and a fiber-optic switch) to be on or off resonance with characteristic spectral features [5,28,30,31] and modulation/demodulation sequences decoding resulting spectroscopic signals, with a multiplex advantage for sensitivity and specificity.

Multiwavelength spectroscopic tailoring of OPO output by injection seeding is readily implemented with a BPM medium in a passive cavity [5,28,30,31,232]. Moreover, a similar approach is also possible in QPM media with grating channels wide enough to allow different noncollinear phase-matching angles for each of the OPO output wavelengths [290,358,359,434]. Such an approach has been used by Yang and Velsko [290] in a wavelength-agile PPLN OPO DIAL sensing system, pumped by a 1 kHz pulsed Nd:YAG laser and injection seeded by two 1.5 μm TDLs;

its 3 µm idler output is rapidly tunable over 400 cm^{-1} (12 THz) by using an acousto-optic deflector to vary the pump-beam angle.

Injection-seeded ns-pulsed OPOs are useful for UV DIAL detection of O_3 in the troposphere [344–346,435,436]. Fix et al. [435] devised such an OPO with intracavity SFG, generating output pulse energies up to 16 mJ in the 281–293 nm range, for DIAL studies of tropospheric O_3. More recently, Darrell Armstrong and Arlee Smith [344–346,436] reported laboratory prototype ns-pulsed UV sources for airborne or satellite-based DIAL remote sensing of O_3. These comprised OPOs pumped at 532 nm (from a frequency-doubled, Q-switched SLM Nd:YAG laser), generating a tunable signal output at ~803 nm. The OPO signal output was then mixed by SFG with additional 532 nm light either inside the OPO cavity or in a subsequent SFG stage, to generate 10 ns pulses at 320 nm. To optimize efficiency, three important characteristics were incorporated in the system design: a pump beam having a high-quality flat-topped spatial profile, an image-rotating nonplanar ring-cavity OPO design [437] capable of generating high-quality large-diameter flat-topped beams, and pulsed injection seeding of the OPO to achieve near-zero cavity buildup time to enhance the SFG efficiency. UV pulse energies approaching 300 mJ with competitive optical conversion efficiencies were projected [436].

Sune Svanberg and coworkers in Lund also developed a frequency-agile OPO system for wide-ranging (220 nm–4.3 µm) DIAL applications [438] and a versatile (deep-UV to mid-IR) mobile OPO/OPA lidar system for atmospheric and other environmental monitoring [439]. These employed fast switching by piezoelectric drivers to facilitate simultaneous multiwavelength DIAL measurements of several spectrally overlapping atmospheric species, with typical optical bandwidths of ~0.2 cm^{-1}.

A miniature near IR laser system for high-resolution three-dimensional lidar was reported by Zayhowski and Wilson [440]. This robustly packaged system incorporated a 1.064 µm passively Q-switched laser [441] with two amplifiers and a multipass KTA OPA [442], which is seeded by a DFB diode laser to generate output at 1.537 µm, which is eye safe (the only spectroscopic aspect of this application). The system [440] is compact, rugged, and portable: qualities that are highly advantageous for airborne lidar-type systems.

2.5.2.3   OPO Applications to Industrial and Environmental Monitoring

Many of the principles that are relevant to the remote sensing of the atmosphere (e.g., by methods such as long-path absorption, lidar, or DIAL) are also applicable to spectroscopic monitoring applications in other settings, such as those associated with the following areas:

- Industrial process control (e.g., by detecting reactive plant streams)
- Inaccessible or hostile media (e.g., furnaces, flames, or other combustion media)
- Environmentally sensitive situations (e.g., natural or manufactured polluting emissions from industrial sites, human communities, or wilderness)
- Some defense and security measures (e.g., screening for explosives or biological agents)

• Biomedical and life-science diagnostics (e.g., human breath analysis correlated with assorted physiological conditions)

A wide range of laser-spectroscopic techniques is applicable in this context [51,386–388]. Tunable OPOs can be involved in many such techniques, as is indicated by Tables 2.4 and 2.5 and by preceding discussion in Sections 2.5.1, 2.5.2.1, and 2.5.2.2. Special issues of some journals [60–71] also indicate trends in OPO-based applications to industrial and environmental sensing. It is beyond the scope of this chapter to be comprehensive. We therefore merely highlight a few selected examples that are representative of OPO applications to spectroscopic sensing of gas-phase or airborne molecular species. Beyond that, readers may find that Tables 2.4 and 2.5 can direct them to a wider range of useful applications. An early OPO-spectroscopic application to gas-flow diagnostics by IR LIF imaging of CO has already been presented in Section 2.1.2 and Figure 2.2 [72–74].

As a specific example, the inspection of Table 2.4 reveals that OPO-spectroscopic sensing of ethane (C_2H_6) and other light alkanes has been a proving ground for CW tunable OPOs, using detection by CRD [130] or PA [131,375,379–381]. C_2H_6 is of interest, because it is produced by plants, animals, and humans via lipid peroxidation of cell membranes [442–445], and it indicates plant stress. Two of these CW OPO-based spectroscopic studies of C_2H_6, by CRD [130] and by PA [375] spectroscopies, have employed single-frequency SLM CW PPLN OPOs with submegahertz optical bandwidths but no ready continuous tuning capability; the OPO idler output wavelength therefore needed to be "parked" (much like a line-tunable CO or CO_2 laser) at a particular position in the spectral profile that could be well characterized (e.g., by FTIR spectroscopy). In this way, subparts ppbv detection sensitivities were achieved for traces of C_2H_6 diluted in N_2 at 1 atm [130,375]). In the same context, the Nd:YAG-laser-pumped CW fan-grating PPLN OPO developed by Bisson et al. [378] was used to record high-quality mode-hop-scanned PA spectra of CH_4 [378], C_2H_6 [131], and C_2H_4 [131]; a 0.11 ppbv detection limit was established for C_2H_6 diluted in N_2 at 1 atm [131]. The transportable, highly sensitive PA spectrometer reported by Müller et al. [131] was based on an advanced CW fan-grating PPLN OPO that is pump resonant (for low threshold) and dual cavity (for spectral agility). In three similar papers, van Herpen et al. [379–381] reported continuous tuning by intracavity étalon in a CW Nd:YAG-pumped SRO containing a PPLN fan grating; as summarized in Table 2.4, this has been applied to PA spectroscopy of C_2H_6 diluted in N_2 at 1 atm with a projected detection limit as low as 0.01 ppbv.

In a more recent spectroscopic application (also concerned with C_2H_6 sensing), Ngai et al. [382] reported a diode laser–pumped CW OPO based on PP MgO:LiNbO$_3$ in a signal-resonant, étalon tuned ring cavity pumped at 1.082 µm by a fiber-laser-amplified diode laser. The idler output of this CW OPO system had a power of up to 300 mW; it was continuously tunable without mode-hops over 5.2 cm^{-1} and had spectral coverage of at least 16.5 cm^{-1} via pump-source tuning. It has been used for quartz-enhanced PA spectroscopy (QEPAS) [446] measurements at ~3.35 µm of a C_2H_6/N_2 mixture in laboratory air; a continuous spectral scan was recorded over a 15.1 cm^{-1} range with a pressure-broadened linewidth of ~0.03 cm^{-1} (0.9 GHz) and attributed to a multicomponent gas mixture comprising 2.2 ppmv C_2H_6, 1.53 ppmv CH_4, and 1.1% H_2O in N_2 and O_2 at a total pressure of 0.2 atm [382].

Even higher sensitivity—0.5 pptv (parts per trillion by volume)—of C_2H_6 in air has subsequently been reported by von Basum et al. [447] with a 3 min integration time. They used a CW singly resonant PPLN OPO operating at ~3 μm and CRD-spectroscopic detection to achieve a minimum detectable absorption coefficient of 1.6×10^{-10} cm^{-1} Hz$^{-1/2}$. Their frequency-tuning capabilities facilitated multigas analysis with simultaneous monitoring of C_2H_6, CH_4, and H_2O vapor in human breath.

More recently, Arslanov et al. [448] have used a fiber-amplified DBR diode laser to pump a CW singly resonant MgO:PPLN OPO with an output wavelength range of 3–4 μm and a capability for rapid (100 THz/s; ~3.3 cm^{-1}/ms) and broad mode-hop-free tuning (150 GHz; 5 cm^{-1}) for wavelength modulation spectroscopy of C_2H_6. A noise-equivalent absorption sensitivity of 1.2×10^{-9} cm^{-1} Hz$^{-1/2}$ was realized. By recording the absorption peak of C_2H_6 at 2996.9 cm^{-1} in 1.3 s, a detection sensitivity of 0.8 ppbv was attained for C_2H_6 in $N_2(g)$. The OPO's broad continuous tunability was demonstrated by covering a spectral range of 35.4 cm^{-1} (1.06 THz) while recording absorption features of C_2H_6, CH_4, and H_2O vapor in three successive 6.5 s spectral scans.

There is much ongoing interest in using tunable CW and ns-pulsed OPOs and other optical parametric devices for spectroscopic sensing in the mid-IR region, particularly beyond the range that is accessible to convenient NLO media such as PPLN [45–47,84,94]. There are various early examples of mid-IR OPOs [46,47,104,258,377,449], but their application to spectroscopy remains formative. For example, a broadly tunable $ZnGeP_2$ (ZGP) OPO, pumped at 2.8 μm by a 100 ns pulsed Er,Cr:YSGG laser and yielding an idler optical bandwidth of ~2 cm^{-1}, has been used [449] for CRD-spectroscopic detection of common explosives (trinitrotoluene [TNT], triacetone triperoxide [TATP], hexogen [RDX], penthrite [PETN], and tetryl) at trace levels; a detection limit of 0.075 ppbv in air is projected for TNT. The idler tuning range (6–10 μm) of this ZGP OPO offers access to the mid-IR "fingerprint" region, which is highly advantageous for many molecular sensing applications.

The extraordinary promise of OP GaAs as an NLO medium [6,7,49,94–107], particularly for spectroscopic sensing in the mid-IR by CW or ns-pulsed optical parametric devices, has already been addressed in Section 2.2.3. Many of the early mid-IR spectroscopic applications of OP GaAs appear to have relied on tunable DFG and OPG/OPA systems. In particular, we note the application of a CW OP GaAs DFG system [101,102] to CRD spectroscopy of N_2O gas (15 ppmv in 1 atm of N_2, with traces of H_2O), in a continuous 25 cm^{-1} spectral scan with ~0.2 cm^{-1} optical bandwidth [103]. Vodopyanov and coworkers subsequently demonstrated the operation of ns-pulsed tunable OP GaAs OPOs in the mid-IR [104] and in wide-ranging mid-IR continua produced by an OP GaAs OPG [105].

Recent mid-IR spectroscopic initiatives in the area of ultrafast synchronously pumped OP GaAs OPOs and their frequency comb applications have already been surveyed in Sections 2.1.2, 2.3.3, and 2.3.5 [75,76,177,178,182–184,191–193].

A particularly innovative OPO-based spectroscopic development at Macquarie University entailed use of injection-seeded ns-pulsed BPM OPOs for dual-line CARS spectroscopy [232], in which a passive-cavity OPO was simultaneously seeded by separate TDLs to generate two adjustable output wavelengths. As already explained in Section 2.4.2.4, these two TDL seeders were set to match Stokes wavelengths that were characteristic of low- and high-J rovibrational Raman peaks in the CARS spectrum, yielding a single-shot coherent Raman thermometric instrument (e.g., for N_2 in furnace air [232]). This dual-line, injection-seeded approach to CARS spectroscopy complemented conventional OPO CARS techniques, either continuously scanned [11,227,232,234,235] or multiwavelength [227,228,234,353,354,450,451], and was the precursor of other proposed [28,30,31] multiwavelength OPO-spectroscopic tailoring strategies for atmospheric, industrial, and environmental spectroscopic sensing.

Although this chapter has focused largely on OPO-based spectroscopic measurements of gas-phase or airborne species, it should not be forgotten that OPOs and other optical parametric devices have a wide range of spectroscopic and imaging applications in biology, medicine, and health sciences, with substantial opportunities for user-friendly OPO-type systems to be marketed. For instance, we cite a key paper on OPO-based biosensing, in which Tiihonen et al. [452] reported a tailored dual-wavelength source of coherent UV light for fluorescence spectroscopy of biomolecules. The UV light source comprised a diode-pumped Nd:YAG laser passively Q-switched by an intracavity Cr:YAG saturable absorber to yield pulses of 2.3 ns FWHM duration at 100 Hz repetition rate and an average power of 130 mW. The astigmatic output beam of the diode-bar pump source was converted into a homogeneous beam profile by means of a "beam-twisting" mode converter to attain 50% conversion efficiency in a PPKTP frequency doubler; the resulting 532 nm output comprised 1.8 ns, 0.65 mJ pulses at 100 Hz with excellent beam quality ($M^2 = 1.3$). This 532 nm pump source drove two separate signal-resonant PPKTP OPO cavities, each containing a Type-I (ooe) BBO SFG crystal. The resulting cascaded parametric UV-generation processes in the two PPKTP/BBO OPO/SFG systems generated 1 ns, 27 µJ output pulses with wavelengths of 293 and 343 nm and ~7% conversion efficiencies with respect to 532 nm. The former wavelength (293 nm) was devised to match the LIF-excitation wavelength of the ubiquitous tryptophan amino-acid residue, while the latter wavelength (343 nm) was chosen for LIF excitation of NADH (the reduced form of nicotinamide adenine dinucleotide—a typical nucleotide that plays a key role in the oxidation of fuel biomolecules). The potential utility of this dual-wavelength UV source was demonstrated [452] by recording dispersed LIF spectra of nonpathogenic bacteria (e.g., *Bacillus thuringiensis* at a concentration of 10 µg/mL in saline solution) and auxiliary background from NADH and other unidentified fluorescent biomolecules. Such an OPO-based dual-wavelength (or perhaps multiwavelength, for higher specificity) approach has been proposed as a way to distinguish naturally occurring bacteria from other pathogens (e.g., biological warfare agents). A further significant OPO-based biomedical sensing and imaging application (coherent Raman microscopy) will be considered in Section 2.5.3.

Finally, we note recent reports [453,454] of an OPO-based stand off detection technique that has the potential for remote sensing of hazardous materials. It employs a broadband mid-IR fs-pulsed OPO [179], with spectral coverage over 2700–3200 cm^{-1} (~3.1–3.7 µm), for optical ablation of a possibly hazardous deposit, together with an FTIR spectrometer to characterize the resulting vapor. In preliminary experiments, stand off spectra were recorded at a 1–2 m range for vaporized H_2O, nitromethane (CH_3NO_2; a simulant of many explosives), and thiodiglycol (relevant to chemical warfare). The results imply that OPO-based active FTIR stand off spectroscopy is promising as a new way to detect industrial pollutants and to identify chemical agents, explosives, or other hazardous materials. It is concluded that "Compared with a blackbody source, a spatially coherent broadband mid-IR light source such as a femtosecond OPO is inherently more suitable for stand-off spectroscopy because of its excellent spatial coherence, enabling its output light to propagate over a long distance without substantial diffraction, and high spectral brightness, which means that the signal is still detectable at a stand-off distance of a few meters even when it has experienced significant loss from highly-scattering real-world surfaces" [453].

2.5.3 COHERENT RAMAN MICROSCOPY: A BIOMEDICAL APPLICATION OF OPOS

Laser-based microscopy is already well established in biomedicine and the life sciences, yielding three-dimensional imaging with fine spatial resolution, high sensitivity, and discrete chemical or biomolecular selectivity. Well-established scanning confocal and multiphoton microscopies apply either to a restricted range of media containing natural endogenous fluorophores (e.g., certain amino acids, such as tryptophan [452]) or to substances that have been labeled with an exogenous fluorophore (which may be toxic, subject to photobleaching, or inconvenient to use). Another approach targets vibrational signature(s) of biomolecules by (spontaneous) linear Raman spectroscopy, but this is limited by weak cross sections.

Coherent Raman spectroscopic sensing, notably by CARS and SRS, has emerged as a promising approach to biomolecule-specific microscopic imaging and microspectroscopy. These two forms of NLO Raman microscopy—CARS and SRS—are now collectively referred to as coherent Raman scattering (CRS) microscopy [455,456]. Moreover, it will be shown later in this section that OPOs play key roles in instrumentation for CRS microscopy.

As in the case of its linear optical precursor, spontaneous Raman microscopy, the chemical specificity of CRS microscopy is derived from intrinsic molecular vibrational characteristics (revealed by Raman spectroscopy), rather than from an electronic fluorophore (which may need to be attached as an exogenic label to biomolecules of interest); this avoids practical complications associated with staining of biological media prior to fluorescence microscopy and simplifies *in vivo* examination of living cells and tissues. As in multiphoton microscopy, the tight focusing used in CRS microscopy provides a fine sectioning capability for three-dimensional biomedical imaging, and the NLO scattering mechanisms offer size selectivity, including subwavelength spatial resolution. This enables observation of biochemical structures and processes at subcellular levels. CRS microscopy can thus address significant challenges in optical diagnostics and sensing, including the characterization of tissues, cells, and biomolecules (e.g., imaging of lipids) and wide-ranging applications (e.g., security screening of biological agents or explosives; microscopic imaging of photoresists and microelectronic circuits).

CARS microscopy [455–465] was introduced several years before its SRS counterpart. The CARS technique offers high sensitivity and collection efficiency, detection wavelengths that are blueshifted from excitation and fluorescent wavelengths, and amenability to three-dimensional imaging. As explained in Section 2.5.1, CARS spectroscopy depends on the third-order NLO susceptibility $\chi^{(3)}$, by means of which two coherent light waves (ω_{pump} and ω_{Stokes}) combine to generate a coherent anti-Stokes wave ($\omega_{AS} = 2\omega_{pump} - \omega_{Stokes}$) when ($\omega_{pump} - \omega_{Stokes}$) matches a molecular Raman-active transition frequency Ω. CARS spectra can be recorded either by tuning ($\omega_{pump} - \omega_{Stokes}$) through Ω or in multiplex mode, where ω_{Stokes} is broadband with resonances at Ω in a continuum of output frequencies ω_{AS}. One of two popular CARS microscopy configurations (F-CARS) [457,458] detects signal in the forward direction. The other (E-CARS) uses *epi*-detection, with CARS output light at ω_{AS} counterpropagating back toward the source of the incident laser light at ω_P and ω_S. For example, mechanisms that allow *epi*-detection [456–460,466] are often less affected by a solvent background signal that complicates F-CARS; E-CARS enables CARS endoscopy applications [466].

Several ongoing challenges for research on CARS microspectroscopy and its applications to microscopic imaging include the following:

- Optimization of CARS epi-detection: Two mechanisms responsible for E-CARS *epi*-detection, in which CARS output light (at ω_{AS}) counterpropagates back toward the source of the incident light (at ω_{pump} and ω_{Stokes}), entail incomplete backward destructive interference, due to scattering either from small objects that are comparable in size to optical wavelengths (λ_{AS}, λ_{pump}, λ_{Stokes}) or from interfaces between media with different $\chi^{(3)}$ values [457–460,466]. A third *epi*-detection mechanism [460,466] involves multiple scattering of CARS light from thick samples (>100 μm), and is often the dominant source of *epi*-scattering from turbid media such as human skin. The optimization of such *epi*-detection mechanisms is highly critical for applications such as CARS endoscopy, in which light is delivered to and from the target by optical fiber [466,467].

- Suppression of nonresonant CARS background: A persistent problem in CARS microscopy is that spectroscopic information contained in the bio-molecule-specific resonant susceptibility $\chi_R^{(3)}(\Omega)$ may be obscured by a nonresonant background, since the CARS signal varies as $| \chi_R^{(3)}(\Omega) + \chi_{NR}^{(3)} |^2$ [456–465]. Various ways to eliminate (or at least reduce) this nonresonant background were surveyed in the corresponding chapter in the second edition of this book [5]; many of these are elaborate and have proved difficult to implement routinely. In an ingenious instance of one of these background-suppression techniques [468], Herman Offerhaus and coworkers at Twente have used a frequency-doubled Nd:YAG laser (delivering ~15 ps pulses with a repetition rate of ~80 MHz) to synchronously pump an LBO OPO, similar to a preceding design [469], in a cascaded phase-preserving chain that generates not only the CARS output wave of prime spectroscopic interest but also a more intense coherent local oscillator wave to enable OH detection of CARS signals at the shot-noise limit. The CARS output (with frequency $\omega_{AS} = 2\,\omega_{pump} - \omega_{Stokes}$) is coherently excited at two frequencies: ω_{pump}, which is effectively AOM shifted by ~20 kHz ($= |\omega_{pump} - \omega_{laser}|$) from the 1064 nm fundamental laser frequency ω_{laser}, and ω_I ($\equiv \omega_{Stokes}$) from the OPO idler output wave (e.g., at ~1578 nm for CARS spectroscopy of CH-stretch vibrations in toluene, for which $\Omega \approx 3060$ cm^{-1}). The OPO, pumped at 532 nm (corresponding to $\omega_P = 2\,\omega_{laser}$), generates a signal output wave at ω_S ($= \omega_P - \omega_I = 2\omega_{laser} - \omega_{Stokes}$), which is phase coherent with the CARS output at ω_{AS} and frequency shifted from it by twice the AOM-shifted frequency ($= 2|\omega_{pump} - \omega_{laser}|$). The OPO signal beam therefore serves effectively as a local oscillator for heterodyne detection and is combined with the CARS beam (e.g., both at ~803 nm) on a fast square-law PD. The AOM-induced beat frequency ($2|\omega_{pump} - \omega_{laser}|$) at ~40 kHz avoids the $1/f$-type noise of the electronic detection system to optimize CARS detection sensitivity for high-contrast CARS microscopy of biomolecular solutes at concentrations below the micromoles per liter limit [468]. Subsequent work by the Twente group has developed other aspects of vibrational phase-contrast CARS microscopy [470–477].

- Trade-offs between duration, power, and so on of laser pulses: There are complicated trade-offs in CARS microscopy between temporal resolution, spectral bandwidth, focal geometry (e.g., CARS phase-matching angles), pulse repetition rate (including scanned imaging speed), peak power for optimal nonlinearity, damage thresholds (both *in vivo* and *in vitro*), spatial resolution, and optical coherence. The potential for optothermal or NLO photolytic damage is much more critical when the target is biological tissue (e.g., *in vivo*) [456–459,464,478,479] than in the case of inert materials. It is important to characterize such trade-offs carefully when developing new, compact, accessible CARS microspectroscopic instruments. There are also prospects for surface-enhanced CARS microscopy [480,481], enabling trace detection of biological and forensic material, such as pathogens in drinking water, bacterial spores (e.g., anthrax), and explosives.

CRS microscopy [455,456,482] is now established as a wide-ranging form of NLO imaging and microspectroscopy. CARS microscopy emerged in 2004 [457,458], but it took almost 5 years before SRS microscopy was recognized [483–487] as a competitive contrast mechanism for microscopy. Both of these forms of CRS microscopy depend on the third-order NLO susceptibility $\chi^{(3)}$ of the target molecules, with two coherent light waves (ω_{pump} and ω_{Stokes}) combining to generate a signal that is resonantly enhanced when the difference frequency ($\omega_{pump} - \omega_{Stokes}$) matches a molecular Raman-active frequency Ω. However, they differ mechanistically [455,456,482,484]. CARS is a parametric process with phase-matching conditions for the detected anti-Stokes wave ($\omega_{AS} = 2\omega_{pump} - \omega_{Stokes}$) that is scattered off a nonlinear optically induced vibrational coherence. On the other hand, SRS is nonparametric and automatically phase matched because it probes loss/gain in the $\omega_{pump}/\omega_{Stokes}$ waves arising from an excitation of vibrational population.

The advantages of SRS microscopy relative to CARS microscopy have been lucidly summarized in table 2 of [482]:

- Insensitivity of SRS to the electronic nonresonant background that has been problematic in CARS microscopy [5,456–465,468]

- Close correspondence of SRS spectral profiles to those of linear Raman spectra, whereas CARS spectral profiles are often affected by interference between resonant and nonresonant CARS signals (which leads to dispersive CARS line shapes that are distorted and more difficult to interpret, and occasionally yield coherent image artifacts)
- Attainability of shot-noise-limited sensitivity in SRS, whereas CARS is more limited by laser-intensity noise
- Absence of spatial coherence and existence of a point-spread function in SRS, avoiding complications in the case of CARS
- Linear relationship of SRS signal strength to the number density of Raman-active modes inside the focal volume, so that SRS has a linear concentration dependence, whereas CARS concentration dependences are more complicated, ranging from linear to quadratic
- Susceptibility of CARS to contamination by two-photon-excited fluorescence, which is avoided in the case of SRS (because a blueshifted CARS beam at ω_{AS} is not generated)

These relative advantages of SRS microscopy are borne out by a representative sample of recent publications [455,456,482–487]—most of them (apart from [483], [485], and, possibly, [484]) reliant on one or more OPOs as a vital part of the SRS microscopy instrumentation. The assets and constraints of OPOs as coherent light sources for CRS microscopy have been surveyed and various aspects of instrument design presented [488].

Advanced laser-scanning microscopes are established research instruments in numerous laboratories, where their microscopic imaging capability has significantly enhanced biomedical diagnostics. However, the laser and detection systems required for high-performance CRS scanning microscopy are typically elaborate and expensive, so that there continues to be room for instrumental simplification [5]. For instance, fiber-based OPOs offer prospects in this regard (as will be considered in Section 2.5.4, where relevant references will be cited).

Experimental and theoretical studies [457–459,478,479] show that the optimum pulse duration for CRS microscopy of living biological samples is ~1–10 ps, using 0.5–500 nJ pulses. Shorter-duration pulses can cause NLO photodamage to *in vivo* targets [479], while light pulses longer than ~10 ns can thermally damage living tissue if the pulse energies (and hence peak powers) are high enough to generate detectable CARS or SRS signals. Such effects are aggravated by the high repetition rates regularly used to enhance CRS imaging efficiency. Moreover, Equation 2.23 [199] indicates that pulse durations shorter than ~2 ps FWHM exceed the FT limit required to match the FWHM spectral linewidth of ~10 cm^{-1} (~300 GHz) for typical Raman bands of molecules in aqueous solution or biological tissue. Likewise, a 10 fs pulse will have an FT-limited optical bandwidth of ~44 THz (~1500 cm^{-1}), which is poorly matched to the resonant portion of a typical CRS spectrum. We note that ps-pulsed tunable OPOs are highly advantageous for CRS microscopy because their optical bandwidth enables virtually all of the light impinging on the target to be concentrated within the characteristic Raman linewidth of a single relevant feature in the vibrational spectrum of particular interest.

Longer pulses (up to ~5 ns) can occasionally be used for CARS microscopy. This was demonstrated in the case of large-area CARS microscopy by Monika Ritsch-Marte, Stefan Bernet, and coworkers in Innsbruck [489,490] using 3 ns optical pulses from a 10 Hz laser/OPO system and a wide-field microscope with a dark-field condensing lens and an intensified charge-coupled device (CCD) camera. We note subsequent work on wide-field CARS microscopy by the Innsbruck group [491–496] and by Daniel Palanker and coworkers at Stanford [497,498].

Significant early research on high-performance scanning CARS microscopy, by Sunney Xie and coworkers at Harvard [457–459], was performed with ps-pulse trains from two separate tunable Ti:sapphire lasers to provide the necessary coherent Raman pump and Stokes waves (at frequencies ω_{pump} and ω_{Stokes}, respectively). This approach was both expensive and technically complicated, in view of the need to ensure that the CARS-excitation pulse trains were coincident temporally as well as spatially within the focal region of the target. The technology to enable tight pulse-train synchronization (reducing the tolerance to ~20 fs, compared with the usual few picoseconds) was developed [499,500] to minimize CARS signal fluctuations and yield enhanced vibrational CARS-microscopic images of living cells and polymer beads. However (returning to the theme of this chapter), research on CARS microscopy [458,460,468,469,499–501] has tended to favor one or more ps-pulsed tunable OPO systems, in which the temporal and spatial relationships between the pump, signal, and idler waves (at ω_P, ω_S, and ω_I) are automatically well defined by the NLO processes in the OPO itself. Similar OPO-based instrumentation has been adopted more recently for SRS microscopy [455,456,482,484,486,487,502–509].

For instance, the LBO OPO [469], mentioned above in the context of background-suppressed CARS detection [468], used a 30 mm Brewster-angled LBO crystal (Type I, NCPM) in a signal-resonant SRO folded cavity with an intracavity Lyot filter to reduce the OPO signal bandwidth. NCPM operation ensured that all parts of the OPO cavity remained fixed during scanning and that CARS measurements entailed no adjustment apart from adjusting the synchronously pumped OPO cavity length to allow for variation in round-trip time. The OPO was pumped by an 80 MHz train of 12 ps pulses at 532 nm (with typical average power of 2 W and OPO threshold of ~0.55 W) via SHG from a passively mode-locked Nd:YVO$_4$ laser generating ~5 W, 15 ps pulses at 1064 nm. The OPO signal output comprised a train of 6.4 ps pulses that could be tuned over the wavelength range 740–930 nm by varying the temperature of the LBO crystal between 105°C and 145°C. With an average 532 nm pump power of 1.2 W, the OPO signal output power exceeded 0.3 W over the full operating range, which was adequate for CARS spectroscopy and microscopy. The tunable signal beam (740–930 nm) of the OPO was combined with the 1064 nm Nd:YVO$_4$ laser fundamental to obtain high-resolution (~2 cm^{-1}) vibrational CARS spectra of molecules in the CH stretch region (2700–3100 cm^{-1}). The straightforward, convenient tunability of the OPO was demonstrated by using laser-scanning CARS microscopy to localize and identify different polymer microparticles of the same size and shape with lateral and axial resolutions less than 0.5 and 1 μm, respectively.

In early research on CARS microscopy [501], Xie and coworkers developed a comparable broadly tunable ps-pulsed PPKTP OPO system that was pumped by an 80 MHz train of 6 ps pulses at 532 nm (with 5 W average power and an OPO threshold as low as ~40 mW for the 924/1254 nm combination of signal/idler wavelengths) from a commercially available mode-locked Nd:YVO$_4$ laser. This PPKTP OPO system generated the two colors for CARS microscopy, with a continuously tunable frequency difference over a broad range of Raman shifts (100–3700 cm^{-1}) by varying the temperature of the single PPKTP crystal. Moreover, the near IR output (900–1300 nm) allowed deep penetration into thick samples and reduced NLO photodamage. This compact single-laser OPO source of tunable picosecond pulses has been used for CARS-microscopic imaging of *in vivo* cell and *ex vivo* tissue targets [501]. Its stable operation, broad tunability with a single NLO crystal, and improved penetration depth made it an optimal source for CARS imaging in chemical and biomedical research. In subsequent developments of CARS microscopy, the Xie research group used the same form of mode-locked Nd:YVO$_4$ laser together with one [460] or two [510] commercially available broadly tunable ps-pulsed LBO OPOs. The second OPO served as a reference source for real-time subtraction of nonresonant CARS background by an FM-CARS technique [510] to improve contrast in laser-scanning vibrational microscopic imaging. Subsequently, a high-power ps-pulsed source for CRS microscopy has been described [511]; it comprises a fiber laser and amplifier, the second harmonic output of which is used to pump an LBO OPO.

More recently, similar OPO-based systems have been used by Xie and coworkers for their investigations of SRS microscopy. Their tunable ps-pulsed LBO OPO design incorporates an electrically tunable Lyot filter to enable intracavity electro-optic frequency modulation for either FM-CARS microscopy or SRS microscopy [487]. Rapid frequency modulation (at >1 MHz) of either the pump (ω_{pump}) or the Stokes (ω_{Stokes}) input radiation is essential to SRS spectroscopy, so that stimulated Raman gain or loss, respectively, can be detected by means of a lock-in amplifier. Such modulation also helps to reduce SRS background signals (in addition to the CARS-type electronic nonresonant background, which is nonexistent in SRS) such as those due to cross-phase modulation, thermal lensing, or two-color two-photon absorption [487]. The OPO system is driven by a mode-locked Nd:YVO$_4$ laser, which has a cavity length of ~3.94 m and generates a train of 7 ps pulses at a 76 MHz repetition rate. A portion of the 1.064 μm laser fundamental is typically used as the coherent Raman Stokes wave (ω_{Stokes}). The remainder is frequency doubled and used to synchronously pump the LBO OPO, which has a cavity length of ~7.88 m (exactly twice that of the laser cavity) and thereby generates two completely independent 5.7 ps output pulse trains with a repetition rate of 38 MHz for use as the tunable Raman pump wave (ω_{pump}); with 3.5 W of 532 nm pump power, the OPO signal output power exceeds 0.75 W [487]. This OPO system has been applied in FM-CARS imaging of individual bacterial cells grown on deuterated carbon sources and in SRS microscopy (free of nonresonant background) of the accumulation of a surface-active compound on mouse skin.

Variants of such a synchronously pumped LBO OPO system have been used in subsequent SRS microscopy investigations [502,505,506]. Multicolor narrowband SRS microscopy has also been demonstrated [507] with a commercially available synchronously pumped LBO OPO adapted to enable rapid line-by-line wavelength tuning; this is achieved by applying stepwise voltages to the Pockels cell in the above-mentioned electro-optically controlled intracavity Lyot filter. This OPO system has been used for SRS-microscopic measurements of polymer beads and of live HeLa cells with moving intracellular lipid droplets.

Several established manufacturers of laser-scanning microscopy equipment have been offering fully operable commercial CARS microscopy systems for several years. At this stage, we are not aware of any commercially available SRS microscopes, although there is sufficient information in the research literature to guide assembly of such a system from readily available laser, OPO, laser-scanning microscope, and other optoelectronic components.

2.5.4 FIBER-BASED OPOS: APPLICATIONS TO COHERENT RAMAN MICROSCOPY

Optical fiber lasers have already been widely used as optical pump sources for various forms of OPO [75,76,106,127,172,180,183,187,220,274,275,382,448]. Likewise, optical fibers enable external control processes such as injection seeding [239–247,309,313,323] and optical feedback [159] in various OPO systems. However, the implementation of an optical fiber to serve as the NLO medium of an OPO itself is still a developing field of research.

The impetus for developing OPOs based on optical fibers is much the same as that for other fiber-optical devices, both active (including lasers) and passive: better beam quality, higher efficiency, compactness, portability, and modularity. Unfortunately, optical fibers are generally unsuitable for second-order OPOs (those based on the second-order NLO susceptibility, $\chi^{(2)}$) because they are centrosymmetric. As a result, fiber-based OPO (FOPO) development has focused on four-wave-mixing (FWM) processes mediated by the third-order NLO susceptibility, $\chi^{(3)}$ [512,513]. The fact that $\chi^{(3)}$ processes are significantly weaker than $\chi^{(2)}$ processes is offset by the small beam sizes and much longer interaction lengths available in optical fibers. Ultrashort pulses, synchronous pumping, and enhancement by SRS [514,515] can be used to lower the threshold and increase the efficiency of a FOPO.

FOPOs most often use a degenerate FWM (DFWM) interaction, in which the pump provides two identical input waves, and signal and idler sidebands are generated above and below the pump frequency ω_P, respectively. Energy conservation then results in the signal and idler frequencies being equally separated in frequency from the pump. The sideband separation is determined by minimizing the phase mismatch (κ) of the four optical waves [512], as follows.

$$\kappa = \beta\left(\omega_P + \Omega\right) + \beta\left(\omega_P - \Omega\right) - 2\beta\left(\omega_P\right) + 2\gamma P \approx 0 \qquad (2.25)$$

where:
   $\beta(\omega)$ is the linear propagation constant of the fiber at frequency ω
   Ω is the sideband-detuning frequency between the pump and signal/idler frequencies ω_S/ω_I
   γ is the NLO optical coefficient (related to $\chi^{(3)}$)
   P is the pump power

The chromatic dispersion D is an important parameter that strongly affects the frequency offset of the signal and idler from the pump and their bandwidth; it is related to the group velocity $v_g = (d\omega/d\beta)$ and to β as follows:

$$D = \frac{d(1/v_g)}{d\lambda} = -\left(\frac{2\pi c}{\lambda^2}\right)\left(\frac{d^2\beta}{d\omega^2}\right) \tag{2.26}$$

In addition, the parametric gain g is defined by

$$g^2 = (\gamma P)^2 - \left(\frac{\kappa}{2}\right)^2 \tag{2.27}$$

Figure 2.13 shows the predicted chromatic-dispersion profile (a) and DFWM gain map (b) for a bare tellurite glass rod/fiber with a diameter of 10 μm [516]. This very simple example is an ideal way to illustrate the importance of dispersion on the FWM interaction. The zero-dispersion wavelength (ZDW) is approximately 2 μm. The fiber has normal dispersion ($D < 0$) at wavelengths shorter than the ZDW and anomalous dispersion ($D > 0$) at wavelengths longer than the ZDW. The two regimes have a profound impact on the DFWM gain shown in Figure 2.13b. In the normal-dispersion regime, the FWM is characterized by small gain bandwidth for the signal and idler and a large frequency separation of the sidebands from the pump. Conversely, in the anomalous-dispersion regime, the signal and idler waves have significant gain over a much broader range of wavelengths, and their frequency separation is relatively small. This DFWM gain map is typical of fibers with dispersion dominated by the intrinsic material dispersion.

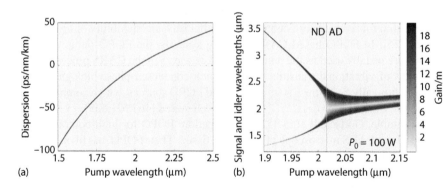

FIGURE 2.13 Simulation of degenerate four-wave mixing in a tellurite glass rod/fiber with a diameter of 10 μm [516]. (a). The chromatic dispersion, D, is negative (i.e., normal dispersion) at wavelengths less than the zero dispersion wavelength (ZDW, ~2.02 μm) and positive (i.e., anomalous dispersion) at wavelengths greater than the ZDW. (b). Normal dispersion (ND) produces narrowband signal and idler waves that are well separated from the pump, while anomalous dispersion (AD) produces broadband gain near the pump. (From White, R. T., et al., Mid-infrared sources based on four-wave mixing in microstructured optical fibres. In *Australian Conference on Optical Fibre Technology (ACOFT)*, *2009*, The Australian Optical Society, 2009, poster 27; http://trove.nla.gov.au/work/165364345?selected version=NBD49050633).

The state of development of FOPOs is comparable to that of bulk-phase second-order ($\chi^{(2)}$) OPOs two decades ago. At that time, OPO performance was limited by various technical problems (e.g., as outlined in Section 2.1.1). In the case of FOPOs, the main obstacle is the difficulty of fabricating long lengths of optical fiber with adequate dispersion uniformity [517]. Standard optical fibers such as those produced in large quantities for the telecommunications industry (e.g., Corning SMF-28) have extremely low structural errors (in terms of refractive indices and core size) over large distances (kilometers) and therefore have correspondingly stable dispersion properties. Unfortunately, their optical properties (such as dispersion, ZDW, nonlinear coefficient) are generally unsuitable for any particular FOPO application. The structural variation over length in specialty fibers such as microstructured optical fibers is much higher and, at this stage, limits the range of dispersion profiles available for efficient FOPO operation. This is particularly true for the narrowband, large frequency shift operation that is common in the normal-dispersion regime, although the problem can be reduced by pumping short (centimeter-scale) fibers with femtosecond pulses [518].

Despite current fiber-fabrication limitations, efficient FOPOs with large tuning ranges have been reported. For example, John Harvey and coworkers in Auckland reported an ns-pulsed FOPO operating in the transition region near the ZDW (1556 nm in their fiber) of a dispersion-shifted silica fiber [519]. They achieved impressive signal and idler tuning ranges of 1300–1500 nm and 1600–1860 nm, respectively, by tuning their 4 ns pump pulses from 1532 to 1556 nm. Subsequent work in Auckland yielded broadly tunable watt-level CW output [520].

In view of their immaturity, FOPOs have not yet been generally adopted as spectroscopic tools. They have, however, found a niche as sources for CARS microscopy of biological tissue [521–523], as already surveyed in Section 2.5.3. All-fiber sources are attractive alternatives to bulk OPOs for clinical deployment because of their potential for reduced cost, compactness, reliability, and flexibility of light delivery [524,525]. In FOPO-based CARS imaging systems, the FOPO pump and one sideband are usually used as the pump and Stokes waves in the CARS process [523]. Linewidths of vibrational transitions for common condensed-phase biological molecules are typically 5–20 cm^{-1}, so that ps-pulsed FOPO sources, which combine high peak power with an appropriate FT limit, are well suited [464,521,525].

For example, Gottschall et al. [521] developed an FOPO for high-contrast spectrally resolved CARS microscopy of biological tissue. Their FOPO, based on a 13 cm length of PCF, generated 180 mW (5.6 kW peak) of signal output at ~780–795 nm. The signal wave and the residual pump wave at ~1032 nm (130 mW; 2.9 kW peak) were used as the CARS pump and Stokes waves, respectively. High-resolution CARS images were recorded at Raman shifts of 2850 cm^{-1} (CH$_2$) and 2930 cm^{-1} (CH$_3$) for a 1×1 mm region in a sample of human perivascular tissue. An image of ~16 million pixels could be collected in 32 s with a 2 μs dwell time. Lipid-filled adipocytes were found to be contrasted in false color against the connective-tissue protein fibers, thereby discriminating lipids from proteins by CARS imaging at two distinct Raman-shift frequencies that could be tuned by slight resonator cavity-length adjustments to optimize the contrast.

In other work, Lamb et al. [522] used a FOPO to record CARS images of mouse tissue, while Zhai et al. [523] recorded CARS images of the myelin sheath of rat spinal cord, which they combined with TPE of fluorescence of axons in the same sample.

It is evident that FOPOs are at a relatively early stage of development and that they have much potential for particular spectroscopic applications, such as coherent Raman microscopy.

2.5.5 Defense Applications of OPOs: Infrared Countermeasures

Defense applications place high demands on laser-based systems in terms of expected performance and reliability as well as the environmental extremes of military operations. Moreover, there are often significant restrictions on the size, weight, and power consumption (SWaP) of the laser devices to fit modern military platforms. Technological maturity is therefore required, especially for mission-critical scenarios. In this section, we consider IR countermeasures—an example of defense applications in which OPO and OPA devices have been widely adopted. This provides further testimony to the technological maturity that such devices have attained over their 40 year history [8,9].

Missiles guided by IR radiation represent a deadly threat in all military domains (air, land, and maritime). In the air domain, MANPADS (Man Portable Air Defense System) devices are particularly problematic because they are relatively inexpensive, are easy to use, and have proliferated worldwide. An IR-guided missile contains an electro-optic subsystem, known as the "seeker"; this detects and locks onto the heat signature of the platform (e.g., an aircraft or other vehicle) and guides the missile toward its target. Over the years, IR-guided missiles have evolved to exploit various subbands within the mid-IR spectral window, the region of the electromagnetic spectrum in which strong emissions from aircraft engines can be easily detected. To be an effective countermeasure, a system ideally needs to operate multiband within the mid-IR region. Early solutions employed flares as IR countermeasures, but these became less effective as the threat evolved. Current state-of-the-art solutions employ DIRCM (Directed InfraRed CounterMeasure) technologies in which intense coherent light (e.g., a laser or OPO beam) is directed from the aircraft to the missile's seeker to confuse its ability to track the aircraft.

A DIRCM is a complex system consisting of several key components: a missile warning sensor to initially detect the incoming missile; an FLIR (Forward-Looking InfraRed) thermal camera to acquire and track the missile; and a jamming laser to generate and transmit a jamming signal to the missile seeker. This all occurs through a high-speed turret and is controlled by a sophisticated system processor. A typical operational scenario for a MANPADS would approximately involve a range of 5 km and a time to impact of 10 s. Such conditions place exacting requirements on design and performance of the DIRCM laser.

The principal spectroscopic requirement of a DIRCM laser source is that it needs to mimic the spectral signature of the target in the IR region. For IR-guided threats, this involves generating output in the 2–5 μm spectral region. Over the years, IR-guided threats have evolved substantially in terms of how the seeker functions and which 2–5 μm subband of wavelengths it is designed to detect and track. Strong atmospheric absorption by CO_2 and H_2O leaves a number of atmospheric transmission windows within the 2–5 μm region that influence the design and performance of both the seeker and the DIRCM laser source. Prior to actual engagement, it can be extremely difficult to know which portion of the 2–5 μm mid-IR region needs to be accessed by the DIRCM for a particular missile encountered on a specific mission. Consequently, the output of a DIRCM laser-based source ideally needs to be multispectral, to cover as many of these spectral transmission windows as possible and therefore as many types of threat as possible. OPO and OPA sources offer appealing ways to generate laser-like radiation over broad swaths within these spectral windows. The ability of an OPO (Figures 2.5c and 2.6a) or OPA (Figure 2.5b) to operate in a free-running manner, so that both signal and idler are able to generate broad spectral output with optical bandwidths of many hundreds of nanometers, makes them the preferred choice for current-generation DIRCM laser sources.

Further required characteristics of such a DIRCM laser-based source are as follows:

- A DIRCM laser source must be able to deposit enough power into the seeker head to jam it, generating intensities that are higher than the thermal signature of the CW-emitting target. Of the typical operating regimes for OPOs shown in Table 2.2, DIRCM laser sources typically use Class B, ns-pulsed OPOs. DIRCM laser architectures can employ OPOs and OPAs in a variety of ways: they can not only be used as the final wavelength-conversion stage for generating the 2–5 μm jamming radiation, but they can also serve as prior frequency-conversion stages within the pump lasers themselves [267,526].
- Emitted light from the DIRCM laser source must have sufficient beam quality to be able to propagate large distances to the seeker, so that the seeker of the incoming IR missile is engaged by the DIRCM laser as early and as far away as possible, and illumination of the seeker is maintained for as long as is required to break the seeker's lock on the target. This places high operational demands on the OPO's beam quality in terms of divergence and pointing stability (so that the DIRCM laser turret can constantly track and illuminate the rapidly approaching seeker with sufficient intensity to cause optical break-lock).
- A DIRCM laser source must be capable of being modulated to confuse the seeker's tracking signal, as high intensity alone may not be enough for it to jam the seeker. The DIRCM beam must be modulated by a custom temporal waveform capable of interfering with the seeker's guidance loop. The interference mechanism creates an error signal in the guidance loop that needs to be corrected if the missile is to hit its intended target. The process of correcting for this error causes the seeker to lose track of its target. The DIRCM pump laser and OPO wavelength-conversion stages need to have a highly adaptable duty cycle while maintaining strict performance requirements for wavelength, optical power, and beam quality, as different missile types require a variety of jamming modulation codes.
- A DIRCM laser source must be highly reliable, because the ultimate goal of the chosen countermeasure system is to be able to protect human life and

expensive military assets. It is impressive that, in the 20 years since the first edition of this book [1], the development of reliable OPO and OPA technology now yields not only routine laboratory instrumentation but also highly critical military devices.

- A DIRCM laser source must have a wide environmental tolerance (e.g., from −40°C to +70°C), because military devices need to operate under harsher environmental constraints than is customary for typical laboratory instrumentation. The conditions of military operations (e.g., in extremes ranging from hot dusty deserts to wet tropics, and aircraft ambient temperatures varying from hot on the tarmac to freezing at high altitude) require a robust laser architecture that can be engineered to meet demanding performance specifications. OPO-based technologies have been found to meet such demands.
- A DIRCM laser source must be configurable to fit within the constraints of the required platform, so that SWaP are major drivers for military capabilities, particularly in the air domain.

OPOs and OPAs have been recognized as a preferred way to develop IR-based countermeasures to heat-seeking missiles. However, there have been relatively few commercial products based on such technologies from which to choose. This has arisen not because the technology has been unsuitable for the application, but rather, as a result of the cost of engineering and of the verification and validation processes that are essential before any new technology can be inserted into expensive military systems that are employed in life-threatening scenarios. The relatively small market also hinders adoption of DIRCM technology.

The first commercial laser-based DIRCM system was developed by Northrop Grumman [527,528]. The DIRCM laser, known as Viper, was first qualified in 2003, and some 2000 units are in service. The Viper laser, originally developed in conjunction with Fibertek Inc., is a diode-pumped Nd:YAG laser, which is frequency converted using a PPLN OPO and has a very low SWaP footprint (~33 cm diameter × 5 cm height and a weight of ~4.5 kg).

Many defense companies are exploring the opportunities of bringing competing DIRCM products to market, and defense agencies around the world are also conducting research to develop more advanced DIRCM laser sources. Consequently, an interesting array of OPO-based DIRCM laser architectures is currently under investigation. The most mature solutions, such as those in the Viper, employ diode-pumped solid-state lasers to pump the final OPO stage. Recent trends are to adopt hybrid (fiber-pumped solid-state) pump lasers, while future directions would suggest that OPOs will be directly fiber pumped with either thulium-ion (Tm^{3+}) or holmium-ion (Ho^{3+}) fiber sources. Key OPO pump wavelengths are ~1 μm in the case of the early systems and ~2 μm for the next-generation solutions.

Of the NLO materials listed in Table 2.1, no single material has been found to suit the entire demands of DIRCM applications. One approach is to employ a cascaded system in which an OPO of one material, such as KTP, is used to pump an OPO or OPA of another material, such as ZGP [267,526]. The preferred approach, which is simpler, is to employ a single conversion stage. The two most common materials of choice for such single-stage DIRCM architectures are the BPM material ZGP (which requires a pump wavelength above 2 μm to avoid increased absorption at shorter wavelengths) and the QPM material PPLN (which has limited ability to operate efficiently around 4 μm). OP GaAs is another very promising material for DIRCM applications, but its widespread use has been held back by the limited supply of material of suitable quality. Several defense agencies have been active either in developing OP GaAs material itself or in evaluating its performance as a means of generating the required DIRCM laser wavelengths. Access to many of those results, however, is still encumbered by the classified nature of defense work. Nevertheless, there are clear indications that OP GaAs has much potential as an OPO material for DIRCM applications. One report has demonstrated an output level of 3 W with 53% efficiency and excellent beam quality ($M^2 = 1.4$) [529]; this OPO device was tempera-ture tunable from 30°C to 60°C and produced signal and idler outputs from 3.8 to 3.6 μm and from 4.5 to 4.9 μm, respectively.

First-generation OPO-based laser sources for DIRCM applications have used conventional diode-pumped solid-state laser sources such as Nd:YAG. This mature technology is suitable for defense applications that entail ~1 μm pumping of simple PPLN-based OPO cavities, such as in the Viper laser. It is also suitable for cas-caded OPO architectures that require ~2 μm pumping of materials such as ZGP and has been demonstrated by using a Type-II degenerate KTP OPO as the 2 μm pump source [267,526].

The maturity of Tm^{3+}-based fiber lasers has provided an attractive route to gener-ating 2 μm pump radiation through the resonant pumping of Ho^{3+}-based solid-state lasers: the so-called hybrid DIRCM pump source, which combines both fiber-laser and solid-state laser technologies. Such efforts have enabled ZGP to become the current material of choice for DIRCM OPOs. Its excellent thermal and mechanical properties and high NLO coefficients deliver highly efficient, high-power OPO oper-ation. A power output of 10.1 W with 59% optical efficiency in the 3–5 μm region and with an M^2 of 1.5 was produced from a Type-I doubly resonant OPO cavity con-sisting of two 12 mm ZGP crystals in a walk-off compensated geometry [530]. The OPO cavity was pumped by a 40 kHz Q-switched 2.1 μm Ho:YAG laser, which was in turn pumped by a 790 nm diode-pumped 1.9 μm Tm^{3+} fiber laser. The output of this 2 μm pumped ZGP OPO highlights the increased performance achievable with such second-generation DIRCM laser architectures compared with more traditional OPOs driven by diode-pumped solid-state lasers, such as the PPLN Viper pumped at ~1 μm.

A significant advantage of OPO systems pumped by fiber lasers over OPOs driven by a diode-pumped solid-state laser is that the former have greater power-scaling potential without sacrificing control over other key performance param-eters, such as beam quality. Perhaps the greatest advantage of OPOs pumped by fiber lasers is their greater "engineerability" for harsh military environments. Using two Tm^{3+} fiber lasers to pump a single Ho:YAG laser, consisting of a sin-gle oscillator using two Ho:YAG rods, researchers have demonstrated repetitive Q-switched operation at 35 kHz; this yields a maximum OPO output power of 27 W in the mid-IR with a conversion efficiency of 62% and $M^2 = 4.0$ [531]. The Q-switched Ho:YAG stage can be pumped by either a CW or a quasi-CW Tm^{3+}

fiber laser, delivering similar average output powers. The latter results in a modulated peak power output at a reduced duty cycle, which can be advantageous for some applications. Under such quasi-CW pumping conditions, a ZGP OPO operating at 1 kHz and 25% duty cycle produced a modulated peak output power of 99 W in the 3–5 µm mid-IR region [531]. This flexibility in the mode of operation of the OPO significantly aids the development of appropriate modulated jam codes for defeating the incoming seeker. At such power levels, the OPO stage is capable of sufficient feedback that it can significantly damage the pump laser, and it becomes necessary to employ an optical isolator between the Ho:YAG pump laser and the OPO. In contrast to the early days of NLO material development for OPOs, in which that material itself was the most fragile component, the optical isolator now limits the achievable mid-IR output power. One solution is to use a ring OPO cavity [532], which removes the requirement for the optical isolator and allows the full power of the pump laser to be used to pump the OPO. A four-mirror ring cavity with two 12 mm ZGP crystals has been used to demonstrate the highest-brightness ZGP OPO with 30 W output power and a beam quality of $M^2 = 1.3$ [533]. Using a similar ring OPO cavity but with a more complex pump architecture, the highest reported output power of a ZGP OPO in the mid-IR is 41.2 W, but with a reduced beam quality of $M^2 < 4.4$ [534].

One direction that research activities into the next generation of OPO sources for DIRCM applications are taking is to examine the replacement of the hybrid pump source with a pulsed all-fiber pump solution. Recent results have demonstrated a ZGP OPO pumped by a monolithic power-scalable 2 µm source based on Tm^{3+}-doped fiber master-oscillator power-amplifier architectures [535]. Such an OPO system produced 3 W with a conversion efficiency of 25%. Two limitations of such systems are the strong absorption feature of ZGP at wavelengths below 2.1 µm and the restriction that Tm^{3+} fiber lasers do not operate efficiently above 2.05 µm. However, longer pump wavelengths are readily available in Ho^{3+}-doped fibers, which operate efficiently at wavelengths above 2.12 µm [536], and this is unlikely to become a long-term problem once pulsed Ho^{3+} fiber lasers become more mature.

As a future trend, the ability to manufacture an efficient monolithic fiber laser–based pump for mid-IR OPOs will be a major factor in the successful engineering of more advanced OPO-based DIRCM solutions. Beyond that is the potential to combine soft and hard glass-fiber technologies that might enable the generation of both pump and OPO stages all within fiber. Such future options would significantly reduce the costly engineering of free-space lasers in favor of monolithic fiber-based solutions with increased reliability, and improved environmental and SWaP capabilities for military applications. Another likely trend will see a greater exploitation of OP GaAs as a third key NLO material for DIRCM-based OPO applications, providing increased flexibility to juggle the competing requirements of wavelength, power, and source modulation. It is also clear from the high-power OPO results currently achieved for DIRCM applications that the power limit has not yet been reached. We should therefore expect to see further improvements in the maximum power achieved for OPO-based DIRCM systems over coming years—an outcome that may ultimately lead to even more power from tunable OPOs and OPAs employed in many spectroscopic applications.

2.5.6 Terahertz Waves from Coherent Optical Parametric Systems

The final case study of this chapter concerns the role of coherent optical parametric systems (OPOs, OPGs, and OPAs) in the generation of terahertz waves (e.g., ~1–3 THz, with wavelengths of ~300–100 μm; also known as the submillimeter waves, between the far-IR and microwave regions). Terahertz radiation offers distinctive opportunities for spectroscopic sensing, with diverse applications to the nondestructive identification, inspection, and imaging of packaged pharmaceutical products, illicit drugs and pathogens, foodstuffs, medical and agricultural substances, explosives and other defense/security materials, and so forth [537–544]. Much of the optoelectronic instrumentation used in this context relies on lasers and nonlinear optics [545–561], with optical parametric devices playing a prominent role. A comprehensive review of terahertz-wave generation by means of lasers has been presented by Kitaev [556]. In this section, we focus primarily on the optical parametric production of tunable coherent terahertz waves in $LiNbO_3$ by stimulated phonon-polariton scattering in the vicinity of that NLO material's A_1-symmetry vibrational mode at ~250 cm^{-1}. This was investigated in early research by Pantell, Puthoff, and coworkers [562–565]. Much more recently, that pre-1975 work has provided a basis for extensive research on coherent optical parametric terahertz-wave generation by Kodo Kawase and coworkers in Japan [336,546–549,557,558,561,566–593] and by Malcolm Dunn and coworkers in Scotland [350,594–598]. Another research group that has published prolifically in this area since 2010 is that of De-Gang Xu and coworkers at Tianjin University in China [599–611]. Further research in this area [612–614] has recently been reported by Andrew Lee, Helen Pask, and one of us (YH) at Macquarie University. The common theme in papers cited by these four research groups entails the development of OPOs, OPGs, or OPAs pumped by an ns-pulsed Q-switched Nd:YAG laser to directly produce coherent tunable terahertz radiation in a single step via stimulated phonon-polariton scattering in NLO crystals of either $LiNbO_3$ or MgO: $LiNbO_3$.

Incidentally, this section of the literature adopts a somewhat confusing convention in which the shorter-wavelength output wave is referred to as the "idler," contrary to the usual convention defined in the context of Equation 2.2.3. To avoid any such confusion, we refer to the two output waves as the "seed wave" (i.e., the conventional signal, typically at ~1.07 μm) and the "terahertz wave" (i.e., the conventional idler, typically at ~2 THz). The three optical frequencies involved in this context are therefore ω_{pump}, ω_{seed}, and ω_{THz}, in descending order of frequency, with ω_{THz} much lower than ω_{pump} and ω_{seed} (which are both typically in the near IR region). As in the context of Equation 2.3, there is an energy-conservation condition ($\omega_{pump} = \omega_{seed} + \omega_{THz}$) as well as corresponding momentum conservation that dictates phase-matching conditions.

Such $LiNbO_3$- or MgO:$LiNbO_3$-based coherent optical parametric systems [546–549,557,558] employ a noncollinear phase-matching geometry to ensure that the generated terahertz wave propagates at a large angle to the 1.064 μm pump and ~1.07 μm seed waves [546–549,557,558,566–570,572–576,593,594], thereby rapidly exiting the NLO crystal, since the terahertz wave is strongly absorbed in this medium. As for any OPG, a terahertz OPG does not need to have an optical cavity;

nevertheless, in generating the terahertz wave, the pump wave is often allowed to propagate back along its incident path in the NLO medium. Corresponding terahertz OPOs typically employ a singly resonant optical cavity for the seed wave, with non-collinear pump and terahertz waves propagating clear of that cavity [546–549,556–558]. Wide, continuous tuning of such a terahertz OPO can be attained by varying the angle between the resonated seed wave and the pump wave. Injection seeding by a narrowband tunable source [336,350,546–549,556–558,574,577,578,587] can reduce the optical bandwidth of the terahertz wave to <100 MHz (<0.003 cm^{-1}), as determined [350,577,578] by recording low-pressure absorption spectra of H_2O vapor at ~1.92 THz (~64 cm^{-1}).

In many of these OPG and OPO designs [336,350,546–549,557,558,572–578,593–597], an Si-prism array is used to enhance out-coupling of the terahertz wave. Less efficient terahertz-wave out-coupling is feasible by means of a monolithic grating [566], a single Si prism [567], or a trapezoidal NLO crystal [569]. In addition, Dunn and coworkers [350,593–597] have devised a compact, noncollinear phase-matched $MgO:LiNbO_3$ OPO system with a novel intersecting-cavity geometry, to locate the NLO medium within the high circulating intracavity field of the pump laser. This allows use of a lower-energy pump laser compared with previous work [546–549,557,558,566–578] and eliminates coupling optics between the pump laser and the OPO. The effective extracavity pump-laser energy required to reach threshold for OPO operation is thus reduced at least ~25-fold, from >18 to ~0.7 mJ/pulse [593]. The intersecting-cavity geometry therefore enables a compact Nd:YAG laser, excited at 808 nm by 20 W, 500 μs pulses from a quasi-CW diode laser, to be used. The observed downconversion efficiency is close to 50% when the OPO is operated at two times above threshold [593]. Moreover, in contrast to conventional intracavity OPGs, the intersecting-cavity geometry incorporates a separate, independently rotatable seed-wave cavity, combining the advantages of wide spectral coverage via angle tuning with rapid walk-off of the terahertz wave. This intersecting-cavity design has been emulated and developed by Lee, Pask et al. [612–614].

Further progress, in the field of coherent terahertz-wave optical parametric systems based on stimulated phonon-polariton scattering, has included the following developments:

- Cryogenic cooling of $LiNbO_3$ [568] or $MgO:LiNbO_3$ [561] can be used to enhance terahertz-wave output from stimulated-polariton OPOs or OPGs.
- High-gain terahertz-wave OPAs have also been used to enhance the output efficiency of terahertz-wave optical parametric systems [561,591,592].
- Various high-power terahertz-wave OPO or OPG system designs have used two $MgO:LiNbO_3$ NLO crystals, set in line [546,557,561,574,577] or at an angle of ~65° [600,601,603,615].
- Use of compact pump lasers has helped to improve the footprint and performance of terahertz-wave OPO/OPG/OPA systems [581,585,587,588,612,613].
- Cherenkov phase matching (in which the velocity of the polarization wave inside the NLO medium exceeds the velocity of the radiated terahertz wave) [556,584,586,596] has enabled high conversion efficiency and wide tunability of monochromatic terahertz waves [584,596].

- Additional terahertz output wavelengths can be produced by cascaded dif-ference-frequency generation in either QPM [596] or BPM [597,614] optical parametric systems.
- BPM NLO media (e.g., bulk $LiNbO_3$ or $MgO:LiNbO_3$) can be replaced by QPM media (e.g., PPLN) [575,596,604]. Novel QPM phase-matching schemes, based on work by Molter et al. [616], have been developed for tera-hertz OPGs, in which the grating-period vector Λ is either perpendicular or at an angle to the propagation direction of a collinear 1.064 μm pump and ~1.07 μm seed-wave beams, and the resulting terahertz waves exit rapidly at steep angles to minimize absorption losses [596].

Optical parametric systems (OPOs, OPGs, and OPAs) that yield coherent tun-able terahertz radiation via stimulated phonon-polariton scattering in $LiNbO_3$, $MgO:LiNbO_3$, or PPLN, as outlined in this section, have much potential for spectros-copy and for nondestructive sensing and imaging. So far, however, it appears that not many applications have actually been realized in this area. The spectroscopic resolu-tion (down to ~100 MHz) of such devices has been demonstrated by several measure-ments of pure rotational molecular absorption spectra of H_2O vapor in the terahertz region [336,350,546–549,557]. Likewise, intracavity stimulated-polariton OPOs and OPGs have been used, respectively, for terahertz spectroscopic measurements of absorption linewidth [350] and self-collisional frequency shifts [595] in $CO(g)$—the molecule that provided our key OPO-spectroscopic benchmarks in Section 2.1.

In more utilitarian applications, stimulated-polariton optical parametric systems have been used for terahertz spectroscopy of bigger molecules such as L-glutamic acid (a key biochemical species) [594], of illicit drugs such as methamphetamines (concealed in paper envelopes and referenced to aspirin) [579], and of explosives such as RDX, PETN, and octogen (HMX) [559]. Within this context of the nonde-structive inspection and identification of unknown (and often concealed) substances, component pattern analysis methods have been developed to facilitate multispectral optical parametric terahertz imaging [579,580].

It should be noted that the foregoing $LiNbO_3$-based OPO and OPG techniques are able to produce coherent tunable terahertz radiation directly in a single NLO process, which is in contrast to other forms of terahertz-wave generation that rely on cascaded NLO processes, such as those entailing a dual-frequency coherent optical source followed by a separate difference-frequency generation stage. It is understood [546] that the mechanism for coherent terahertz generation enhanced by stimulated-polariton scattering is attributable to a combination of second-order and third-order NLO processes. The former is an optical parametric process that is described in terms of the second-order NLO susceptibility $\chi^{(2)}$; it arises from elec-tronic polarization and has a functional dependence on the three optical fields with frequencies ω_{pump}, ω_{seed}, and ω_{THz}. The latter (which is believed [546] to make a sub-stantial contribution to terahertz-wave production) arises from the third-order NLO susceptibility $\chi^{(3)}$ as a result of ionic polarization effects after energy absorbed by electronic processes has been transferred by the nuclei to create phonons; this term depends on the vibrational coordinate Q_0 (for the polariton mode in the ionic $LiNbO_3$ crystal) as well as the three optical fields at ω_{pump}, ω_{seed}, and ω_{THz}. The single-step advantage of LiNbO$_3$-based OPO and OPG techniques arises from the fact that the relevant NLO susceptibilities, $\chi^{(2)}$ and $\chi^{(3)}$, are resonantly enhanced when the optical difference frequency ($\omega_{pump} - \omega_{seed}$) is in the vicinity of the vibrational frequency for the material's A_1-symmetry phonon-polariton mode. Conveniently (in the particular case of LiNbO$_3$), this occurs when ($\omega_{pump} - \omega_{seed}$), which equals ω_{THz}, falls in the range of ~1–3 THz. Stimulated phonon-polariton scattering then yields the seed wave at ω_{seed} and facilitates direct, single-step optical parametric production of a coherent terahertz wave at ω_{THz}; this has angle tuned phase-matching conditions and is amenable to further enhancement by injection seeding at ω_{seed}.

Optical parametric conversion based on stimulated phonon-polariton scattering in LiNbO$_3$ is just one of many forms of laser- and NLO-based optoelectronic instrumentation for the generation of tunable coherent terahertz waves that are suitable for spectroscopic sensing and imaging [545–561]. In particular, Kitaev [556] has comprehensively reviewed many such forms of terahertz-wave generation, including terahertz lasers (e.g., entailing population inversion in optically pumped molecules or some semiconductor media) as well as large-scale free-electron lasers and synchrotron sources, We therefore need to mention only a few techniques that resemble (or compete with) the direct stimulated-polariton optical parametric approaches that have been considered in detail above.

Closely related difference-frequency generation of terahertz waves, in which a DFG stage produces terahertz waves by NLO conversion of two incident pump frequencies (typically IR and tunable), requires two separate lasers or dual-frequency output from a single OPO source, with phase-matching conditions virtually identical to those for a terahertz OPO or OPG. In the ns-pulsed context, Kawase and coworkers have reported several such two-stage DFG approaches for generation of terahertz or subterahertz waves; for instance:

- A dual-signal-wave OPO, comprising a series pair of PPLN gratings pumped by a Nd:YAG laser, was used [557,571,575] with a phase-matched DAST (4-dimethylamino-N-methyl-4-stilbazolium tosylate) DFG crystal to yield terahertz-wave output at ~100–150 μm (3–2 THz).
- Nearly degenerate signal outputs at 1300 nm and ~1300–1314 nm from a two-crystal Nd:YAG-pumped PPKTP OPO were used [618] with a PPLN DFG stage to yield subterahertz (millimeter-wave) difference frequencies at ~0.34 or ~0.26 THz (depending on choice of PPLN grating period Λ), and higher-order QPM outputs in the terahertz range.
- Subsequently [589], the same two-crystal Nd:YAG-pumped PPKTP OPO was used with a new configurationally locked polyene (OH1) DFG crystal as a widely tunable (~0.3–3 THz; ~1–0.1 mm) source of coherent terahertz waves that has proved to perform more efficiently than the abovementioned organic DFG material DAST [571,575].

In the context of ps- and fs-pulsed optical parametric devices, Vodopyanov and coworkers have shown that OP GaAs has much potential for terahertz-wave generation [106,107,554,555,619–624]. An early device of this type generated an average output power of 1 mW at 2.8 THz with an optical bandwidth of ~300 GHz

($\sim$10 cm^{-1}) and a ps-pulse repetition rate of 50 MHz, by DFG of the signal and idler waves of a near-degenerate, synchronously pumped doubly resonant OPO [620]. Such terahertz-generating DFG processes effectively approach the limit of optical rectification—one of the most primitive of the second-order ($\chi^{(2)}$-based) NLO processes [86,556]. Other ps- and fs-pulsed terahertz-generating optical parametric devices based on PPLN have been studied by the research groups of Beigang [626–629] and Reid [164,165,630].

In a particularly significant advance, Kiessling and coworkers have recently reported CW operation of an OP GaAs intracavity DFG system [631,632]. Closely spaced PPLN OPO signal and idler intracavity light fields resonating at wavelengths of $\sim$2 µm are converted to a backward-propagating terahertz wave via parametric difference-frequency generation in an OP GaAs crystal that is located inside the same doubly resonant OPO cavity. A frequency-tuning range of 1–4.5 THz, a sub-10 MHz linewidth, a Gaussian beam profile, and >25 µW of CW output power have been demonstrated. This progress (in an area where successful applications had hitherto been confined to picosecond systems) should enable future high-resolution (sub-Doppler) OPO-spectroscopic applications in the terahertz region, provided that narrowband CW terahertz output powers can be scaled up into the milliwatt range [631,632]. Incidentally, the context of this research has been introduced [631] with reference to early high-resolution pure rotational spectroscopy of CO(g) [633]—our key OPO-spectroscopic benchmark molecule, as in Section 2.1—below its Doppler limit, using a tunable narrowband (<20 kHz) backward-wave oscillator operating in the subterahertz region.

The above intracavity combination of a CW PPLN OPO OP GaAs DFG system is derived from exploratory work by Kiessling and coworkers on CW terahertz OPO systems [633–636]. Their early work [634] used a singly resonant bow-tie OPO cavity, pumped at 1.03 µm by a CW Yb:YAG solid-state laser and containing a dual-grating MgO:PPLN NLO crystal with two successive QPM regions to generate a pair of signal waves at $\sim$1.4 µm; their difference frequency at 0.64–0.85 THz was then demonstrated by means of external ion-irradiated InGaAs photomixers. In subsequent research [634], a singly resonant multigrating MgO:PPLN OPO was used to deliver CW single-frequency idler output at 2.33–5.32 µm as well as additional cascaded optical parametric forward and backward idler waves that are able to yield tunable phase-matched frequencies around 3.5 and 1.5 THz, respectively. These findings were combined [636] in a CW terahertz OPO emitting a coherent diffraction-limited beam tunable from 1.3 to 1.7 THz with power levels exceeding 1 µW; this entailed simultaneous phase matching of two intracavity parametric processes in a single MgO:PPLN crystal inside a signal-resonant optical cavity where cascaded NLO processes generated backward-propagating terahertz radiation. A later CW terahertz PPLN OPO design by the same group [637] used a high-finesse build up cavity for the 1.03 µm pump laser and was tunable over 1.2–2.9 THz with a few microwatts of terahertz output power. Elsewhere [638], a higher-power CW terahertz source, emitting up to 2 mW of power at 1 or 1.9 THz (but with unspecified terahertz linewidth and tunability), employed a dual-color vertical external-cavity surface-emitting laser and intracavity DFG in slanted PPLN.

Backward-propagating DFG and OPO processes are crucial to assorted terahertz-generation strategies discussed in this section (e.g., in the domain of CW terahertz OPOs [631,632,634–637]). It should be noted that the prospect of a backward OPO was first proposed by Harris in 1966 [639], more than 40 years before such a device—a mirrorless OPO—was convincingly demonstrated in 2007 [640,641]. Backward OPOs were originally envisaged [639] as BPM devices that would operate in the mid-IR (in view of the dispersion properties of available birefringent NLO materials). They were subsequently discussed actively as a theoretical possibility [642,643] in the context of DFG—which is effectively their nonparametric NLO precursor. However, those predictions were not realized until it was possible to write QPM gratings of very fine pitch (e.g., Λ <1 µm) on flux-grown PPKTP [644,645], thereby facilitating the necessary phase-matching conditions for a backward OPO (with copropagating signal and pump waves and a counterpropagating idler wave) [641] or for backward SHG (with counterpropagating fundamental and second-harmonic waves) [645].

A backward OPO relies on parametric interaction of counterpropagating optical waves to automatically establish distributed feedback and thereby realize novel sources of coherent tunable radiation. Such an OPO can be "mirrorless" because it does not require alignment or any optical components other than the second-order NLO medium itself [639,641]. The originally demonstrated mirrorless OPO [641] comprised a PPKTP QPM grating with $\Lambda = 0.8$ µm, pumped at ~0.82 µm by a focused 1 kHz train of 47 ps pulses from a Ti:sapphire regenerative amplifier; this yielded signal and idler waves at ~1.14 and ~2.94 µm with pulse energies of ~16 and ~6 µJ, respectively. The spectral profile of the OPO signal output was essentially a wavelength-shifted replica of the pump-laser spectrum, which had a FWHM optical bandwidth of ~300 GHz (~10 cm^{-1}); by contrast, the backward-propagating OPO idler output had an optical bandwidth, ~3 GHz (~0.1 cm^{-1}), that was two orders of magnitude narrower. This spectral property resulted in generation of narrowband idler radiation from a free-running OPO requiring no resonator mirrors or adjustable optics (such as intracavity grating, étalon, or injection seeder) [639,641]. The signal and idler frequencies were also remarkably insensitive to temperature variations (compared with a conventional copropagating PPKTP OPO), so that the narrowband idler frequency was temperature stable and amenable to high-precision mid-IR temperature tuning.

At the risk of meandering too far from the central theme of terahertz OPOs, we note that backward (mirrorless) OPOs have been likened to the NLO equivalent of a distributed-feedback (DFB) laser, which also does not require conventional mirrors [639]. Several other DFB-based OPO wavelength-control strategies (the first two of which have already been discussed in Section 2.4.2) may also be noted in this context:

- An ns-pulsed tunable PPLN OPO [294], in which a permanent phase-conjugate grating is written in PPLN by UV light to provide DFB operation
- Our ns-pulsed SAT OPO design [248,249], in which dynamic, adjustment-free DFB-type operation of an ns-pulsed narrowband SLM-tunable PPKTP OPO is achieved by using CW tunable seed radiation (e.g., at ~840 nm) to

write a wavelength-selective Bragg grating in a photorefractive crystal (e.g., $Rh:BaTiO_3$)

- A compact tunable ns-pulsed PPKTP OPO [646] incorporating a volume Bragg grating retroreflector [647] and delivering signal output at ~760 nm with a tuning range of ~2.6 THz (~87 cm^{-1}) and an optical bandwidth of ~130 GHz (~4.3 cm^{-1})

Finally, as is the case in the mid-IR, the spectroscopic potential of terahertz-wave optical parametric devices is challenged by the development of quantum cascade lasers (QCLs) [550,553,556,560]. However, the utility of all terahertz semiconductor lasers (including p-Ge lasers as well as QCLs [556]) is complicated by the need for them to be cryogenically cooled. Nevertheless, "a source of fresh hope" was recognized in 2007 [551] as a result of developments [552] in which a QCL emitting at dual mid-IR wavelengths of 7.6 and 8.7 μm produced terahertz output at ~60 μm (~5 THz) via intracavity difference-frequency generation in coupled AlInAs/InGaAs quantum wells engineered to have a giant NLO susceptibility $\chi^{(2)}$ for the DFG process [648]. This system required a cryogenic operating temperature of ~80 K, but the authors [552] were optimistic at that time that further developments would enable operation at thermoelectric-cooler temperatures. Subsequent developments [648–654] appear to have justified that optimism, as spectroscopically useful monolithic DFG-based terahertz QCLs operating at room temperature become an increasingly realistic prospect.

2.6 CONCLUSION: OPO-SPECTROSCOPIC PREDICTIONS REALIZED

The subject area of this chapter on spectroscopic applications of tunable OPOs has grown enormously, in both scientific and technological terms, since the first edition of this book [1] was published. This is demonstrated by the number of our selectively cited references, which trebled during the approximately 15 years that separate the first (1995) [1] and second (2009) [5] editions of this book and has increased by a further ~70% during the subsequent 5 years leading to this third edition. The first edition [1] was written at a time when spectroscopic applications of ns-pulsed tunable OPOs had recently undergone a resurgence, after a period (approximately 1975–1985, say) of relatively low activity compared with developments in the 10 years following the initial realization (50 years ago!) of an OPO [250]. Since approximately 1985, the spectroscopic utility of OPOs (whether CW or pulsed in the nanosecond and ultrafast time domains) has helped to promote virtually unabated continuation of that resurgence to the present day. As new technologies (e.g., mid-IR QCLs) become increasingly available as convenient, compact substitutes for CW and ns-pulsed OPOs, other forms of OPO-based spectroscopy (e.g., highly coherent ultrafast OPOs and frequency combs) have emerged to take their place.

In updating our previously published versions [1,5] of this chapter, we have aimed to preserve its original function as a primer for those wanting to know about the basics of tunable OPO principles and techniques, with particular emphasis on ns-pulsed systems and their spectroscopic applications. At the same time as retaining a historical perspective, we have aimed to provide a (highly selective) survey of state-of-the-art developments in tunable OPOs in the context of spectroscopic applications. As in the second edition [5], this has proved to be a challenging task. We have needed to cover the key roles that ultrafast-pulsed and CW OPOs have assumed over the last 20 years or so, and to provide perspectives on $\chi^{(2)}$- and $\chi^{(3)}$-based NLO wavelength-conversion devices in general (e.g., see Figure 2.5): OPGs, OPAs, and DFGs, in addition to OPOs themselves.

As in previous editions [1,5], this chapter is far from comprehensive, so that its scope allows no more than a superficial, biased sampling of the many things that have happened and are happening in the field of OPO-based spectroscopy, with a sufficiently representative list of references for detailed bibliographic purposes. Our personal research interests (e.g., on the use of linear or nonlinear atomic and molecular spectroscopy to verify the performance of injection-seeded ns-pulsed SLM-tunable OPOs, as in most of Section 2.4 and much of Section 2.5) are unashamedly represented in the chosen topics. Moreover, most of the examples cited concern rovibrational spectroscopy (either IR or Raman) and bypass much important OPO-based research in the visible and UV regions (e.g., LIF-based biosensing and biomolecular imaging). Nevertheless, an attempt has been made to deal, at least cursorily, with areas of the subject in which our expertise may not be well established. The chapter focuses at first on how tunable OPOs work (e.g., see Tables 2.1 and 2.2 and Figures 2.6 through 2.10) and how spectroscopic measurements can be used to test their performance (e.g., see Tables 2.3 through 2.5 and Figure 2.11), before moving on to selected examples where spectroscopy itself is a central motivation. How to optimize the performance of CW, ns-pulsed or ps/fs-pulsed OPOs for spectroscopic purposes remains a pervasive theme throughout this chapter. Since the second edition [5], additional emerging fields have been selectively surveyed, notably fiber-based OPOs (Section 2.5.4), OPO-based defense countermeasures (Section 2.5.5), and terahertz OPOs (Section 2.5.6).

To conclude, it is fascinating to reflect on a number of early predictions concerning OPO-spectroscopic applications that have ultimately been successfully realized, as follows.

- OPOs as an established technology for spectroscopy and other applications: In the 50th year of established OPO technology [250], we note the prescient remark in Stephen Harris's 1969 review [8]: "within a few years, narrow-band tunable sources will be available over the entire spectral region from 0.2 μ to greater than 100 μ. ... Such sources are likely to have significant impact on many types of excited state spectroscopy, optical pumping, semiconductor studies, and photochemistry." This chapter provides ample evidence that his foresight has been well and truly fulfilled.
- CO(g) as an OPO-spectroscopic benchmark: As noted in Sections 2.1.1, 2.1.2, 2.3.5, 2.5.1, 2.5.2, and 2.5.6 (and specifically illustrated in Figures 2.1 through 2.3), measurements of the diatomic molecule CO have provided a series of significant OPO-spectroscopic benchmarks since 1975, when Robert Byer declared prophetically that "the use of parametric oscillator sources for molecular spectroscopy should increase rapidly" [10].

- Injection seeding as a convenient means of OPO-spectroscopic tuning: The first demonstration (in 1969 by Bjorkholm and Danielmeyer) [305] of an injection-seeded OPO and a subsequent rate-equation model (in 1979 by Cassedy and Jain) [307] for injection seeding of an ns-pulsed OPO have provided the basis of an OPO wavelength-control approach as an alternative to intracavity gratings or étalons. Injection seeding by an independent narrowband tunable source has been particularly useful in our OPO-spectroscopic research at Macquarie University, as explained in Sections 2.4.2 and 2.4.3.

- QPM NLO media: As discussed in Section 2.2.1, the possibility of QPM as an alternative to BPM was portrayed in 1962 by Armstrong et al. in figure 10a of their seminal NLO-theory paper [85]. However, it took another ~30 years before the QPM concept was realized practically in the form of PP NLO materials such as PPLN and PPKTP, tailored for specific wavelengths by periodic structuring of ferroelectric domains. It should be evident throughout this chapter that, over the last approximately 20 years [91], such QPM media have greatly enhanced the efficiency, stability, durability, tunability, spectral quality, versatility, and compactness of OPOs suitable for spectroscopy over a wide range of the IR, UV, and terahertz regions. (Incidentally, the NLO community was much quicker to take up the second QPM strategy suggested in Figure 10b of [85], which entails periodic total internal reflection and Fresnel birefringence; this approach was first demonstrated in 1966 by Boyd and Patel [655] and then in 1998 by Komine et al. [656] [in both cases via SHG of pulsed IR laser radiation in plane-parallel slabs of GaAs or ZnSe]. It has subsequently been explored by Rosencher and coworkers [657–661] in the contexts of DFG [tunable between 8 and 13 μm] of signal and idler waves from a Nd:YAG-pumped pulsed $LiNbO_3$ OPO [657–659] and $4 \rightarrow 2$ μm SHG of pulsed OPO idler radiation [660,661], using NLO media such as GaAs or ZnSe. As far as we know, this periodic total-internal-reflection QPM approach has not been successfully used to phase match an OPO—presumably because of unacceptable reflection losses that it would entail.)

- Fresh prospects from OPOs based on OP GaAs: OP GaAs may be regarded as a further outcome of the 1962 proposal of QPM materials by Armstrong et al. [85]. As explained in Section 2.2.3, OP GaAs shows great promise as a NLO medium for various forms of coherent wavelength conversion (SHG, DFG, continuum generation, and particularly OPOs and OPGs in the mid-IR, far-IR, and terahertz regions) due to its large NLO coefficient, its advantageous phase-matching dispersion relationships, its wide-ranging IR transparency over 0.9–17 μm, its high laser-damage threshold, and its high thermal conductivity. A number of OPO-spectroscopic breakthroughs depending on OP GaAs, particularly by Vodopyanov and coworkers, have been outlined in Sections 2.1.2, 2.2.3, 2.3.3, 2.3.5, 2.5.2, 2.5.5, and 2.5.6. It seems likely that OP GaAs will have an increasing impact on OPO applications in spectroscopy and far beyond, provided that its commercial availability (limited at present by the complications of its fabrication and, perhaps, by national strategic issues) can be improved.

- The long-awaited realization of backward OPOs: Backward-propagating DFG and OPO processes are crucial to assorted terahertz-generation strategies discussed above (e.g., in the domain of CW terahertz OPOs [631,631,634–637]). It should be noted that the prospect of a backward OPO was first proposed by Harris in 1966 [639], more than 40 years before such a device—a mirrorless OPO—was convincingly demonstrated in 2007 [640,641]. Backward OPOs were originally envisaged [8,639] as BPM devices that would operate in the mid-IR (in view of the dispersion properties of the birefringent NLO materials that were then available), but they have subsequently been facilitated by QPM devices. Their prospects were later considered theoretically [642,643] in the already realized context of DFG—effectively, their nonparametric NLO precursor.

- "Good-bye to Ti: and Dye?": As mentioned in Section 2.1.1, this mid-1990s advertising slogan was in circulation at a time when it seemed possible that OPOs would displace both Ti:sapphire and dye lasers as the preferred source of tunable coherent radiation for many applications, particularly spectroscopy. While the slogan may be true with regard to the apparent decline of dye lasers, it is certainly not valid for Ti:sapphire. Meanwhile, it is apparent that OPOs themselves are likely to be displaced from areas of application where they were once preferred. This is particularly valid in the case of QCLs, which have become commercially available and are now increasingly used for finely tunable mid-IR spectroscopic applications [44,388,662–666] in which NLO systems (based on OPO, OPG, and DFG devices) had previously been dominant. The potential of QCLs as tunable sources of coherent terahertz radiation has been briefly surveyed at the end of Section 2.5.6, although the utility of terahertz QCLs is at present limited by the need to provide cryogenics for such devices. It is in the nature of cutting-edge technology and scientific frontiers that one form of instrument may eventually be superseded by another. However, in the case of tunable OPOs, this chapter provides many encouraging indications that OPO-spectroscopic applications still have a long way to go as new devices, innovative techniques, and fresh experimental challenges emerge.

ACKNOWLEDGMENTS

The chapter has been significantly influenced by the work of other researchers in this field, with whom we have worked, copublished, communicated, met at conferences, or merely enjoyed virtual contact through the optical physics literature. Such colleagues are too numerous to name explicitly, other than by citing some of their published work. We specifically acknowledge financial support from the Australian Research Council (ARC) and from Macquarie University, including its MQ Photonics Research Centre (and the ARC Special Research Centre for Lasers and Applications, from which MQ Photonics evolved).

REFERENCES

1. Orr, B. J., M. J. Johnson, and J. G. Haub, Spectroscopic applications of pulsed tunable optical parametric oscillators. In F. J. Duarte (Ed.), *Tunable Laser Applications*, 1st edn, Chapter 2, pp. 11–82, Marcel-Dekker, New York, 1995.
2. Stuke, M. (Ed.), *Dye Lasers: 25 Years*, Springer, Berlin, 1992.
3. Duarte, F. J. (Ed.), *High-Power Dye Lasers*, Springer, Berlin, 1992.
4. Segal, D. M., *J. Mod. Opt.* 40: 965–966, 1993; this is a book review of [3].
5. Orr, B. J., Y. He, and R. T. White, Spectroscopic applications of pulsed tunable optical parametric oscillators. In F. J. Duarte (Ed.), *Tunable Laser Applications*, 2nd edn, Chapter 2, pp. 15–95, CRC Press, New York, 2009.
6. Sorokina, I. T. and K. L. Vodopyanov (Eds), *Solid-State Mid-Infrared Sources*, Springer, Berlin, 2003.
7. Ebrahim-Zadeh, M. and I. T. Sorokina (Eds), *Mid-Infrared Coherent Sources and Applications* (NATO Science for Peace and Security Series B: Physics and Biophysics), Springer, Berlin, 2007.
8. Harris, S. E., Tunable optical parametric oscillators, *Proc. IEEE* 57: 2096–2113, 1969.
9. Byer, R. L., Parametric oscillators. In R. G. Brewer and A. Mooradian (Eds), *Laser Spectroscopy*, pp. 77–101, Plenum, New York, 1973.
10. Byer, R. L., Optical parametric oscillators. In H. Rabin and C. L. Tang (Eds), *Quantum Electronics: A Treatise*, Volume I, Part B, Chapter 9, pp. 578–702, Academic, New York, 1975.
11. Byer, R. L. and R. L. Herbst, Parametric oscillation and mixing. In Y.-R. Shen (Ed.), *Nonlinear Infrared Generation*, Chapter 3, pp. 81–137, Springer, Berlin, 1977.
12. Brosnan, S. J. and R. L. Byer, Optical parametric oscillator threshold and linewidth studies, *IEEE J. Quantum Elect.* QE-15: 415–431, 1979.
13. Sackett, P. (US Air Force Cambridge Research Laboratory), cited in [10] as a private communication to R. L. Byer (1972).
14. Henningsen, T., M. Garbuny, and R. L. Byer, Remote detection of CO by parametric tunable laser, *Appl. Phys. Lett.* 24: 242–244, 1974.
15. Kildal, H. and R. L. Byer, Comparison of laser methods for the remote detection of atmospheric pollutants, *Proc. IEEE* 59: 1644–1663, 1971.
16. Leone, S. R. and C. B. Moore, *V–V* energy transfer in HCl with tunable optical parametric oscillator excitation, *Chem. Phys. Lett.* 19: 340–344, 1973.
17. Michael, D. W., K. Kolenbrander, and J. M. Lisy, New cavity design for a $LiNbO_3$ optical parametric oscillator, *Rev. Sci. Instrum.* 57: 1210–1212, 1986.
18. Minton, T. K., S. A. Reid, H. L. Kim, and J. D. McDonald, A scanning, single-mode, $LiNbO_3$ optical parametric oscillator, *Opt. Commun.* 69: 289–293, 1989.
19. Bosenberg, W. R., W. S. Pelouch, and C. L. Tang, High-efficiency and narrow-linewidth operation of a two-crystal β-BaB_2O_4 optical parametric oscillator, *Appl. Phys. Lett.* 55: 1952–1954, 1989.
20. Bosenberg, W. R. and D. R. Guyer, Single-frequency optical parametric oscillator, *Appl. Phys. Lett.* 61: 387–389, 1992.
21. Bosenberg, W. R. and D. R. Guyer, Broadly tunable, single-frequency optical parametric frequency-conversion system, *J. Opt. Soc. Am. B* 10: 1716–1722, 1993.
22. Fix, A., T. Schröder, and R. Wallenstein, The optical parametric oscillators of beta-bariumborate and lithiumborate: New sources of powerful tunable laser radiation in the ultraviolet, visible and near infrared, *Laser Optoelektronik* 23(3): 106–110, 1991.
23. Tang, C. L., W. R. Bosenberg, T. Ukachi, R. J. Lane, and L. K. Cheng, Optical parametric oscillators, *Proc. IEEE* 80: 365–374, 1992.

24. Dmitriev, V. G., G. G. Gurzayan, and D. N. Nikogosyan, *Handbook of Nonlinear Optical Crystals*, 3rd edn, Springer, New York, 1999.
25. Nikogosyan, D. N., *Nonlinear Optical Crystals: A Complete Survey*, Springer, New York, 2005.
26. Smith, A. V., *SNLO Nonlinear Optics Code*, Windows-based free public domain software downloadable from http://www.as-photonics.com/snlo.
27. Koechner, W., *Solid-State Laser Engineering*, 6th edn, Springer, New York, 2006.
28. Orr, B. J., IR lidar applications in air monitoring. In R. A. Meyers (Ed.), *Encyclopedia of Analytical Chemistry: Applications, Theory and Instrumentation*, Volume 3, pp. 2007–2032, Wiley, Chichester, 2000.
29. Baxter, G. W., M. A. Payne, B. D. W. Austin, C. A. Halloway, J. G. Haub, Y. He, A. P. Milce, J. W. Nibler, and B. J. Orr, Spectroscopic diagnostics of chemical processes: Applications of optical parametric oscillators, *Appl. Phys. B.* 71: 651–663, 2000.
30. He, Y., P. Wang, R. T. White, and B. J. Orr, Spectroscopic applications of optical parametric oscillators, *Opt. Photonics News* 13(5): 56–60 and 76, 2002.
31. Orr, B. J., Optical parametric devices: Overview. In R. D. Guenther, D. G. Steel, and L. Bayvel (Eds), *Encyclopedia of Modern Optics*, pp. 43–51, Elsevier Physics, Oxford, 2004.
32. Orr, B. J. and Y. He, Tunable nonlinear-optical devices for laser-spectroscopic sensing. In P. E. Powers (Ed.), *Nonlinear Frequency Generation and Conversion: Materials, Devices, and Applications IX, Proc. SPIE* 7582: 75820J/1–75820J/14, 2010.
33. Orr, B. J. and Y. He, Cavity-based absorption spectroscopy techniques. In M. Baudelet (Ed.), *Laser Spectroscopy for Sensing: Fundamentals, Techniques and Applications*, Chapter 6, pp. 167–207, Woodhead Publishing Series in Electronic and Optical Materials, Number 43, Woodhead, Cambridge, 2014.
34. Tang, C. L., Optical parametric processes in nonlinear optics, *Int. J. Nonlinear Opt. Phys.* 3: 205–224, 1994.
35. Barnes, N. P., Optical parametric oscillators. In F. J. Duarte (Ed.), *Tunable Lasers Handbook*, Chapter 7, pp. 293–348, Academic, San Diego, 1995.
36. Sutherland, R. L., Optical parametric generation, amplification, and oscillation. In R. L. Sutherland (Ed.), *Handbook of Nonlinear Optics—Optical Engineering Series*, Volume 52, Chapter 3, pp. 111–206, Marcel Dekker, New York, 1996.
37. Piskarskas, A. P., Optical parametric generators: Tunable, powerful and ultrafast, *Opt. Photonics News*, 8(7): 24–28 and 55, 1997.
38. Dixon, G. J., Periodically poled lithium niobate shines in the IR, *Laser Focus World* 33(5): 105–111, 1997.
39. Tang, C. L., Tutorial on optical parametric processes and devices, *J. Nonlinear Opt. Phys. Mater.* 6: 535–547, 1997.
40. Byer, R. L., Quasi-phasematched nonlinear interactions and devices, *J. Nonlinear Opt. Phys. Mater.* 6: 549–592, 1997.
41. Dunn, M. H. and M. Ebrahim-Zadeh, Parametric generation of tunable light from continuous-wave to femtosecond pulses, *Science* 286: 1513–1517, 1999.
42. Dunn, M. H. and M. Ebrahim-Zadeh, Optical parametric oscillators. In D. M. Finlayson and B. D. Sinclair (Eds), *Advances in Lasers and Applications*, Chapter 4, pp. 61–82, Institute of Physics, London, 1999.
43. Ebrahim-Zadeh, M. and M. H. Dunn, Optical parametric oscillators. In M. Bass, J. M. Enoch, E. W. Van Stryland, and W. L. Wolfe (Eds), *Handbook of Optics, Vol. IV, Fiber Optics and Nonlinear Optics*, Chapter 22, pp. 22.1–22.73, McGraw-Hill, New York, 2001.
44. Curl, R. F. and F. K. Tittel, Tunable infrared laser spectroscopy, *Ann. Rep. Prog. Chem., Sec. C: Phys. Chem.* 98: 219–272, 2002.

45. Vodopyanov, K. L., OPOs target the longwave infrared, *Laser Focus World* 37(5): 225–232, 2002.
46. Vodopyanov, K. L., Pulsed mid-IR optical parametric oscillators. In I. T. Sorokina and K. L. Vodopyanov (Eds), *Solid-State Mid-Infrared Sources*, Chapter 4, pp. 141–178, Springer, Berlin, 2003.
47. Ebrahim-Zadeh, M., Mid-infrared and continuous-wave optical parametric oscillators. In I. T. Sorokina and K. L. Vodopyanov (Eds), *Solid-State Mid-Infrared Sources*, Chapter 5, pp. 179–218, Springer, Berlin, 2003.
48. Ebrahim-Zadeh, M., Parametric light generation, *Phil. Trans. Roy. Soc. London Ser. A: Math. Phys. Eng. Sci.* 361: 2731–2750, 2003.
49. Hum, D. S. and M. M. Fejer, Quasi-phasematching, *Comptes Rendus Physique* 8: 180–198, 2007.
50. Pasiskevicius, V., G. Strömqvist, F. Laurell, and C. Canalias, Quasi-phase matched nonlinear media: Progress towards nonlinear optical engineering, *Opt. Mater.* 34: 513–523, 2012.
51. Demtröder, W., *Laser Spectroscopy*, Volume 1 (Basic Principles) and Volume 2 (Experimental Techniques), 4th edn, Springer, Berlin, 2008.
52. Sigrist, M. W., High resolution infrared laser spectroscopy and gas sensing applications. In M. Quack and F. Merkt (Eds), *Handbook of High-Resolution Spectroscopy*, Volume 2, pp. 1129–1152, Wiley-VCH, Chichester (From MW to IR and UV Spectroscopy), 2011.
53. Svelto, O., S. Longhi, G. D. Valle, G. Huber, S. Kück, M. Pollnau, H. Hillmer, T. Kusserow, R. Engelbrecht, F. Rohlfing, J. Kaiser, A. Peterson, R. Malz, G. Marowsky, K. Mann, P. Simon, C. K. Rhodes, F. J. Duarte, A. Borsutzky, J. A. L'huillier, M. W. Sigrist, H. Wächter, E. Saldin, E. Schneidmiller, M. Yurkov, R. Sauerbrey, J. Hein, M. Gianella, J. Helmcke, K. Midorikawa, F. Riehle, S. Steinberg, and H. Brand, Lasers and coherent light sources. In F. Träger (Ed.), *Springer Handbook of Lasers and Optics*, 2nd edn, Chapter 11, pp. 641–1046, Springer, Berlin, 2012; note section 11.9, Optical parametric oscillators, pp. 863–882.
54. Svanberg, S. and W. Demtröder, Optical and spectroscopic techniques. In F. Träger (Ed.), *Springer Handbook of Lasers and Optics*, 2nd edn, Chapter 13, pp. 1097–1169, Springer, Berlin, 2012.
55. Arslanov, D. D., M. Spunei, J. Mandon, S. M. Cristescu, S. T. Persijn, and F. J. M. Harren, Continuous-wave optical parametric oscillator based infrared spectroscopy for sensitive molecular gas sensing, *Laser Photon. Rev.* 7: 188–206, 2013.
56. Tittel, F. K., R. Lewicki, R. Lascola, and S. McWhorter, Emerging infrared laser absorption spectroscopic techniques for gas analysis. In W. M. Geiger and M. W. Raynor (Eds), *Trace Analysis of Specialty and Electronic Gases*, Chapter 4, pp. 71–109, Wiley, Hoboken, NJ, 2013.
57. Ebrahim-Zadeh, M., S. C. Kumar, A. Esteban-Martin, and G. K. Samanta, Breakthroughs in photonics 2012: Breakthroughs in optical parametric oscillators, *IEEE Photonics J.* 5: 0700105/1–0700105/5, 2013.
58. Peng, J., Developments of mid-infrared optical parametric oscillators for spectroscopic sensing: A review, *Opt. Eng.* 53: 061613, 2014; http://opticalengineering.spiedigitallibrary.org/article.aspx?articleid=1838804.
59. Baudelet, M. (Ed.), *Laser Spectroscopy for Sensing: Fundamentals, Techniques and Applications*, Woodhead Publishing Series in Electronic and Optical Materials, Number 43, Woodhead, Cambridge, 2014.
60. Byer, R. L. and A. Piskarskas (Eds), Optical parametric oscillation and amplification, feature issue of *J. Opt. Soc. Am. B* 10: 1656–1791, 1993.
61. Byer, R. L. and A. Piskarskas (Eds), Optical parametric oscillation and amplification, feature issue of *J. Opt. Soc. Am. B* 10: 2148–2238, 1993.

62. Bosenberg, W. R. and R. C. Eckardt (Eds), Optical parametric devices, feature issue of *J. Opt. Soc. Am. B* 12: 2084–2322, 1995.
63. Ebrahim-Zadeh, M., R. C. Eckardt, and M. H. Dunn (Eds), Optical parametric devices and processes, feature issue of *J. Opt. Soc. Am. B* 16: 1477–1602, 1999.
64. Schiller, S. and J. Mlynek (Eds), Continuous-wave optical parametric oscillators, special issue of *Appl. Phys. B* 66: 661–764, 1998.
65. Berger, V. and E. Rosencher (Eds), Optical parametric sources for the infrared/Sources optiques paramétriques pour l'infrarouge, special issue of *Comptes Rendus Physique* 8: 1099–1224, 2007.
66. Boulanger, B., S. T. Cundiff, D. J. Gauthier, M. Karlsson, Y.-Q. Lu, R. A. Norwood, D. Skryabin, and T. Taira, Focus issue introduction: Nonlinear optics, *Opt. Express* 19: 23561–23566, 2011; www.osapublishing.org/oe/abstract.cfm?URI = oe-19-23-23561.
67. Byer, R. L., 50 years of nonlinear optics, Tunable sources from OPOs to coherent x-rays. In *Nonlinear Optics*, OSA Technical Digest (CD) (Optical Society of America, 2011), paper NWB2; accessible via a link on page 23563 in Boulanger, B., S. T. Cundiff, D. J. Gauthier, M. Karlsson, Y.-Q. Lu, R. A. Norwood, D. Skryabin, and T. Taira, Focus issue introduction: Nonlinear optics, *Opt. Express* 19: 23561–23566, 2011.
68. Tittel, F. K. (Ed.), Environmental trace gas detection using laser spectroscopy, special issue of *Appl. Phys. B* 67: 273–527, 1998.
69. Richter, D., A. Fried, and F. K. Tittel (Eds), Trends in laser sources, spectroscopic techniques and their applications to trace-gas detection, special issue of *Appl. Phys. B* 75: 143–403, 2002.
70. Tittel, F. K. and A. A. Kosterev (Eds), Optics: Trends in laser sources, spectroscopic techniques and their applications to trace-gas detection, special issue of *Appl. Phys. B* 85: 171–477, 2006.
71. Henderson, A., P. Roper, R. D. Mead, J. R. Gord, G. J. Fiechtner, and G. E. Tietz, Carbon monoxide absorption spectroscopy using a diode-pumped continuous wave optical parametric oscillator. In T. Li (Ed.), *Laser Applications to Chemical and Environmental Analysis*, Volume 36 of *OSA Trends in Optics and Photonics Series* (OSA, Washington DC, 2000), paper PD3; http://www.osapublishing.org/abstract. cfm?URI = LACEA-2000-PD3.
72. Kirby, B. J. and R. K. Hanson, Planar laser-induced fluorescence imaging of carbon monoxide using vibrational (infrared) transitions, *Appl. Phys. B* 69: 505–507, 1999.
73. Kirby, B. J. and R. K. Hanson, Imaging of CO and CO_2 using infrared planar laser-induced fluorescence, *Proc. Combus. Inst.* 28: 253–259, 2000.
74. Kirby, B. J. and R. K. Hanson, Linear excitation schemes for IR planar-induced fluorescence imaging of CO and CO_2, *Appl. Opt.* 41: 1190–1201, 2002.
75. Haakestad, M. W., T. P. Lamour, N. Leindecker, A. Marandi, and K. L. Vodopyanov, Intra-cavity trace molecular detection with a broadband mid-IR frequency comb source, *J. Opt. Soc. Am. B* 30: 631–640, 2013.
76. Vodopyanov, K. L., Massively-parallel intra-cavity trace molecular detection in the mid-infrared using broadband frequency combs, *Proc. SPIE* 8993 (Quantum Sensing and Nanophotonic Devices XI): 899303/1–899303/8, 2014.
77. Shen, Y. R., *The Principles of Nonlinear Optics*, Wiley, New York, 1984 (reprinted in the Wiley Classics Series, 2003).
78. Yariv, A., *Quantum Electronics*, 3rd edn, Wiley, New York, 1989.
79. Butcher, P. N. and D. Cotter, *The Elements of Nonlinear Optics*, Cambridge University Press, Cambridge, 1990.
80. Boyd, R. W., *Nonlinear Optics*, 2nd edn, Academic, New York, 2003.
81. Tang, C. L., Spontaneous and stimulated parametric processes. In H. Rabin and C. L. Tang (Eds), *Quantum Electronics: A Treatise*, Volume I, Part A, Chapter 6, pp. 419–446, Academic, New York, 1975.

82. Mandel, L. and E. Wolf, *Optical Coherence and Quantum Optics*, Cambridge University Press, Cambridge, 1995.

83. Zeilinger, A., *Dance of the Photons: From Einstein to Quantum Teleportation*, Farrar, Straus and Giroux, New York, 2010.

84. Fischer, C. and M. W. Sigrist, Mid-IR difference-frequency generation. In I. T. Sorokina and K. L. Vodopyanov (Eds), *Solid-State Mid-Infrared Sources*, Chapter 3, pp. 97–141, Springer, Berlin, 2003.

85. Armstrong, J. A., N. Bloembergen, J. Ducuing, and P. S. Pershan, Interaction between light waves in a nonlinear dielectric, *Phys. Rev.* 127: 1918–1939, 1962.

86. Franken, P. A. and J. F. Ward, Optical harmonics and nonlinear phenomena, *Rev. Mod. Phys.* 35: 23–39, 1963.

87. Miller, R. C., D. A. Kleinman, and A. Savage, Quantitative studies of optical harmonic generation in CdS, $BaTiO_3$, and KH_2PO_4 type crystals, *Phys. Rev. Lett.* 11: 146–149, 1963.

88. Fejer, M. M., G. A. Magel, D. H. Jundt, and R. L. Byer, Quasi-phase matched second harmonic generation: Tuning and tolerances, *IEEE J. Quantum Elect.* 28: 2631–2654, 1992.

89. Yamada, M., N. Nada, M. Saitoh, and K. Watanabe, First-order quasi-phase matched $LiNbO_3$ waveguide periodically poled by applying an external yield for efficient blue second harmonic generation, *Appl. Phys. Lett.* 62: 435–436, 1993.

90. Burns, W. K., W. McElhanon, and L. Goldberg, Second harmonic generation in field poled, quasi-phase-matched, bulk $LiNbO_3$, *IEEE Photon. Technol. Lett.* 6: 252–254, 1994.

91. Myers, L. E., R. C. Eckardt, M. M. Fejer, R. L. Byer, W. R. Bosenberg, and J. W. Pierce, Quasi-phase-matched optical parametric oscillators in bulk periodically poled $LiNbO_3$, *J. Opt. Soc. Am. B* 12: 2102–2110, 1995.

92. Houé, M. and P. D. Townsend, An introduction to methods of periodic poling for second harmonic generation, *J. Phys. D* 28: 1747–1763, 1995.

93. Miller, R. C., Optical second harmonic generation in piezoelectric crystals, *Appl. Phys. Lett.* 5: 17–19, 1964.

94. Schunemann, P. G., Improved NLO crystals for mid-IR laser applications, *Proc. SPIE.* 6455 (Nonlinear Frequency Generation and Conversion: Materials, Devices, and Applications VI): 64550R/1–64550R/7, 2007.

95. Skauli, T., K. L. Vodopyanov, T. J. Pinguet, A. Schober, O. Levi, L. A. Eyres, M. M. Fejer, B. Gerard, L. Becouarn, E. Lallier, and G. Arisholm, Measurement of nonlinear coefficient of orientation-patterned GaAs and demonstration of highly efficient second harmonic generation, *Opt. Lett.* 27: 628–630, 2002.

96. Skauli, T., P. S. Kuo, K. L. Vodopyanov, T. J. Pinguet, O. Levi, L. A. Eyres, J. S. Harris, M. M. Fejer, B. Gerard, L. Becouarn, and E. Lallier, Improved dispersion relations for GaAs and applications to nonlinear optics, *J. Appl. Phys.* 94: 6447–6455, 2003.

97. Ebert, C. B., L. A. Eyres, M. M. Fejer, and J. S. Harris, MBE growth of antiphase GaAs films using GaAs/Ge/GaAs heteroepitaxy, *J. Cryst. Growth* 201–202: 187–193, 1999.

98. Eyres, L. A., P. J. Tourreau, T. J. Pinguet, C. B. Ebert, J. S. Harris, M. M. Fejer, L. Becouarn, B. Gerard, and E. Lallier, All-epitaxial fabrication of thick, orientation-patterned GaAs films for nonlinear optical frequency conversion, *Appl. Phys. Lett.* 79: 904–906, 2001.

99. Bliss, D. F., C. Lynch, D. Weyburne, K. O'Hearn, and J. S. Bailey, Epitaxial growth of thick GaAs on orientation-patterned wafers for nonlinear optical applications, *J. Cryst. Growth* 287: 673–678, 2006.

100. Yu, X., L. Scaccabarozzi, A. C. Lin, M. M. Fejer, and J. S. Harris, Growth of GaAs with orientation-patterned structures for nonlinear optics, *J. Cryst. Growth* 301–302: 163–167, 2007.

101. Kulp, T. J., S. E. Bisson, R. P. Bambha, T. A. Reichardt, U. B. Goers, K. W. Aniolek, D. A. V. Kliner, B. A. Richman, K. M. Armstrong, R. Sommers, R. Schmitt, P. E. Powers, O. Levi, T. Pinguet, M. Fejer, J. P. Koplow, L. Goldberg, and T. G. McRae. The application of quasi-phasematched parametric light sources to practical infrared chemical sensing systems, *Appl. Phys. B* 75: 317–327, 2002.

102. Levi, O., T. J. Pinguet, T. Skauli, L. A. Eyres, K. R. Parameswaran, J. S. Harris, M. M. Fejer, T. J. Kulp, S. E. Bisson, B. Gerard, E. Lallier, and L. Becouarn. Difference frequency generation of 8-μm radiation in orientation-patterned GaAs, *Opt. Lett.* 27: 2091–2093, 2002.

103. Bisson, S. E., T. J. Kulp, O. Levi, J. S. Harris, and M. M. Fejer, Long-wave IR chemical sensing based on difference frequency generation in orientation-patterned GaAs, *Appl. Phys. B* 85: 199–206, 2006.

104. Vodopyanov, K. L., O. Levi, P. S. Kuo, T. J. Pinguet, J. S. Harris, M. M. Fejer, J. S. Harris, B. Gerard, L. Becouarn, and E. Lallier, Optical parametric oscillation in quasi-phase-matched GaAs, *Opt. Lett.* 29: 1912–1914, 2004.

105. Kuo, P. S., K. L. Vodopyanov, M. M. Fejer, D. M. Simanovskii, X. Yu, J. S. Harris, D. Bliss, and D. Weyburne, Optical parametric generation of a mid-infrared continuum in orientation-patterned GaAs, *Opt. Lett.* 31: 71–73, 2006.

106. Imeshev, G., M. E. Fermann, K. L. Vodopyanov, M. M. Fejer, X. Yu, J. S. Harris, D. Bliss, and C. Lynch, High-power source of THz radiation based on orientation-patterned GaAs pumped by a fiber laser, *Opt. Express* 14: 4439–4444, 2006.

107. Vodopyanov, K. L., M. M. Fejer, X. Yu, J. S. Harris, Y.-S. Lee, W. C. Hurlbut, V. G. Kozlov, D. Bliss, and C. Lynch, Terahertz-wave generation in quasi-phase-matched GaAs, *Appl. Phys. Lett.* 89: 141119/1–141119/3, 2006.

108. Myers, L. E., R. C. Eckardt, M. M. Fejer, R. L. Byer, and W. R. Bosenberg, Multigrating quasi-phase-matched optical parametric oscillators in periodically poled LiNbO$_3$, *Opt. Lett.* 21: 591–593, 1996.

109. Eckardt, R. C., C. D. Nabors, W. J. Kozlovsky, and R. L. Byer, Optical parametric oscillator frequency tuning and control, *J. Opt. Soc. Am. B* 8: 646–667, 1991; see also an erratum in *J. Opt. Soc. Am. B* 12: 2322, 1995.

110. Henderson, A. J., M. J. Padgett, J. Zhang, W. Sibbett, and M. H. Dunn, Continuous frequency tuning of a CW optical parametric oscillator through tuning of its pump source, *Opt. Lett.* 20: 1029–1031, 1995.

111. Scheidt, M., B. Beier, R. Knappe, K.-J. Boller, and R. Wallenstein, Diode-laser-pumped continuous-wave KTP optical parametric oscillator, *J. Opt. Soc. Am. B* 12: 2087–2094, 1995.

112. Lindsay, I. D., G. A. Turnbull, M. H. Dunn, and M. Ebrahim-Zadeh, Doubly-resonant continuous-wave optical parametric oscillator pumped by a single-mode laser diode, *Opt. Lett.* 23: 1889–1891, 1998.

113. Schiller, S., K. Schneider, and J. Mlynek, Theory of an optical parametric oscillator with resonant pump and signal, *J. Opt. Soc. Am. B* 16: 1512–1524, 1999.

114. Yang, S. T., R. C. Eckardt, and R. L. Byer, Continuous-wave singly resonant optical parametric oscillator pumped by a single-frequency resonantly doubled Nd:YAG laser, *Opt. Lett.* 18: 971–973, 1993.

115. Schneider, K., P. Kramper, S. Schiller, and J. Mlynek, Toward an optical synthesizer: A single-frequency parametric oscillator using periodically poled LiNbO$_3$, *Opt. Lett.* 22: 1293–1295, 1997.

116. Schneider, K. and S. Schiller, Narrow-linewidth, pump-enhanced singly-resonant optical parametric oscillator pumped at 532 nm, *Appl. Phys. B* 65: 775–777, 1997.

117. Oshman, M. K. and S. E. Harris, Theory of optical parametric oscillation internal to the laser cavity, *IEEE J. Quantum Elect.* QE-4: 491–502, 1968.

118. Turnbull, G. A., M. H. Dunn, and M. Ebrahim-Zadeh, Continuous-wave, intra-cavity optical parametric oscillators: An analysis of power characteristics, *Appl. Phys. B* 66: 701–710, 1998.

119. Ebrahim-Zadeh, M., G. A. Turnbull, T. J. Edwards, D. J. M. Stothard, I. D. Lindsay, and M. H. Dunn, Intra-cavity continuous-wave singly resonant optical parametric oscillators, *J. Opt. Soc. Am. B* 16: 1499–1511, 1999.

120. Colville, F. G., M. H. Dunn, and M. Ebrahim-Zadeh, Continuous-wave, singly resonant intra-cavity parametric oscillator, *Opt. Lett.* 22: 75–77, 1997.

121. Turnbull, G. A., T. J. Edwards, M. H. Dunn, and M. Ebrahim-Zadeh, Continuous-wave singly resonant intra-cavity optical parametric oscillator based on periodically-poled LiNbO$_3$, *Electron. Lett.* 33: 1817–1818, 1997.

122. Stothard, D. J. M., M. Ebrahim-Zadeh, and M. H. Dunn, Low-pump-threshold, continuous-wave, singly resonant optical parametric oscillator, *Opt. Lett.* 23: 1895–1897, 1997.

123. Bosenberg, W. R., A. Drobshoff, J. I. Alexander, L. E. Myers, and R. L. Byer, Continuous-wave singly resonant optical parametric oscillator based on periodically poled LiNbO$_3$, *Opt. Lett.* 21: 713–715, 1996.

124. Bosenberg, W. R., A. Drobshoff, J. I. Alexander, L. E. Myers, and R. L. Byer, 93% pump depletion, 3.5-W continuous-wave, singly resonant optical parametric oscillator, *Opt. Lett.* 21: 1336–1338, 1996.

125. Powers, P. E., T. J. Kulp, and S. E. Bisson, Continuous tuning of a continuous-wave periodically poled lithium niobate optical parametric oscillator by use of a fan-out grating design, *Opt. Lett.* 23: 159–161, 1998.

126. Klein, M. E., D. H. Lee, J.-P. Meyn, K.-J. Boller, and R. Wallenstein, Singly resonant continuous-wave optical parametric oscillator pumped by a diode laser, *Opt. Lett.* 24: 1142–1144, 1999.

127. Gross, P., M. E. Klein, T. Walde, K.-J. Boller, M. Auerbach, P. Wessels, and C. Fallnich, Fiber-laser-pumped continuous-wave singly-resonant optical parametric oscillator, *Opt. Lett.* 27: 418–420, 2002.

128. Turnbull, G. A., D. McGloin, I. D. Lindsay, M. Ebrahim-Zadeh, and M. H. Dunn, Extended mode-hop-free tuning using a dual-cavity, pump-enhanced optical parametric oscillator, *Opt. Lett.* 25: 341–343, 2000.

129. Lindsay, I. D., C. Petridis, M. H. Dunn, and M. Ebrahim-Zadeh, Continuous-wave pump-enhanced singly-resonant optical parametric oscillator pumped by an external-cavity diode laser, *Appl. Phys. Lett.* 78: 871–873, 2000.

130. Popp, A., F. Müller, F. Kühnemann, S. Schiller, G. von Basum, H. Dahnke, P. Hering, and M. Mürtz, Ultra-sensitive mid-infrared cavity leak-out spectroscopy using a CW optical parametric oscillator, *Appl. Phys. B.* 75: 751–754, 2002.

131. Müller, F., A. Popp, F. Kühnemann, and S. Schiller, Transportable, highly sensitive photoacoustic spectrometer based on a continuous-wave dual-cavity optical parametric oscillator, *Opt. Express* 11: 2820–2825, 2003.

132. Stothard, D. J. M., P.-Y. Fortin, A. Carleton, M. Ebrahim-Zadeh, and M. H. Dunn, Comparison of continuous-wave optical parametric oscillators based on periodically poled LiNbO$_3$ and periodically poled RbTiOAsO$_4$ pumped internal to a high-power Nd:YVO$_4$ laser, *J. Opt. Soc. Am. B* 20: 2102–2108, 2003.

133. Reid, D. T., G. T. Kennedy, A. Miller, W. Sibbett, and M. Ebrahim-Zadeh, Widely tunable near- to mid-infrared femtosecond and picosecond optical parametric oscillators using periodically poled LiNbO$_3$ and RbTiOAsO$_4$, *IEEE J. Sel. Top. Quantum Electron.* 4: 238–248, 1998.

134. Sibbett, W., D. T. Reid, and M. Ebrahim-Zadeh, Versatile femtosecond laser sources for time-resolved studies: Configurations and characterizations, *Phil. Trans. Roy. Soc. London Ser. A* 356(1736): 283–296, 1998.

135. Reid, D. T., J. Sun, T. P. Lamour, and T. I., Ferreiro, Advances in ultrafast optical para- metric oscillators, *Laser Phys. Lett.* 8: 8–15, 2011.

136. Edelstein, D. C., E. S. Wachman, and C. L. Tang, Broadly tunable high repetition rate femtosecond optical parametric oscillator, *Appl. Phys. Lett.* 54: 1728–1730, 1989.

137. Pelouch, W. S., P. E. Powers, and C. L. Tang, Ti:sapphire-pumped, high-repetition-rate femtosecond optical parametric oscillator, *Opt. Lett.* 17: 1070–1072, 1992.

138. Nebel, A., C. Fallnich, R. Beigang, and R. Wallenstein, Noncritically phase-matched continuous-wave mode-locked singly resonant optical parametric oscillator synchro- nously pumped by a Ti:sapphire laser, *J. Opt. Soc. Am. B* 10: 2195–2200, 1993.

139. Chung, J. and A. E. Siegman, Singly resonant continuous-wave mode-locked $KTiOPO_4$ optical parametric oscillator pumped by a Nd:YAG laser, *J. Opt. Soc. Am. B* 10: 2201– 2210, 1993.

140. Grässer, C., D. Wang, R. Beigang, and R. Wallenstein, Singly resonant optical paramet- ric oscillator of $KTiOPO_4$ synchronously pumped by the radiation from a continuous- wave mode-locked Nd:YLF laser, *J. Opt. Soc. Am. B* 10: 2218–2221, 1993.

141. Dudley, J. M., D. T. Reid, M. Ebrahim-Zadeh, and W. Sibbett, Characteristics of a non- critically phase-matched Ti:sapphire-pumped femtosecond optical parametric oscilla- tor, *Opt. Commun.* 104: 419–430, 1994.

142. McCahon, S. W., S. A. Anson, D.-J. Jang, and T. F. Boggess, Generation of 3–4-µm femtosecond pulses from a synchronously pumped, critically phase-matched $KTiOPO_4$ optical parametric oscillator, *Opt. Lett.* 22: 2309–2311, 1995.

143. Fallnich, C., B. Ruffing, T. Herrmann, A. Nebel, R. Beigang, and R. Wallenstein, Experimental investigation and numerical simulation of the influence of resonator- length detuning on the output power, pulse duration and spectral width of a CW mode- locked picosecond optical parametric oscillator, *Appl. Phys. B.* 60: 427–436, 1995.

144. Nebel, A., H. Frost, R. Beigang, and R. Wallenstein, Visible femtosecond pulses by second-harmonic generation of a CW mode-locked KTP optical parametric oscillator, *Appl. Phys. B.* 60: 453–458, 1995.

145. French, S., M. Ebrahim-Zadeh, and A. Miller, High-power, high-repetition-rate pico- second optical parametric oscillator for the near- to mid-infrared, *Opt. Lett.* 21: 131– 133, 1996.

146. Burr, K. C., C. L Tang, M. A. Arbore, and M. M. Fejer, Broadly tunable mid-infrared femtosecond optical parametric oscillator using all-solid-state-pumped periodically poled lithium niobate, *Opt. Lett.* 22: 1458–1460, 1997.

147. Reid, D. T., C. McGowan, W. Sleat, M. Ebrahim-Zadeh, and W. Sibbett, Compact, efficient 344-MHz repetition-rate femtosecond optical parametric oscillator, *Opt. Lett.* 22: 525–527, 1997.

148. Reid, D. T., Z. Penman, M. Ebrahim-Zadeh, W. Sibbett, H. Karlsson, and F. Laurell, Broadly tunable infrared femtosecond optical parametric oscillator based on periodi- cally poled $RbTiOAsO_4$, *Opt. Lett.* 22: 1397–1399, 1997.

149. McGowan, C., D. T. Reid, Z. E. Penman, M. Ebrahim-Zadeh, W. Sibbett, and D. H. Jundt, Femtosecond optical parametric oscillator based on periodically poled lithium niobate, *J. Opt. Soc. Am. B* 15: 694–701, 1998.

150. Kennedy, G. T., D. T. Reid, A. Miller, M. Ebrahim-Zadeh, H. Karlsson, G. Arvidsson, and F. Laurell, Near- to mid-infrared picosecond optical parametric oscillator based on periodically poled $RbTiOAsO_4$, *Opt. Lett.* 23: 503–505, 1998.

151. Penman, Z. E., P. Loza-Alvarez, D. T. Reid, M. Ebrahim-Zadeh, W. Sibbett, and D. H. Jundt, All-solid state mid-infrared femtosecond optical parametric oscillator based on periodically-poled lithium niobate, *Opt. Commun.* 146: 147–150, 1998.

152. Lefort, L., K. Peuch, G. W. Ross, Y. P. Svirko, and D. C. Hanna, Optical paramet- ric oscillation out to 6.3 µm in periodically poled lithium niobate under strong idler absorption, *Appl. Phys. Lett.* 73: 1610–1612, 1998.

153. Penman, Z. E., C. McGowan, P. Loza-Alvarez, D. T. Reid, M. Ebrahim-Zadeh, W. Sibbett, and D. H. Jundt, Femtosecond optical parametric oscillators based on periodically poled lithium niobate, *J. Mod. Opt.* 45: 1285–1294, 1998.

154. Loza-Alvarez, P., D. T. Reid, M. Ebrahim-Zadeh, W. Sibbett, H. Karlsson, P. Henriksson, G. Arvidsson, and F. Laurell, Periodically poled RbTiOAsO$_4$ femtosecond optical parametric oscillator tunable from 1.38 to 1.58 μm, *Appl. Phys. B.* 146: 177–180, 1999.

155. Loza-Alvarez, P., C. T. A. Brown, D. T. Reid, W. Sibbett, and M. Missey, High repetition-rate ultrashort-pulse optical parametric oscillator continuously tunable from 2.8 to 6.8 μm, *Opt. Lett.* 24: 1523–1525, 1999.

156. Marzenell, S., R. Beigang, and R. Wallenstein, Synchronously pumped femtosecond optical parametric oscillator based on AgGaSe$_2$ tunable from 2 μm to 8 μm, *Appl. Phys. B* 69: 423–428, 1999.

157. Ebrahim-Zadeh, M., P. J. Phillips, and S. Das, Low-threshold, mid-infrared optical parametric oscillation in periodically poled LiNbO$_3$ synchronously pumped by a Ti:sapphire laser, *Appl. Phys. B.* 72: 793–801, 2001.

158. Maus, M., E. Rousseau, M. Cotlet, G. Schweitzer, J. Hofkens, M. Van der Auweraer, F. C. De Schryver, and A. Krueger, New picosecond laser system for easy tunability over the whole ultraviolet/visible/near infrared wavelength range based on flexible harmonic generation and optical parametric oscillation, *Rev. Sci. Instrum.* 72: 36–40, 2001.

159. Sudmeyer, T., J. Aus der Au, R. Paschotta, U. Keller, P. G. R. Smith, G. W. Ross, and D. C. Hanna, Novel ultrafast parametric systems: High repetition rate single-pass OPG and fibre-feedback OPO, *J. Phys. D: Appl. Phys.* 34: 2433–2439, 2001.

160. Hoyt, C. W., M. Sheik-Bahae, and M. Ebrahim-Zadeh, High-power picosecond optical parametric oscillator based on periodically poled lithium niobate, *Opt. Lett.* 27: 1543–1545, 2002.

161. Artigas, D. and D. T. Reid, High idler conversion in femtosecond optical parametric oscillators, *Opt. Commun.* 210: 113–120, 2002.

162. Tillman, K. A., D. T. Reid, D. Artigas, J. Hellstrom, V. Pasiškevičius, and F. Laurell, Low-threshold, high-repetition-frequency femtosecond optical parametric oscillator based on chirped-pulse frequency conversion, *J. Opt. Soc. Am. B* 20: 1309–1316, 2003.

163. Tillman, K. A., D. T. Reid, D. Artigas, J., and T. Y. Jiang, Idler-resonant femtosecond tandem optical parametric oscillator tuning from 2.1 μm to 4.2 μm, *J. Opt. Soc. Am. B* 21: 1551–1558, 2004.

164. Tillman, K. A., R. R. J. Maier, D. T. Reid, and E. D. McNaghten, Mid-infrared absorption spectroscopy across a 14.4 THz spectral range using a broadband femtosecond optical parametric oscillator, *Appl. Phys. Lett.* 85: 3366–3368, 2004.

165. Tillman, K. A., R. R. J. Maier, D. T. Reid, and E. D. McNaghten, Mid-infrared absorption spectroscopy of methane using a broadband femtosecond optical parametric oscillator based on aperiodically poled lithium niobate, *J. Opt. A: Pure Appl. Opt.* 7: S408–S414, 2005.

166. Tillman, K. A., D. T. Reid, R. R. J. Maier, and E. D. McNaghten, Mid-infrared absorption spectroscopy of methane across a 14.4-THz spectral range using a broadband femtosecond optical parametric oscillator based on aperiodically poled lithium niobate, *Proc. SPIE* 5989 (Technologies for Optical Countermeasures II; Femtosecond Phenomena II; and Passive Millimetre-Wave and Terahertz Imaging II): 59890U/1–59890U/9, 2005.

167. Kornaszewski, L. W., N. Gayraud, J. M. Stone, W. N. MacPherson, A. K. George, J. C. Knight, D. P. Hand, and D. T. Reid, Mid-infrared methane detection in a photonic bandgap fiber using a broadband optical parametric oscillator, *Opt. Express* 15: 11219–11224, 2007.

168. Ebrahim-Zadeh, M., Efficient ultrafast frequency conversion sources for the visible and ultraviolet based on BiB$_3$O$_6$, *IEEE J. Sel. Top. Quantum Electron.* 13: 679–691, 2007.

169. Gayraud, N., L. W. Kornaszewski, J. M. Stone, J. C. Knight, and D. T. Reid, Mid-infrared gas sensing using a photonic bandgap fiber, *Appl. Opt.* 47: 1269–1277, 2008.

170. Sun, J. H., B. J. S. Gale, and D. T. Reid, Control of the carrier-envelope phases of a synchronously pumped femtosecond optical parametric oscillator and its applications, *Chinese Sci. Bull.* 53: 642–651, 2008.

171. Adler, F., K. C. Cossel, M. J. Thorpe, I. Hartl, M. E. Fermann, and J. Ye, Phase-stabilized, 1.5 W frequency comb at 2.8–4.8 μm, *Opt. Lett.* 34: 1330–1332, 2009.

172. Lamour, T. P., L. Kornaszewski, J. H. Sun, and D. T. Reid, Yb:fiber-laser-pumped high-energy picosecond optical parametric oscillator, *Opt. Express* 17: 14229–14234, 2009.

173. Sun, J. H. and D. T. Reid, Coherent synthesis of visible-region optical pulses by using an optical parametric oscillator and a laser, *Proc. SPIE* 7431 (Time and Frequency Metrology II): 743103/1–743103/8, 2009.

174. Ferreiro, T. I., J. H. Sun, and D. T. Reid, Locking the carrier-envelope-offset frequency of an optical parametric oscillator without f–$2f$ self-referencing, *Opt. Lett.* 35: 1668–1670, 2010.

175. Lamour, T. P., J. H. Sun, and D. T. Reid, Wavelength stabilization of a synchronously pumped optical parametric oscillator: Optimizing proportional-integral control, *Rev. Sci. Instrum.* 81: 053101/1–053101/6, 2010.

176. Adler, F., P. Maslowski, A. Foltynowicz, K. C. Cossel, T. C. Briles, I. Hartl, and J. Ye, Mid-infrared Fourier transform spectroscopy with a broadband frequency comb, *Opt. Express* 18: 21861–21872, 2010.

177. Leindecker, N., A. Marandi, R. L. Byer, and K. L. Vodopyanov, Broadband degenerate OPO for mid-infrared frequency comb generation, *Opt. Express* 19: 6296–6302, 2011.

178. Vodopyanov, K. L., E. Sorokin, I. T. Sorokina, and P. G. Schunemann, Mid-IR frequency comb source spanning 4.4–5.4 μm based on subharmonic GaAs optical parametric oscillator, *Opt. Lett.* 36: 2275–2277, 2011.

179. Zhang, Z. W., J. H. Sun, T. Gardiner, and D. T. Reid, Broadband conversion in an Yb:KYW-pumped ultrafast optical parametric oscillator with a long nonlinear crystal, *Opt. Express* 19: 17127–17132, 2011.

180. Lamour, T. P. and D. T. Reid, 650-nJ pulses from a cavity-dumped Yb:fiber-pumped ultrafast optical parametric oscillator, *Opt. Express* 19: 17557–17562, 2011.

181. Zhang, Z. W., C. L. Gu, J. H. Sun, C. Y. Wang, T. Gardiner, and D. T. Reid, Asynchronous midinfrared ultrafast optical parametric oscillator for dual-comb spectroscopy, *Opt. Lett.* 37: 187–189, 2012.

182. Leindecker, N., A. Marandi, K. L. Vodopyanov, and R. L. Byer, Broadband mid-IR subharmonic OPOs for molecular spectroscopy, *Proc. SPIE* 8240 (Nonlinear Frequency Generation and Conversion: Materials, Devices, and Applications XI): 82400X/1–82400X/7, 2012.

183. Leindecker, N., A. Marandi, R. L. Byer, K. L. Vodopyanov, J. Jiang, I. Hartl, M. Fermann, and P. G. Schunemann, Octave-spanning ultrafast OPO with 2.6–6.1 μm instantaneous bandwidth pumped by femtosecond Tm-fiber laser, *Opt. Express* 20: 7046–7053, 2012.

184. Marandi, A., N. C. Leindecker, V. Pervak, R. L. Byer, and K. L. Vodopyanov, Coherence properties of a broadband femtosecond mid-IR optical parametric oscillator operating at degeneracy, *Opt. Express* 20: 7255–7262, 2012.

185. Ricciardi, I., E. De Tommasi, P. Maddaloni, S. Mosca, A. Rocco, J.-J. Zondy, M. De Rosa, and P. De Natale, Frequency comb-referenced singly-resonant OPO for sub-Doppler spectroscopy, *Opt. Express* 20: 9178–9186, 2012.

186. McCracken, R. A., J. H. Sun, C. G. Leburn, and D. T. Reid, Broadband phase coherence between an ultrafast laser and an OPO using lock-to-zero CEO stabilization, *Opt. Express* 20: 16269–16274, 2012.

187. Gu, C., M. Hu, L. Zhang, J. Fan, Y. Song, C. Wang, and D. T. Reid, High average power, widely tunable femtosecond laser source from red to mid-infrared based on an Yb-fiber-laser-pumped optical parametric oscillator, *Opt. Lett.* 38: 1820–1822, 2013.

188. Zhang, Z. W., T. Gardiner, and D. T. Reid, Mid-infrared dual-comb spectroscopy with an optical parametric oscillator, *Opt. Lett.* 38: 3148–3150, 2013.

189. Zhang, Z. W., D. T. Reid, S. C. Kumar, M. Ebrahim-Zadeh, P. G. Schunemann, K. T. Zawilski, and C. R. Howle, Femtosecond-laser pumped CdSiP$_2$ optical parametric oscillator producing 100 MHz pulses centered at 6.2 μm, *Opt. Lett.* 38: 5110–5113, 2013.

190. Foltynowicz, A., P. Maslowski, A. Fleisher, B. Bjork, and J. Ye, Cavity-enhanced optical frequency comb spectroscopy in the mid-infrared application to trace detection of hydrogen peroxide, *Appl. Phys. B* 110: 163–175, 2013.

191. Lee, K. F., J. Jiang, C. Mohr, J. Bethge, M. E. Fermann, N. Leindecker, K. L. P. G. Schunemann, and I. Hartl, Carrier envelope offset frequency of a doubly resonant, non-degenerate, mid-infrared GaAs optical parametric oscillator, *Opt. Lett.* 38: 1191–1193, 2013.

192. Ingold, K. A., A. Marandi, C. W. Rudy, K. L. Vodopyanov, and R. L. Byer, Fractional-length sync-pumped degenerate optical parametric oscillator for 500-MHz 3-μm mid-infrared frequency comb generation, *Opt. Lett.* 39: 900–903, 2014.

193. Lee, K. F., N. Granzow, M. A. Schmidt, W. Chang, L. Wang, Q. Coulombier, J. Troles, N. Leindecker, K. L. Vodopyanov, P. G. Schunemann, M. E. Fermann, P. S. Russell, and I. Hartl. Midinfrared frequency combs from coherent supercontinuum in chalcogenide and optical parametric oscillation, *Opt. Lett.* 39: 2056–2059, 2014.

194. Reid, D. T., Z. W. Zhang, and C. R. Howle, Active FTIR-based standoff detection in the 3–4 micron region using broadband femtosecond optical parametric oscillators, *Proc. SPIE* 9073 (Chemical, Biological, Radiological, Nuclear, and Explosives—CBRNE—Sensing XV): 907302/1–907302/7, 2014.

195. Danielius, R., A. Piskarskas, A. Stabinis, G. P. Banfi, P. Di Trapani, and R. Righini, Traveling-wave parametric generation of widely tunable, highly coherent femtosecond light pulses, *J. Opt. Soc. Am. B* 10: 2222–2231, 1993; see also an erratum in *J. Opt. Soc. Am. B* 12: 2321, 1995.

196. Cerullo, G. and S. De Silvestri, Ultrafast optical parametric amplifiers, *Rev. Sci. Instrum.* 74: 1–18, 2003.

197. Dubietis, A., R. Butkus, and A. P. Piskarskas, Trends in chirped pulse optical parametric amplification, *IEEE J. Sel. Top. Quantum Electron.* 12: 163–172, 2006.

198. Tiihonen, M., V. Pasiškevičius, and F. Laurell, Broadly tunable picosecond narrow-band pulses in a periodically-poled KTiOPO$_4$ parametric amplifier, *Opt. Express* 14: 8728–8736, 2006.

199. Siegman, A. E., *Lasers*, University Science, Mill Valley, CA, 1986.

200. Stowe, M. C., Thorpe, M. J., Pe'er, A., Ye, J., Stalnaker, J. E., Gerginov, V., and Diddams, S. A., Direct frequency comb spectroscopy, *Adv. Atom. Mol. Opt. Phys.* 55: 1–60, 2008.

201. Salour, M. M. and C. Cohen-Tannoudji, Observation of Ramsey's interference fringes in the profile of Doppler-free two-photon resonances, *Phys. Rev. Lett.* 38: 757–760, 1977.

202. Teets, R., J. Eckstein, and T. W. Hänsch, Coherent two-photon excitation by multiple light pulses, *Phys. Rev. Lett.* 38: 760–764, 1977.

203. Udem, Th. and F. Riehle, Frequency combs applications and optical frequency standards, *Rivista del Nuovo Cimento* 30: 563–606, 2007.

204. Diddams, S. A., The evolving optical frequency comb [Invited], *J. Opt. Soc. Am. B* 27: B51–B62, 2010.

205. Jones, D. J., S. A. Diddams, J. K. Ranka, A. Stentz, R. S. Windeler, J. L. Hall, and S. T. Cundiff, Carrier-envelope phase control of femtosecond mode-locked lasers and direct optical frequency synthesis, *Science* 288: 635–639, 2000.

206. Schibli, T. R., I. Hartl, D. C. Yost, M. J. Martin, A. Marcinkevičius, M. E. Fermann, and J. Ye, Optical frequency comb with submillihertz linewidth and more than 10 W average power, *Nat. Photon.* 2: 355–359, 2008.

207. Hagemann, C., C. Grebing, C. Lisdat, S. Falke, T. Legero, U. Sterr, F. Riehle, M. Martin, and J. Ye, Ultrastable laser with average fractional frequency drift rate below 5×10^{-19}/ s, *Opt. Lett.* 39: 5102–5105, 2014.

208. Adler, F., M. J. Thorpe, K. C. Cossel, and J. Ye, Cavity-enhanced direct frequency comb spectroscopy: Technology and applications, *Ann. Rev. Anal. Chem.* 3: 175–205, 2010.

209. Foltynowicz, A., P. Masłowski, T. Ban, F. Adler, K. C. Cossel, T. C. Briles, and J. Ye, Optical frequency comb spectroscopy, *Faraday Discuss.* 150: 23–31, 2011.

210. Masłowski, P., K. C. Cossel, A. Foltynowicz, and J. Ye, Cavity-enhanced direct frequency comb spectroscopy. In G. Gagliardi and H.-P. Loock (Eds), *Cavity-Enhanced Spectroscopy and Sensing*, Chapter 8, pp. 271–321, Springer, Berlin, 2014.

211. Thorpe, M. J., K. D. Moll, R. J. Jones, B. Safdi, and J. Ye, Broadband cavity ring-down spectroscopy for sensitive and rapid molecular detection, *Science* 311: 1595–1599, 2006.

212. Thorpe, M. J., D. D. Hudson, K. D. Moll, J. Lasri, and J. Ye, Cavity-ringdown molecular spectroscopy based on an optical frequency comb at 1.45–1.65 micrometers, *Opt. Lett.* 32: 307–309, 2007.

213. Thorpe, M. J., D. Balslev-Clausen, M. S. Kirchner, and J. Ye, Cavity-enhanced optical frequency comb spectroscopy: Application to human breath analysis, *Opt. Express.* 16: 2387–2397, 2008.

214. Thorpe, M. J. and J. Ye, Cavity-enhanced direct frequency comb spectroscopy, *Appl. Phys. B* 91: 397–414, 2008.

215. Thorpe, M. J., F. Adler, K. C. Cossel, M. H. G. de Miranda, and J. Ye, Tomography of a supersonically cooled molecular jet using cavity-enhanced direct frequency comb spectroscopy, *Chem. Phys. Lett.* 468: 1–8, 2009.

216. Cossel, K. C., F. Adler, K. A. Bertness, M. J. Thorpe, J. Feng, M. W. Raynor, and J. Ye, Analysis of trace impurities in semiconductor gas via cavity-enhanced direct frequency comb spectroscopy, *Appl. Phys. B.* 100: 917–924, 2010.

217. Foltynowicz, A., T. Ban, P. Masłowski, F. Adler, and J. Ye, Quantum-noise-limited optical frequency comb spectroscopy, *Phys. Rev. Lett.* 107: 233002/1–233002/5, 2011.

218. Nugent-Glandorf, L., T. Neely, F. Adler, A. J. Fleisher, K. C. Cossel, B. Bjork, T. Dinneen, J. Ye, and S. A. Diddams, Mid-infrared virtually imaged phased array spectrometer for rapid and broadband trace gas detection, *Opt. Lett.* 37: 3285–3287, 2012.

219. Fleisher, A. J., B. J. Bjork, T. Q. Bui, K. C. Cossel, M. Okumura, and J. Ye, Mid-infrared time-resolved frequency comb spectroscopy of transient free radicals, *J. Phys. Chem. Lett.* 5: 2241–2246, 2014.

220. Hartl, I., A. Marcinkevicius, M. E. Fermann, T. R. Schibli, D. C. Yost, D. D. Hudson, and J. Ye, Cavity-enhanced similariton Yb-fiber laser frequency comb: 3×10^{14} W/cm^2 peak intensity at 136 MHz, *Opt. Lett.* 32: 2870–2872, 2007.

221. Inaba, H., T. Ikegami, F.-L. Hong, Y. Bitou, A. Onae, T. R. Schibli, K. Minoshima, and H. Matsumoto, Doppler-free spectroscopy using a continuous-wave optical frequency synthesizer, *Appl. Opt.* 45: 4910–4915, 2006.

222. Inaba, H., T. Ikegami, F.-L. Hong, A. Onae, Y. Koga, T. R. Schibli, K. Minoshima, H. Matsumoto, S. Yamadori, O. Tohyama, and S.-I. Yamaguchi. Phase locking of a continuous-wave optical parametric oscillator to an optical frequency comb for optical frequency synthesis, *IEEE J. Quantum Elect.* 40: 929–936, 2004.

223. Vaernewijck, X. D. D., K. Didriche, C. Lauzin, A. Rizopoulos, M. Herman, and S. Kassi, Cavity enhanced FTIR spectroscopy using femto OPO absorption source, *Mol. Phys.* 109: 2173–2179, 2011.

224. Jin, Y. W., S. M. Cristescu, F. J. M. Harren, and J. Mandon, Two-crystal mid-infrared optical parametric oscillator for absorption and dispersion dual-comb spectroscopy, *Opt. Lett.* 39: 3270–3273, 2014.

225. Haub, J. G., M. J. Johnson, B. J. Orr, and R. Wallenstein, A continuously tunable, injection-seeded β-barium borate optical parametric oscillator: Spectroscopic applications, *Appl. Phys. Lett.* 58: 1718–1720, 1991.

226. Fix, A., T. Schröder, R. Wallenstein, J. G. Haub, M. J. Johnson, and B. J. Orr, A tunable β-barium borate optical parametric oscillator: Operating characteristics with and without injection seeding, *J. Opt. Soc. Am. B* 10: 1744–1750, 1993.

227. Haub, J. G., M. J. Johnson, and B. J. Orr, Spectroscopic and nonlinear-optical applications of a tunable β-barium borate optical parametric oscillator, *J. Opt. Soc. Am. B* 10: 1765–1777, 1993.

228. Johnson, M. J., J. G. Haub, H.-D. Barth, and B. J. Orr, Rotationally resolved coherent anti-Stokes Raman spectroscopy by using a tunable optical parametric oscillator, *Opt. Lett.* 18: 441–443, 1993.

229. Johnson, M. J., J. G. Haub, and B. J. Orr, Continuously tunable, narrowband operation of an injection-seeded ring-cavity optical parametric oscillator: Spectroscopic applications, *Opt. Lett.* 20: 1277–1279, 1995.

230. Haub, J. G., M. J. Johnson, A. J. Powell, and B. J. Orr, Bandwidth characteristics of a pulsed optical parametric oscillator: Application to degenerate four-wave mixing spectroscopy, *Opt. Lett.* 20: 1637–1639, 1995.

231. Haub, J. G., R. M. Hentschel, M. J. Johnson, and B. J. Orr, Controlling the performance of a pulsed optical parametric oscillator: A survey of techniques and spectroscopic applications, *J. Opt. Soc. Am. B* 12: 2128–2141, 1995.

232. Baxter, G. W., M. J. Johnson, J. G. Haub, and B. J. Orr, OPO CARS: Coherent anti-Stokes Raman spectroscopy using tunable optical parametric oscillators injection-seeded by external-cavity diode lasers, *Chem. Phys. Lett.* 251: 211–218, 1996.

233. Baxter, G. W., J. G. Haub, and B. J. Orr, Back conversion in a pulsed optical parametric oscillator: Evidence from injection-seeded sidebands, *J. Opt. Soc. Am. B* 14: 2723–2730, 1997.

234. Baxter, G. W., H.-D. Barth, and B. J. Orr, Laser spectroscopy with a pulsed, narrowband infrared optical parametric oscillator system: A practical, modular approach, *Appl. Phys. B* 66: 653–657, 1998.

235. Baxter, G. W., Y. He, and B. J. Orr, A pulsed optical parametric oscillator, based on periodically poled lithium niobate (PPLN), for high-resolution spectroscopy, *Appl. Phys. B* 67: 753–756, 1998.

236. He, Y., G. W. Baxter, and B. J. Orr, Locking the cavity of a pulsed PPLN optical parametric oscillator to the wavelength of a CW injection-seeder by an "intensity-dip" method, *Rev. Sci. Instrum.* 70: 3203–3213, 1999.

237. He, Y. and B. J. Orr, Tunable single-mode operation of a pulsed optical parametric oscillator pumped by a multi-mode laser, *Appl. Opt.* 40: 4836–4848, 2001.

238. He, Y. and B. J. Orr, Cavity ringdown spectroscopy: New approaches and outcomes, *J. Chinese Chem. Soc. (Taiwan)* 48: 591–601, 2001.

239. White, R. T., Y. He, B. J. Orr, M. Kono, and K. G. H. Baldwin, Pulsed injection-seeded optical parametric oscillator with low frequency chirp for high-resolution spectroscopy, *Opt. Lett.* 28: 1248–1250, 2003.

240. White, R. T., Y. He, B. J. Orr, M. Kono, and K. G. H. Baldwin, Control of frequency chirp in nanosecond-pulsed laser spectroscopy. 1. Optical-heterodyne chirp analysis techniques, *J. Opt. Soc. Am. B* 21: 1577–1585, 2004.

241. White, R. T., Y. He, B. J. Orr, M. Kono, and K. G. H. Baldwin, Control of frequency chirp in nanosecond-pulsed laser spectroscopy. 2. A long-pulse optical parametric oscillator for narrow optical bandwidth, *J. Opt. Soc. Am. B* 21: 1586–1594, 2004.

242. White, R. T., Y. He, B. J. Orr, M. Kono, and K. G. H. Baldwin, Transition from single-mode to multimode operation of an injection-seeded pulsed optical parametric oscillator, *Opt. Express* 12: 5655–5660, 2004.

243. Kono, M., K. G. H. Baldwin, Y. He, R. T. White, and B. J. Orr, Heterodyne-assisted pulsed spectroscopy with a nearly Fourier-transform limited, injection-seeded optical parametric oscillator, *Opt. Lett.* 30: 3413–3415, 2005.

244. Kono, M., K. G. H. Baldwin, Y. He, R. T. White, and B. J. Orr, CHAPS: A new precision laser-spectroscopic technique, *J. Opt. Soc. Am. B* 23: 1181–1189, 2006.

245. White, R. T., Y. He, B. J. Orr, M. Kono, and K. G. H. Baldwin, Control of frequency chirp in nanosecond-pulsed laser spectroscopy. 3. Spectrotemporal dynamics of an injection-seeded optical parametric oscillator, *J. Opt. Soc. Am. B* 24: 2601–2609, 2007.

246. He, Y., M. Kono, R. T. White, M. J. Sellars, K. G. H. Baldwin, and B. J. Orr, Coherent heterodyne-assisted pulsed spectroscopy: Sub-Doppler two-photon spectra of krypton, characterizing a tunable nonlinear-optical ultraviolet light source, *Appl. Phys. B* 99: 609–612, 2010.

247. Kono, M., Y. He, K. G. H. Baldwin, and B. J. Orr, Sub-Doppler two-photon spectroscopy of 33 Rydberg levels in atomic xenon excited at 205–213 nm: Diverse isotopic and hyperfine structure, *J. Phys. B* 46: 035401/1–035401/16, 2013.

248. He, Y. and B. J. Orr, Narrowband tuning of an injection-seeded pulsed optical parametric oscillator based on a self-adaptive, phase-conjugate cavity mirror, *Opt. Lett.* 29: 2169–2171, 2004.

249. He, Y. and B. J. Orr, Self-adaptive, narrowband tuning of a pulsed optical parametric oscillator and a continuous-wave diode laser via phase-conjugate photorefractive cavity reflectors: Verification by high-resolution spectroscopy, *Appl. Phys. B.* 96: 545–560, 2009.

250. Giordmaine, J. A. and R. C. Miller, Tunable coherent parametric oscillation in $LiNbO_3$ at optical frequencies, *Phys. Rev. Lett.* 14: 973–976, 1965.

251. Ebrahim-Zadeh, M., A. J. Henderson, and M. H. Dunn, An excimer-pumped β-BaB_2O_4 optical parametric oscillator tunable from 354 nm to 2.370 μm, *IEEE J. Quantum Elec.* 26: 1241–1252, 1990.

252. Myers, L. E. and W. R. Bosenberg, Periodically poled lithium niobate and quasi-phase-matched optical parametric oscillators, *IEEE J. Quantum Elect.* 33: 1663–1672, 1997.

253. Bäder, U., J. Bartschke, I. Klimov, A. Borsutzky, and R. Wallenstein, Optical parametric oscillator of quasi-phase-matched $LiNbO_3$ pumped by a compact high repetition rate single-frequency passively Q-switched Nd:YAG laser, *Opt. Commun.* 147: 95–98, 1998.

254. Hellstrom, J., V. Pasiškevičius, F. Laurell, and H. Karlsson, Efficient nanosecond optical parametric oscillators based on periodically poled KTP emitting in the 1.8–2.5 μm spectral range, *Opt. Lett.* 24: 1233–1235, 1999.

255. Chen, Y.-H., Y.-Y. Lin, C.-H. Chen, and Y.-C. Huang, Monolithic quasi-phase-matched nonlinear crystal for simultaneous laser Q switching and parametric oscillation in a Nd:YVO$_4$ laser, *Opt. Lett.* 30: 1045–1047, 2005.

256. Cho, K.-H., B. K. Rhee, Y. Sasaki, and H. Ito, Pulsed intra-cavity optical parametric oscillator with high average power based on periodically poled $LiNbO_3$, *J. Nonlinear Opt. Phys. Mater.* 14: 383–389, 2005.

257. Tsai, L. Y., Y. F. Chen, S.-T. Lin, Y.-Y. Lin, and Y.-C. Huang, Compact efficient passively Q-switched Nd:GdVO$_4$/PPLN/Cr^{4+}:YAG tunable intra-cavity optical parametric oscillator, *Opt. Express.* 13: 9543–9547, 2005.

258. Zhang, X., B. Yao, Y. Wang, Y. Ju, and Y. Zhang, Middle-infrared intra-cavity periodically poled MgO:LiNbO$_3$ optical parametric oscillator, *Chinese Opt. Lett.* 5: 426–427, 2007.

259. Gorelik, P. V., F. N. C. Wong, D. Kolker, and J.-J. Zondy, Cascaded optical parametric oscillation with a dual-grating periodically poled lithium niobate crystal, *Opt. Lett.* 31: 2039–2041, 2006.

260. Isyanova, Y., G. A. Rines, D. Welford, and P. F. Moulton, Tandem OPO source generating 1.5–10-µm wavelengths. In S. Payne and C. Pollack (Eds), *Advanced Solid State Lasers*, Volume 1, *OSA Trends in Optics and Photonics* (Optical Society of America, 1996), paper OP10; http://www.osapublishing.org/abstract.cfm?URI=ASSL-1996-OP10.

261. Isyanova, Y., A. Dergachev, D. Welford, and P. F. Moulton, Multi-wavelength, 1.5–10-µm tunable, tandem OPO. In M. Fejer, H. Injeyan, and U. Keller (Eds), *Advanced Solid State Lasers*, Volume 26, *OSA Trends in Optics and Photonics* (Optical Society of America, 1999), paper WB4; http://www.osapublishing.org/abstract.cfm?URI=ASSL-1999-WB4.

262. Ganikhanov, F., T. Caughey, and K. L. Vodopyanov, Narrow-linewidth middle-infrared ZnGeP$_2$ optical parametric oscillator, *J. Opt. Soc. Am. B* 18: 818–822, 2001.

263. Henriksson, M., M. Tiihonen, V. Pasiškevičius, and F. Laurell, ZnGeP$_2$ parametric oscillator pumped by a linewidth-narrowed parametric 2 µm source, *Opt. Lett.* 31: 1878–1880, 2006.

264. Henriksson, M., M. Tiihonen, V. Pasiškevičius, and F. Laurell, Mid-infrared ZGP OPO pumped by near-degenerate narrowband type-I PPKTP parametric oscillator, *Appl. Phys. B* 88: 37–41, 2007.

265. Henriksson, M., L. Sjöqvist, M. Tiihonen, V. Pasiškevičius, and F. Laurell, Tandem OPO systems for mid-infrared generation using quasi phase-matching and volume Bragg gratings, *Proc. SPIE* 6738 (Technologies for Optical Countermeasures IV): 673805/1–673805/11, 2007.

266. Henriksson, M., L. Sjöqvist, M. Tiihonen, V. Pasiškevičius, and F. Laurell, Tandem PPKTP and ZGP OPO for mid-infrared generation, *Proc. SPIE* 7115 (Technologies for Optical Countermeasures V): 71150O/1–71150O/10, 2008.

267. Lancaster, D. G., Efficient Nd:YAG pumped mid-IR laser based on cascaded KTP and ZGP optical parametric oscillators and a ZGP parametric amplifier, *Opt. Commun.* 282: 272–275, 2009.

268. Agnesi, A., E. Piccinini, G. C. Reali, and C. Solcia, Efficient all-solid-state tunable source based on a passively Q-switched high-power Nd:YAG laser, *Appl. Phys. B.* 65: 303–305, 1997.

269. Karlsson, H., M. Olson, G. Arvidsson, F. Laurell, U. Bäder, A. Borsutzky, R. Wallenstein, S. Wickström, and M. Gustafsson, Nanosecond optical parametric oscillator based on large-aperture periodically poled RbTiOAsO$_4$, *Opt. Lett.* 24: 330–332, 1999.

270. Conroy, R. S., C. F. Rae, M. H. Dunn, B. D. Sinclair, and J. M. Ley, Compact, actively Q-switched optical parametric oscillator, *Opt. Lett.* 24: 1614–1616, 1999.

271. Baxter, G. W., P. Schlup, and I. T. McKinnie, Efficient, single frequency, high repetition rate, PPLN OPO pumped by a prelase Q-switched diode-pumped Nd:YAG laser, *Appl. Phys. B.* 70: 301–304, 2000.

272. Elder, I. F. and J. A. C. Terry, Efficient conversion into the near- and mid-infrared using a PPLN OPO, *J. Opt. A* 2: L19–L23, 2000.

273. Hansson, G. and D. D. Smith, Mid-infrared-wavelength generation in 2-µm pumped periodically poled lithium niobate, *Appl. Opt.* 37: 5743–5746, 1998.

274. Britton, P. E., D. Taverner, K. Puech, D. J. Richardson, P. G. R. Smith, G. W. Ross, and D. C. Hanna, Optical parametric oscillation in periodically poled lithium niobate driven by a diode-pumped Q-switched erbium fiber laser, *Opt. Lett.* 23: 582–584, 1998.

275. Britton, P. E., H. L. Offerhaus, D. J. Richardson, P. G. R. Smith, G. W. Ross, and D. C. Hanna, Parametric oscillator directly pumped by a 1.55-μm erbium-fiber laser, *Opt. Lett.* 24: 975–977, 1999.

276. Nakamura, K., T. Hatanaka, and H. Ito, High output energy quasi-phase-matched optical parametric oscillator using diffusion-bonded periodically poled and single domain LiNbO3, *Jap. J. Appl. Phys. 2: Lett* 40: L337–L339, 2001.

277. Zhang, B., J. Yao, H. Zhang, D. Xu, P. Wang, X. Li, and X. Ding, Angle-tuned signal-resonated optical parametric oscillator based on periodically poled lithium niobate, *Chinese Opt. Lett.* 1: 346–349, 2003.

278. Chiang, A.-C., T.-D. Wang, Y.-Y. Lin, C.-W. Lau, Y.-H. Chen, B.-C. Wong, Y.-C. Huang, J.-T. Shy, Y.-P. Lan, Y.-F. Chen, and P.-H. Tsao. Pulsed optical parametric generation, amplification, and oscillation in monolithic periodically poled lithium niobate crystals, *IEEE J. Quantum Elect.* 40: 791–799, 2004.

279. Balachninaite, O., R. Grigonis, V. Sirutkaitis, and R. C. Eckardt, A coherent spectrophotometer based on a periodically poled lithium niobate optical parametric oscillator, *Opt. Commun.* 248: 15–25, 2005.

280. Zhang, X.-B., B.-Q. Yao, Y.-L. Ju, and Y.-Z. Wang, A 2.048-μm Tm,Ho:GdVO₄ laser pumped doubly resonant optical parametric oscillator based on periodically poled lithium LiNbO₃, *Chinese Phys. Lett.* 24: 1953–1954, 2007.

281. Baumgartner, R. A. and R. L. Byer, Remote SO₂ measurements at 4 μm with a continuously tunable source, *Opt. Lett.* 2: 163–165, 1978.

282. Baumgartner, R. A. and R. L. Byer, Continuously tunable ir lidar with applications to remote measurements of SO₂ and CH₄, *Appl. Opt.* 17: 3555–3561, 1978.

283. Endemann, M. and R. L. Byer, Remote single-ended measurements of atmospheric temperature and humidity at 1.77 μm using a continuously tunable source, *Opt. Lett.* 5: 452–454, 1978.

284. Brassington, D. J., Differential absorption lidar measurements of atmospheric water vapor using an optical parametric oscillator source, *Appl. Opt.* 21: 4411–4416, 1982.

285. Gloster, L. A. W., I. T. McKinnie, Z. X. Jiang, T. A. King, J. M. Boon-Engering, W. E. van der Veer, and W. Hogervorst, Narrow-band β-BaB₂O₄ optical parametric oscillator in a grazing-incidence configuration, *J. Opt. Soc. Am. B* 12: 2117–2121, 1995.

286. Boon-Engering, J. M., L. A. W. Gloster, W. E. van der Veer, I. T. McKinnie, T. A. King, and W. Hogervorst, Highly efficient single-longitudinal-mode β-BaB₂O₄ optical parametric oscillator with a new cavity design, *Opt. Lett.* 20: 2087–2089, 1995.

287. Huisken, F., M. Kaloudis, J. Marquez, Y. L. Chuzavkov, S. N. Orlov, Y. N. Polivanov, and V. V. Smirnov, Single-mode KTiOPO₄ optical parametric oscillator, *Opt. Lett.* 20: 2306–2308, 1995.

288. Schlup, P., S. D. Butterworth, and I. T. McKinnie, Efficient single-frequency pulsed periodically poled lithium niobate optical parametric oscillator, *Opt. Commun.* 154: 191–195, 1998.

289. Schlup, P., I. T. McKinnie, and S. D. Butterworth, Single-mode, singly resonant, pulsed periodically poled lithium niobate optical parametric oscillator, *Appl. Opt.* 38: 7398–7401, 1999.

290. Yang, S. T. and S. P. Velsko, Frequency-agile kilohertz repetition-rate optical parametric oscillator based on periodically poled lithium niobate, *Opt. Lett.* 24: 133–135, 1999.

291. Yu, C.-S. and A. H. Kung, Grazing-incidence periodically poled LiNbO₃ optical parametric oscillator, *J. Opt. Soc. Am. B* 16: 2233–2238, 1999.

292. Liang, G.-C., H.-H. Liu, A. H. Kung, A. Mohacsi, A. Miklos, and P. Hess, Photoacoustic trace detection of methane using compact solid-state lasers, *J. Phys. Chem. A* 104: 10179–10183, 2000.

293. Miklos, A., C.-H. Lim, W.-W. Hsiang, G.-C. Liang, A. H. Kung, A. Schmohl, and P. Hess, Photoacoustic measurement of methane concentrations with a compact pulsed optical parametric oscillator, *Appl. Opt.* 41: 2985–2993, 2002.

294. Chiang, A. C., Y. Y. Lin, T. D. Wang, Y. C. Huang, and J. T. Shy, Distributed-feedback optical parametric oscillation by use of a photorefractive grating in periodically poled lithium niobate, *Opt. Lett.* 27: 1815–1817, 2002.

295. Haidar, S., Y. Sasaki, E. Niwa, K. Masumoto, and H. Ito, Electro-optic tuning of a periodically poled $LiNbO_3$ optical parametric oscillator and mixing its output waves to generate mid-IR tunable from 9.4 to 10.5 µm, *Opt. Commun.* 229: 325–330, 2004.

296. Scherer, J. J., D. Voelkel, D. J. Rakestraw, J. B. Paul, C. P. Collier, R. J. Saykally, and A. O'Keefe, Infrared cavity ringdown laser absorption spectroscopy (IR-CRLAS), *Chem. Phys. Lett.* 245: 273–280, 1995.

297. Scherer, J. J., D. Voelkel, and D. J. Rakestraw, Infrared cavity ringdown laser absorption spectroscopy (IR-CRLAS) in low pressure flames, *Appl. Phys. B* 64: 699–705, 1997.

298. Busch, K. W. and M. A. Busch (Eds), *Cavity-Ringdown Spectroscopy: An Ultratrace-Absorption Measurement Technique*, Vol. 720 of ACS Symposium Series, American Chemical Society, Washington, DC, 1999.

299. Berden, G., R. Peeters, and G. Meijer, Cavity ring-down spectroscopy: Experimental schemes and application, *Int. Rev. Phys. Chem.* 19: 565–607, 2000.

300. Richman, B. A., K. W. Aniolek, T. J. Kulp, and S. E. Bisson, Continuously tunable, single-longitudinal-mode, pulsed mid-infrared optical parametric oscillator based on periodically poled lithium niobate, *J. Opt. Soc. Am. B* 17: 1233–1239, 2000.

301. Raffy, J., T. Debuisschert, and J.-P. Pocholle, Widely tunable optical parametric oscillator with electrical wavelength control, *Opt. Lett.* 22: 1589–1591, 1997.

302. Aniolek, K. W., P. E. Powers, T. J. Kulp, B. A. Richman, and S. E. Bisson, Cavity ringdown laser absorption spectroscopy with a 1 kHz mid-infrared periodically poled lithium niobate optical parametric generator/optical parametric amplifier, *Chem. Phys. Lett.* 302: 555–562, 1999.

303. Aniolek, K. W., R. L. Schmitt, T. J. Kulp, B. A. Richman, S. E. Bisson, and P. E. Powers, Microlaser-pumped periodically poled lithium niobate optical parametric generator-optical parametric amplifier, *Opt. Lett.* 25: 557–559, 2000.

304. Wu, S., V. A. Kapinus, and G. A. Blake, A nanosecond optical parametric generator/amplifier seeded by an external cavity diode laser, *Opt. Commun.* 159: 74–79, 1999.

305. Bjorkholm, J. E. and H. G. Danielmeyer, Frequency control of a pulsed optical parametric oscillator by radiation injection, *Appl. Phys. Lett.* 15: 171–173, 1969.

306. Kreuzer, L. B., Single mode oscillation of a pulsed singly resonant optical parametric oscillator, *Appl. Phys. Lett.* 15: 263–265, 1969.

307. Cassedy, E. S. and M. Jain, A theoretical study of injection tuning of optical parametric oscillators, *IEEE J. Quantum Elect.* QE-15: 1290–1301, 1979.

308. Fan, Y. X., R. C. Eckardt, R. L. Byer, J. Nolting, and R. Wallenstein, Visible BaB_2O_4 optical parametric oscillator pumped at 355 nm by a single-axial-mode pulsed source, *Appl. Phys. Lett.* 53: 2014–2016, 1988.

309. Hovde, D. C., J. H. Timmermans, G. Scoles, and K. K. Lehmann, High power injection seeded optical parametric oscillator, *Opt. Commun.* 86: 294–300, 1991.

310. Huisken, F., A. Kulcke, D. Voelkel, C. Laush, and J. M. Lisy, New infrared injection-seeded optical parametric oscillator with high energy and narrow bandwidth output, *Appl. Phys. Lett.* 62: 805–807, 1993.

311. Fix, A., R. Feldbausch, M. Inguscio, G. M. Tino, and R. Wallenstein, Injection-seeded single longitudinal mode optical parametric oscillator of beta-barium-borate. In P. L. Knight and P. L. Kelley (Eds), *International Conference on Quantum Electronics Technical Digest Series, 1992*, Volume 9, pp. 528–529, XVIII International Quantum Electronics Conference, 1992; conference edition: ISBN 3-900-538-33-6.

312. Fix, A., R. Feldbausch, and R. Wallenstein, Tuning, output, and spectral characteristics of seeded and unseeded Nd:YAG laser-pumped optical parametric oscillators of beta-barium-borate. In Volume 11 of *1993 OSA Technical Digest Series*, paper CWD2, pp. 244–246, *Conference on Lasers and Electro-Optics, 1993*, Optical Society of America, Washington, DC, 1993; www.osapublishing.org/conference.cfm?meetingid=18&yr=1993.

313. Milton, M. J. T., T. D. Gardiner, G. Chourdakis, and P. T. Woods, Injection seeding of an infrared optical parametric oscillator with a tunable diode laser, *Opt. Lett.* 19: 281–283, 1994.

314. Raymond, T. D., W. J. Alford, A. V. Smith, and M. S. Bowers, Frequency shifts in injection-seeded optical parametric oscillators with phase mismatch, *Opt. Lett.* 19: 1520–1522, 1994.

315. Smith, A. V., W. J. Alford, T. D. Raymond, and M. S. Bowers, Comparison of a numerical model with measured performance of a seeded, nanosecond KTP optical parametric oscillator, *J. Opt. Soc. Am. B* 12: 2253–2267, 1995.

316. Boon-Engering, J. M., W. E. van der Veer, J. W. Gerritsen, and W. Hogervorst, Bandwidth studies of an injection-seeded β-barium borate optical parametric oscillator, *Opt. Lett.* 20: 380–382, 1995.

317. Bourdon, P., M. Péalat, and V. I. Fabelinsky, Continuous-wave diode-laser injection-seeded β-barium borate optical parametric oscillator: A reliable source for spectroscopic studies, *Opt. Lett.* 20: 474–476, 1995.

318. Fröchtenicht, R., M. Kaloudis, M. Koch, and F. Huisken, Vibrational spectroscopy of small water complexes embedded in large liquid helium clusters, *J. Chem. Phys.* 105: 6128–6140, 1996.

319. Srinivasan, N., T. Kimura, H. Kiriyama, M. Yamanaka, Y. Izawa, S. Nakai, and C. Yamanaka, Bandwidth narrowing of an all-solid-state optical parametric oscillator amplifier system, *Jpn. J. Appl. Phys.* 35: 3457–3458, 1996.

320. Fix, A. and R. Wallenstein, Spectral properties of pulsed nanosecond optical parametric oscillators: Experimental investigation and numerical analysis, *J. Opt. Soc. Am. B* 13: 2484–2497, 1996.

321. Plusquellic, D. F., O. Votava, and D. J. Nesbitt, Absolute frequency stabilization of an injection-seeded optical parametric oscillator, *Appl. Opt.* 35: 1464–1472, 1996.

322. Votava, O. J., R. Fair, D. F. Plusquellic, E. Riedle, and D. J. Nesbitt, High-resolution vibrational overtone studies of HOD and H_2O with single-mode, injection-seeded ring optical parametric oscillators, *J. Chem. Phys.* 107: 8854–8865, 1997.

323. Milton, M. J. T., T. D. Gardiner, F. Molero, and J. Galech, Injection-seeded optical parametric oscillator for range-resolved DIAL measurements of atmospheric methane, *Opt. Commun.* 142: 153–160, 1997.

324. Voelkel, D., Yu. L. Chuzavkov, J. Marquez, S. N. Orlov, Yu. N. Polivanov, V. V. Smirnov, and F. Huisken, Infrared degenerate four-wave mixing and resonance-enhanced stimulated Raman scattering in molecular gases and free jets, *Appl. Phys. B.* 65: 93–99, 1997.

325. Borsutzky, A., Frequency control of pulsed optical parametric oscillators, *Quantum Semiclass. Opt.* 9: 191–207, 1997.

326. Bourdon, P. and M. Péalat, Coherent anti-Stokes Raman scattering spectroscopy using an optical parametric oscillator, *Quantum Semiclass. Opt.* 9: 269–278, 1997.

327. Ehret, G., A. Fix, V. Weiss, G. Poberaj, and T. Baumert, Diode-laser-seeded optical parametric oscillator for airborne water vapor DIAL application in the upper troposphere and lower stratosphere, *Appl. Phys. B* 67: 427–431, 1998.

328. Fix, A., V. Weiss, and G. Ehret, Injection-seeded optical parametric oscillator for airborne water vapour DIAL, *Pure Appl. Opt.* 7: 837–852, 1998.

329. Schlup, P., N. A. Russell, I. T. Mckinnie, S. D. Butterworth, A. L. Oien, and D. M. Warrington, Efficient, single frequency, injection-seeded collinear and noncollinear BBO OPOs, *Proc. SPIE.* 3265 (Solid State Lasers VII): 285–294, 1998.

330. Fair, J. R., O. Votava, and D. J. Nesbitt, OH stretch overtone spectroscopy and transition dipole alignment of HOD, *J. Chem. Phys.* 108: 72–80, 1998.

331. Alford, W. J., R. J. Gehr, R. L. Schmitt, A. V. Smith, and G. Arisholm, Beam tilt and angular dispersion in broad-bandwidth, nanosecond optical parametric oscillators, *J. Opt. Soc. Am. B* 16: 1525–1532, 1999.

332. Haidar, S. and H. Ito, Injection-seeded optical parametric oscillator for efficient difference frequency generation in mid-IR, *Opt. Commun.* 171: 171–176, 1999.

333. Brown, A. J. W., High energy, tunable, single frequency optical parametric oscillator system. In M. Fejer, H. Injeyan, and U. Keller (Eds), *Advanced Solid State Lasers*, Volume 26, *OSA Trends in Optics and Photonics* (Optical Society of America, 1999), paper WC6; http://www.osapublishing.org/abstract.cfm?URI = ASSL-1999-WC6.

334. Votava, O., D. F. Plusquellic, T. L. Myers, and D. J. Nesbitt, Bond-breaking in quantum state selected clusters: Inelastic and nonadiabatic intracluster collision dynamics in Ar–$H_2O \rightarrow Ar + H(^2S) + OH(^2\Pi^{\pm}_{1/2,3/2};N)$, *J. Chem. Phys.* 112: 7449–7460, 2000.

335. Isyanova, Y. and P. F. Moulton, Injection-seeded, pump-enhanced, tunable KTA OPO. In H. Injeyan, U. Keller, and C. Marshall (Eds), *Advanced Solid State Lasers*, Volume 34, *OSA Trends in Optics and Photonics* (Optical Society of America, 2000), paper TuA7; http://www.osapublishing.org/abstract.cfm?URI = ASSL-2000-TuA7.

336. Imai, K., K. Kawase, J.-I. Shikata, H. Minamide, and H. Ito, Injection-seeded terahertz-wave parametric oscillator, *Appl. Phys. Lett.* 78: 1026–1028, 2001.

337. Vasa, N. J., K. Saito, K. Ikuta, Y. Oki, and M. Maeda, Development of a compact light source at 1.67 μm for methane leak detection using DIAL, *Proc. SPIE* 4153 (Lidar Remote Sensing for Industry and Environment Monitoring): 471–479, 2001.

338. Fitzpatrick, J. A. J., O. V. Chekhlov, J. M. F. Elks, C. M. Western, and S. H. Ashworth, An injection seeded narrow bandwidth pulsed optical parametric oscillator and its application to the investigation of hyperfine structure in the PF radical, *J. Chem. Phys.* 115: 6920–6930, 2001.

339. Chekhlov, O. V., J. A. J. Fitzpatrick, O. V. Chekhlov, K. N. Rosser, C. M. Western, and S. H. Ashworth, An all solid-state narrow bandwidth optical parametric oscillator and its applications to the high resolution spectroscopy of free radicals, *J. Mod. Opt.* 49: 865–876, 2002.

340. Poberaj, G., A. Fix, A. Assion, M. Wirth, C. Kiemle, and G. Ehret, Airborne all-solid-state DIAL for water vapor measurements in the tropopause region: System description and assessment of accuracy, *Appl. Phys. B* 75: 165–172, 2002.

341. Fitzpatrick, J. A. J., O. V. Chekhlov, C. M. Western, and S. H. Ashworth, Sub-Doppler spectroscopy of the PH radical: Hyperfine structure in the A $^3\Pi$ state, *J. Chem. Phys.* 118: 4539–4545, 2003.

342. Klingenberg, H. H. and P. Mahnke, Wavelength switching in the acceptance bandwidth of a dual-injection-seeded optical parametric oscillator, *Proc. SPIE* 5481 (Wavefront Transformation and Laser Beam Control): 108–114, 2004.

343. Kulatilaka, W. D., T. N. Anderson, T. L. Bougher, and R. P. Lucht, Development of injection-seeded, pulsed optical parametric generator/oscillator systems for high-resolution spectroscopy, *Appl. Phys. B* 80: 669–680, 2005.

344. Armstrong, D. J. and A. V. Smith, All solid-state high-efficiency source for satellite-based UV ozone DIAL, *Proc. SPIE* 5653 (Lidar Remote Sensing for Industry and Environmental Monitoring V): 1–15, 2005.

345. Armstrong, D. J. and A. V. Smith, High efficiency intra-cavity sum-frequency-generation in a self-seeded image-rotating nanosecond optical parametric oscillator, *Proc. SPIE* 5710 (Nonlinear Frequency Generation and Conversion: Materials, Devices, and Applications IV): 1–8, 2005.

346. Armstrong, D. J. and A. V. Smith, Efficient all-solid-state UV lidar sources: From 100s of millijoules to 100s of microjoules, *Proc. SPIE* 5887 (Lidar Remote Sensing for Environmental Monitoring VI): 588703/1–588703/8, 2005.

347. Smith, A. V., Bandwidth and group-velocity effects in nanosecond optical parametric amplifiers and oscillators, *J. Opt. Soc. Am. B* 22: 1953–1965, 2005.

348. Mahnke, P., H. H. Klingenberg, A. Fix, and M. Wirth, Dependency of injection seeding and spectral purity of a single resonant KTP optical parametric oscillator on the phase matching condition, *Appl. Phys. B* 89: 1–7, 2007.

349. Amediek, A., A. Fix, M. Wirth, and G. Ehret, Development of an OPO system at 1.57 μm for integrated path DIAL measurement of atmospheric carbon dioxide, *Appl. Phys. B* 92: 295–302, 2008.

350. Walsh, D., D. J. M. Stothard, T. J. Edwards, P. G. Browne, C. F. Rae, and M. H. Dunn, Injection-seeded intra-cavity terahertz optical parametric oscillator, *J. Opt. Soc. Am. B* 26: 1196–1202, 2009.

351. Mahnke, P. and M. Wirth, Real-time quantitative measurement of the mode beating of an injection-seeded optical parametric oscillator, *Appl. Phys. B* 99: 141–148, 2010.

352. Velarde, L., D. P. Engelhart, D. Matsiev, J. LaRue, D. J. Auerbach, and A. M. Wodtke, Generation of tunable narrow bandwidth nanosecond pulses in the deep ultraviolet for efficient optical pumping and high resolution spectroscopy, *Rev. Sci. Instrum.* 821: 063106/1–063106/10, 2010.

353. Thariyan, M. P., V. Ananthanarayanan, A. H. Bhuiyan, S. V. Naik, J. P. Gore, and R. P. Lucht, Dual-pump CARS temperature and major species concentration measurements in counter-flow methane flames using narrowband pump and broadband Stokes lasers, *Combust. Flame* 157: 1390–1399, 2010.

354. Thariyan, M. P., A. H. Bhuiyan, S. E. Meyer, S. V. Naik, J. P. Gore, and R. P. Lucht, Dual-pump coherent anti-Stokes Raman scattering system for temperature and species measurements in an optically accessible high-pressure gas turbine combustor facility, *Measure. Sci. Technol.* 22: 015301/1–015301/12, 2011.

355. Fix, A., C. Buedenbender, M. Wirth, M. Quatrevalet, A. Amediek, C. Kiemle, and G. Ehret, Optical parametric oscillators and amplifiers for airborne and spaceborne active remote sensing of CO_2 and CH_4, *Proc. SPIE* 8182 (Lidar Technologies, Techniques, and Measurements for Atmospheric Remote Sensing VII): 818206/1–818206/10, 2011.

356. Refaat, T. F., S. Ismail, A. R. Nehrir, J. W. Hair, J. H. Crawford, I. Leifer, and T. Shuman, Performance evaluation of a 1.6-μm methane DIAL system from ground, aircraft and UAV platforms, *Opt. Express* 21: 30415–30432, 2013.

357. Abdullin, U. A., G. P. Dzhotyan, Yu. E. D'yakov, B. V. Zhdanov, V. I. Pryalkin, V. B. Sobolev, and A. I. Kholodnykh, Investigation of the spectral and energy characteristics of a pulsed optical parametric oscillator operating in the regime of external signal injection, *Sov. J. Quantum Electron.* 14: 538–543, 1984.

358. Smilgevičius, V., A. Stabinis, A. Piskarskas, V. Pasiškevičius, J. Hellström, S. Wang, and F. Laurell, Noncollinear optical parametric oscillator with periodically poled KTP, *Opt. Commun.* 173: 365–369, 2000.

359. Russell, S. M., P. E. Powers, M. J. Missey, and K. L. Schepler, Broadband mid-infrared generation with two-dimensional quasi-phase-matched structures, *IEEE J. Quantum Elect.* 37: 877–887, 2001.

360. Fischer, B., S. Sternklar, and S. Weiss, Photorefractive oscillators, *IEEE J. Quantum Elect.* 25: 550–569, 1989.

361. Partovi, A., J. Millerd, E. M. Garmire, M. Ziari, W. H. Steier, S. B. Trivedi, and M. B. Klein, Photorefractivity at 1.5 μm in CdTe:V, *Appl. Phys. Lett.* 57: 846–848, 1990.

362. Godard, A., G. Pauliat, G. Roosen, P. Graindorge, and P. Martin, Relaxation of the alignment tolerances of a 1.55-μm extended-cavity semiconductor laser by use of an intra-cavity photorefractive filter, *Opt. Lett.* 26: 1955–1957, 2001.

363. He, Y. and B. J. Orr, Robust tunable single-frequency operation of a diode laser by a self-pumped phase-conjugate reflector and a high-finesse filter, *Opt. Lett.* 33: 2368–2370, 2008.

364. He, Y. and B. J. Orr, Narrowband tuning of a pulsed optical parametric oscillator by wavelength-selective feedback. In *Conference on Lasers and Electro-Optics/ Quantum Electronics and Laser Science Conference*, Technical Digest, Optical Society of America, 2003, paper CTuM16; http://www.osapublishing.org/abstract. cfm?URI=CLEO-2003-CTuM16.

365. Fee, M. S., K. Danzmann, and S. Chu, Optical heterodyne measurement of pulsed lasers: Toward high-precision pulsed spectroscopy, *Phys. Rev. A* 45: 4911–4924, 1992.

366. Gangopadhyay, S., N. Melikechi, and E. E. Eyler, Optical phase perturbations in nanosecond pulsed amplification and second-harmonic generation, *J. Opt. Soc. Am. B* 11: 231–241, 1994.

367. Bergeson, S. D., K. G. H. Baldwin, T. B. Lucatorto, T. J. McIlrath, C. H. Cheng, and E. E. Eyler, Doppler-free two-photon spectroscopy in the vacuum ultraviolet: Helium 1 ^{1}S–2 ^{1}S transition, *J. Opt. Soc. Am. B* 17: 1599–1606, 2000.

368. Melikechi, N., S. Gangopadhyay, and E. E. Eyler, Phase dynamics in nanosecond pulsed dye laser amplification, *J. Opt. Soc. Am. B* 11: 2402–2411, 1994.

369. Smith, A. V., R. J. Gehr, and M. S. Bowers, Numerical models of broad-bandwidth nanosecond optical parametric oscillators, *J. Opt. Soc. Am. B* 16: 609–619, 1999.

370. Arisholm, G., G. Rustad, and K. Stenersen, Importance of pump-beam group velocity for backconversion in optical parametric oscillators, *J. Opt. Soc. Am. B* 18: 1882–1890, 2001.

371. Anstett, G., A. Borsutzky, and R. Wallenstein, Investigation of the spatial beam quality of pulsed ns-OPOs, *Appl. Phys. B* 76: 541–545, 2003.

372. Anstett, G., M. Nitmann, and R. Wallenstein, Experimental investigation and numerical simulation of the spatio-temporal dynamics of the light pulses in nanosecond optical parametric oscillators, *Appl. Phys. B* 79: 305–313, 2004.

373. Anstett, G. and R. Wallenstein, Experimental investigation of the spectro-temporal dynamics of the light pulses of Q-switched Nd:YAG lasers and nanosecond optical parametric oscillators, *Appl. Phys. B* 79: 827–836, 2004.

374. Mahnke, P. and H. H. Klingenberg, Observation and analysis of mode competition in optic parametric oscillators, *Appl. Phys. B* 78: 171–177, 2004.

375. Vodopyanov, K. L., J. P. Maffetone, I. Zwieback, and W. Ruderman, AgGaS$_2$ optical parametric oscillator continuously tunable from 3.9 to 11.3 μm, *Appl. Phys. Lett.* 75: 1204–1206, 1999.

376. Kühnemann, F., K. Schneider, A. Hecker, A. A. E. Martis, W. Urban, S. Schiller, and J. Mlynek, Photoacoustic trace gas detection using a CW single-frequency parametric oscillator, *Appl. Phys. B* 66: 741–745, 1998.

377. Vodopyanov, K. L., J. P. Maffetone, I. Zwieback, and W. Ruderman, AgGaS$_2$ optical parametric oscillator continuously tunable from 3.9 to 11.3 μm, *Appl. Phys. Lett.* 75: 1204–1206, 1999.

378. Bisson, S. E., K. M. Armstrong, T. J. Kulp, and M. Hartings, Broadly tunable, mode-hop-tuned CW optical parametric oscillator based on periodically poled lithium niobate, *Appl. Opt.* 40: 6049–6055, 2001.

379. van Herpen, M., S. te Lintel Hekkert, S. E. Bisson, and F. J. M. Harren, Wide single-mode tuning of a 3.0–3.8-μm, 700-mW, continuous-wave Nd:YAG-pumped optical parametric oscillator based on periodically poled lithium niobate, *Opt. Lett.* 27: 640–642, 2002.

380. van Herpen, M. M. J. W., S. Li, S. E. Bisson, S. te Lintel Hekkert, and F. J. M. Harren, Tuning and stability of a continuous-wave mid-infrared high-power single resonant optical parametric oscillator, *Appl. Phys. B* 75: 329–333, 2002.

381. van Herpen, M. M. J. W., S. Li, S. E. Bisson, and F. J. M. Harren, Photoacoustic trace gas detection of ethane using a continuously tunable, continuous-wave optical parametric oscillator based on periodically poled lithium niobate, *Appl. Phys. Lett.* 81: 1157–1159, 2002.

382. Ngai, A. K. Y., S. T. Persijn, I. D. Lindsay, A. A. Kosterev, P. Gross, C. J. Lee, S. M. Cristescu, F. K. Tittel, K.-J. Boller, and F. J. M. Harren, Continuous wave optical parametric oscillator for quartz-enhanced photoacoustic trace gas sensing, *Appl. Phys. B.* 89: 123–128, 2007.

383. Petelski, T., R. S. Conroy, K. Bencheikh, J. Mlynek, and S. Schiller, All-solid-state, tunable, single-frequency source of yellow light for high-resolution spectroscopy, *Opt. Lett.* 26: 1013–1015, 2001.

384. Kovalchuk, E. V., D. Dekorsy, A. I. Lvovsky, C. Braxmeier, J. Mlynek, A. Peters, and S. Schiller, High-resolution Doppler-free molecular spectroscopy with a continuous-wave optical parametric oscillator, *Opt. Lett.* 26: 1430–1432, 2001.

385. Kulatilaka, W. D., T. N. Anderson, T. L. Bougher, and R. P. Lucht, Development of injection-seeded, pulsed optical parametric generator/oscillator systems for high-resolution spectroscopy, *Appl. Phys. B.* 80: 669–680, 2005.

386. Svanberg, S., *Atomic and Molecular Spectroscopy*, 4th edn, Springer, New York, 2004.

387. Sigrist, M. W. (Ed.), *Air Monitoring by Spectroscopic Techniques*, Wiley, New York, 1994.

388. Tittel, F. K., D. Richter, and A. Fried, Mid-infrared laser applications in spectroscopy. In I. T. Sorokina and K. L. Vodopyanov (Eds), *Solid-State Mid-Infrared Sources*, Chapter 11, pp. 445–510, Springer, Berlin, 2003.

389. Eckbreth, A. C., *Laser Diagnostics for Combustion Temperature and Species*, Abacus, Cambridge, MA, 1988.

390. Nibler, J. W. and G. A. Pubanz, Coherent Raman spectroscopy of gases. In R. J. H. Clark and R. E. Hester (Eds), *Advances in Non-Linear Spectroscopy*, pp. 1–49, Wiley, New York, 1988.

391. Greenhalgh, D. A., Quantitative CARS spectroscopy. In R. J. H. Clark and R. E. Hester (Eds), *Advances in Non-Linear Spectroscopy*, pp. 193–251, Wiley, New York, 1988.

392. Harvey, A. B. (Ed.), *Chemical Applications of Nonlinear Raman Spectroscopy*, Academic, New York, 1981.

393. Farrow, R. L. and D. J. Rakestraw, Detection of trace molecular species using degenerate four-wave mixing, *Science* 257: 1894–1900, 1992.

394. Vander Wal, R. L., B. E. Holmes, J. B. Jeffries, P. M. Danehy, R. L. Farrow, and D. J. Rakestraw, Detection of HF using infrared degenerate four-wave mixing, *Chem. Phys. Lett.* 191: 251–258, 1990.

395. Germann, G. J., A. McIlroy, T. Dreier, R. L. Farrow, and D. J. Rakestraw, Detection of polyatomic molecules using infrared degenerate four-wave mixing, *Ber. Bunsenges. Phys. Chem.* 97: 1630–1634, 1993.

396. Germann, G. J., R. L. Farrow, and D. J. Rakestraw, Infrared degenerate four-wave mixing spectroscopy of polyatomic molecules: CH_4 and C_2H_2, *J. Opt. Soc. Am. B* 12: 25–32, 1995.

397. Eyler, E. E., D. E. Chieda, M. C. Stowe, M. J. Thorpe, T. R. Schibli, and J. Ye, Prospects for precision measurements of atomic helium using direct frequency comb spectroscopy, *Eur. Phys. J. D* 48: 43–55, 2008.

398. Herrmann, M., M. Haas, U. D. Jentschura, F. Kottmann, D. Leibfried, G. Saathoff, Ch. Gohle, A. Ozawa, V. Batteiger, S. Knünz, N. Kolachevsky, H. A. Schüssler, T. W. Hänsch, and Th. Udem, Feasibility of coherent xuv spectroscopy on the 1S–2S transition in singly ionized helium, *Phys. Rev A.* 79: 052505/1–052505/15, 2009.

399. Kandula, D. Z., C. Gohle, T. J. Pinkert, W. Ubachs, and K. S. E. Eikema, Extreme ultraviolet frequency comb metrology, *Phys. Rev. Lett.* 105: 063001/1–063001/4, 2010.

400. Pinkert, T. J., D. Z. Kandula, C. Gohle, I. Barmes, J. Morgenweg, and K. S. E. Eikema, Widely tunable XUV frequency comb generation, *Opt. Lett.* 36: 2026–2028, 2011.

401. D. Z. Kandula, Ch. Gohle, T. J. Pinkert, W. Ubachs, and K. S. E. Eikema, XUV frequency comb metrology on the ground state of helium, *Phys. Rev. A* 84: 062512/1–062512/16, 2011.

402. Yost, D. C., A. Cingöz, T. K. Allison, A. Ruehl, M. E. Fermann, I. Hartl, and J. Ye, Power optimization of XUV frequency combs for spectroscopy applications [Invited], *Opt. Express* 19: 23483–23493, 2011.

403. Falcone, R. W., J. R. Willison, J. F. Young, and S. E. Harris, Measurement of the He ls2s $^1S_0$ isotopic shift using a tunable VUV anti-Stokes light source, *Opt. Lett.* 3: 162–163, 1978.

404. Weiser, P. S., D. A. Wild, and E. J. Bieske, Infrared spectra of $Cl^--(C_2H_2)_n$ $(1 < n \leq 9)$ anion clusters: Spectroscopic evidence for solvent shell closure, *J. Chem. Phys.* 110: 9443–9449, 1999.

405. Wild, D. A., P. J. Milley, Z. M. Loh, P. S. Weiser, and E. J. Bieske, Infrared spectra of $Br^--(C_2H_2)_n$ complexes, *Chem. Phys. Lett.* 323: 49–54, 2000.

406. Wild, D. A., P. J. Milley, Z. M. Loh, P. P. Wolynec, P. S. Weiser, and E. J. Bieske, Structural and energetic properties of the $Br^--C_2H_2$ anion complex from rotationally resolved mid-infrared spectra and *ab initio* calculations, *J. Chem. Phys.* 113: 1075–1089, 2000.

407. Weiser, P. S., D. A. Wild, and E. J. Bieske, Infrared spectra of $I^--(C_2H_2)_n$ $(1 \leq n \leq 4)$ anion complexes, *Chem. Phys. Lett.* 299: 303–308, 1999.

408. Bieske, E. J., Infrared investigations of negatively charged complexes and clusters, *Int. Rev. Phys. Chem.* 22: 129–151, 2003.

409. Orr, B. J., Spectroscopy and energetics of the acetylene molecule: Dynamical complexity alongside structural simplicity, *Int. Rev. Phys. Chem.* 25: 655–718, 2006.

410. Payne, M. A., A. P. Milce, M. J. Frost, and B. J. Orr, Symmetry-breaking collisional energy transfer in the $4\nu_{CH}$ rovibrational manifold of acetylene: Spectroscopic evidence of a quasi-continuum of background states, *Chem. Phys. Lett.* 324: 48–56, 2000.

411. Payne, M. A., A. P. Milce, M. J. Frost, and B. J. Orr, Rovibrational energy transfer in the $4\nu_{CH}$ manifold of acetylene viewed by IR-UV double resonance spectroscopy. 4. Collision-induced quasi-continuous background effects, *J. Phys. Chem. A* 110: 3307–3319, 2006.

412. Hinkley, E. D. (Ed.), *Laser Monitoring of the Atmosphere*, Springer, New York, 1976.

413. Grant, W. B. and R. T. Menzies, A survey of laser and selected optical systems for remote measurement of pollutant gas concentrations, *J. Air Pollut. Cont. Assoc.* 33: 187–194, 1983.

414. Killinger, D. K. and A. Mooradian (Eds), *Optical and Laser Remote Sensing*, Springer, New York, 1983.

415. Killinger, D. K. and N. Menyuk, Laser remote sensing of the atmosphere, *Science* 235: 37–45, 1987.

416. Grant, W. B., Laser remote sensing techniques. In L. J. Radziemski, R. W. Solarz, and J. A. Paisner (Eds), *Laser Spectroscopy and Its Applications*, Chapter 8, pp. 565–621, Marcel Dekker, New York, 1987.

417. Sigrist, M. W., Introduction to environmental sensing. In M. W. Sigrist (Ed.), *Air Monitoring by Spectroscopic Techniques*, Chapter 1, pp. 1–26, Wiley, New York, 1994.

418. Platt, U., Differential optical absorption spectroscopy (DOAS). In M. W. Sigrist (Ed.), *Air Monitoring by Spectroscopic Techniques*, Chapter 2, pp. 27–84, Wiley, New York, 1994.

419. Svanberg, S., Differential absorption LIDAR (DIAL). In M. W. Sigrist (Ed.), *Air Monitoring by Spectroscopic Techniques*, Chapter 3, pp. 85–161, Wiley, New York, 1994.

420. Grant, W. B., LIDAR for atmospheric and hydrospheric studies. In F. J. Duarte (Ed.), *Tunable Laser Applications*, 1st edn, Chapter 7, pp. 213–305, Marcel-Dekker, New York, 1995.

421. Grant, W. B., E. V. Browell, R. T. Menzies, K. Sassen, and C.-Y. She (Eds), *Selected Papers on Laser Applications in Remote Sensing*, SPIE Optical Engineering, Bellingham, WA, 1997, MS141.

422. Grant, W. B., LIDAR Bibliography, *Optics Journal*, Optical Society of America, Washington, DC, 2006; http://www.opticsjournal.com/lidarbibliography.htm; also http://lidarmax.altervista.org/englidar/download/tutorial_Lidar/LIDARBibliography.pdf.

423. Ehret, G., C. Kiemle, W. Renger, and G. Simmet, Airborne remote sensing of tropospheric water vapor with a near-infrared differential absorption lidar system, *Appl. Opt.* 32: 4534–4551, 1993.

424. Kiemle, C., M. Wirth, A. Schäfler, A. Fix, S. Rahm, A. Dörnbrack, and G. Ehret, Water vapour and wind profiles from collocated airborne lidars during COPS 2007, *Proc. SPIE* 6750 (Lidar Technologies, Techniques, and Measurements for Atmospheric Remote Sensing III): 67500P/1–67500P/9, 2007.

425. Schwarzer, H., A. Börner, A. Fix, B. Günther, H.-W. Hübers, M. Raugust, F. Schrandt, and M. Wirth, Development of a wavelength stabilized seed laser system for an airborne water vapour lidar experiment, *Proc. SPIE* 6681 (Lidar Remote Sensing for Environmental Monitoring VIII): 66810H/1–66810H/8, 2007.

426. Flentje, H., A. Dörnbrack, A. Fix, G. Ehret, and E. Hólm, Evaluation of ECMWF water vapor fields by airborne differential absorption lidar measurements: A case study between Brazil and Europe, *Atmos. Chem. Phys.* 7: 5033–5042, 2008.

427. Kiemle, C., M. Wirth, A. Fix, G. Ehret, U. Schumann, T. Gardiner, C. Schiller, N. Sitnikov, and G. Stiller, First airborne water vapor lidar measurements in the tropical upper troposphere and mid-latitudes lower stratosphere: Accuracy evaluation and intercomparisons with other instruments, *Atmos. Chem. Phys.* 8: 5245–5261, 2008.

428. Wirth, M., A. Fix, P. Mahnke, H. Schwarzer, F. Schrandt, and G. Ehret, The airborne multi-wavelength water vapor differential absorption lidar WALES: System design and performance, *Appl. Phys. B* 96: 201–213, 2009.

429. Ehret, G., C. Kiemle, M. Wirth, A. Amediek, A. Fix, and S. Houweling, Space-borne remote sensing of CO_2, CH_4, and N_2O by integrated path differential absorption lidar: A sensitivity analysis, *Appl. Phys. B* 96: 593–608, 2008.

430. Livrozet, M. J., F. Elsen, J. Wüppen, J. Löhring, C. Büdenbender, A. Fix, B. Jungbluth, and H.-D. Hoffmann, Feasibility and performance study for a space-borne 1645 nm OPO for French-German satellite mission MERLIN, *Proc. SPIE* 8959 (Solid State Lasers XXIII: Technology and Devices): 89590G/1–89590G/7, 2014.

431. Amediek, A., A. Fix, M. Wirth, and G. Ehret, Development of an OPO system at 1.57 µm for integrated path DIAL measurement of atmospheric carbon dioxide, *Appl. Phys. B* 92: 295–302, 2008.

432. Fix, A., C. Büdenbender, M. Wirth, M. Quatrevalet, A. Amediek, C. Kiemle, and G. Ehret, Optical parametric oscillators and amplifiers for airborne and spaceborne active remote sensing of CO_2 and CH_4, *Proc. SPIE* 8182 (Solid State Lasers XXIII: Technology and Devices): 818206/1–818206/10, 2011.

433. Löhring, J., J. Luttmann, R. Kasemann, M. Schlösser, J. Klein, H.-D. Hoffmann, A. Amediek, C. Büdenbender, A. Fix, M. Wirth, M. Quatrevalet, and G. Ehret, INNOSLAB-based single-frequency MOPA for airborne lidar detection of CO_2 and methane, *Proc. SPIE* 8959 (Solid State Lasers XXIII: Technology and Devices): 89590J/1–89590J/8, 2014.

434. Henderson, S. W., T. J. Carrig, P. Gatt, D. D. Smith, and C. P. Hale, Tunable single-frequency near IR lasers for DIAL applications, *Proc. SPIE* 4153 (Lidar Remote Sensing for Industry and Environment Monitoring): 443–454, 2001.

435. Fix, A., M. Wirth, A. Meister, G. Ehret, M. Pesch, and D. Weidauer, Tunable ultraviolet optical parametric oscillator for differential absorption lidar measurements of tropospheric ozone, *Appl. Phys. B* 75: 153–163, 2002.

436. Armstrong, D. J. and A. V. Smith, All solid-state high-efficiency tunable UV source for airborne or satellite-based ozone DIAL systems, *IEEE J. Sel. Top. Quantum Electron.* 13: 721–731, 2007.

437. Smith, A. V. and D. J. Armstrong, Nanosecond optical parametric oscillator with 90 degree image rotation: Design and performance, *J. Opt. Soc. Am. B* 19: 1801–1814, 2002.

438. Weibring, P., J. N. Smith, H. Edner, and S. Svanberg, Development and testing of a frequency-agile optical parametric oscillator for differential absorption lidar, *Rev. Sci. Instrum.* 74: 4478–4484, 2003.

439. Weibring, P., H. Edner, and S. Svanberg, Versatile mobile lidar system for environmental monitoring, *Appl. Opt.* 42: 3583–3594, 2003.

440. Zayhowski, J. J. and A. L. Wilson, Miniature eye-safe laser system for high-resolution three-dimensional lidar, *Appl. Opt.* 46: 5951–5956, 2007.

441. Zayhowski, J. J., Periodically poled lithium niobate optical parametric amplifiers pumped by high-power passively Q-switched microchip lasers, *Opt. Lett.* 22: 169–171, 1997.

442. Jeys, T. H., Multipass optical parametric amplifier, *Opt. Lett.* 21: 1229–1231, 1996.

443. Elstner, E. F. and J. R. Konze, Effects of point freezing on ethylene and ethane production by sugar beet leaf disks, *Nature* 263: 351–352, 1976.

444. Knutson, M. D., G. J. Handelman, and F. E. Viteri, Methods for measuring ethane and pentane in expired air from rats and humans, *Free Rad. Biol. Med.* 28: 514–519, 2000.

445. Kühnemann, F., Photoacoustic trace gas detection in plant biology. In P. Hering, J. P. Lay, and S. Stry (Eds), *Laser in Environmental and Life Science*, Chapter 16, Springer, Berlin, 2003.

446. Kosterev, A. A., F. K. Tittel, D. V. Serebryakov, A. L. Malinovsky, and I. V. Morozov, Applications of quartz tuning forks in spectroscopic gas sensing, *Rev. Sci. Instrum.* 76: 043105/1–043105/9, 2005.

447. von Basum, G., D. Halmer, P. Hering, M. Mürtz, S. Schiller, F. Müller, A. Popp, and F. Kühnemann, Parts per trillion sensitivity for ethane in air with an optical parametric oscillator cavity leak-out spectrometer, *Opt. Lett.* 29: 797–799, 2004.

448. Arslanov, D. D., M. Spunei, A. K. Y. Ngai, S. M. Cristescu, I. D. Lindsay, S. T. Persijn, K. J. Boller, and F. J. M. Harren, Rapid and sensitive trace gas detection with continuous wave optical parametric oscillator-based wavelength modulation spectroscopy, *Appl. Phys. B* 103: 223–228, 2011.

449. Todd, M. W., R. A. Provencal, T. G. Owano, B. A. Paldus, A. Kachanov, K. L. Vodopyanov, M. Hunter, S. L. Coy, J. I. Steinfeld, and J. T. Arnold, Application of mid-infrared cavity-ringdown spectroscopy to trace explosives detection using a broadly tunable (6–8 µm) optical parametric oscillator, *Appl. Phys. B* 75: 367–376, 2002.

450. Brüggemann, D., J. Hertzberg, B. Wies, Y. Waschke, R. Noll, K.-F. Knoche, and G. Herziger, Test of an optical parametric oscillator (OPO) as a compact and fast tunable Stokes source in coherent anti-Stokes Raman spectroscopy (CARS), *Appl. Phys. B* 55: 378–380, 1992.

451. Hertzberg, J., D. Brüggemann, and B. Wies, Optical parametric oscillator (OPO) — compact and fast tunable Stokes source in CARS spectroscopy. In E. M. Castellucci, R. Righini, and P. Foggi (Eds), *Coherent Raman Spectroscopy: Applications and New Developments*, pp. 15–20, World Scientific, Singapore, 1993.

452. Tiihonen, M., V. Pasiškevičius, and F. Laurell, Tailored UV-laser source for fluorescence spectroscopy of biomolecules, *Opt. Lasers Eng.* 45: 444–449, 2007.

453. Zhang, Z., R. J. Clewes, C. R. Howle, and D. T. Reid, Active FTIR-based stand-off spectroscopy using a femtosecond optical parametric oscillator, *Opt. Lett.* 39: 6005–6008, 2014.

454. Reid, D. T., Z. Zhang, and C. R. Howle, Active FTIR-based standoff detection in the 3–4 micron region using broadband femtosecond optical parametric oscillators, *Proc. SPIE* 9073 (Chemical, Biological, Radiological, Nuclear, and Explosives Sensing XV): 907302/1–907302/7, 2014.

455. Cheng, J.-X., and X. S. Xie (Eds), *Coherent Raman Scattering Microscopy* (Series in Cellular and Clinical Imaging), CRC Press, New York, 2012.

456. Alfonso-Garcia, A., R. Mittal, E. S. Lee, and E. O. Potma, Biological imaging with coherent Raman scattering microscopy: A tutorial, *J. Biomed. Opt.* 19: 071407/1–I071407/13, 2014.

457. Cheng, J.-X. and X. S. Xie, Coherent anti-Stokes Raman scattering microscopy: Instrumentation, theory, and applications, *J. Phys. Chem. B* 108: 827–840, 2004.

458. Potma, E. O. and X. S. Xie, CARS microscopy for biology and medicine, *Opt. Photon. News* 14(11): 40–45, November 2004.

459. Volkmer, A., Vibrational imaging and microspectroscopies based on coherent anti-Stokes Raman scattering microscopy, *J. Phys. D: Appl. Phys.* 38: R59–R81, 2005.

460. Evans, C. L., E. O. Potma, M. Puoris'haag, D. Côté, C. P. Lin, and X. S. Xie, Chemical imaging of tissue *in vivo* with video-rate coherent anti-Stokes Raman scattering microscopy, *Proc. Natl. Acad. Sci. (USA)* 102: 16807–16812, 2005.

461. Rodriguez, L. G., S. J. Lockett, and G. R. Holtom, Coherent anti-Stokes Raman scattering microscopy: A biological review, *Cytometry* 69A: 779–791, 2006.

462. Cheng, J.-X., Coherent anti-Stokes Raman scattering microscopy, *Appl. Spectrosc.* 61: 197A–208A, 2007.

463. Müller, M. and A. Zumbusch, Coherent anti-Stokes Raman scattering microscopy, *Chem. Phys. Chem.* 8: 2156–2170, 2007.

464. Evans, C. L. and X. S. Xie, Coherent anti-Stokes Raman scattering microscopy: Chemical imaging for biology and medicine, *Ann. Rev. Anal. Chem.* 1: 883–909, 2008.

465. Le, T. T., S. Yue, and J.-X. Cheng, Shedding new light on lipid biology by CARS microscopy, *J. Lipid Res.* 51: 3091–3102, 2010.

466. Légaré, F., C. L. Evans, F. Ganikhanov, and X. S. Xie, Towards CARS endoscopy, *Opt. Express* 14: 4427–4432, 2006.

467. Wang, H., T. B. Huff, and J.-X. Cheng, Coherent anti-Stokes Raman scattering imaging with photonic crystal fiber delivered laser source, *Opt. Lett.* 31: 1417–1419, 2006.

468. Jurna, M., J. P. Korterik, C. Otto, and H. L. Offerhaus, Shot noise limited heterodyne detection of CARS signals, *Opt. Express* 15: 15207–15213, 2007.

469. Jurna, M., J. P. Korterik, H. L. Offerhaus, and C. Otto, Noncritical phase-matched lithium triborate optical parametric oscillator for high resolution coherent anti-Stokes Raman scattering spectroscopy and microscopy, *Appl. Phys. Lett.* 89: 251116/1–251116/3, 2006.

470. Jurna, M., J. P. Korterik, C. Otto, J. L. Herek, and H. L. Offerhaus, Vibrational phase contrast microscopy by use of coherent anti-Stokes Raman scattering, *Phys. Rev. Lett.* 103: 043905/1–043905/4, 2009.

471. Jurna, M., E. T. Garbacik, J. P. Korterik, C. Otto, J. L. Herek, and H. L. Offerhaus, Vibrational phase contrast CARS microscopy for quantitative analysis, *Proc. SPIE* 7569 (Multiphoton Microscopy in the Biomedical Sciences X): 75690F/1–75690F/9, 2010.

472. Orsel, K., E. T. Garbacik, M. Jurna, J. P. Korterik, C. Otto, J. L. Herek, and H. L. Offerhaus, Heterodyne interferometric polarization coherent anti-Stokes Raman scattering (HIP-CARS) spectroscopy, *J. Raman Spectrosc.* 41: 1678–1681, 2010.

473. Jurna, M., E. T. Garbacik, J. P. Korterik, J. L. Herek, C. Otto, and H. L. Offerhaus, Visualizing resonances in the complex plane with vibrational phase contrast coherent anti-Stokes Raman scattering, *Anal. Chem.* 82: 7656–7659, 2010.

474. Jurna, M., J. L. Herek, and H. L. Offerhaus, Implementation of vibrational phase contrast coherent anti-Stokes Raman scattering microscopy, *Appl. Opt.* 50: 1839–1842, 2011.

475. Garbacik, E. T., J. P. Korterik, C. Otto, S. Mukamel, J. L. Herek, and H. L. Offerhaus, Background-free nonlinear microspectroscopy with vibrational molecular interferometry, *Phys. Rev. Lett.* 107: 253902/1–253902/4, 2011.

476. Garbacik, E. T., J. P. Korterik, C. Otto, S. Mukamel, J. L. Herek, and H. L. Offerhaus, Background-free nonlinear microspectroscopy with vibrational molecular interferometry, *Proc. SPIE* 8226 (Multiphoton Microscopy in the Biomedical Sciences XII): 822605/1–822605/7, 2012.

477. Garbacik, E. T., J. P. Korterik, C. Otto, J. L. Herek, and H. L. Offerhaus, Epi-detection of vibrational phase contrast coherent anti-Stokes Raman scattering, *Opt. Lett.* 39: 5814–5817, 2014.

478. Yakovlev, V. V., Advanced instrumentation for non-linear Raman microscopy, *J. Raman Spectrosc.* 34: 957–964, 2003.

479. Fu, Y., H. Wang, R. Shi, and J.-X. Cheng, Characterization of photodamage in coherent anti-Stokes Raman scattering microscopy, *Opt. Express* 14: 3942–3951, 2006.

480. Hayazawa, N, T. Ichimura, M. Hashimoto, Y. Inouye, and S. Kawata, Amplification of coherent anti-Stokes Raman scattering by a metallic nanostructure for a high resolution vibration microscopy, *J. Appl. Phys.* 95: 2676–2681, 2004.

481. Koo, T.-W., S. Chan, and A. A. Berlin, Single-molecule detection of biomolecules by surface-enhanced coherent anti-Stokes Raman scattering, *Opt. Lett.* 30: 1024–1026, 2005.

482. Min, W., C. W. Freudiger, S. Lu, and X. S. Xie, Coherent nonlinear optical imaging: Beyond fluorescence microscopy, *Ann. Rev. Phys. Chem.* 62: 507–530, 2011.

483. Ploetz, E., S. Laimgruber, S. Berner, W. Zinth, and P. Gilch, Femtosecond stimulated Raman microscopy, *Appl. Phys. B* 87: 389–393, 2007.

484. Freudiger, C. W., W. Min, B. G. Saar, S. Lu, G. R. Holtom, C. He, J. C. Tsai, J. X. Kang, and X. S. Xie, Label-free biomedical imaging with high sensitivity by stimulated Raman scattering microscopy, *Science* 322: 1857–1861, 2008.

485. Nandakumar, P., A. Kovalev, and A. Volkmer, Vibrational imaging based on stimulated Raman scattering microscopy, *New J. Phys.* 11: 033026–033035, 2009.

486. Ozeki, Y., F. Dake, S. Kajiyama, K. Fukui, and K. Itoh, Analysis and experimental assessment of the sensitivity of stimulated Raman scattering microscopy, *Opt. Express* 17: 3651–3658, 2009.

487. Saar, B. G., G. R. Holtom, C. W. Freudiger, C. Ackermann, W. Hill, and X. S. Xie, Intra-cavity wavelength modulation of an optical parametric oscillator for coherent Raman microscopy, *Opt. Express* 17: 12532–12539, 2009.

488. Brustlein, S., P. Ferrand, N. Walther, S. Brasselet, C. Billaudeau, D. Marguet, and H. Rigneault, Optical parametric oscillator-based light source for coherent Raman scattering microscopy: Practical overview, *J. Biomed. Opt.* 16: 021106/1–021106/10, 2011.

489. Heinrich, C., S. Bernet, and M. Ritsch-Marte, Wide-field coherent anti-Stokes Raman scattering microscopy, *Appl. Phys. Lett.* 84: 816–818, 2004.

490. Heinrich, C., C. Meusburger, S. Bernet, and M. Ritsch-Marte, CARS microscopy in a wide-field geometry with nanosecond pulses, *J. Raman Spectrosc.* 37: 675–679, 2006.

491. Heinrich, C., S. Bernet, and M. Ritsch-Marte, Nanosecond microscopy with spectroscopic resolution, *New J. Phys.* 8: 36/1–36/8, 2006.

492. Heinrich, C., A. Hofer, A. Ritsch, C. Ciardi, S. Bernet, and M. Ritsch-Marte, Selective imaging of saturated and unsaturated lipids by wide-field CARS-microscopy, *Opt. Express* 16: 2699–2708, 2008.

493. Heinrich, C., A. Hofer, S. Bernet, and M. Ritsch-Marte, Coherent anti-Stokes Raman scattering microscopy with dynamic speckle illumination, *New J. Phys.* 10: 023029/1–023029/9, 2008.

494. Jesacher, A., C. Roider, S. Khan, G. Thalhammer, S. Bernet, and M. Ritsch-Marte, Contrast enhancement in widefield CARS microscopy by tailored phase matching using a spatial light modulator, *Opt. Lett.* 36: 2245–2247, 2011.

495. Berto, P., A. Jesacher, C. Roider, S. Monneret, H. Rigneault, and M. Ritsch-Marte, Wide-field vibrational phase imaging in an extremely folded box-CARS geometry, *Opt. Lett.* 38: 709–711, 2013.

496. Garbacik, E. T., J. P. Korterik, C. Otto, J. L. Herek, and H. L. Offerhaus, Epi-detection of vibrational phase contrast coherent anti-Stokes Raman scattering, *Opt. Lett.* 39: 5814–5817, 2014.

497. Toytman, I., K. Cohn, T. Smith, D. Simanovskii, and D. Palanker, Wide-field coherent anti-Stokes Raman scattering microscopy with non-phase-matching illumination, *Opt. Lett.* 32: 1941–1943, 2007.

498. Toytman, I., D. Simanovskii, and D. Palanker, On illumination schemes for wide-field CARS microscopy, *Opt. Express* 17: 7339–7347, 2009.

499. Jones, D. J., E. O. Potma, J.-X. Cheng, B. Burfeindt, Y. Pang, J. Ye, and X. S. Xie, Synchronization of two passively mode-locked, picosecond lasers within 20 fs for coherent anti-Stokes Raman scattering microscopy, *Rev. Sci. Instrum.* 73: 2843–2848, 2002.

500. Potma, E. O., D. J. Jones, J.-X. Cheng, X. S. Xie, and J. Ye, High-sensitivity coherent anti-Stokes Raman scattering microscopy with two tightly synchronized picosecond lasers, *Opt. Lett.* 27: 1168–1170, 2002.

501. Ganikhanov, F., S. Carrasco, X. S. Xie, M. Katz, W. Seitz, and D. Kopf, Broadly tunable dual-wavelength light source for coherent anti-Stokes Raman scattering microscopy, *Opt. Lett.* 31: 1292–1294, 2006.

502. Saar, B. G., C. W. Freudiger, J. Reichman, C. M. Stanley, G. R. Holtom, and X. S. Xie, Video-rate molecular imaging *in vivo* with stimulated Raman scattering, *Science* 330: 1368–1370, 2010.

503. Saar, B. G., Y. Zeng, C. W. Freudiger, Y.-S. Liu, M. E. Himmel, X. S. Xie, and S.-Y. Ding, Label-free, real-time monitoring of biomass processing with stimulated Raman scattering microscopy, *Angew. Chem. Int. Ed.* 49: 5476–5479, 2010.

504. Slipchenko, M. N., H. Chen, D. R. Ely, Y. Jung, M. T. Carvajal, and J.-X. Cheng, Vibrational imaging of tablets by *epi*-detected stimulated Raman scattering microscopy, *Analyst* 135: 2613–2619, 2010.

505. Saar, B. G., L. R. Contreras-Rojas, X. S. Xie, and R. H. Guy, Imaging drug delivery to skin with stimulated Raman scattering microscopy, *Mol. Pharm.* 8: 969–975, 2011.

506. Saar, B. G., R. S. Johnston, C. W. Freudiger, X. S. Xie, and E. J. Seibel, Coherent Raman scattering fiber endoscopy, *Opt. Lett.* 36: 2396–2398, 2011.

507. Kong, L., M. Ji, G. R. Holtom, D. Fu, C. W. Freudiger, and X. S. Xie, Multicolor stimulated Raman scattering microscopy with a rapidly tunable optical parametric oscillator, *Opt. Lett.* 38: 145–147, 2013.

508. Mittal, R., M. Balu, T. Krasieva, E. O. Potma, L. Elkeeb, C. B. Zachary, and P. Wilder-Smith, Evaluation of stimulated Raman scattering microscopy for identifying squamous cell carcinoma in human skin, *Lasers Surg. Med.* 45: 496–502, 2013.

509. Zhang, D., P. Wang, M. N. Slipchenko, and J.-X. Cheng, Fast vibrational imaging of cells and tissues by stimulated Raman scattering microscopy, *Acc. Chem. Res.* 47: 2282–2290, 2014.

510. Ganikhanov, F., C. L. Evans, B. G. Saar, and X. S. Xie, High-sensitivity vibrational imaging with frequency modulation coherent anti-Stokes Raman scattering (FM CARS) microscopy, *Opt. Lett.* 31: 1872–1874, 2006.

511. Kieu, K., B. G. Saar, G. R. Holtom, X. S. Xie, and F. W. Wise, High-power picosecond fiber source for coherent Raman microscopy, *Opt. Lett.* 34: 2051–2053, 2009.

512. Marhic, M. E., *Fiber Optical Parametric Amplifiers, Oscillators and Related Devices*, Cambridge University Press, Cambridge, 2008.

513. Sharping, J. E., Microstructure fiber based optical parametric oscillators, *IEEE J. Lightwave Tech.* 26: 2184–2191, 2008.

514. Xu, Y., S. Murdoch, R. Leonhardt, and J. Harvey, Raman-assisted continuous-wave tunable all-fiber optical parametric oscillator, *J. Opt. Soc. Am. B* 26: 1351–1356, 2009.

515. Li, Z., C. Lu, H-Y. Tam, and P. K. A. Wai, Continuous-wave pumped, all-fiber optical parametric oscillator assisted by stimulated Raman scattering, *Opt. Commun.* 282: 2906–2908, 2009.

516. White, R. T., W. Q. Zhang, S. Afshar Vahid, and T. M. Monro, Mid-infrared sources based on four-wave mixing in microstructured optical fibres. In *Australian Conference on Optical Fibre Technology (ACOFT), 2009*, The Australian Optical Society, 2009, poster 27; http://trove.nla.gov.au/work/165364345?selectedversion=NBD49050633.

517. Chen, J. S. Y., S. G. Murdoch, R. Leonhardt, and J. D. Harvey, Effect of dispersion fluctuations on widely tunable optical parametric amplification in photonic crystal fibers, *Opt. Express* 14: 9491–9501, 2006.

518. Sharping, J. E., M. A. Foster, A. L. Gaeta, J. Lasri, O. Lyngnes, and K. Vogel, Octave-spanning, high-power microstructure-fiber-based optical parametric oscillators, *Opt. Express* 15: 1474–1479, 2007.

519. Wong, G. K. L., S. G. Murdoch, R. Leonhardt, and J. D. Harvey, High-conversion-efficiency widely-tunable all-fiber optical parametric oscillator, *Opt. Express* 15: 2947–2952, 2007.

520. Xu, Y. Q., K. F. Mak, and S. G. Murdoch, Multiwatt level output powers from a tunable fiber optical parametric oscillator, *Opt. Lett.* 36: 1966–1968, 2011.

521. Gottschall, T., T. Meyer, M. Baumgartl, B. Dietzek, J. Popp, J. Limpert, and A. Tünnermann, Fiber-based optical parametric oscillator for high resolution coherent anti-Stokes Raman scattering (CARS) microscopy, *Opt. Express* 22: 21921–21928, 2014.

522. Lamb, E. S., S. Lefrancois, M. Ji, W. J. Wadsworth, X. Sunney Xie, and F. W. Wise, Fiber optical parametric oscillator for coherent anti-Stokes Raman scattering microscopy, *Opt. Lett.* 38: 4154–4157, 2013.

523. Zhai, Y.-H., C. Goulart, J. E. Sharping, H. Wei, S. Chen, W. Tong, M. N. Slipchenko, D. Zhang, and J.-X. Cheng, Multimodal coherent anti-Stokes Raman spectroscopic imaging with a fiber optical parametric oscillator, *Appl. Phys. Lett.* 98: 191106/1–191106/3, 2011.

524. Andresen, E. R., C. K. Nielsen, J. Thøgersen, and S. R. Keiding, Fiber laser-based light source for coherent anti-Stokes Raman scattering microspectroscopy, *Opt. Express* 15: 4848–4856, 2007.

525. Meyer, T., M. Chemnitz, M. Baumgartl, T. Gottschall, T. Pascher, C. Matthäus, B. F. M. Romeike, B. R. Brehm, J. Limpert, A. Tünnermann, M. Schmitt, B. Dietzek, and J. Popp, Expanding multimodal microscopy by high spectral resolution coherent anti-Stokes Raman scattering imaging for clinical disease diagnostics, *Anal. Chem.* 85: 6703–6715, 2013.

526. Karaganov, V., M. Law, M. Kaesler, D. G. Lancaster, and M. R. G. Taylor, Engineering development of a directed IR countermeasure laser, *Proc. SPIE* 5615 (Technologies for Optical Countermeasures): 48–53, 2004.

527. Northrop Grumman Corp., Viper™ Mid-IR Laser, Brochure DS-252-BAS-1104-A; www.northropgrumman.com/Capabilities/ViperMidIRLaser/Documents/viper.pdf.

528. Overton, G., Photonics applied: Defense: IR countermeasures aim for safer flights, *Laser Focus World* 47(8): 35–43, August, 2011; www.laserfocusworld.com/articles/print/volume-47/issue-8/features/photonics-applied-defense-ir-countermeasures-aim-for-safer-flights.html.

529. Grisard, A., F. Gutty, E. Lallier, and B. Gérard, Compact fiber laser-pumped mid-infrared source based on orientation-patterned gallium arsenide. In D. H. Titterton and M. A. Richardson (Eds), *Technologies for Optical Countermeasures VII, Proc. SPIE* 7836: 783606/1–783606/7, 2010.

530. Hemming, A., J. Richards, S. Bennetts, A. Davidson, N. Carmody, P. Davies, L. Corena, and D. Lancaster, A high power hybrid mid-IR laser source, *Opt. Commun.* 283: 4041–4045, 2010.

531. Hemming, A., J. Richards, A. Davidson, N. Carmody, S. Bennetts, N. Simakov, and J. Haub, 99 W mid-IR operation of a ZGP OPO at 25% duty cycle, *Opt. Express* 21: 10062–10069, 2013.

532. Lippert, E., H. Fonnum, G. Arisholm, and K. Stenerson, A 22-watt mid-infrared optical parametric oscillator with V-shaped 3-mirror ring resonator, *Opt. Express* 18: 26475–26483, 2010.

533. Hemming, A., J. Richards, A. Davidson, N. Carmody, N. Simakov, M. Hughes, P. Davies, S. Bennetts, and J. Haub, A high power mid-IR ZGP ring OPO. In *Technical Digest of 2013 Conference on Lasers and Electro-Optics, CLEO 2013* (Optical Society of America, 2013), paper CW1B.7; http://www.osapublishing.org/abstract.cfm?URI=CLEO_SI-2013-CW1B.7.

534. Yao, B.-Q., Y.-J. Shen, X.-M. Duan, T.-Y. Dai, Y.-L. Ju, and Y.-Z. Wang, A 41-W $ZnGeP_2$ optical parametric oscillator pumped by a Q-switched Ho:YAG laser, *Opt. Lett.* 39: 6589–6592, 2014.

535. Simakov, N., A. Davidson, A. Hemming, S. Bennetts, M. Hughes, N. Carmody, P. Davies, and J. Haub, Mid-Infrared generation in $ZnGeP_2$ pumped by a monolithic, power scalable 2-μm source. In *Fiber Lasers IX: Technology, Systems, and Applications*, *Proc. SPIE* 8237: 82373K/1–82373K/6, 2012.

536. Hemming, A., N. Simakov, J. Haub, and A. Carter, A review of recent progress in holmium-doped silica fibre sources, *Opt. Fib. Technol.* 20: 621–630, 2014.

537. Mittleman, D. (Ed.), *Sensing with Terahertz Radiation*, Springer, Berlin, 2003.

538. Chamberlain, J. M., Where optics meets electronics: Recent progress in decreasing the terahertz gap, *Philos. Trans. Roy. Soc. London A* 362: 199–213, 2004.

539. Federici, J. F., B. Schulkin, F. Huang, D. Gary, R. Barat, F Oliveira, and D. Zimdars, THz imaging and sensing for security applications—Explosives, weapons and drugs, *Semicond. Sci. Technol.* 20: S266–S280, 2005.

540. Chan, W. L., J. Diebel, and D. M. Mittleman, Imaging with THz radiation, *Rep. Prog. Phys.* 70: 1325–1379, 2007.

541. Zeitler, J. A., P. F. Taday, D. A. Newnham, M. Pepper, K. C. Gordon, and T. Rades, Terahertz pulsed spectroscopy and imaging in the pharmaceutical setting—A review, *J. Pharm. Pharmacol.* 59: 209–223, 2007.

542. Lee, Y.-S., *Principles of Terahertz Science and Technology*, Springer, Berlin, 2009.

543. Jepsen, P. U., D. G. Cooke, and M. Koch, Terahertz spectroscopy and imaging — Modern techniques and applications, *Laser Photon. Rev.* 5: 124–166, 2011; see also erratum in *Laser Photon. Rev.* 5: 418, 2012.

544. El Haddad, J., B. Bousquet, L. Canioni, and P. Mounaix, Review in terahertz spectral analysis, *Trends Anal. Chem.* 44: 98–105, 2013; http://www.sciencedirect.com/science/article/pii/S0165993613000022.

545. Ding, Y.-J. and I. B. Zotova, Coherent and tunable terahertz oscillators, generators, and amplifiers, *J. Nonlinear Opt. Phys. Mater* 11: 75–97, 2002.

546. Kawase, K., J.-I. Shikata, and H. Ito, Terahertz wave parametric source, *J. Phys. D: Appl. Phys.* 35: R1–R14, 2002.

547. Kawase, K., J.-I. Shikata, and H. Ito, Narrow-linewidth tunable terahertz-wave sources using nonlinear optics. In I. T. Sorokina and K. L. Vodopyanov (Eds), *Solid-State Mid-Infrared Sources*, Chapter 9, pp. 397–423, Springer, Berlin, 2003.

548. Kawase, K., Y. Ogawa, H. Minamide, and H. Ito, Terahertz parametric sources and imaging applications, *Semicon. Sci. Tech.* 20: S258–S265, 2005.

549. Dobroiu, A., C. Otani, and K. Kawase, Terahertz-wave sources and imaging applications, *Measure. Sci. Tech.* 17: R161–R174, 2006.

550. Tonouchi, M., Cutting-edge terahertz technology, *Nat. Photon.* 1: 97–105, 2007.

551. Linfield, E., Terahertz applications—A source of fresh hope, *Nat. Photon.* 1: 257–258, 2007.

552. Belkin, M. A., F. Capasso, A. Belyanin, D. L. Sivco, A. Y. Cho, D. C. Oakley, C. J. Vineis, and G. W. Turner, Terahertz quantum-cascade-laser source based on intra-cavity difference-frequency generation, *Nat. Photon.* 1: 288–292, 2007.

553. Williams, B. S., Terahertz quantum-cascade lasers, *Nat. Photon.* 1: 517–525, 2007.

554. Vodopyanov, K. L., Tunable THz sources based on quasi-phase-matched gallium arsenide. In M. Ebrahim-Zadeh and I. T. Sorokina (Eds), *Mid-Infrared Coherent Sources and Applications* (NATO Science for Peace and Security Series B: Physics and Biophysics), Chapter II-9, pp. 419–441, Springer, Berlin, 2007.

555. Vodopyanov, K. L., Optical THz-wave generation with periodically-inverted GaAs, *Laser Photon. Rev.* 2: 11–25, 2008.

556. Kitaeva, G. Kh. Terahertz generation by means of optical lasers, *Laser Phys. Lett.* 5: 559–576, 2008.

557. Suizu, K. and K. Kawase, Monochromatic-tunable terahertz-wave sources based on nonlinear frequency conversion using lithium niobate crystal, *IEEE J. Sel. Top. Quantum Electron.* 14: 295–306, 2008.

558. Hayashi, S. and K. Kawase, Terahertz-wave parametric sources. In K. Y. Kim (Ed.), *Recent Optical and Photonic Technologies*, Chapter 6, pp. 109–124, InTechOpen, Croatia, 2010; http://www.intechopen.com/books/recent-optical-and-photonic-technologies/terahertz.

559. Palka, N., T. Trzcinski, and M. Szustakowski, Terahertz spectra of explosives measured by optical parametric oscillator-based system and time domain spectroscopy, *Acta Phys. Pol.* 122: 946–949, 2012.

560. Dean, P., A. Valavanis, J. Keeley, K. Bertling, Y. L. Lim, R. Alhathlool, A. D. Burnett, L. H. Li, S. P. Khanna, D. Indjin, T. Taimre, A. D. Rakić, E. H. Linfield, and A. G. Davies, Terahertz imaging using quantum cascade lasers—A review of systems and applications, *J. Phys. D: Appl. Phys.* 47: 374008/1–374008/22, 2014.

561. Hayashi, S.-I., K. Nawata, T. Taira, J.-I. Shikata, K. Kawase, and H. Minamide, Ultrabright continuously tunable terahertz-wave generation at room temperature, *Scient. Rep.* 4: 5045/–5045/5, 2014.

562. Puthoff, H. E., R. H. Pantell, B. G. Huth, and M. A. Chacon, Near-forward Raman scattering in LiNbO$_3$, *J. Appl. Phys.* 39: 2144–2146, 1968.

563. Yarborough, J. M., S. S. Sussman, H. E. Puthoff, R. H. Pantell, and B. C. Johnson, Efficient, tunable optical emission from LiNbO$_3$ without a resonator, *Appl. Phys. Lett.* 15: 102–105, 1969.

564. Johnson, B. C., H. E. Puthoff, J. SooHoo, and S. S. Sussman, Power and linewidth of tunable stimulated far-infrared emission in LiNbO$_3$, *Appl. Phys. Lett.* 18: 181–183, 1971.

565. Piestrup, M. A., R. N. Fleming, and R. H. Pantell, Continuously tunable submillimeter wave source, *Appl. Phys. Lett.* 26: 418–421, 1975.

566. Kawase, K., M. Sato, T. Taniuchi, and H. Ito, Coherent tunable THz-wave generation from LiNbO$_3$ with monolithic grating coupler, *Appl. Phys. Lett.* 68: 2483–2485, 1996.

567. Kawase, K., M. Sato, K. Nakamura, T. Taniuchi, and H. Ito, Unidirectional radiation of widely tunable THz wave using a prism coupler under noncollinear phase matching condition, *Appl. Phys. Lett.* 71: 753–755, 1997.

568. Shikata, J., K. Kawase, M. Sato, K. Nakamura, T. Taniuchi, and H. Ito, Enhancement of terahertz-wave output from LiNbO$_3$ optical parametric oscillators by cryogenic cooling, *Opt. Lett.* 24: 202–204, 1999.

569. Morikawa, A., K. Kawase, J.-I. Shikata, T. Taniuchi, and H. Ito, Parametric THz-wave generation using trapezoidal LiNbO$_3$, *Proc. SPIE* 3828 (Terahertz Spectroscopy and Applications II): 302–310, 1999.

570. Shikata, J.-I., K. Kawase, K.-I. Karino, T. Taniuchi, and H. Ito, Tunable terahertz-wave parametric oscillators using $LiNbO_3$ and $MgO:LiNbO_3$ crystals, *IEEE Trans. Micro. Theo. Tech.* 48: 653–661, 2000.

571. Kawase, K., T. Hatanaka, H. Takahashi, K. Nakamura, T. Taniuchi, and H. Ito, Tunable terahertz-wave generation from DAST crystal by dual signal-wave parametric oscillation of periodically poled lithium niobate, *Opt. Lett.* 25: 1714–1716, 2000.

572. Kawase, K., J. Shikata, H. Minamide, K. Imai, and H. Ito, Arrayed silicon prism coupler for a THz-wave parametric oscillator, *Appl. Opt.* 40: 1423–1426, 2001.

573. Kawase, K., K. Imai, K. Kawase, and H. Ito, A frequency-agile terahertz-wave parametric oscillator, *Opt. Express* 8: 699–704, 2001.

574. Kawase, K., J.-I. Shikata, K. Imai, and H. Ito, Transform-limited, narrow-linewidth, THz wave parametric generator, *Appl. Phys. Lett.* 78: 2819–2821, 2001.

575. Ito, H., T. Hatanaka, S. Haidar, K. Nakamura, K. Kawase, and T. Taniuchi, Periodically poled $LiNbO_3$ OPO for generating mid-IR to terahertz waves, *Ferroelectrics* 253: 95–104, 2001.

576. Sato, A., K. Kawase, H. Minamide, S. Wada, and H. Ito, Tabletop terahertz-wave parametric generator using a compact, diode-pumped Nd:YAG laser, *Rev. Sci. Instrum.* 72: 3501–3504, 2001.

577. Kawase, K., H. Minamide, K. Imai, J.-I. Shikata, and H. Ito, Injection-seeded terahertz-wave parametric generator with wide tunability, *Appl. Phys. Lett.* 80: 195–197, 2002.

578. Imai, K., K. Kawase, H. Minamide, and H. Ito, Achromatically injection-seeded terahertz-wave parametric generator, *Opt. Lett.* 27: 2173–2175, 2002.

579. Kawase, K., K. Y. Ogawa, Y. Watanabe, and H. Inoue, Non-destructive terahertz imaging of illicit drugs using spectral fingerprints, *Opt. Express* 11: 2549–2554, 2003.

580. Kawase, K., Y. Ogawa, and Y. Watanabe, Component pattern analysis of chemicals using multispectral THz-imaging system, *Proc. SPIE* 5354 (Terahertz and Gigahertz Electronics and Photonics III): 63–70, 2006.

581. Hayashi, S., H. Minamide, T. Ikari, Y. Ogawa, J.-I. Shikata, H. Ito, C. Otani, and K. Kawase, Output power enhancement of a palmtop terahertz-wave parametric generator, *Appl. Opt.* 46: 117–123, 2007.

582. Kawase, K. and S.-I. Hayashi, Terahertz wave parametric generation and applications, *Proc. SPIE* 6772 (Terahertz Physics, Devices, and Systems II): 677202/1–677202/5, 2007.

583. Shibuya, T., T. Akiba, K. Suizu, H. Uchida, C. Otani, and K. Kawase, Terahertz-wave generation using a 4-dimethylamino-N-methyl-4-stilbazolium tosylate crystal under intra-cavity conditions, *Appl. Phys. Express* 1: 042002/1–042002/3, 2008.

584. Suizu, K., K. Koketsu, T. Shibuya, T. Tsutsui, T. Akiba, and K. Kawase, Extremely frequency-widened terahertz wave generation using Cherenkov-type radiation, *Opt. Express* 17: 6676–6681, 2009.

585. Hayashi, S.-I., T. Shibuya, H. Sakai, T. Taira, C. Otani, Y. Ogawa, and K. Kawase, Tunability enhancement of a terahertz-wave parametric generator pumped by a microchip Nd:YAG laser, *Appl. Opt.* 48: 2899–2902, 2009.

586. Kawase, K., K. Suizu, S. Hayashi, and T. Shibuya, Nonlinear optical terahertz wave sources, *Opt. Spectros.* 108: 841–845, 2010.

587. Nakagomi, Y., K. Suizu, T. Shibuya, and K. Kawase, Multi-mode laser-pumped injection-seeded terahertz-wave parametric generator, *Jpn. J. Appl. Phys.* 49: 102701/1–102701/3, 2010.

588. Hayashi, S.-I., K. Nawata, H. Sakai, T. Taira, H. Minamide, and K. Kawase, High-power, single-longitudinal-mode terahertz-wave generation pumped by a microchip Nd:YAG laser, *Opt. Express* 20: 2881–2886, 2012.

589. Uchida, H., S. R. Tripathi, K. Suizu, T. Shibuya, T. Osumi, and K. Kawase, Widely tunable broadband terahertz radiation generation using a configurationally locked polyene 2-[3-(4-hydroxystyryl)-5,5-dimethylcyclohex-2-enylidene] malononitrile crystal via difference frequency generation, *Appl. Phys. B* 111: 489–493, 2013.

590. Murate, K., Y. Taira, S. R. Tripathi, S.-I. Hayashi, K. Nawata, H. Minamide, and K. Kawase, A high dynamic range and spectrally flat terahertz spectrometer based on optical parametric processes in LiNbO$_3$, *IEEE Trans. Terahertz Sci. Tech.* 4: 523–526, 2014.

591. Taira, Y., S. R. Tripathi, K. Murate, S.-I. Hayashi, K. Nawata, H. Minamide, and K. Kawase, A terahertz wave parametric amplifier with a gain of 55 dB, *IEEE Trans. Terahertz Sci. Tech.* 4: 753–755, 2014.

592. Tripathi, S. R., Y. Taira, S.-I. Hayashi, K. Nawata, K. Murate, H. Minamide, and K. Kawase, Terahertz wave parametric amplifier, *Opt. Lett.* 39: 1649–1652, 2014.

593. Edwards, T. J., D. Walsh, M. B. Spurr, C. F. Rae, M. H. Dunn, and P. G. Browne, Compact source of continuously and widely-tunable terahertz radiation, *Opt. Express* 14: 1582–1589, 2006.

594. Edwards, T. J., D. Walsh, M. B. Spurr, P. G. Browne, C. F. Rae, and M. H. Dunn, Compact and coherent source of widely tunable THz radiation, *Proc. SPIE* 6402 (Optics and Photonics for Counterterrorism and Crime Fighting II): 64020C/1–64020C/8, 2006.

595. Stothard, D. J. M., T. J. Edwards, D. Walsh, C. L. Thomson, C. F. Rae, M. H. Dunn, and P. G. Browne, Line-narrowed, compact, and coherent source of widely tunable terahertz radiation, *Appl. Phys. Lett.* 92: 141105/1–141105/3, 2008.

596. Walsh, D. A., P. G. Browne, M. H. Dunn, and C. F. Rae, Intra-cavity parametric generation of nanosecond terahertz radiation using quasi-phase-matching, *Opt. Express* 18: 13951–13963, 2010.

597. Thomson, C. L., and M. H. Dunn, Observation of a cascaded process in intra-cavity terahertz optical parametric oscillators based on lithium niobate, *Opt. Express* 21: 17647–17658, 2013.

598. Zhong, K., J.-Q. Yao, D.-G. Xu, Z. Wang, Z.-Y. Li, H.-Y. Zhang, and P. Wang, Enhancement of terahertz wave difference frequency generation based on a compact walk-off compensated KTP OPO, *Opt. Commun.* 283: 3520–3524, 2010.

599. Li, Z.-Y., J.-Q. Yao, D.-G. Xu, K. Zhong, P.-B. Bing, and J.-L. Wang, Study on the generation of high-power terahertz wave from surface-emitted THz-wave parametric oscillator with MgO:LiNbO$_3$ crystal, *Proc. SPIE* 7854 (Infrared, Millimeter Wave, and Terahertz Technologies): 78543H/1–78543H/9, 2010.

600. Li, Z.-Y., J.-Q. Yao, D. Lu, D.-G. Xu, J.-L. Wang, and P.-B. Bing, High-power terahertz radiation based on a compact eudipleural THz-wave parametric oscillator, *Chin. Phys. Lett.* 28: 064209/1–064209/4, 2011.

601. Li, Z.-Y., J.-Q. Yao, D.-G. Xu, K. Zhong, J.-L. Wang, and P.-B. Bing, High-power terahertz radiation from surface-emitted THz-wave parametric oscillator, *Chin. Phys. B* 20: 054207/1–054207/5, 2011.

602. Li, Z.-Y., P.-B. Bing, J.-Q. Yao, D.-G. Xu, and K. Zhong, High-powered tunable terahertz source based on a surface-emitted terahertz-wave parametric oscillator, *Opt. Eng.* 51: 091605/1–091605/4, 2012.

603. Li, Z.-Y., P.-B. Bing, D.-G. Xu, and J.-Q. Yao, High-power tunable terahertz generation from a surface-emitted THz-wave parametric oscillator based on two MgO:LiNbO$_3$ crystals, *Optik* 124: 4884–4886, 2013.

604. Xu, D.-G., W. Shi, K. Zhong, Y.-Y. Wang, P.-X. Liu, and J.-Q. Yao, Widely tunable THz generation in QPM-GaAs crystal pumped by a near-degenerate dual-wavelength KTP OPO at around 2.127 μm, *Proc. SPIE* 8604 (Nonlinear Frequency Generation and Conversion: Materials, Devices, and Applications XII): 86040E/1–86040E/6, 2013.

605. Xu, D.-G., H. Zhang, H. Jiang, Y.-Y. Wang, C.-M. Liu, H. Yu, Z.-Y. Li, W. Shi, and J.-Q. Yao, High energy terahertz parametric oscillator based on surface-emitted configuration, *Chin. Phys. Lett.* 30: 024212/1–024212/4, 2013.

606. Wang, Y.-Y., D.-G. Xu, H. Jiang, K. Zhong, and J.-Q. Yao, A high-energy, low-threshold tunable intra-cavity terahertz-wave parametric oscillator with surface-emitted configuration, *Laser Phys.* 23: 055406/1–055406/5, 2013.

607. Liu, P.-X., D.-G. Xu, J-Q. Li, C. Yan, Z.-X. Li, Y.-Y. Wang, and J.-Q. Yao, Monochromatic Cherenkov THz source pumped by a singly resonant optical parametric oscillator, *IEEE Photon. Tech. Lett.* 26: 494–496, 2014.

608. Liu, P.-X., D.-G. Xu, Y. Li, X.-Y. Zhang, Y.-Y. Wang, J.-Q. Yao, and Y.-C. Wu, Widely tunable and monochromatic terahertz difference frequency generation with organic crystal DSTMS, *Europhys. Lett.* 106: 60001/1–60001/5, 2014.

609. Li, Z.-Y., P.-B. Bing, S. Yuan, D.-G. Xu, and J.-Q. Yao, Investigation on terahertz parametric oscillators using GaP crystal with a noncollinear phase-matching scheme, *J. Mod. Opt.* 62: 302–306, 2015.

610. Li, Z.-Y., P.-B. Bing, S. Yuan, D.-G. Xu, and J.-Q. Yao, Investigation on terahertz parametric oscillators using quasi-phase-matching GaP crystal, *Mod. Phys. Lett. B* 29: 1450258/1–1450258/10, 2015.

611. Wang, Y.-Y., Z.-X. Li, J.-Q. Li, C. Yan, T.-N. Chen, D.-G. Xu, W. Shi, H. Feng, and J.-Q. Yao, Energy scaling of a tunable terahertz parametric oscillator with a surface emitted configuration, *Laser Phys.* 24: 125402/1–125402/5, 2014.

612. Lee, A. J., Y. He, and H. M. Pask, Frequency-tunable THz source based on stimulated polariton scattering in Mg:LiNbO$_3$, *IEEE J. Quantum Elect.* 49: 357–364, 2013.

613. Lee, A. J. and H. M. Pask, Continuous wave, frequency-tunable terahertz laser radiation generated via stimulated polariton scattering, *Opt. Lett.* 39: 442–445, 2014.

614. Lee, A. J. and H. M. Pask, Cascaded stimulated polariton scattering in a Mg:LiNbO$_3$ terahertz laser, *Opt. Express* 23: 8687–8698, 2015.

615. Ikari, T., R. Guo, H. Minamide, and H. Ito, Energy scalable terahertz-wave parametric oscillator using surface-emitted configuration, *J. European Opt. Soc.: Rap. Pub.* 5: 10054/1–10054/4, 2010.

616. Molter, D., M. Theuer, and R. Beigang, Nanosecond terahertz optical parametric oscillator with a novel quasi phase matching scheme in lithium niobate, *Opt. Express* 17: 6623–6628, 2009.

617. Ito, H., K. Suizu, T. Yamashita, T. Sato, and A. Nawahara, Random frequency accessible broad tunable terahertz-wave source using phase-matched 4-dimethylamino-N-methyl-4-stilbazolium tosylate crystal, *Jpn. J. Appl. Phys.* 46: 7321–7324, 2007.

618. Suizu, K., T. Shibuya, S. Nagano, T. Akiba, K. Edamatsu, H. Ito, and K. Kawase, Pulsed high peak power millimeter wave generation via difference frequency generation using periodically poled lithium niobate, *Jpn. J. Appl. Phys.* 46: L982–L984, 2007.

619. Lee, Y.-S., W. C. Hurlbut, K. L. Vodopyanov, M. M. Fejer, and V. G. Kozlov, Generation of multi-cycle intra-cavity terahertz-wave generation in a synchronously pumped optical parametric oscillator using quasi-phase-matched GaAs, *Appl. Phys. Lett.* 89: 181104/1–181104/3, 2006.

620. Schaar, J. E., K. L. Vodopyanov, and M. M. Fejer, Intra-cavity terahertz-wave generation in a synchronously pumped optical parametric oscillator using quasi-phase-matched GaAs, *Opt. Lett.* 32: 1284–1286, 2007.

621. Schaar, J. E., K. L. Vodopyanov, P. S. Kuo, M. M. Fejer, X. Yu, A. Lin, J. S. Harris, D. Bliss, C. Lynch, V. G. Kozlov, and W. C. Hurlbut, Terahertz sources based on intra-cavity parametric down-conversion in quasi-phase-matched gallium arsenide, *IEEE J. Sel. Top. Quantum Electron.* 14: 354–362, 2008.

622. Vodopyanov, K. L. and Y. H. Avetisyan, Optical terahertz wave generation in a planar GaAs waveguide, *Opt. Lett.* 33: 2314–2316, 2008.

623. Vodopyanov, K. L., W. C. Hurlbut, and V. G. Kozlov, Photonic THz generation in GaAs via resonantly enhanced intra-cavity multispectral mixing, *Appl. Phys. Lett.* 99: 041104/1–041104/3, 2011.

624. Tekavec, P. F., W. C. Hurlbut, V. G. Kozlov, and K. L. Vodopyanov, Terahertz generation from quasi-phase matched gallium arsenide using a type II ring cavity optical parametric oscillator, *Proc. SPIE* 8261 (Terahertz Technology and Applications V): 82610V/1–82610V/9, 2012.

625. Kiessling, J., K. Buse, K. L. Vodopyanov, and I. Breunig, Continuous-wave optical parametric source for terahertz waves tunable from 1 to 4.5 THz frequency, *Proc. SPIE* 8964 (Nonlinear Frequency Generation and Conversion: Materials, Devices, and Applications XIII): 896408/1–896408/8, 2014.

626. Weiss, C., G. Torosyan, Y. Avetisyan, and R. Beigang, Generation of tunable narrowband surface-emitted terahertz radiation in periodically poled lithium niobate, *Opt. Lett.* 26: 563–565, 2001.

627. Weiss, C., G. Torosyan, J.-P. Meyn, R. Wallenstein, R. Beigang, and Y. Avetisyan, Tuning characteristics of narrowband THz radiation generated via optical rectification in periodically poled lithium niobate, *Opt. Express* 8: 497–502, 2001.

628. L'huillier, J. A., G. Torosyan, M. Theuer, Y. Avetisyan, and R. Beigang, Generation of THz radiation using bulk, periodically and aperiodically poled lithium niobate— Part 1: Theory, *Appl. Phys. B* 86: 185–196, 2007.

629. L'huillier, J. A., G. Torosyan, M. Theuer, C. Rau, Y. Avetisyan, and R. Beigang, Generation of THz radiation using bulk, periodically and aperiodically poled lithium niobate—Part 2: Experiments, *Appl. Phys. B* 86: 197–208, 2007.

630. Tillman, K. A., D. T. Reid, R. R. J. Maier, and E. D. McNaghten, Mid-infrared absorption spectroscopy of methane across a 14.4-THz spectral range using a broadband femtosecond optical parametric oscillator based on aperiodically poled lithium niobate, *Proc. SPIE* 5989 (Technologies for Optical Countermeasures II; Femtosecond Phenomena II; and Passive Millimetre-Wave and Terahertz Imaging II): 59890U/1–59890U/9, 2005.

631. Kiessling, J., I Breunig, P. G. Schunemann, K Buse, and K. L. Vodopyanov, High power and spectral purity continuous-wave photonic THz source tunable from 1 to 4.5 THz for nonlinear molecular spectroscopy, *New J. Phys.* 15: 105014/1–105014/11, 2013.

632. Kiessling, J., K. Buse, K. L. Vodopyanov, and I. Breunig, Continuous-wave optical parametric source for terahertz waves tunable from 1 to 4.5 THz frequency, *Proc. SPIE* 8964 (Nonlinear Frequency Generation and Conversion: Materials, Devices, and Applications XIII): 896408/1–896408/8, 2014.

633. Winnewisser, G., S. P. Belov, Th. Klaus, and R. Schieder, Sub-Doppler measurements on the rotational transitions of carbon monoxide, *J. Molec. Spectrosc.* 184: 468–472, 1997.

634. Breunig, I., J. Kiessling, R. Sowade, B. Knabe, and K. Buse, Generation of tunable continuous-wave terahertz radiation by photomixing the signal waves of a dual-crystal optical parametric oscillator, *New J. Phys.* 10: 073003/1–073003/6, 2008.

635. Kiessling, J., R. Sowade, I. Breunig, K. Buse, and V. Dierolf, Cascaded optical parametric oscillations generating tunable terahertz waves in periodically poled lithium niobate crystals, *Opt. Express* 17: 87–91, 2009.

636. Sowade, R., I. Breunig, I. C. Mayorga, J. Kiessling, C. Tulea, V. Dierolf, and K. Buse, Continuous-wave optical parametric terahertz source, *Opt. Express* 17: 22303–22310, 2009.

637. Kiessling, J., F. Fuchs, K. Buse, and I. Breunig, Pump-enhanced optical parametric oscillator generating continuous wave tunable terahertz radiation, *Opt. Lett.* 36: 4374–4376, 2011.

638. Scheller, M., J. M. Yarborough, J. V. Moloney, M. Fallahi, M. Koch, and S. W. Koch, Room temperature continuous wave milliwatt terahertz source, *Opt. Express* 18: 27112–27117, 2010.

639. Harris, S. E., Proposed backward wave oscillation in the infrared, *Appl. Phys. Lett.* 9: 114–116, 1966.

640. Khurgin, J. B., Optical parametric oscillator: Mirrorless magic, *Nat. Photon.* 1: 446–447, 2007.

641. Canalias, C. and V. Pasiškevičius, Mirrorless optical parametric oscillator, *Nat. Photon.* 1: 459–462, 2007.

642. Ding, Y. J. and J. B. Khurgin, Backward optical parametric oscillators and amplifiers, *IEEE J. Quantum Elect.* 32: 1574–1582, 1996.

643. Su, H., S.-C. Ruan, and Y. Guo, Generation of mid-infrared wavelengths larger than 4.0 μm in a mirrorless counterpropagating configuration, *J. Opt. Soc. Am. B* 23: 1626–1629, 2006.

644. Canalias, C., V. Pasiškevičius, R. Clemens, and F. Laurell, Submicron periodically poled flux-grown KTiOPO$_4$, *Appl. Phys. Lett.* 82: 4233–4235, 2003.

645. Canalias, C., V. Pasiškevičius, M. Fokine, and F. Laurell, Backward quasi-phase-matched second-harmonic generation in submicrometer periodically poled flux-grown KTiOPO$_4$, *Appl. Phys. Lett.* 86: 181105/1–181105/3, 2003.

646. Jacobsson, B., C. Canalias, V. Pasiškevičius, and F. Laurell, Narrowband and tunable ring optical parametric oscillator with a volume Bragg grating, *Opt. Lett.* 32: 3278–3280, 2007.

647. Hellström, J. E., B. Jacobsson, V. Pasiškevičius, and F. Laurell, Finite beams in reflective volume Bragg gratings: Theory and experiments, *IEEE J. Quantum Elect.* 44: 81–89, 2008.

648. Belkin, M. A., K. Vijayraghavan, A. Vizbaras, A. Jiang, F. Demmerle, G. Boehm, R. Meyer, M. C. Amann, A. Matyas, R. Chashmahcharagh, P. Lugli, C. Jirauschek, and Z. R. Wasilewski, THz quantum cascade lasers for operation above cryogenic temperatures, *Proc. SPIE* 8640 (Novel In-Plane Semiconductor Lasers XII): 864014/1–864014/6, 2013.

649. Vijayraghavan, K., Y. Jiang, M. Jang, A. Jiang, K. Choutagunta, A. Vizbaras, F. Demmerle, G. Boehm, M. C. Amann, and M. A. Belkin, Broadly tunable terahertz generation in mid-infrared quantum cascade lasers, *Nat. Commun.* 4: 3021/1–3021/7, 2013.

650. Jiang, A., A. Matyas, K. Vijayraghavan, C. Jirauschek, Z. R. Wasilewski, and M. A. Belkin, Experimental investigation of terahertz quantum cascade laser with variable barrier heights, *J. Appl. Phys.* 115: 163103/1–163103/5, 2014.

651. Vijayraghavan, K., M. Jang, A. Jiang, X. Wang, M. Troccoli, and M. A. Belkin, *IEEE Photon. Technol. Lett.* 26: 391–394, 2014.

652. Lee, J., M. Tymchenko, C. Argyropoulos, P.-Y. Chen, F. Lu, F. Demmerle, G. Boehm, M. C. Amann, A. Alu, and M. A. Belkin, Giant nonlinear response from plasmonic metasurfaces coupled to intersubband transitions, *Nature* 511 (7507): 65–69, 2014.

653. Jung, S., A. Jiang, Y. Jiang, K. Vijayraghavan, X. Wang, M. Troccoli, and M. A. Belkin, Broadly tunable monolithic room-temperature terahertz quantum cascade laser sources, *Nat. Commun.* 5: 4267, 2014.

654. Jiang, Y., K. Vijayraghavan, S. Jung, F. Demmerle, G. Boehm, M. C. Amann, and M. A. Belkin, External cavity terahertz quantum cascade laser sources based on intra-cavity frequency mixing with 1.2–5.9 THz tuning range, *J. Opt.* 16: 094002/1–094002/9, 2014.

655. Boyd, G. D. and C. K. N. Patel, Enhancement of optical second-harmonic generation by reflection phase matching in ZnSe and GaAs, *Appl. Phys. Lett.* 8: 313–315, 1966.

656. Komine, H., W. H. Long, Jr., J. W. Tully, and E. A. Stappaerts, Quasi-phase matched second-harmonic generation by use of a total internal-reflection phase shift in gallium arsenide and zinc selenide plates, *Opt. Lett.* 23: 661–663, 1998.

657. Haïdar, R., Ph. Kupecek, E. Rosencher, R. Triboulet, and Ph. Lemasson, Quasi-phase-matched difference frequency generation (8–13 μm) in an isotropic semiconductor using total reflection, *Appl. Phys. Lett.* 82: 1167–1169, 2003.

658. Haïdar, R., Ph. Kupecek, E. Rosencher, R. Triboulet, and Ph. Lemasson, New mid-infrared optical sources based on isotropic semiconductors (zinc selenide and gallium arsenide) using total internal reflection quasi-phase-matching, *Proc. SPIE* 5136 (Solid State Crystals 2002: Crystalline Materials for Optoelectronics): 335–343, 2003.

659. Haïdar, R., N. Forget, Ph. Kupececk, and E. Rosencher, Fresnel phase matching for three-wave mixing in isotropic semiconductors, *J. Opt. Soc. Am. B* 21: 1522–1534, 2004.

660. Raybaut, M., A. Godard, A. Toulouse, C. Lubin, and E. Rosencher, Nonlinear reflection effects on Fresnel phase matching, *Appl. Phys. Lett.* 92: 121112/1–121112/3, 2008.

661. Raybaut, M., A. Godard, A. Toulouse, C. Lubin, and E. Rosencher, Fresnel phase matching: Exploring the frontiers between ray and guided wave quadratic nonlinear optics, *Opt. Express* 16: 18457–18478, 2008.

662. Kosterev, A., G. Wysocki, Y. Bakhirkin, S. So, R. Lewicki, M. Fraser, F. Tittel, and R. F. Curl, Application of quantum cascade lasers to trace gas analysis, *Appl. Phys. B* 90: 165–176, 2008.

663. Tittel, F. K., G. Wysocki, A. A. Kosterev, and Y. A. Bakhirkin, Semiconductor laser based trace gas sensor technology: Recent advances. In M. Ebrahim-Zadeh and I. T. Sorokina (Eds), *Mid-Infrared Coherent Sources and Applications* (NATO Science for Peace and Security Series B: Physics and Biophysics), Chapter III.1, pp. 467–493, Springer, Berlin, 2007.

664. Taubman, M. S., T. L. Myers, B. D. Cannon, and R. M. Williams, Stabilization, injection and control of quantum cascade lasers, and their application to chemical sensing in the infrared, *Spectrochim. Acta A* 60: 3457–3468, 2004.

665. Young, C., S.-S. Kim, and B. Mizaikoff, Chemical sensing using quantum cascade lasers. In M. Lackner (Ed.), *Lasers in Chemistry* (Probing Matter). Volume 1, Chapter 4, pp. 77–108, Wiley-VCH, Chichester, 2008.

666. Curl, R. F., F. Capasso, C. Gmachl, A. A. Kosterev, B. McManus, R. Lewicki, M. Pusharsky, G. Wysocki, and F. K. Tittel, Quantum cascade lasers in chemical physics, *Chem. Phys. Lett.* 487: 1–18, 2010.

3 Solid-State Organic Dye Lasers

Angel Costela, I. García-Moreno, and R. Sastre

CONTENTS

3.1 INTRODUCTION

From the mid-1960s, dye lasers have been attractive sources of coherent tunable visible radiation because of their unique operational flexibility [1,2]. Dye lasers can emit both pulsed and continuous-wave forms, can be pumped with a wide variety of excitation sources, and exhibit an inherent ability to yield high pulse energies and high average powers. Hundreds of dyes have been demonstrated to lase measurably, covering the range from the ultraviolet to the near infrared. The introduction of wavelength-selective elements in the laser cavity allows narrow-linewidth operation and tunability, and the large gain bandwidth of these molecules makes possible the generation of ultrashort pulses. The versatile nature of these lasers has resulted in their applicability to a wide range of different fields, from basic science, such as physics, chemistry, and spectroscopy, to medicine and industry.

Organic dyes are fluorescent molecules with high molecular weights, characterized by containing extended systems of conjugated double bonds. In a dye laser, these molecules are dissolved in an organic solvent or incorporated into a solid matrix. A simplified diagram of the rather complex energy level structure of an organic dye is shown in Figure 3.1. When pumped with visible or ultraviolet light, higher vibrational levels of the first excited electronic singlet state S_1 of the dye molecules are populated. After fast radiationless relaxation, the excited dye molecules accumulate in the lowest vibrational level of S_1, which constitutes the upper level of the laser transition. Laser emission depopulates this level into higher-lying vibrational–rotational levels of the ground electronic state S_0. Finally, nonradiative processes remove molecules from the lower level of the laser transition. Competing with the radiative depopulation of S_1, there are radiationless transitions into the lower triplet state T_1. This

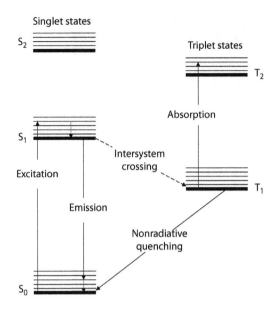

Singlet states

S_2

Triplet states

T_2

Absorption

S_1

Intersystem
crossing

Excitation

T_1

Emission

Nonradiative
quenching

S_0

FIGURE 3.1 Schematic energy-level diagram for a typical dye molecule.

intersystem crossing process populates the lower metastable triplet state and could cause considerable losses if the triplet–triplet absorption bands overlap the lasing band, inhibiting or even halting the lasing process. The triplet losses can be reduced by adding small quantities of appropriate triplet quenchers. These losses are not very important under pulsed excitation with nanosecond pulses because the usual inter-system crossing rates are not fast enough to build up an appreciable triplet population in the nanosecond time domain.

The levels shown schematically in Figure 3.1 are spaced closely enough to form a continuum due to line-broadening mechanisms. Thus, the different fluorescent lines overlap, and absorption and fluorescence spectra consist of a broad continuum, as illustrated in Figure 3.2. Although dyes have been demonstrated to lase in the solid, liquid, or gas phase, it is in the liquid and solid phases that dyes have made a signifi-cant impact as laser media. From the early days of the development of dye lasers, attempts were made to incorporate the dye molecules into solid hosts, and the first solid-state dye lasers (SSDLs) were demonstrated by Soffer and McFarland in 1967 [3] and by Peterson and Snavely in 1968 [4] with pulsed laser and flashlamp pump-ing, respectively. Over the next decade, a variety of materials and pumping arrange-ments were tried for the operation of dyes in the solid state, but the lasing efficiencies were low, and the dye molecules experienced fast photodegradation, with the result that the laser emission faded rather quickly [5]. Thus, liquid solutions of dyes in organic solvents, in which the active medium can be obtained with high optical qual-ity and cooled by simply using a flow system, became the standard media for dye lasers. Nevertheless, this approach was never fully satisfactory because of the seri-ous inconveniences evidenced by the liquid dye lasers, mainly related to the need to handle large volumes of messy and sometimes toxic liquids. In addition, continuous

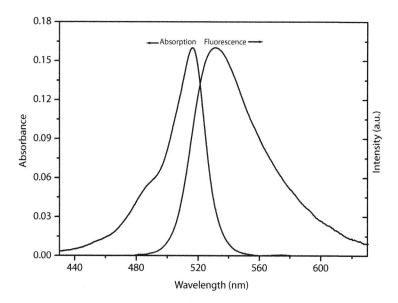

FIGURE 3.2   UV/VIS absorption and fluorescence spectra of the laser dye pyrromethene 567 in methanol solution.

circulation of the solution requires pumps and the design of complex and bulky cells, which, together with the large dye/solvent reservoirs, increases the size and cost of these dye laser systems and has restricted their use outside the laboratory.

The problems posed by liquid dye lasers stimulated further consideration of the SSDL approach, and in the early 1990s the development of improved host materials with higher laser-damage resistance [5,6] and the synthesis of new high-performance laser dyes [7–9] spurred a renaissance in the field of SSDLs. The 1990s witnessed a great deal of activity in the field, and, as a result, significant advances were made toward the development of practical, tunable SSDLs [2,10]. In recent years, approaches involving the use of new polymeric formulations, organic–inorganic hybrid materials, polymeric media with dispersed silica nanoparticles, or silicon-modified organic matrices as host materials for laser dyes are resulting in SSDLs that are fully competitive with their liquid counterparts. These promising results have been obtained with dyes emitting in the green to red spectral region. Much less work has been done with dyes emitting in the blue region, and the results obtained in solid state are still far from the performance of the same dyes in liquid solution.

In this chapter, we present an overview of the main recent developments of SSDLs and outline the state of the art in the field. The focus will be on those developments that could lead to the practical implementation of SSDL in the short term. Thus, we shall concentrate mainly on the results obtained using dyes with emission in the spectral region from the green to the red. SSDL narrow-linewidth oscillators are discussed in Chapter 4, and medical applications of dye lasers are described in Chapter 8.

3.2 MATERIALS

The basic requirements imposed on a solid matrix to be used as host for lasing dye molecules are high optical quality with a low level of scattering, transparency at both pump and lasing wavelengths, high damage threshold to laser radiation, and good thermal and photochemical stability. A simple technology for doping the matrix material with different classes of organic dyes is also desirable. Thus, in the development of materials for tunable solid-state lasers, the problems to be addressed are the design and optimization of solid matrices with the required properties, the selection or design of dyes with the desirable characteristics, and the development of the appropriate fabrication technology.

Over the years, a variety of materials have been tried as solid hosts for lasing dyes: from mixtures of solvents at low temperature, gelatin, or organic molecular crystals, to inorganic glasses, transparent polymers, and organic–inorganic hybrid materials [5,10]. From work done over the last decade, it is becoming apparent that properly modified polymeric formulations and advanced hybrid materials are well-positioned candidates for developing efficient and stable SSDLs.

3.2.1 ORGANIC POLYMERS

Polymers have been tried as solid hosts for lasing dyes from the early days of SSDLs. These materials exhibit some features that make them very attractive in this application: good chemical compatibility with organic dyes; excellent optical homogeneity, important to avoid interference in the gain medium due to microscopic variation of the refractive index; adaptability to inexpensive fabrication techniques; and ease in modifying in a controlled way relevant characteristics, such as free volume, chemical composition, molecular weight, microstructure, or viscoelasticity. The main limitations of polymers as materials for SSDL are related to photodegradation processes, due to the low power-damage threshold of the matrix, as well as to thermal lensing effects due to the relatively high values of $\partial n/\partial T$ in these media [11].

A great part of the damage caused by laser radiation in the polymeric materials used in the early studies on SSDL, three decades ago, was due to the presence of absorbing centers in the material, such as molecular impurities and foreign absorbing inclusions. The first significant improvements in the laser-damage threshold of organic polymers came from the generalized use of processes such as distillation, sonication, and microfiltration in the preparation of the materials. Optical uniformity of the polymer matrix, avoiding or minimizing the intrinsic anisotropy developed during polymerization, requires strict control of the polymerization rate and the thermal conditions during the polymerization step.

There was soon enough evidence to establish that the resistance to laser damage depended on the viscoelastic properties of the matrix. This opened a new way to enhance the laser resistance of the material and led to two different approaches in the search for improved materials, which can be called *external* and *internal plasticization*. External plasticization of the polymer is achieved by adding different low-molecular-weight additives. It reduces the induced elastic limit of the polymer to below the brittle-fracture point, improving the laser resistance by several orders of magnitude [12]. The low-molecular-weight additives have some mobility in the polymer matrix and can migrate and leach out over time, with unpredictable effects. This problem can be overcome by using internal plasticization: copolymerization of the matrix basic compound with aliphatic acrylic comonomers [13].

By using the former approach, Maslyukov et al. [14] demonstrated, in 1995, lasing efficiencies in the range 40%–60% with matrices of modified poly(methyl methacrylate) (MPMMA) doped with rhodamine dyes and pumped longitudinally at 532 nm. The useful lifetime or normalized photostability of the samples (defined as the number of pump pulses that produce a 50% drop in the laser output) was 15,000 pulses at a pump repetition rate of 3.33 Hz. The internal plasticization approach was followed by Costela et al., who, also in 1995, demonstrated laser action with efficiency of 21% using the dye rhodamine 6G (Rh6G) dissolved in a copolymer of 2-hydroxyethyl methacrylate (HEMA) and methyl methacrylate (MMA) under transversal pumping at 337 nm [13]. In this case, the useful lifetime of the samples was 4500 pulses (20 GJ/mol, in terms of total input energy per mole of dye molecule when the output energy is down to 50% of its initial value). Comparative studies on the laser performance of Rh6G incorporated either in copolymers of HEMA and MMA or in MPMMA were carried out by Giffin et al. in 1999 [15]. When longitudinally pumped, under identical experimental conditions, the MPMMA materials demonstrated higher efficiency, but the copolymer formulation exhibited superior normalized photostability (up to 240 GJ/mol).

When organic polymers are used as hosts for lasing dyes, the interesting possibility arises of covalently binding the chromophore to the main chain of the polymer. One important mechanism of dye degradation when incorporated into polymeric matrices seems to be the thermal destruction of the dye due to poor thermal dissipation in the polymer host. When the dye is a part of the polymer chain, additional channels are open for the dissipation, along the polymer backbone, of the absorbed pump energy that is not converted into emission, with a corresponding increase in the laser photostability [16]. This effect is more important when a spacing group is introduced between the chromophore and the polymerizable double bonds incorporated into the dye molecule, so that the pendant group of the chromophore is distant from the polymeric main chain, resulting in no direct interaction between the excited dye group and the macromolecule chains. Using this approach, Costela et al. demonstrated, in 1996, an increase of the useful lifetime to 12,000 pulses when the Rh6G chromophore was linked covalently to the polymeric chains [16].

At the beginning of the 1990s, the rhodamine dyes, with emission in the yellow-red region of the spectrum, were known to give excellent laser results in liquid solution. Thus, they were an obvious first choice in any attempt to develop a dye laser in the solid state. The promising results obtained in solid state with rhodamine dyes notwithstanding, a line of research aiming to obtain more efficient and stable laser dyes was vigorously pursued. As a result, a new class of laser dyes with reduced triplet–triplet absorption over the lasing spectral region was synthesized and characterized by Boyer and coworkers during the late 1980s and early 1990s ([17] and references therein). These dyes are dipyrromethene.BF_2 (PM.BF_2) complexes (Figure 3.3), with emission covering the spectral region from the green-yellow to the red, depending on the substituents on the chromophore. They are ionic and highly polar laser dyes, have high fluorescence quantum yields and low triplet extinction coefficients over the laser action spectral region, and exhibit good solubility in many solvents, including alcohols and MMA. These dyes have been demonstrated to lase with good performance both in liquid solution and when incorporated into solid hosts, and some of them outperform the most widely employed laser dye, Rh6G, considered in those days the benchmark for efficiency and photostability [10].

One disadvantage of the dipyrromethene dyes is the presence of amine aromatic groups in their structure (Figure 3.3), which renders them vulnerable to photochemical reactions with oxygen and makes these dyes relatively unstable in air-saturated solutions [17]. In 1999, Ahmad and colleagues showed that this problem could be dealt with by incorporating quenchers of singlet oxygen in the liquid and solid solutions of the pyrromethene (PM) dyes [18]: when the singlet oxygen quencher 1,4-diazobicy-clo (2,2,2) octane (DABCO) was present, the photostability of dye PM567 doubled, while the lasing efficiency remained about the same. In this way, laser conversion efficiencies in the range 60%–70% were obtained for longitudinal pumping at 532 nm of PM567 dissolved in PMMA with DABCO as the additive. The useful lifetime was 550,000 pulses, corresponding to a normalized photostability of 270 GJ/mol, at a 2 Hz repetition rate. A substantial increase in the photostability of PM567, of up to 350 GJ/mol, was also achieved by the addition of coumarin C540A laser dye, as coumarin reduces the effectiveness of *in situ* oxygen degradation of PM567 [19].

As pointed out, by the mid-1990s, studies with rhodamine dyes had demonstrated that, when the dyes were incorporated into polymer hosts, lasing efficiencies and photostability depended on the viscoelastic properties of the medium. In particular, studies carried out by our group showed that for each dye there is an optimum copolymer formulation that results in the best matrix/dye combination [10]. A next logical step was to extend our research to the new, high-performance dipyrromethene dyes and probe their lasing properties when incorporated into appropriate polymers. We began by using commercial PM dyes and, after characterizing their photophysical and lasing properties in a variety of solvents, proceeded to incorporate them into carefully chosen polymeric formulations, to gather information on the polymer parameters and structure composition that optimized the laser operation. Next, we proceeded to synthesize new PM.BF$_2$ complexes and demonstrated that with

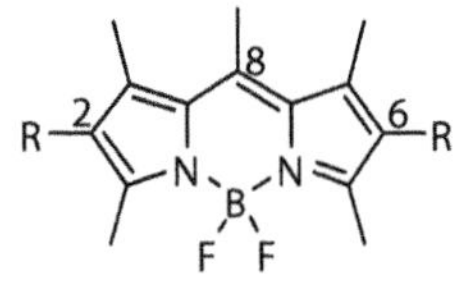

Dye	R
PM567	Et
PM597	*t*-Bu
PM580	*n*-Bu

FIGURE 3.3   Molecular structures of some commercial dipyrromethene.BF$_2$ complexes. Et: C$_2$H$_5$; Bu: CH$_3$(CH$_2$)$_3$.

appropriate chemical modifications in the pyrromethene chromophore, new dyes could be obtained that outperformed the commercially available laser dyes.

In our studies, the solid samples were typically rods, 10 mm in diameter and 10 mm in length, with a cut along the axis of the cylinder defining a lateral flat surface. Pumping geometry was transversal, with the pump radiation (typically nanosecond pulses from a frequency-doubled Nd:YAG laser, 532 nm) being focused onto the lateral flat surface of the samples [19]. The dyes were incorporated into PMMA or into a variety of copolymers of MMA with different acrylic and methacrylic monomers (Figure 3.4). MMA was chosen as the pivotal component in the formulations developed, because the excellent optical transparency and relatively high laser resistance of PMMA make this material an obligatory reference in any strategy directed toward improving laser performance in polymeric SSDLs.

In a first study, commercial dye PM567 was dissolved in homopolymer PMMA and copolymers of MMA with a number of linear and cross-linking acrylic and methacrylic monomers in different vol./vol. proportions [20]. In this way, the polarity and rigidity of the final material were carefully controlled. It was found that an important parameter governing the lasing performance of the dye in polymeric materials is the polymer-free volume, which is controlled by the degree of cross-linking. As the degree of cross-linking in the material increases, the polymer-free volume decreases, which induces a significant reduction of rotational and vibrational molecular freedom. As a result, nonradiative decay of excited dye molecules is prevented, leading to a significant increase of the emission quantum yield of the dye. For a certain concentration of the cross-linking monomer, the free volume available within the polymeric matrix will be completely occupied by the dye. Increasing the degree of cross-linking beyond this point will result in the dye molecules being

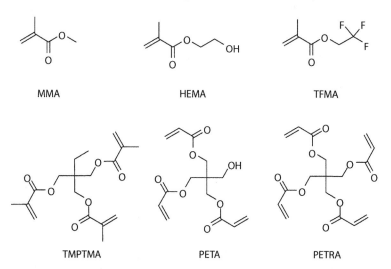

FIGURE 3.4 Molecular structures of some monomers used in solid-state dye lasers: methyl methacrylate (MMA), 2-hydroxyethyl methacrylate (HEMA), 2,2,2,-trifluoroethyl methacrylate (TFMA), trimethylolpropane trimethacrylate (TMPTMA), pentaerythritol triacrylate (PETA), and pentaerythritol tetraacrylate (PETRA).

partially excluded from the shrinking free volume, and dimers and higher aggregates, with their deleterious effect on laser operation, will be formed. Thus, for any given dye, there will be an optimum degree of cross-linking that optimizes the dye-lasing performance. This effect is illustrated in Table 3.1, which lists relevant laser parameters for solid solutions of dye PM567 in homopolymer PMMA and copolymers of MMA with cross-linking monomers having three (TMPTMA, PETA) and four (PETRA) polymerizable double bonds in lateral chains attached to the same carbon atom (Figure 3.4).

The complexity of the mechanisms involved in the laser action of dyes in a solid matrix can be appreciated from the results obtained in matrices containing the monomers TMPTMA and PETA. Both monomers are triple functionalized, so that when copolymerized with MMA in the same vol./vol. ratio, they determine the same degree of cross-linking. On the other hand, PETA is acrylic, which results in increased plasticity of the resulting polymer (i.e., an increased mobility of the local segments between the cross-linking points of the resulting macromolecular net), and incorporates in its structure a hydroxyl group, which should result in a more polar polymer. As a result, the photostability of PM567 in the matrix containing PETA is lower than in the matrix containing TMPTMA.

Figure 3.5 illustrates the effect on the lasing photostability of the dye of modifying the relative proportions of monomers in a given copolymer. In terms of the accumulated absorbed pump energy per mole of dye molecule, laser emission from dye PM567 dissolved in COP(MMA-PETRA 95:5) matrix remained at 70% of its initial value after absorption of 90 GJ/mol. It should be noticed that the evolution of the laser output with the number of pump pulses shown in Figure 3.5 was obtained at a repetition rate of 5 Hz, whereas the results in Table 3.1, which show faster degradation, were obtained at 10 Hz repetition rate. Thus, when the pump repetition rate increases, so does the degradation rate. It seems that at high repetition rate, the dissipation channels for the energy released to the medium as heat are not fast enough, and as a result the thermal degradation of the dye is enhanced. This interpretation

TABLE 3.1
Laser Parameters[a] for Dye PM567 Dissolved in Homopolymer PMMA and Cross-Linked Copolymers (COP)

Material	λ_{max}^{a} (nm)	$\Delta\lambda^{a}$ (nm)	Eff[a] (%)	$I_{30\,000}$ (%)[b]
PMMA	562	7	12	16
COP(MMA-TMPTMA 95:5)	564	5	19	20
COP(MMA-PETA 95:5)	568	5	21	12
COP(MMA-PETRA 95:5)	564	6	18	80

[a] λ_{max}: peak of the laser emission; $\Delta\lambda$: FWHM of the laser emission; Eff: energy-conversion efficiency. Dye concentration 1.5×10^{-3} M. Pump energy and repetition rate: 5.5 mJ and 10 Hz, respectively. FWHM, full width at half maximum.

[b] Intensity of the laser output after n pump pulses in the same position of the sample referred to initial intensity I_0, I_n (%) = $(I_n/I_0) \times 100$.

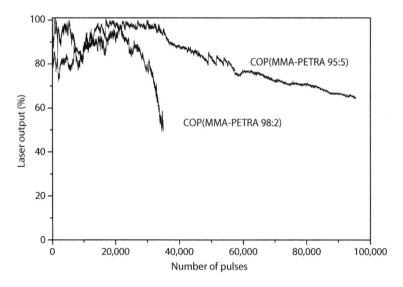

FIGURE 3.5 Normalized laser output as a function of the number of pump pulses for PM567 dissolved in copolymers of MMA and PETRA. Dye concentration: 1.5×10^{-3} M. Pumping at 532 nm with 5.5 mJ pulses at 5 Hz repetition rate. (From Costela, A. et al., *Phys. Chem. Phys.,* 5, 4745–4763, 2003. Reproduced by permission of the PCCP Owner Societies.)

was confirmed in studies on the effect of heat load on the stability of polymeric dye lasers, in which the capability of each material to dissipate the heat generated in the sample as a consequence of the pump energy excitation was characterized by photothermal deflection spectroscopy [21,22]. These studies demonstrated that the accumulation of heat into the material increases significantly for pumping repetition rates higher than 1 Hz.

Recently, Jiang and coworkers have demonstrated slope efficiency of 51.63% and normalized photostability of 180.7 GJ/mol for PM567 doped into modified copolymers of MMA and HEMA with organic modifying additive methanol under 5 Hz pumping [23]. With dye PM580 incorporated into MPMMA with methanol, both broadband and narrowband laser emission was demonstrated, with slope efficiencies of 66.0% and 42.7%, respectively [24]. The lifetime performance depended on the laser operating wavelength and pump intensity. At the central emission wavelength of 562.5 nm, the emission remained almost constant over 20,000 shots when pumped by 0.48 J/cm² at 1 Hz. Increasing the pump fluence to 1.43 J/cm² resulted in the output energy decreasing to 47.5% of its initial output value after 20,000 shots at 1 Hz. Thus, when operating at low pump laser intensity, a solid-state dye sample based on MPMMA doped with PM580 could be used to obtain a stable narrowband dye seed laser.

Earlier studies to improve the lasing performance of the PM dyes had demonstrated that their photophysical and lasing properties depend on their molecular structure, and that adequate substituents in the molecular core can enhance the laser action [25,26]. Pursuing this approach, we studied the effect of introducing a number of substitutions at the 8 position of the PM567 molecule while maintaining the four methyl groups in the 1, 3, 5, and 7 positions and the ethyl groups in positions 2 and 6. In particular, we synthesized analogues of PM567 (Figure 3.6) in which the methyl group at position 8 was replaced by a methacryloyloxypolymethylene or an acetoxypolymethylene chain with n methylenes, resulting in monomeric dyes PnMA and their model compounds PnAc, and analogues in which the substituents at position 8 were p-(methacryloyloxypolymethylene)phenyl or p-(acetoxypolymethylene)phenyl groups with one or three methylene groups (dyes PArnMA and PArnAc, respectively). The model dyes (PnAc and PArnAc) were dissolved in different polymeric matrices, whereas the monomer dyes (PnMA and PArnMA) were bonded covalently to the polymeric chains.

With dyes PnAc and PnMA, lasing efficiencies of up to 40% were obtained, whereas the maximum efficiency obtained with dye PM567 in the same materials and under the same experimental conditions was 30% [27]. Some of the most relevant results obtained with these dyes incorporated into different polymeric formulations are shown in Table 3.2. The highest photostabilities were reached in cross-linked materials with the chromophores linked covalently to the polymer chains. In some of them, the laser output remained stable or dropped by less than 15% after 100,000 pump pulses in the same position of the sample at a 10 Hz repetition rate. Figure 3.7 shows those materials for which the laser output remained stable or decreased by less than 10% after 60,000 pump pulses. Figure 3.8 compares the evolution of the laser output with the number of pump pulses of a monomer dye linked covalently to the polymer matrix, the corresponding model dye dissolved in the same material, and PM567 incorporated into homopolymer PMMA. The figure clearly shows an improvement in photostability in the covalently bonded material. We estimate for material TERP[P5MA-(MMA-PETRA 95:5)] in Figure 3.8 an accumulated absorbed pump energy per mole of dye molecule of 180 GJ/mol after 95,000 pump pulses at 10 Hz repetition rate, with the laser emission still remaining at 88% of its initial value.

With dyes PArnAc and PArnMA, the lasing efficiencies were lower, of the order of 20%, but the laser emission remained at about the initial level after 100,000 pump pulses at 10 Hz repetition rate with the chromophores linked covalently to the polymeric chains (Table 3.2) [28].

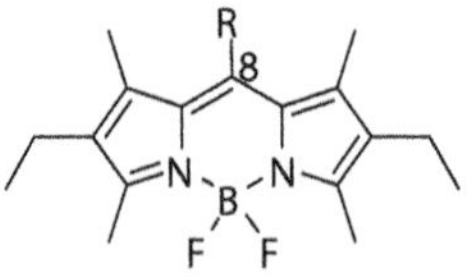

	R	n
PM567	-Me	-
PnAc	-(CH$_2$)$_n$OCOMe	1,3,5,10,15
PnMA	-(CH$_2$)$_n$OCOMe=CH$_2$	1,3,5,10,15
P1ArnAc	◯ (CH$_2$)$_n$OCOMe	1,3
P1ArnMA	◯ (CH$_2$)$_n$OCOMe=CH$_2$	1,3

FIGURE 3.6 Molecular structures of modified dipyrromethene.BF$_2$ complexes. Me: CH$_3$.

TABLE 3.2

Laser Parameters[a] for Model (PnAc, PArnAc) and Monomeric (PnMA, PArnMA) Dyes in Copolymers (COP) and Terpolymers (TERP)

Material	λ_{max}[a] (nm)	$\Delta\lambda$[a] (nm)	Eff[a] (%)	Laser Output[b]	
				$I_{60,000}$ (%)	$I_{100,000}$ (%)
P1Ac/COP(MMA-PETRA 95:5)	591	12	27	107	—
COP(P3 MA-MMA)	569	6	34	100	—
TERP[P3 MA-(MMA-HEMA 7:3)]	569	4	37	87	—
TERP[P3 MA-(MMA-TMPTMA 95:5)]	565	5	28	112	133
COP(P3MA-MMA)	568	5	36	75	—
P5Ac/COP(MMA-HEMA 7:3)	565	6	39	83	—
TERP[P5MA-(MMA-TFMA 7:3)]	565	9	38	80	70
TERP[P5MA-(MMA-PETA 95:5)]	562	5	23	87	—
P10Ac/COP(MMA-TFMA 7:3)	561	8	40	50	—
TERP[P10MA-(MMA-HEMA 7:3)]	566	5	27	80	—
P10Ac/COP(MMA-PETRA 95:5)	563	10	34	87	—
TERP[P10MA-(MMA-PETA 95:5)]	563	5	28	101	
COP(PAr1MA/MMA)	558	9	20		96
COP(PAr3MA/MMA)	555	9	16		96

[a] λ_{max}: peak of the laser emission; $\Delta\lambda$: FWHM of the laser emission; Eff: energy conversion efficiency. Dye concentration: 1.5×10^{-3} M. FWHM, full width at half maximum.

[b] Intensity of the dye laser output after n pump pulses in the same position of the sample referred to initial intensity I_0, $I_n(\%) = (I_n/I_0) \times 100$. Pump energy and repetition rate: 5.5 mJ and 10 Hz, respectively.

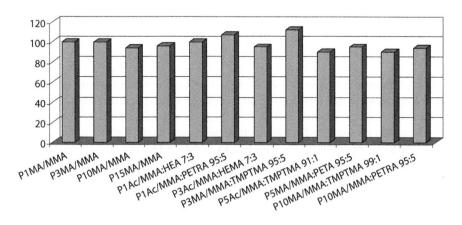

FIGURE 3.7 Percent intensity (referred to initial intensity) of the laser output from a number of newly synthesized dipyrromethene.BF$_2$ dyes incorporated into linear and cross-linked copolymers of MMA, after 60,000 pump pulses at the same position of the sample. PnAc/MMA-monomer: model dyes dissolved in copolymer; PnMA-MMA-monomer: monomer dyes linked covalently to polymeric chains, producing terpolymers with the indicated MMA-monomer proportion. Pump energy and repetition rate: 5.5 mJ/pulse and 10 Hz, respectively.

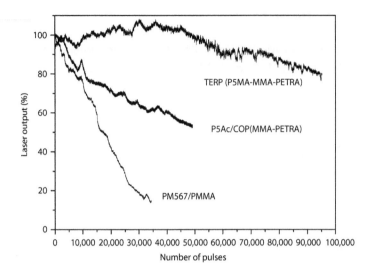

FIGURE 3.8 Evolution of the normalized laser output of monomer dye P5MA linked covalently to polymer matrix with composition MMA-PETRA 95:5, model dye P5Ac dissolved in the same matrix, and dye PM567 dissolved in PMMA.

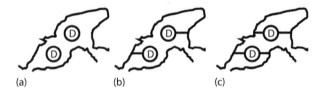

FIGURE 3.9 Representation of dye molecules D dissolved into a polymeric framework (a), and the same chromophore covalently bonded to the same polymer through one bond (b) or through two bonds (c).

Further improvements in photostability were obtained by double cross-linking of the chromophore to the polymeric chains (Figure 3.9). In this case, instead of incorporating one methacryloyloxypolymethylene group at position 8 in dye PM567, two polymerizable methacryloyloxypolymethylene groups were attached to positions 2 and 6 of PM567 dye (Figure 3.3, with R: Et-CH$_2$OCOC(Me)=CH$_2$). The copolymer of this new dye with MMA exhibited lasing efficiency of 37% with the laser emission remaining at 67% of the initial output after 400,000 pump pulses at 30 Hz repetition rate, corresponding to an accumulated absorbed pump energy of 950 GJ/mol [29].

Bichromatic laser emission was obtained from some of the aforementioned analogues, both monomeric and model compounds, of dye PM567 incorporated into solid polymeric matrices [30]. Depending on dye concentration, matrix structure, dye–matrix interaction, and pump fluence, two peaks separated by 10–14 nm appear in the laser emission spectral band. This unusual feature could be explained in terms of reabsorption/reemission effects and spectral broadening of the S$_0$–S$_1$ transition. The short-wavelength emission corresponds to the usual homogeneous

S_0–S_1 transition and dominates at low dye concentration. The long-wavelength emission appears when reabsorption/reemission and inhomogeneous broadening dominate, so that gain at the vibrational shoulder competes advantageously with that of the short-wavelength mode.

Over recent years, a number of modifications of the molecular structure of the PM chromophore system with adequate substituents have been tried, giving rise to new dyes of this family with a good balance between efficiency and photostability [31–35]. In particular, efficiencies of over 50% with stable laser emission for more than 100,000 pulses under repeated transversal pumping at 10 Hz were demonstrated for derivatives of PM567 and PM597 in which fluorine atoms were replaced by carboxylate or cyano groups, respectively, incorporated into PMMA matrices [34,35]. Emission displaced toward longer wavelengths was obtained from diiodinated [36] and chlorinated [37] PM dyes, or by using energy transfer processes in multichromophoric systems incorporating two donor and one acceptor PM dyes [38]. The matrix material was PMMA. Energy transfer processes in cassettes based on PM and rhodamine pairs resulted in efficient and photostable laser emission in poly(2-hydroxyethyl methacrylate) (PHEMA) matrices [39].

Improvements in the lasing properties of gain media based on dyes PM567 and PM597 have been demonstrated by using polymers with fluorine atoms incorporated into their structure [40]. The presence of fluorine atoms in the polymer matrix results in high thermal stability and enhanced chemical resistance compared with nonfluorinated analogues, as a result of the bond energy of C–F (116 kcal/mol) being higher than that of C–H (99 kcal/mol), as well as the low polarity and relatively small size of the fluorine atom [41]. Fluorine-modified organic matrices were prepared, in which the total fluorine content was varied, adding to MMA different volumetric proportions of monomers with three (TFMA, Figure 3.4), five (PFMA, as in Figure 3.4 but with end group CF_2–CF_3), and seven (HFMA, as in Figure 3.4 with end group CF_2–CF_2–CF_3) fluorine atoms. Lasing efficiencies of up to 35% (PM567) and 42% (PM597) were obtained under transversal pumping. The highest photostability was recorded for PM597 dissolved in an MMA–HFMA 7:3 copolymer, with the laser output remaining at the initial level after 500,000 pump pulses in the same position of the sample at 30 Hz repetition rate, corresponding to an accumulated pump energy of 12,300 GJ/mol (Figure 3.10).

Some efforts have been made recently to extend the tuning range of SSDLs to the red-edge spectral region (600–750 nm), within what is often termed the *optical window*. The potential advantages of emission in this spectral region are the nearness to the second low-loss window of typical polymer optical fibers (a window that lies at 650 nm [42]), and significant reduction of the background signal in biological applications because of the lower autoabsorption and autofluorescence of biomolecules, low light scattering, and deep penetration of the light at these wavelengths in biological systems [43]. Fan et al. [44] demonstrated laser emission at 650 nm from dye LDS698 incorporated into MPMMA. Under longitudinal pumping, normalized photostability of 102 GJ/mol with slope efficiency of 13.5% was obtained. At about the same time, photosensitive materials based on a variety of commercial dyes with emission in this red-edge region (sulforhodamine B, perylene red, rhodamine 640, LDS698, LDS722, LDS730) incorporated into different linear, cross-linked,

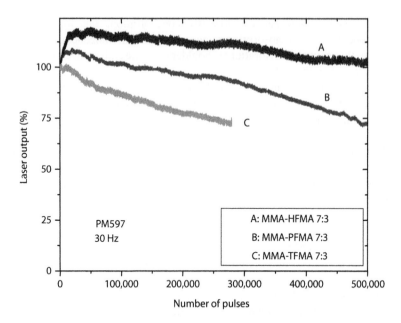

FIGURE 3.10 Evolution of the normalized laser output of PM597 in copolymers of MMA with fluorinated monomers at 30 Hz repetition rate. Dye concentration: 7×10^{-4} M. Pumping at 532 nm with 3.5 mJ pulses.

fluorinated, and silylated polymeric matrices were designed and synthesized [45–48]. Some results are summarized in Table 3.3, which shows data on lasing efficiency, peak of the laser emission, and laser photostability (with respect to initial intensity) after 100,000 pump pulses in the same position of the sample. Lasing efficiencies ranged from 20% for the styryl dyes to 46% for the xanthene chromophores, under transversal pumping at 532 nm. For the sake of clarity, in Figure 3.11, the actual evolution of the laser output with the number of pump pulses at 10 Hz repetition rate is shown graphically for some of the materials. For comparison with the results reported in [44], the normalized photostability of dye LDS698 in Table 3.3 was 3920 GJ/mol. When these materials were placed in a grazing-incidence grating tunable resonator, tunable laser emission was obtained with linewidths of the order of 0.15 cm^{-1} and a tuning range of up to 70 nm, continuously covering the region from 575 to 750 nm (Table 3.3 and Figure 3.12).

Some potential important applications of SSDLs, such as photodynamic therapy or treatment of port-wine stains and other vascular anomalies, would require the laser energy to be applied in high-repetition rate pulses. Thus, we prepared solid laser samples in the form of coin-sized disks, 2 mm thick, consisting of dyes Rh6G or PM567 incorporated into polymeric matrices, and pumped them longitudinally with the green line of a copper-vapor laser at an average power of up to 800 mW and repetition rate of up to 1 kHz [49]. With PM567 dissolved in COP(MMA-PETA 95:5), 290 mW average power (37% lasing efficiency) at peak wavelength of 550 nm was obtained. The laser output decreased to 150 mW (52% of the initial power) after 30 min irradiation time at 1 kHz (1.8×10^6 shots) and to 32 mW (11% of the initial

TABLE 3.3
Laser Properties[a] of Sulforhodamine B, Perylene Red, Rhodamine 640, LDS698, LDS722, and LDS730 Incorporated into Different Linear, Cross-linked, Fluorinated, and Silylated Polymeric Matrices

Dye	$c^a \times 10^4$ (M)	Material	$\lambda_{max}{}^a$ (nm)	Eff[a] (%)	$I_{100,000}$ (%)[b]	Tuning range (nm)
SulRhB	6	COP[(HEMA-MMA 7:3)-PETRA 9:1]	608	46	99	575–645
PerRed	5	COP(MMA-TFMA 7:3)	618	21	95	605–655
Rh640	6	COP (HEMA-PETA 9:1)	640	36	79	620–660
LDS698	4	PHEMA	660	21	55	635–695
LDS722	4	COP(HEMA-TMSPMA 8:2)	674	23	55	650–720
LDS730	8	COP(HEMA-TMSPMA 7:3)	730	20	100	690–750

Note: Structure of TMSPMA, see Figure 3.19.

[a] c: dye concentration; λ_{max}: peak of the laser emission; Eff: energy-conversion efficiency.

[b] Intensity of the laser output after n pump pulses in the same position of the sample referred to initial intensity I_0, I_n (%) = $(I_n/I_0) \times 100$. Pump energy and repetition rate: 5.5 mJ and 10 Hz, respectively.

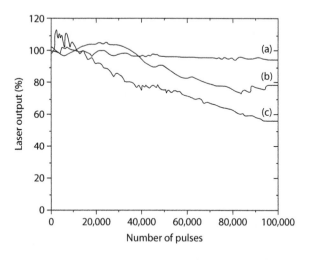

FIGURE 3.11 Evolution of the normalized laser output of (a) perylene red in COP(MMA-TFMA 7:3), (b) rhodamine 640 in COP(MEMA-PETRA 9:1), and (c) LDS722 in COP(HEMA-TMSPMA 8:2). Pump wavelength, pulse duration, energy, and repetition rate are 532 nm, 12 ns, 5.5 mJ/pulse, and 10 Hz, respectively. Structure of TMSPMA, see Figure 3.19. (García-Moreno, I. et al., Materials for reliable solid state dye laser at the red spectral edge. *Adv. Funct. Mat.* 2009. 19. 2547–2552. Copyright Wiley-VCH Verlag GmbH & Co. KGaA. Reproduced with permission.)

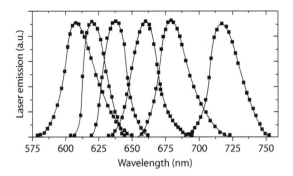

FIGURE 3.12 Tunable laser emission over the red-edge spectral region from the materials shown in Table 3.3. The solid lines are for ease of viewing only.

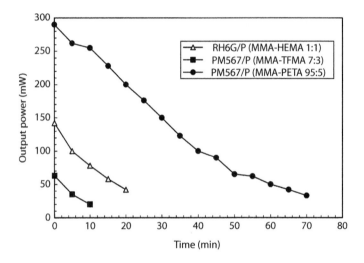

FIGURE 3.13 Evolution of the output power as a function of time of PM567 and Rh6G in different polymeric media when pumped with a copper-vapor laser at 1 kHz repetition rate. (Reprinted from Costela, A. et al., *Appl. Phys. Lett.*, 79, 452–454, 2001. Copyright 2001, AIP Publishing LLC. With permission.)

power) after 70 min operation (4.2×10^6 shots) (Figure 3.13). Output power of up to 1 W at 6.2 kHz was obtained for short periods of time. When the pump repetition rate was increased to 10 kHz, by using as pump source a diode-pumped, Q-switched, frequency-doubled Nd:YLF laser (emission at 527 nm), the output power of Rh6G/COP(MMA-HEMA 1:1) decreased to half the initial value after about 6.6 min (or about 4.0 million shots). In the case of PM567/COP(MMA-PETRA 95:5), the output power decreased to half the initial value after about 7.8 min (Figure 3.14) [50].

A high-repetition rate (16 kHz) laser emission, tunable in the wavelength range 605–635 nm, based on rhodamine B dye incorporated into a copolymer of MMA and MAA (methacrylic acid) was demonstrated by Kytina et al. [51]. The

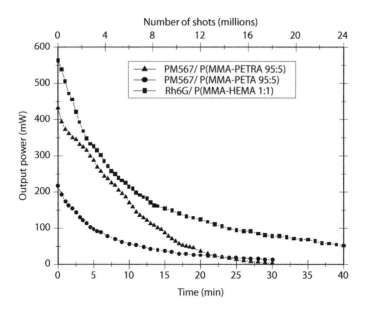

FIGURE 3.14 Evolution of the output power as a function of time of PM567 and Rh6G in different polymeric media when pumped with an Nd:YLF (second harmonic) laser at 10 kHz repetition rate. (Reprinted from *Opt. Commun.*, 218, Abedin, K. M. et al., 10 kHz repetition rate solid-state dye laser pumped by diode-pumped solid-state laser, 359–363, Copyright (2003), with permission from Elsevier.)

disk-shaped polymer gain medium (94 mm diameter, thickness 20 mm) was rotated at a frequency of 42 Hz and pumped transversely with radiation from a copper-vapor laser. Lasing efficiency of 15% (output power 1.5 W) was obtained. The laser output remained stable for 4 h, within 3% accuracy, in a cyclic operation mode with duty cycle 1/6 (1 min operation, 10 s pause). In permanently pumping mode (no pause in pumping with the copper-vapor laser), the maximum operation time (decrease of the output power of the dye laser to 70% of its initial value) was about 2 h for optimized transmission of the laser cavity output mirror.

The use of PMMA solid host incorporating pyrromethene dyes as laser amplifier has been reported. A 25 mm diameter, 7 mm thickness sample of dye pyrromethene 650 (PM650) in PMMA rendered a single-pass gain of 500 at 616 nm [52]. Up to 62% amplifier efficiency was observed in disks (25 mm diameter, 3 mm thickness) of PM567 dispersed in a modified PMMA matrix incorporating small amounts of PETRA and DABCO [53]. The photodegradation rate was found to be reduced substantially by an increase in the rate of stimulated emission, indicating an important role played by excited-state reactions in photodegradation.

In 2006, a continuous-wave (CW) SSDL tunable from 565 to 615 nm was reported [54]. The laser medium consisted of a thin film (thickness between 50 and 100 μm) of Rh6G dissolved in a photopolymer sandwiched between two digital versatile disc (DVD) substrates. The resonator design was a folded cavity, derived from conventional liquid solvent dye laser geometry. The dye laser disk was rotated (50–100 Hz) and translated perpendicularly to the rotation axis (100–300 μm/s) by a combined motor-translation stage unit. Lasing threshold was 550 mW and slope efficiency 2%. Using one disk, 30 min lasing operation was achieved before irreversible photodegradation. An improved and more sophisticated device showing both excellent long- and short-time power stability was presented recently [55]. In the improved design, the thickness of the disk was significantly larger (3 mm), the dye was perylene orange, and the polymer host material was PMMA. An output power of 800 mW around 575 nm with a spectral width of less than 3 GHz, tunability over 30 nm, and a nearly circular mode profile with an M^2 better than 1.4 was obtained. The excellent power stability provides CW laser output over hours without noticeable power loss. The device, including pump laser, could be integrated in a compact housing with dimensions $60 \times 40 \times 20$ cm^3.

3.2.2 ORGANIC–INORGANIC HYBRID MATERIALS

Silicate-based inorganic–organic hybrid polymers are *a priori* good candidates for laser matrices, since, due to their inorganic Si–O–Si backbone, they present improved thermal and mechanical properties compared with common organic polymers. These hybrid materials are prepared from organosilane precursors by sol–gel processing in combination with organic cross-linking of polymerizable monomers [56].

In one approach, the porous structure of a sol–gel inorganic matrix is filled with organic molecules by immersing the bulk in a solution containing laser dye, polymerizable monomer, and catalyst or photoinitiator. In a subsequent step, organic polymerization is started by ultraviolet irradiation or heating, and an interpenetrating polymer incorporating the laser dye is formed.

Hybrids can also be obtained from organically modified silicon alkoxides. In this method, both organic and inorganic networks are obtained in a two-step reaction. An initial inorganic network is formed by polycondensation of the silicon alkoxide. In a second step, organic polymerization is initiated, thermally or photochemically, via free radicals. The possibility of selecting different organic:inorganic ratios as well as the choice of the reaction conditions allows materials with a wide range of properties to be obtained. Materials obtained in this way are usually called organically modified ceramics (ORMOCERs) or organically modified silanes (ORMOSILs).

The first studies on laser emission from dyes incorporated into inorganic and inorganic–organic matrices prepared using sol–gel techniques were carried out in the late 1980s, and showed this to be a promising approach. In 1995, Rahn and King [57] carried out a direct comparison study of laser performance of dyes Rh6G, PM567, perylene red, and perylene orange in organic, inorganic, and hybrid hosts. They found that the nonpolar perylene dyes had better performance in partially organic hosts, whereas the ionic rhodamine and pyrromethene dyes performed best in the inorganic sol–gel glass host. The most promising combinations of dye and host for efficiency and photostability were found to be perylene orange in polycom glass and Rh6G in sol–gel glass. Nevertheless, lasing efficiencies and photostabilities were modest in all cases.

In 2002, Ahmad and colleagues demonstrated high efficiency and photostability for xanthene dyes in wet and dried sol–gel phases, but not for pyrromethene laser dyes [58]. In the next couple of years, lasing slope efficiencies of 79% and 60%

were reported for dyes PM567 and PM597, respectively, incorporated via the sol–gel technique into ORMOSIL host matrices (PM567) [59] and hybrid xerogel matrices (PM597) [60]. These efficiencies were obtained under longitudinal pumping at 532 nm in optimized laser cavities. The useful lifetime for PM567 was 60,000 pulses, 50 GJ/mol in normalized photostability, at a pump repetition rate of 2 Hz and pump fluence of 0.1 J/cm^2, in samples of 4 mm thickness [59]. For PM597, the laser emission dropped to 50% of the initial value after 210,000 pump pulses, when pumped with 1.8 mJ pulses at 10 Hz repetition rate [60]. Under the same irradiation conditions, PM567 in xerogel matrix exhibited a slope efficiency of 80% and a useful lifetime of 180,000 pulses.

With dye perylene red incorporated into ORMOSIL matrices, slope efficiencies of up to 53% with normalized photostabilities of 24 GJ/mol were obtained with samples of 4 mm thickness at a pump fluence of 0.1 J/cm^2 and 2 Hz repetition rate [59]. By codoping perylene red with an optimized coumarin dye concentration, the slope efficiency of perylene red in ORMOSIL matrix increased by a factor of 2, whereas the slope efficiency of PM567 was only marginally increased [61].

Under transversal pumping, slope efficiencies of 32% [62], 43%, and 20% [56] have been obtained for dyes PM567, PM597, and Rh6G, respectively, incorporated into ORMOSIL glass samples and placed in an optimized laser cavity consisting of a full reflector and a 50% broadband reflector as output coupler. Pumped by 1 mJ (20 mJ/cm^2) pulses, the useful lifetime of PM597 in ORMOSIL was 12,000 pulses, which increased to 22,000 pulses when the dye was incorporated into composite glass [62].

Beginning in 2002, our group carried out a detailed investigation on the laser performance of rhodamine and pyrromethene dyes incorporated into organic–inorganic hybrid materials. For inorganic components, we used tetraethoxysilane (TEOS) and tetramethoxysilane (TMOS) (Figure 3.15) in different weight proportions. The organic part was composed of MMA or MMA–HEMA. The synthesis route of the

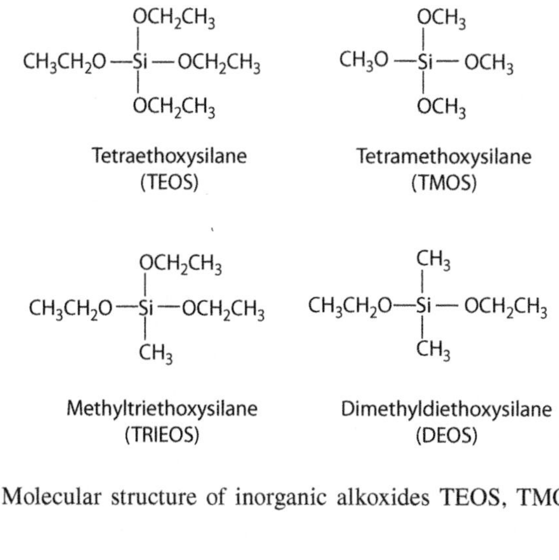

FIGURE 3.15 Molecular structure of inorganic alkoxides TEOS, TMOS, TRIEOS, and DEOS.

hybrid materials was based on the *in situ* and simultaneous hydrolysis–condensation of the inorganic component during the free radical copolymerization of the organic monomers. The geometry of the samples was as previously described (10×10 mm rods with a lateral cut defining a flat surface), and the pumping arrangement was transversal.

The lasing stability of TMOS-based hybrid matrices was significantly worse than in the materials based on TEOS, evidencing the influence of the size of the lateral substituent group of the alkoxide on the laser properties of the resulting material. When Rh6G is used as gain medium, both the lasing efficiency and the photostability first increase with the proportion of the inorganic component, peaking at compositions with 10%–15% (wt%) proportions of TEOS. With pumping at 532 nm, laser efficiencies of up to 26% and laser emission with no sign of degradation, albeit with some oscillations, were obtained after 100,000 pump pulses in the same position of the sample at 10 Hz repetition rate [63]. Higher proportions of the alkoxide in the sample result in a drastic decrease in both efficiency and useful lifetime or stability of the laser emission. It is clear that the presence of the inorganic component in the matrix plays an important role in the photochemical degradation of the dye. The pump radiation leads to a fraction of the dye molecules being converted into active species (radicals, triplets) which, in turn, react with nearby dye molecules, impurities, oxygen, radicals, and groups from the polymer chains or any other active species present in the material. An increase in the proportion of the inorganic alkoxide in the material leads to an increase in the remanent acidity of the medium, which could boost these reactive processes. In addition, because the photochemical mechanism is at least bimolecular, the process can be highly dependent on the microstructure and flexibility of the polymeric chains in these materials. Thus, to optimize the photostability of the dye/hybrid system, a compromise must be reached between the enhancement of thermal dissipation in the material and the increase in the photochemical destruction of the dye by carefully controlling the inorganic–organic matrix composition.

When the pyrromethene dye PM567 was used as gain medium, the laser operation was optimized in matrices with 5% content of TEOS [64]. The lasing efficiency was 26%, and, after an initial decrease, the laser output stabilized and remained at 70% of its initial value after 60,000 pump pulses in the same position of the sample (Figure 3.16).

The presence of the inorganic component in the hybrid matrices increases the rigidity and fragility of the resulting materials. A possible way to decrease the rigidity of the materials while maintaining, or even increasing, the proportion of the inorganic component is by decreasing the functionality of the inorganic compounds, selecting double- and triple-functionalized alkoxides instead of the usual tetrafunctionalized ones, TEOS and TMOS. Pursuing this idea, we prepared hybrid matrices in which the inorganic compounds were trifunctional methyltriethoxysilane (TRIEOS) and difunctional dimethyldiethoxysilane (DEOS) (Figure 3.15), and we performed a systematic study of the influence on the laser action of the composition and structure of these new hybrid matrices [65–67]. DEOS, with only two reactive positions, leads to rapidly growing linear chains, inducing broad inorganic domains less miscible with the organic components, which is detrimental to the

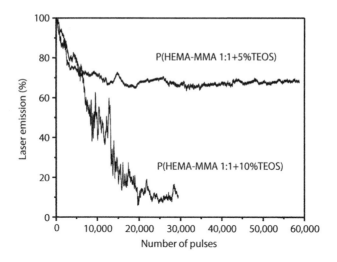

FIGURE 3.16 Normalized laser output as a function of the number of pump pulses for PM567 (1.5×10^{-3} M) in hybrid matrices. Pump energy and repetition rate: 5.5 mJ/pulse and 10 Hz, respectively. (Reprinted from *Chem. Phys. Lett.*, 369, Costela, A. et al., Enhancement of laser properties of pyrromethene 567 dye incorporated into new organic-inorganic hybrid materials, 656–661, Copyright (2003), with permission from Elsevier.)

optical transparency of the samples. TRIEOS, on the other hand, results in a material with better structural and morphological uniformity, without phase separation at the nanometric scale. Laser operation with no decrease in the laser output after 100,000 pump pulses in the same position of the sample at 10 Hz repetition rate was obtained with Rh6G (in matrices with 20% content of TRIEOS), and PM597 (in matrices with 15% TRIEOS, Figure 3.17).

Trying to further improve the photostability of the laser dyes when incorporated into solid hosts, we next synthesized new hybrid materials with improved thermo-optical and mechanical properties based on silica aerogels. These are sponge-like glasses characterized by an extremely high porosity (80%–99%) with easily accessible mesopores (20–100 nm) filled with air. The open pore structure of these materials forms an amorphous inorganic three-dimensional network of low density, which, under appropriate conditions, can be filled with adequate polymeric formulations incorporating a laser dye.

When using silica aerogels filled with fluorinated modified polymers, lasing efficiencies of up to 37% were obtained with dye PM567 [68,69]. Laser emission with a drop of only 10% after 10^6 pulses in the same position of the sample at 10 Hz repetition rate was demonstrated in nonfluorinated polymers, although this emission exhibited a rather irregular behavior with some strong fluctuations. In fluorinated samples, laser emission stable over 100,000 pump pulses was obtained by pumping at 10 Hz with pulses of 5.5 mJ (Figure 3.18; compare with Figure 3.16). By pumping with 3.5 mJ/pulse, the laser emission remained stable over 100,000 pulses at 30 Hz repetition rate.

Over recent years, some more attempts have been made to improve the laser performance of dyes in sol–gel glass and organic–inorganic hybrid materials. Thus,

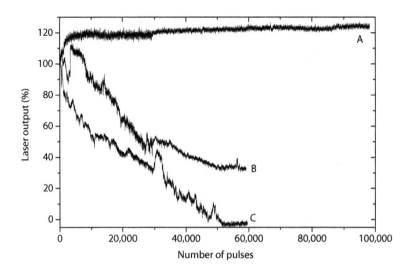

FIGURE 3.17 Normalized laser output as a function of the number of pump pulses for PM597 $(6 \times 10^{-4}\ M)$ in hybrid matrices of P(HEMA-MMA 1:1) with different wt% proportions of TRIEOS: (a) 15% and 10 Hz, (b) 15% and 30 Hz, and (c) 5% and 30 Hz. Pump energy: 5.5 mJ/ pulse. Initial lasing efficiency: 23%. (Reprinted with permission from García-Moreno, I. et al., *J. Phys. Chem. B*, 109, 21618–21626, 2005. Copyright 2005, American Chemical Society.)

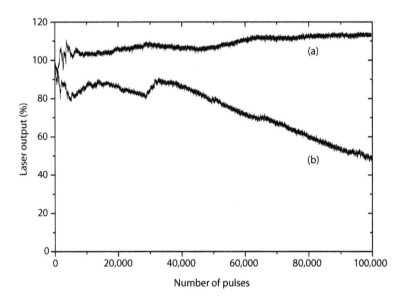

FIGURE 3.18 Normalized laser output as a function of the number of pump pulses for PM567 $(1.5 \times 10^{-3}\ M)$ incorporated into (a) silica aerogel filled with the copolymer COP(MMA:TFMA 7:3) and (b) organic matrix without silica aerogel. Pump energy and repetition rate: 5.5 mJ/pulse and 10 Hz, respectively. (Reprinted from *Chem. Phys. Lett.*, 427, García, O. et al., Efficient optical materials based on fluorinated-polymeric silica aerogels, 375–378, Copyright (2006), with permission from Elsevier.)

rhodamine B was incorporated into polymer, sol–gel glass, and organic–inorganic hybrid hosts, and its laser behavior in the different materials was evaluated [70]. The polymer used was glycidyl methacrylate (GMA), and the inorganic component was TEOS. Relatively high efficiencies (of up to 48% in the hybrid material) were obtained under transversal pumping at 532 nm. The lasing efficiency was consistently higher in hybrid matrix than in sol–gel glass (37.6%) and polymer (33.2%) hosts. Nevertheless, the photostabilities were not as good, and the higher photostability (decrease of the emission to 30% of its initial value after 30,000 pump pulses at 10 Hz and 15 mJ/pulse pumping) was reached in the polymer host, attributed to covalent bonding of the dye to GMA.

Two different approaches to obtaining new mesoporous sol–gel materials specifically designed to incorporate Rh6G were developed by de Queiroz et al. [71]. The first is based on SiO_2 and phenyl-modified silica xerogel, and the second uses mesoporous sodium aluminosilicate glasses. The dye dispersion in the silica xerogels results in high quantum yields (up to 87%), with no substantial decrease in efficiency when dye concentration is increased. On the other hand, sodium aluminosilicate samples exhibit a drastic decrease in quantum yield at concentrations higher than 10^{-4} M. As a result, only the sodium aluminosilicate samples containing 2.1×10^{-5} moles of Rh6G per host formula unit exhibited laser action, while the silicate xerogels worked well with Rh6G concentrations of up to 10^{-3} M. Although emission photostabilities were not high, with a half-life of 6560 pulses under transverse pumping with pulses of 2 m at 10 Hz repetition rate, the emission linewidths remained rather stable during operation, and the ability of the silicate xerogels to host high concentrations of dye makes these materials interesting candidates for biological applications.

3.2.3 SILICON-MODIFIED ORGANIC MATRICES

Despite the good results obtained with the hybrid materials, these compounds present their own problems, such as a complex and lengthy synthesis process, fragility that makes mechanization and polishing of the final material difficult, and sometimes optical inhomogeneity caused by refractive index mismatch between organic and inorganic parts. A possible way to avoid these problems while maintaining the combined advantages of polymer and inorganic materials would be to use organic compounds with silicon atoms directly incorporated into their structure. Thus, the matrix would remain organic, which means plasticity and a relatively more simple synthesis procedure, but with improved thermal properties due to the presence of the silicon atoms. Following this approach, we incorporated dyes PM567 and PM597 into copolymers of MMA or HEMA with 3-(trimethoxysilyl)propyl methacrylate (TMSPMA, Figure 3.19) and into terpolymers of MMA, HEMA, and TMSPMA,

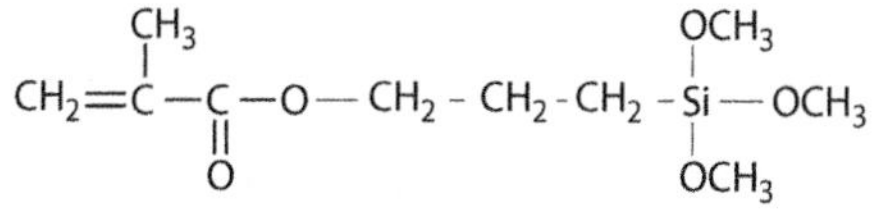

TMSPMA

FIGURE 3.19 Molecular structure of monomer 3-TMSPMA.

and proceeded to study the photophysical, structural, and laser properties of these novel materials [72,73].

A highly photostable laser operation was obtained with the silicon-modified organic matrices, with lasing efficiencies of up to 34% with PM567 and up to 42% with PM597 under transversal pumping at 532 nm in nonoptimized laser cavities. At 10 Hz repetition rate, formulations were found with no sign of degradation in the laser output after 100,000 pump pulses in the same position of the sample for both PM567 and PM567 dyes. This corresponds to an accumulated pump energy absorbed by the system per mole of dye molecules of 518 and 1295 GJ/mol for PM567 and PM597, respectively. When the pump repetition rate increased to 30 Hz, the dye PM567 exhibited a steady decrease in the laser output, which was rather drastic in the samples with the highest content of silicon (Figure 3.20). Dye PM597 was much more stable, and in all but one of the formulations the laser emission remained stable after 100,000 pump pulses at 30 Hz repetition rate (Figure 3.20; compare with Figure 3.17b and c), corresponding to an accumulated pump energy of 2472 GJ/mol. In two selected matrices, COP(MMA:TMSPMA 1:1) and COP(HEMA:TMSPMA 1:1), the laser emission of the dye PM597 remained stable after 700,000 pump pulses in the same position of the sample at 30 Hz repetition rate (Figure 3.21), corresponding to an accumulated pump energy absorbed per mole of dye molecules of 17,300 GJ/mol. By incorporating an acetoxymethyl substituent at position 8 in the PM597 chromophore, the laser emission of the resulting dye, in COP(HEMA:TMSPMA 7:3) matrix, was displaced from 577 to 607 nm, tunable over the range 585–625 nm [74]. The lasing efficiency was 42%, and the output remained at 90% of the initial value after 100,000 pump pulses at 30 Hz (accumulated pump energy: 3137 GJ/mol).

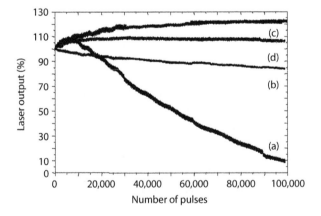

FIGURE 3.20   Normalized laser output as a function of the number of pump pulses for dye PM567 in (a) COP(MMA:TMSPMA 3:7) and (b) COP(HEMA:TMSPMA 7:3), and for dye PM597 in (c) COP(HEMA:TMSPMA 7:3) and (d) TERP(MMA:HEMA:TMSPMA 5:5:10). Dye concentration: 1.5×10^{-3} M (PM567) and 6×10^{-4} M (PM597). Pump energy and repetition rate: 3.5 mJ/pulse and 30 Hz, respectively. (Reprinted from Costela, A. et al., *J. Appl. Phys.*, 101, 073110, 2007. Copyright 2007, AIP Publishing LLC. With permission.)

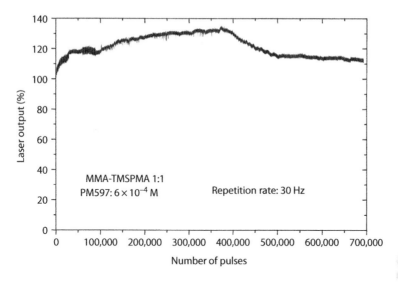

FIGURE 3.21 Normalized laser output as a function of the number of pump pulses in the same position of the sample for dye PM597 in silicon-modified organic matrix.

3.2.4 POLYMERS WITH NANO- AND MICRO-PARTICLES

Recently, Duarte and James [75,76] demonstrated a class of dye-doped, organic–inorganic, solid-state gain media that exhibit lower $|\partial n/\partial T|$ values and improved optical homogeneity than previous composite gain media. The solid matrix consisted of silica nanoparticles uniformly dispersed in PMMA. Using Rh6G as laser dye and a longitudinal pumping scheme, laser conversion efficiencies of 63% were obtained. The laser beam exhibited near-TEM_{00} profile with a beam divergence of 1.9 mrad (~ 1.3 times the diffraction limit). In Chapter 4, the use of these media in SSDL is discussed in detail.

The effect of incorporating dielectric-oxide microparticles into both solid host materials and liquid solutions has been investigated by Ahmad [77]. In particular, PMMA samples containing β-alumina microparticles with diameter less than 0.2 μm, doped with PM567 and Rh6G, were prepared. In these conditions, the photostability of the samples was greatly enhanced: when using samples 8 mm long doped with a PM567 dye concentration of 3.4×10^{-4} M and longitudinal pumping at 2 Hz repetition rate and pump fluence of 0.16 J/cm^2, the number of pulses for the conversion efficiency to fall to half of its initial value is seen to increase from 200,000 without microparticles to 400,000 for samples containing microparticles. The addition of both DABCO and microparticles results in an increase in the operational lifetime to 600,000 pulses, corresponding to a total absorbed pump energy of 365 GJ/mol. When the dye was Rh6G, the addition of microparticles to a solid PMMA sample resulted in proportionally the same enhancement of the photostability as with PM567.

In Section 2.3, it was shown that the use of polymeric hosts with a certain silicon content to increase the thermal conductivity of the polymer resulted in reduced dye degradation. In this way, the dye-lasing photostabilities were significantly enhanced with respect to those of the nonsilylated polymers. Nevertheless, the lasing efficiencies were somewhat lower than those obtained with some hybrid materials, and although the photostabilities increased with the silicon content, the presence of silicon in the polymer backbone was accompanied by a decrease in the glass transition temperature, which eventually renders soft materials inappropriate for polishing. The results of Duarte and James discussed in Section 3.2.4 showed that the design and synthesis of materials with silica incorporated at molecular level might overcome the abovementioned problems. Thus, the approach of implementing polymer matrices incorporating nanoparticles based on polyhedral oligomeric silsesquioxanes (POSS) was explored [78]. These compounds have a compact hybrid structure with a well-defined cage-like inorganic core made up of silicon and oxygen $(SiO_{1.5})_n$ externally surrounded by nonreactive or reactive polymerizable organic ligands, R (Figure 3.22). The type and number of substituents control the interactions between the organic ligand and the medium, defining the compatibility and thus the final properties of the POSS-modified systems. The reduced size of the POSS nanoparticles (1 nm) should avoid, in principle, any optical inhomogeneities. If the functional groups are polymerizable, the POSS cages will be bonded directly to the polymer chains, giving place to an organic–inorganic hybrid network (Figure 3.23) with enhanced thermal, mechanical, and physical properties.

Surprisingly, these enhanced properties led to the best laser performance reported to date for different dye-doped solid matrices, for both rhodamine and pyrromethene dyes [78,79]. With efficiencies as high as 60% for PM567 dye doped into a copolymer COP(MMA:8MMAPOSS 87:13), the laser emission remained unchanged after 8.5×10^5 pulses at 30 Hz repetition rate (Figure 3.24, curve A) and 5.5 mJ/pulse transversal pumping, corresponding to an estimated accumulated absorbed pump energy of 4768 GJ/mol. As a comparison, the same dye in PMMA with no POSS provided an efficiency of 39%, and the laser emission dropped to one-third of the initial value after just 1×10^5 pulses at the lower repetition rate of 10 Hz (Figure 3.24, curve B). The presence of POSS nanoparticles was found to enhance the laser action of dyes of very different families, both polar (Rh6G, rhodamine 640, sulforhodamine B, LDS772, LDS730) and nonpolar (perylene red, pyrromethene 567, pyrromethene 597) with respect to the effectiveness recorded in pure organic solvents and polymeric solutions pumped under the same experimental conditions (Figure 3.25) [80]. In this way, dye-doped POSS solutions could be defined as a kind of universal gain

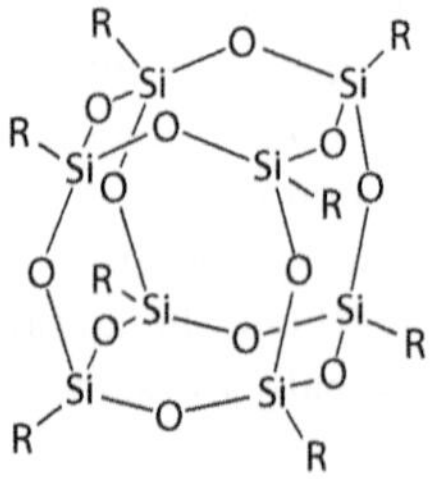

FIGURE 3.22   Structure of octameric POSS. R = H or organic group.

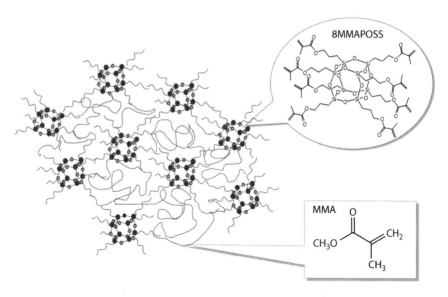

FIGURE 3.23 Schematic representation of copolymer network formed by 8MMAPOSS (octa[propyl methacryl] polyhedral oligomeric silsesquioxane) and MMA.

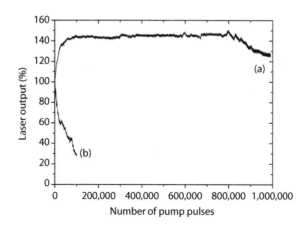

FIGURE 3.24 Normalized laser output as a function of the number of pump pulses in the same position of the sample for dye PM567 in: (a) COP(MMA:8MMAPOSS 87:13) pumped at 30 Hz and (b) pure PMMA pumped at 10 Hz. Pump energy: 5.5 mJ/pulse. (Reprinted with permission from García, O. et al., *J. Phys. Chem. C*, 112, 14710–14713, 2008. Copyright [2008], American Chemical Society.)

media to optimize the laser action that has overcome the dye/host specificity imposed up to now, which has represented one of the most important limitations of these laser systems from an application point of view.

Detailed experimental and theoretical studies seem to indicate that the remarkable improvement in the laser performance of dye-doped POSS systems was a direct consequence of scattering processes [80,81]. The dispersion of POSS nanoparticles

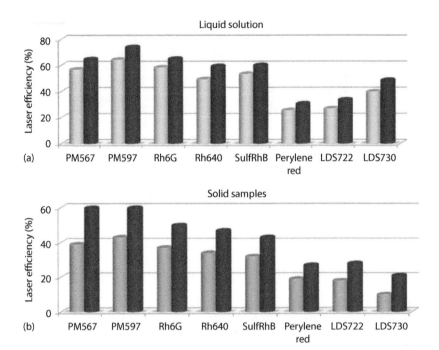

FIGURE 3.25 Laser efficiency of different dyes in the presence (black bars) and absence (gray bars) of 8MMAPOSS nanoparticles in liquid solution (a) and in solid samples (b) under transversal pumping at 532 nm with 6 ns half width at half maximum, 5.5 mJ pulses. The solvents in the liquid solutions were ethyl acetate (PM567, PM597, perylene red) and ethanol (LDS722, LDS730). The composition of the polymeric matrices was PMMA (PM567, PM597, perylene red), copolymer MMA:HEMA 1:1 (Rh6 G, Rh640, SulfRhB), and PHEMA (LDS722, LDS730). In the solutions and solid matrices with POSS, the proportion of 8MMAPOSS nanoparticles was 13 wt%. Dye concentration was: 1.5×10^{-3} M (PM567), 4×10^{-4} M (Rh6G, SulfRhB, LDS722), 5×10^{-4} M (Rh640, perylene red), 6×10^{-4} M (PM597), and 8×10^{-4} M (LDS730).

at a molecular level defines highly homogeneous materials that, when doped with laser dyes, allow coherent laser emission, but, in addition and despite their nanometer size, the POSS particles sustain a weak optical scattering that helps lasing by elongating the light path inside the gain media, thus providing an extra feedback, a phenomenon central to the process called *incoherent random lasing* or *lasing with intensity feedback* [82]. In this way, the laser action in systems based on dye-doped POSS materials is significantly enhanced in both liquid and solid phases [78–80].

The unique chemical and optical properties exhibited by POSS nanoparticles led us to design new hybrid photonic systems based on POSS labeled with fluorescent dyes as pendant groups on their rigid inorganic cores [83]. In particular, we synthesized new hybrid organic–inorganic dyes based on azide-functionalized POSS as the inorganic part and a derivative of PM567 as the organic component. By using a copolymer of MMA with 13% weight ratio of 8MMAPOSS doped with hybrid dye, lasing performance remained at the same level previously demonstrated with PM657 dye simply dissolved in the POSS-containing matrix; lasing efficiency was now 56%, and the laser output remained stable, without any sign of degradation, after 400,000 pump pulses of 5.5 mJ/pulse at 30 Hz repetition rate. These new hybrid systems based on dye-linked POSS nanoparticles may be used as new alternative sources of photonic materials for optoelectronic devices, competing with dendronized or grafted polymers.

Recently, Valiev et al. [84] demonstrated lasing efficiencies as high as 85% for PM567 in pure PMMA with 8MMAPOSS additives, under transversal pumping with pump power density of 54 mW/cm^2. Nevertheless, under pumping at 10 Hz repetition rate, the lasing efficiency dropped during the first minutes of irradiation, stabilizing finally at the 50% efficiency level and remaining there after 140,000 pump pulses. Although the initial lasing efficiencies were lower, when the dye was incorporated into PMMA media with careful purification of initial methylmethacrylate and initiator of polymerization, the long-term operation remained at the same level as when the matrix incorporated 8MMAPOSS, demonstrating that proper purification of the initial substances can result in operating lifetime characteristics of media based on purely polymeric materials highly competitive with those of the matrices with 8MMAPOSS additives.

3.3   APPLICATIONS

The unique operational flexibility of dye lasers has resulted in applications in many fields in science and technology. Their capability of providing coherent, tunable, narrow-linewidth radiation spanning the visible spectrum has made them an invaluable tool in high-resolution atomic and molecular spectroscopy. Isotope separation, remote sensing, and photochemistry are examples of applied fields in which dye lasers have been successfully utilized. In the life sciences, dye lasers have found applications in biology, studying biomedical reaction kinetics of biological molecules, and in medicine, in cancer photodynamic therapy, dermatology, and the treatment of vascular lesions. The medical applications of dye lasers are considered in detail in Chapter 8.

We have already mentioned the problems posed by liquid dye lasers, which have seriously restricted their use outside the laboratory. SSDLs are much more appropriate for use in industrial and medical environments, but the photodegradation problems exhibited by these systems for many years were an insurmountable handicap for any practical use. As shown in this chapter, the technology of SSDLs has greatly improved over the last decade, and new dyes and hosts with performance comparable to that of liquid dye lasers have been developed. These improved SSDL systems, stable, cheap, and user friendly, offer a promising alternative to liquid dye lasers as practical sources of coherent, tunable laser radiation.

REFERENCES

1. Duarte, F. J. and L. W. Hillman (Eds), *Dye Laser Principles*, Academic, New York, 1990.
2. Duarte, F. J. and A. Costela, Dye lasers. In R. D. Guenther, D. G. Steel, and L. Bayvel (Eds), *Encyclopedia of Modern Optics*, pp. 400–414, Elsevier, New York, 2004.

3. Soffer, B. H. and B. B. McFarland, Continuously tunable, narrow-band organic dye lasers, *Appl. Phys. Lett.* 10: 266–267, 1967.

4. Peterson, O. G. and B. B. Snavely, Stimulated emission from flashlamp-excited organic dyes in polymethyl methacrylate, *Appl. Phys. Lett.* 12: 238–240, 1968.

5. O'Connell, R. M. and T. T. Saito, Plastics for high-power laser applications: A review, *Opt. Eng.* 22: 393–399, 1983.

6. Zink, J. I., B. Dunn, R. B. Kaner, E. T. Knobbe, and J. McKiernan, Inorganic sol-gel glasses as matrices for nonlinear optical materials. In S. R. Marder, J. E. Sohn, and G. D. Stucky (Eds), *Materials for Nonlinear Optics*, pp. 541–552, ACS Symposium Series, American Chemical Society, Washington, DC, 1991.

7. Pavlopoulos, T. G., M. Shah, and J. H. Boyer, Efficient laser action from 1,3,5,7,8-pentamethylpyrromethene-BF$_2$ complex and its disodium 2,6-disulfonate derivative, *Opt. Commun.* 70: 425–427, 1989.

8. Pavlopoulos, T. G., J. H. Boyer, M. Shah, K. Thangaraj, and M.-L. Soong, Laser action from 2,6,8-position trisubstituted 1,3,5,7-tetramethylpyrromethene-BF$_2$ complexes: Part 1, *Appl. Opt.* 29: 3585–3586, 1990.

9. Pavlopoulos, T. G., J. H. Boyer, K. Thangaraj, G. Sathyamoorthi, M. Shah, and M.-L. Soong, Laser dye spectroscopy of some pyrromethene-BF$_2$ complexes, *Appl. Opt.* 31: 7089–7094, 1992.

10. Costela, A., I. García-Moreno, and R. Sastre, Materials for solid-state dye lasers. In H. S. Nalwa (Ed.), *Handbook of Advanced Electronic and Photonic Materials and Devices*, Volume 7, Chapter 4, Academic, San Diego, CA, 2001.

11. Duarte, F. J., A. Costela, I. García-Moreno, and R. Sastre, Measurements of $\partial n/\partial T$ in solid-state dye laser gain media, *Appl. Opt.* 39: 6522–6523, 2000.

12. Dyumaev, K. M., A. A. Manenkov, A. P. Maslyukov, A. G. Matyushin, V. S. Nechitailo, and A. M. Prokhorov, Transparent polymers: A new class of optical materials for lasers, *Sov. J. Quantum Electron.* 13: 503–507, 1983.

13. Costela, A., F. Florido, I. García-Moreno, R. Duchowicz, F. Amat-Guerri, J. M. Figuera, and R. Sastre, Solid-state dye lasers based on copolymers of 2-hydroxyethyl methacrylate and methyl methacrylate doped with Rhodamine 6G, *Appl. Phys. B* 60: 383–389, 1995.

14. Maslyukov, A., S. Sokolov, M. Kaivola, K. Nyholm, and S. Popov, Solid-state dye laser with modified poly(methyl methacrylate)-doped active elements, *Appl. Opt.* 34: 1516–1518, 1995.

15. Giffin, S. M., W. J. Wadsworth, I. T. McKinnie, A. D. Woolhouse, G. J. Smith, and T. G. Haskell, Efficient, high photostability, high brightness, co-polymer solid state dye lasers, *J. Mod. Optic.* 46: 1941–1945, 1999.

16. Costela, A., I. García-Moreno, J. M. Figuera, F. Amat-Guerri, R. Mallavia, M. D. Santa-María, and R. Sastre, Solid-state dye lasers based on modified Rhodamine 6G dyes copolymerized with methacrylic monomers, *J. Appl. Phys.* 80: 3167–3173, 1996.

17. Pavlopoulos, T. G., Scaling of dye lasers with improved laser dyes, *Prog. Quant. Electron.* 26: 193–224, 2002.

18. Ahmad, M., M. D. Rahn, and T. A. King, Singlet oxygen and dye triplet-state quenching in solid-state dye lasers consisting of pyrromethene 567-doped poly(methyl methacrylate), *Appl. Opt.* 38: 6337–6342, 1999.

19. Ahmad, M., T. A. King, D.-K. Ko, B. H. Cha, and J. Lee, Highly photostable laser solution and solid-state media based on mixed pyrromethene and coumarin, *Opt. Laser Technol.* 34: 445–448, 2002.

20. Costela, A., I. García-Moreno, and R. Sastre, Polymeric solid-state dye lasers: Recent developments, *Phys. Chem. Phys.* 5: 4745–4763, 2003.

21. Duchowicz, R., B. Scaffardi, A. Costela, I. García-Moreno, R. Sastre, and A. Acuña, Photothermal characterization and stability analysis of polymeric dye lasers, *Appl. Opt.* 39: 4959–4963, 2000.

22. Duchowicz, R., B. Scaffardi, A. Costela, I. García-Moreno, R. Sastre, and A. Acuña, Photothermal analysis of polymeric dye laser materials excited at different pump rates, *Appl. Opt.* 42: 1029–1035, 2003.

23. Jiang, Y., R. Fan, Y. Xia, and D. Chen, Highly efficient and photostable solid-state dye lasers based on modified copolymers doped with PM567, *Opt. Commun.* 284: 1959–1962, 2011.

24. Jiang, Y., R. Fan, Y. Xia, and D. Chen, Tunable solid-state laser based on modified polymethyl methacrylate with methanol doped with pyrromethene 580, *Appl. Opt.* 50: 1302–1306, 2011.

25. López Arbeloa, T., F. López Arbeloa, I. López Arbeloa, I. García-Moreno, A. Costela, R. Sastre, and F. Amat-Guerri, Correlations between photophysics and lasing properties of dipyrromethene-BF_2 dyes in solution, *Chem. Phys. Lett.* 299: 315–321, 1999.

26. Liang, F., H. Zeng, Z. Sun, Y. Yuan, Z. Yao, and Z. Xu, Eight-position substitution effects on laser action of the 1,3,5,7-tetramethyl-2,6-diethyl pyrromethene–BF_2 complexes, *J. Opt. Soc. Am. B* 18: 1841–1845, 2001.

27. Alvarez, M., F. Amat-Guerri, A. Costela, I. García-Moreno, C. Gómez, M. Liras, and R. Sastre, Linear and cross-linked polymeric solid-state dye lasers based on 8-substituted alkyl analogues of pyrromethene 567, *Appl. Phys. B* 80: 993–1006, 2005.

28. García-Moreno, I., A. Costela, L. Campo, R. Sastre, F. Amat-Guerri, M. Liras, F. López Arbeloa, et al., 8-Phenyl-substituted Dipyrromethene. BF_2 complexes as highly efficient and photostable laser dyes, *J. Phys. Chem. A* 108: 3315–3323, 2004.

29. García-Moreno, I. F. Amat-Guerri, M. Liras, A. Costela, L. Infantes, R. Sastre, F. López Arbeloa, et al., Structural changes in the BODIPY Dye PM567 enhancing the laser action in liquid and solid media, *Adv. Funct. Mat.* 17: 3088–3098, 2007.

30. Alvarez, M., A. Costela, I. García-Moreno, F. Amat-Guerri, M. Liras, R. Sastre, F. López Arbeloa, et al., Bichromatic laser emission from dipyrromethene dyes incorporated into solid polymeric media, *J. Appl. Phys.* 101: 113110, 2007.

31. Liras, M., J. Bañuelos Prieto, M. Pintado-Sierra, F. López Arbeloa, I. García-Moreno, A. Costela, L. Infantes, et al., Synthesis, photophysical properties, and laser behavior of 3-Amino and 3-Acetamido BODIPY dyes, *Org. Lett.* 9: 4183–4186, 2007.

32. Alvarez, M., A. Costela, I. García-Moreno, F. Amat-Guerri, M. Liras, R. Sastre, F. López Arbeloa, et al., Photophysical and laser emission studies of 8-polyphenylene-substituted BODIPY dyes in liquid solution and in solid polymeric matrices, *Photochem. Photobiol. Sci.* 7: 802–813, 2008.

33. Bañuelos Prieto, J., A. R. Agarrabeitia, I. García-Moreno, I. López Arbeloa, A. Costela, L. Infantes, M. E. Pérez-Ojeda, et al., Controlling optical properties and function of BODIPY by using asymmetric substitution effects, *Chem. Eur. J.* 16: 14094–14105, 2010.

34. Durán-Sampedro, G., A. R. Agarrabeitia, L. Cerdán, M. E. Pérez-Ojeda, A. Costela, I. García-Moreno, I. Esnal, et al., Carboxylates versus fluorines: Boosting the emission properties of commercial BODIPYs in liquid and solid media, *Adv. Funct. Mat.* 23: 4195–4205, 2013.

35. Durán-Sampedro, G., I. Esnal, A. R. Agarrabeitia, J. Bañuelos Prieto, L. Cerdán, I. García-Moreno, A. Costela, et al., First highly efficient and photostable *E*- and *C*-4,4-difluoro-4-bora-3a,4a,-diaza-*s*-indacene (BODIPY) as dye lasers in the liquid phase, thin films, and solid-state rods, *Chem. Eur. J.* 20: 2646–2653, 2014.

36. Pérez-Ojeda, M. E., C. Thivierge, M. Martín, A. Costela, K. Burgess, and I. García-Moreno, Highly efficient and photostable photonic materials from diiodinated BODIPY laser dyes, *Opt. Mat. Express.* 1: 243–251, 2011.

37. Durán-Sampedro, G., A. R. Agarrabeitia, I. García-Moreno, A. Costela, J. Bañuelos, T. Arbeloa, I. López Arbeloa, et al., Chlorinated BODIPYs: Surprisingly efficient and highly photostable laser dyes, *Eur. J. Org. Chem.* 6335–6350, 2012.

38. Xiao, Y., D. Zhang, X. Qian, A. Costela, I. García-Moreno, M. Martín, M. E. Pérez-Ojeda, et al., Unprecedent laser action from energy transfer in multichromophoric BODIPY cassettes, *Chem. Commun.* 47: 11513–11515, 2011.

39. Gartzia-Rivero, L., H. Yu, J. Bañuelos, I. López Arbeloa, A. Costela, I. García-Moreno, and Y. Xiao, Photophysical and laser properties of cassettes based on a BODIPY and rhodamine pair, *Chem. Asian J.* 8: 3133–3141, 2013.

40. García, O., R. Sastre, D. del Agua, A. Costela, I. García-Moreno, F. López Arbeloa, J. Bañuelos Prieto, et al., Laser and physical properties of BODIPY chromophores in new fluorinated polymeric materials, *J. Phys. Chem. C.* 111: 1508–1516, 2007.

41. Iezzi, R. A., Fluoropolymers for architectural applications. In J. Scheirs (Ed.), *Modern Fluoropolymers*, pp. 271–300, John Wiley, Chichester, 1997.

42. Ramon, M. C., M. Ariu, R. Xia, D. D. C. Bradley, M. S. Reilly, C. Marinelli, C. N. Morgan, et al., A characterization of Rhodamine 640 for optical amplification: Collinear pump and signal gain properties in solutions, thin-film polymer dispersions, and waveguides, *J. Appl. Phys.* 97: 073517, 2005.

43. Umezawa, K., Y. Nakamura, H. Makino, D. Citterio, and K. Suzuki, Bright, color-tunable fluorescent dyes in the visible–near-infrared region, *J. Am. Chem. Soc.* 130: 1550–1551, 2008.

44. Fan, R., Y. Xia, and D. Chen, Solid state dye lasers based on LDS 698 doped in modified polymethyl methacrylate, *Opt. Express.* 16: 9804–9810, 2008.

45. García-Moreno, I., A. Costela, M. Pintado-Sierra, V. Martín, and R. Sastre, Efficient red-edge materials photosensitized by rhodamine 640, *J. Phys. Chem. B* 113: 10611–10618, 2009.

46. García-Moreno, I., A. Costela, M. Pintado-Sierra, V. Martín, and R. Sastre, Enhanced laser action of Perylene-Red doped polymeric materials, *Opt. Express.* 17: 12777–12784, 2009.

47. García-Moreno, I., A. Costela, V. Martín, M. Pintado-Sierra, and R. Sastre, Materials for reliable solid state dye laser at the red spectral edge, *Adv. Funct. Mat.* 19: 2547–2552, 2009.

48. Martin, V., A. Costela, M. Pintado-Sierra, and I. García-Moreno, Sulforhodamine B doped polymeric matrices. A high efficient and stable solid-state dye laser, *J. Photochem. Photobiol. A: Chem.* 219: 265–272, 2011.

49. Costela, A., I. García-Moreno, R. Sastre, D. W. Coutts, and C. E. Webb, High-repetition-rate polymeric solid-state dye lasers pumped by a copper-vapor laser, *Appl. Phys. Lett.* 79: 452–454, 2001.

50. Abedin, K. M., M. Álvarez, A. Costela, I. García-Moreno, O. García, R. Sastre, D. W. Coutts, et al., 10 kHz repetition rate solid-state dye laser pumped by diode-pumped solid-state laser, *Opt. Commun.* 218: 359–363, 2003.

51. Kytina, I. G., V. G. Kytin, and K. Lips, High power polymer dye laser with improved stability, *Appl. Phys. Lett.* 84: 4902–4904, 2004.

52. Lam, S. Y. and M. J. Damzen, Characterisation of solid-state dyes and their use as tunable laser amplifiers, *Appl. Phys. B.* 77: 577–584, 2003.

53. Ray, A. K., S. Kumar, N. V. Mayekar, S. Sinha, S. Kundu, S. Chattopadhyay, and K. Dasgupta, Role of the stimulated-emission rate in the photostability of solid-state dye lasers, *Appl. Opt.* 44: 7814–7822, 2005.

54. Bornemann, R., U. Lemmer, and E. Thiel, Continuous-wave solid-state dye laser, *Opt. Lett.* 31: 1669–1671, 2006.

55. Bronemann, R., E. Thiel, and P. Haring Bolívar, High-power solid-state cw dye laser, *Opt. Express.* 19: 26382–26393, 2011.

56. Reisfeld, R., A. Weiss, T. Saraidarov, E. Yariv, and A. A. Ishchenko, Solid-state lasers based on inorganic-organic hybrid materials obtained by combined sol-gel polymer technology, *Polym. Adv. Technol.* 15: 291–301, 2004.

57. Rahn, M. D. and T. A. King, Comparison of laser performance of dye molecules in sol-gel, polycom, ormosil, and poly(methyl methacrylate) host media, *Appl. Opt.* 34: 8260–8271, 1995.

58. Ahmad, M., T. A. King, D.-K. Ko, B. H. Cha, and J. Lee, Performance and photostability of xanthene and pyrromethene laser dyes in sol-gel phases, *J. Phys. D: Appl. Phys.* 35: 1473–1476, 2002.

59. Yang, Y., M. Wang, G. Qian, Z. Wang, and X. Fan, Laser properties and photostabilities of laser dyes doped in ORMOSILs, *Opt. Mater.* 24: 621–628, 2004.

60. Nhung, T. H., M. Canva, T. T. A. Dao, F. Chaput, A. Brun, N. D. Hung, and J. P. Boilot, Stable doped hybrid sol-gel materials for solid-state dye laser, *Appl. Opt.* 42: 2213–2218, 2003.

61. Yang, Y., J. Zou, H. Rong, G. D. Qian, Z. Y. Wang, and M. Q. Wang, Influence of various coumarin dyes on the laser performance of dyes co-doped into ORMOSILs, *Appl. Phys. B* 86: 309–313, 2007.

62. Yariv, E. and R. Reisfeld, Lasing properties of pyrromethene dyes in sol-gel glasses, *Opt. Mater.* 13: 49–54, 1999.

63. Costela, A., I. García-Moreno, C. Gómez, O. García, L. Garrido, and R. Sastre, Highly efficient and stable doped hybrid organic-inorganic materials for solid-state dye lasers, *Chem. Phys. Lett.* 387: 496–501, 2004.

64. Costela, A., I. García-Moreno, C. Gómez, O. García, and R. Sastre, Enhancement of laser properties of pyrromethene 567 dye incorporated into new organic-inorganic hybrid materials, *Chem. Phys. Lett.* 369: 656–661, 2003.

65. Costela, A., I. García-Moreno, C. Gómez, O. García, and R. Sastre, Environment effects on the lasing photostability of Rhodamine 6G incorporated into organic-inorganic hybrid materials, *Appl. Phys. B.* 78: 629–634, 2004.

66. Costela, A., I. García-Moreno, O. García, D. del Agua, and R. Sastre, Structural influence of the inorganic network in the laser performance of dye-doped hybrid materials, *Appl. Phys. B* 80: 749–755, 2005.

67. García-Moreno, I., A. Costela, A. Cuesta, O. García, D. del Agua, and R. Sastre, Synthesis, structure, and physical properties of hybrid nanocomposites for solid-state dye lasers, *J. Phys. Chem. B* 109: 21618–21626, 2005.

68. Costela, A., I. García-Moreno, C. Gómez, O. García, R. Sastre, A. Roig, and E. Molins, Polymer-filled nanoporous silica aerogels as hosts for highly stable solid-state dye lasers, *J. Phys. Chem. B* 109: 4475–4480, 2005.

69. García, O., R. Sastre, D. del Agua, A. Costela, I. García-Moreno, and A. Roig, Efficient optical materials based on fluorinated-polymeric silica aerogels, *Chem. Phys. Lett.* 427: 375–378, 2006.

70. Al-Shamiri, H. A. S. and M. T. H. Abou Kana, Laser performance and photostability of Rhodamine B in solid host matrices, *Appl. Phys. B* 101: 129–135, 2010.

71. de Queiroz, T. B., M. B. S. Botelho, L. De Boni, H. Eckert, and A. S. S. de Camargo, Strategies for reducing dye aggregation in luminescent host-guest systems: Rhodamine 6G incorporated in new mesoporous sol-gel hosts, *J. Appl. Phys.* 113: 113508, 2013.

72. Costela, A., I. García-Moreno, D. del Agua, O. García, and R. Sastre, Highly photostable solid-state dye lasers based on silicon-modified organic matrices, *J. Appl. Phys.* 101: 073110, 2007.

73. Susdorf, T., D. del Agua, A. Tyagi, A. Penzkofer, O. García, R. Sastre, A. Costela, et al., Photophysical characterization of pyrromethene 597 laser dye in silicon-containing organic matrices, *Appl. Phys. B* 86: 537–545, 2007.

74. Costela, A., I. García-Moreno, M. Pintado-Sierra, F. Amat-Guerri, R. Sastre, M. Liras, F. López Arbeloa, et al., New analogues of the BODIPY dye PM597: Photophysical and lasing properties in liquid solutions and in solid polymeric matrices, *J. Chem. Phys. A* 113: 8118–8124, 2009.

75. Duarte, F. J. and R. O. James, Tunable solid-state lasers incorporating dye-doped, polymer-nanoparticle gain media, *Opt. Lett.* 28: 2088–2090, 2003.
76. Duarte, F. J. and R. O. James, Spatial structure of dye-doped polymer nanoparticle gain media, *Appl. Opt.* 43: 4088–4090, 2004.
77. Ahmad, M., Enhanced photostability of photoluminescent dye-doped solutions and polymers with the addition of dielectric-oxide micro-particles, *Opt. Commun.* 271: 457–461, 2007.
78. García, O., R. Sastre, I. García-Moreno, V. Martín, and A. Costela, New laser hybrid materials based on POSS copolymers, *J. Phys. Chem. C* 112: 14170–14173, 2008.
79. Sastre, R., V. Martín, L. Garrido, J. L. Chiara, B. Trastoy, O. García, A. Costela, et al., Dye-doped polyhedral oligomeric silsesquioxane (POSS)-modified polymeric matrices for highly efficient and photostable solid-state lasers, *Adv. Funct. Mat.* 19: 3307–3316, 2009.
80. Costela, A., I. García-Moreno, L. Cerdán, V. Martín, O. García, and R. Sastre, Dye-doped POSS solutions: Nanomaterials for laser emission, *Adv. Mat.* 21: 4163–4166, 2009.
81. Cerdán, L., A. Costela, I. García-Moreno, V. Martín, and M. E. Pérez-Ojeda, Laser efficiency enhancement due to non-resonant feedback in dye-doped hybrid materials: Theoretical insights and experiment, *IEEE J. Quantum Elect.* 47: 907–919, 2013.
82. Takeda, S. and M. Obara, Extremely selective modal oscillation of random lasing induced by strong multiple scattering, *Appl. Phys. B* 94: 443–450, 2009.
83. Pérez-Ojeda, M. E., B. Trastoy, I. López Arbeloa, J. Bañuelos, A. Costela, I. García-Moreno, and J. L. Chiara, Click assembly of dye-functionalized octasilsesquioxanes for highly efficient and photostable photonic systems, *Chem. Eur. J.* 17: 13258–13268, 2011.
84. Valiev, R. R., E. N. Telminov, T. A. Solodova, E. N. Ponyavina, R. M. Gadirov, G. V. Mayer, and T. N. Kopylova, Lasing of pyrromethene 567 in solid matrices, *Chem. Phys. Lett.* 588: 184–187, 2013.

4 Organic Dye-Doped Polymer-Nanoparticle Tunable Lasers

F. J. Duarte and R. O. James

CONTENTS

4.1 INTRODUCTION

The first broadly tunable laser was the organic dye laser. The dye laser was discovered in 1966 by Sorokin and Lankard [1] and Schäfer et al. [2]. Dye-doped polymer (DDP) gain media for tunable lasers were introduced shortly afterwards by Soffer and McFarland [3] and Peterson and Snavely [4]. However, due to initial difficulties with laser medium optical inhomogeneities and thermal problems, these media were relegated to the archives, with the exception of some sporadic interest (see, e.g., [5]), until the 1990s [6].

Using a highly homogeneous DDP medium named *modified poly(methyl methacrylate)* (MPMMA), Duarte [7] reported, for the first time, on single-transverse-mode beams and narrow-linewidth emission in 1994. The gain medium used by Duarte was developed by researchers in the former Soviet Union [8]. This research on narrow-linewidth solid-state dye lasers was an extension of an earlier effort involving silicate gain media [9]. These reports, in addition to further efforts in the United States and abroad (see, e.g., [10,11]), reenergized the interest in solid-state dye lasers worldwide. This interest and progress can be followed in various reviews [12–14] and in Chapter 3 on solid-state dye lasers by Costela et al. [15]. As of 2007, solid-state dye laser research activity had been reported in more than 30 laboratories around the world.

As already mentioned, the early polymeric matrices presented difficulties in optical homogeneity and thermal dissipation. To solve the $\partial n/\partial T$ problem, researchers introduced hybrid organic–inorganic matrices in which the inorganic portion is silica based.

Examples of such materials include the dye-doped organically modified silicate (ORMOSIL) [6], tetraethoxysilane [7,9], and silica–polymer nanocomposites [16].

An important coherence phenomenon, reported by Duarte and Pope [16], in these organic–inorganic matrices manifested itself due to minute refractive index differences, which caused internal interference that resulted in laser beam inhomogeneities.

Thus, by 2003, the choice for laser researchers consisted of proven highly homogeneous DDP gain media, with poor $\partial n/\partial T$ characteristics, which limit pulse repetition frequencies (prfs), or organic–inorganic alternatives with improved thermal characteristics but exhibiting refractive index conditions that result in internal interference or laser beam inhomogeneities. One alternative to neutralize the laser beam inhomogeneities was reported by Duarte and James [17]. This consisted of dispersing nearly uniform nanoparticle distributions in the DDP matrices. The role of the nanoparticle distribution is to improve the $\partial n/\partial T$ factor without introducing the conditions necessary for internal interference at the lasing wavelength. This was achieved by the near-uniform distribution of the nanoparticles, as will be explained in detail later in the chapter. This new gain medium was called *dye-doped polymer nanoparticle* (DDPN) gain medium.

This chapter first describes the tunable laser resonators and oscillators to which this class of efficient DDP gain media, including functional distributions of silica nanoparticles, is applicable, and then proceeds to present the laser and interference experiments used to characterize these gain media. A detailed material synthesis section follows, and a discussion on nanoparticle distributions, invisible to laser wavelengths in the visible spectrum, is also included.

A brief literature survey indicates that DDPN gain media [17] have attracted the interest of researchers working on dye-doped organic–inorganic gain media [18–21], dye codoped solid-state gain media [22,23], nanocomposite materials for optical devices [24], DDP films [25], photostability of solid-state organic gain media [26], polymeric networks [27], DDP fibers [28], holographic media [29], and microcavity lasers [30,31]. Albeit, so far, DDPN gain media have been demonstrated using rhodamine 6G dye [17], other dyes such as pyrromethenes [32] are attractive candidates to dope these new tunable solid-state laser media.

4.2 TUNABLE LASER OSCILLATOR REVIEW

The narrow-linewidth tunable laser oscillators, or resonators, used to demonstrate the capabilities of solid-state dye lasers have been reviewed in [33,34] and are explained here and in Chapter 5 as applied to semiconductor lasers. For completeness, the architecture and performance of these oscillators are briefly outlined here.

The first multiple-prism grating narrow-linewidth solid-state dye laser oscillators were introduced by Duarte in 1994 [7]. These included the multiple-prism Littrow (MPL) grating oscillator and the hybrid multiple-prism near grazing-incidence (HMPGI) grating oscillator. Experiments yielding improved performance of these oscillators [35] led eventually to an optimized HMPGI grating oscillator [36] and an optimized MPL grating oscillator [37]. These oscillators are depicted in Figures 4.1 and 4.2, respectively. In Table 4.1, the emission characteristics of these high-performance oscillators are tabulated. It should be noted that all these experiments were performed in the nanosecond pulse time domain using rhodamine 6G–doped MPMMA gain media. The most salient characteristics are single-transverse-mode beam characteristics and widely tunable single-longitudinal-mode emission in the $350 \leq \Delta v \leq 375$ MHz range. In the wavelength domain, at $\lambda \approx 590$ nm, these line-widths correspond to the $0.00040 \leq \Delta \lambda \leq 0.00043$ nm range. The beam divergence

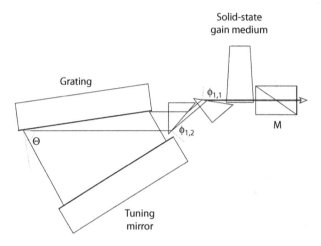

FIGURE 4.1 Solid-state HMPGI grating laser oscillator. (Reprinted from *Opt. Laser Technol.*, 29, Duarte, F. J., Multiple-prism near-grazing-incidence grating solid-state dye laser oscillator, 513–516, Copyright (1997), with permission from Elsevier.)

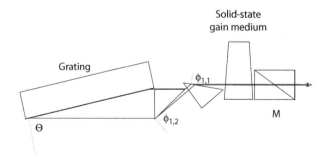

FIGURE 4.2 Optimized solid-state MPL grating laser oscillator. (Reproduced from Duarte, F. J., Multiple-prism grating solid-state dye laser oscillator: Optimized architecture, *Appl. Opt.* 38: 6347–6349, 1999. With permission of Optical Society of America.)

TABLE 4.1
Performance of Narrow-Linewidth Solid-State Dye Laser Oscillators

Gain Medium[a]	Oscillator Architecture	$\Delta\theta$ (mrad)	$\Delta\nu$ (MHz)	Δt^b (ns)	Tuning Range (nm)	ASE[c]	Eff. (%)	References
MPMMA	HMPGI	2.3	375	6	565–610	$\sim 10^{-7}$	3–4[d]	[36]
MPMMA	MPL	2.2	350	3	550–603	$\sim 10^{-6}$	$\sim 5^e$	[37]
HEMA:MMA	MPL	3.5	650	105	564–602	$\sim 10^{-4}$	~ 2	[38]

[a] Belonging to the DDP class.
[b] At full width half-maximum (FWHM).
[c] Amplified spontaneous emission as defined in [39].
[d] Excitation performed with a coumarin 125 dye laser at $\lambda \approx 532$ nm.
[e] Excitation performed with a coumarin 125 dye laser at $\lambda \approx 525$ nm.

for the optimized MPL grating oscillator was measured to be ~ 1.5 times the diffraction limit, with similar characteristics observed for the HMPGI grating oscillator.

An additional oscillator architecture was introduced by Duarte et al. [38] in experiments aimed at demonstrating narrow-linewidth long-pulse lasing in solid-state dye laser oscillators. In these experiments, the linewidths achieved were $\Delta\nu \approx 650$ MHz in pulses as long as $\Delta t \approx 105$ ns. The architecture of this MPL grating oscillator is illustrated in Figure 4.3. An additional novelty in these experiments was the use of a rhodamine 6G–doped 2-hydroxyethyl methacrylate (HEMA):methyl methacrylate (MMA) matrix as the gain medium.

As might have become apparent in the previous discussion, besides tunability, the two most important parameters in the description and characterization of narrow-linewidth tunable laser oscillators are beam divergence ($\Delta\theta$) and laser linewidth ($\Delta\lambda$). These two parameters are intimately related via the cavity linewidth equation [33,34,40]:

$$\Delta\lambda \approx \Delta\theta_R \left(MR\nabla_\lambda\Theta_G \pm R\nabla_\lambda\Phi_P \right)^{-1} \tag{4.1}$$

where:

    R is the number of intracavity return passes

    M is the overall beam magnification provided by the multiple-prism beam expander

    $\nabla_\lambda\Theta_G$ is the grating dispersion in either near grazing-incidence configuration or Littrow configuration

    $\nabla_\lambda\Phi_P$ is the return-pass multiple-prism dispersion

All these quantities are described in detail in the cited references and in Chapter 5. Since, by design, the multiple-prism dispersion can be reduced to $\nabla_\lambda\Phi_P \approx 0$, Equation 4.1 can be expressed simply as

$$\Delta\lambda \approx \Delta\theta_R \left(MR\nabla_\lambda\Theta_G \right)^{-1} \tag{4.2}$$

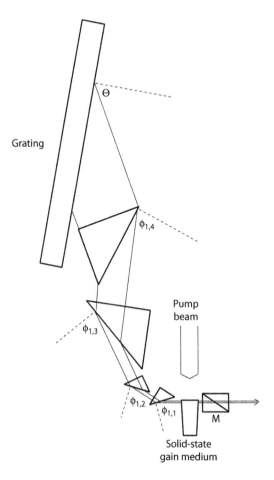

Grating

$\phi_{1,4}$

$\phi_{1,3}$

Pump
beam

$\phi_{1,2}$ $\phi_{1,1}$
M

Solid-state
gain medium

FIGURE 4.3 Long-pulse MPL grating laser oscillator. (Reproduced from Duarte, F. J., T. S. Taylor, A. Costela, I. García-Moreno, and R. Sastre, Long-pulse narrow-linewidth dispersive solid-state dye laser oscillator, *Appl. Opt.* 37: 3987–3989, 1998. With permission of Optical Society of America.)

where the beam divergence is given by [34,40]

$$\Delta\theta_R \approx \frac{\lambda}{\pi w}\left(1+\left(\frac{L_R}{B_R}\right)^2+\left(\frac{LA_R}{B_R}\right)^2\right)^{-1} \tag{4.3}$$

In this equation, w is the beam waist, $L_R=(\pi w^2/\lambda)$ is known as the Rayleigh length, and A_R and B_R are the corresponding multiple-return-pass propagation matrix elements [34,40].

The designer can engineer the cavity so that the term in parentheses becomes close to unity. This can be accomplished when using liquid gain media; however, in organic solid-state gain media, thermal lensing effects prevent reaching the diffraction limit value of the beam divergence. In an optimized dispersive oscillator design [37], the measured beam divergence is

$$\Delta\theta_R \approx \frac{3}{2}\left(\frac{\lambda}{\pi w}\right) \tag{4.4}$$

This is accomplished under experimental conditions that result in $R \approx 3$ [40]. Also, it should be indicated that either Equation 4.1 or 4.3 provides only an upper limit estimate of the linewidth, so that the measured $\Delta\lambda$ is below the theoretical value [33,34]. This discussion is very pertinent to the subject at hand, since the main objective of introducing silica nanoparticles into the gain medium is to modify $\partial n / \partial T$ and thus reduce thermal lensing effects.

A useful observation, at this stage, is that the diffraction-limited expression of the beam divergence:

$$\Delta\theta \approx \frac{\lambda}{\pi w} \tag{4.5}$$

can be derived from the Heisenberg uncertainty principle [34,41]:

$$\Delta p \Delta x \approx h \tag{4.6}$$

which can also be expressed as [34]

$$\Delta\lambda\Delta x \approx \lambda^2 \tag{4.7}$$

$$\Delta v \Delta x \approx c \tag{4.8}$$

and

$$\Delta v \Delta t \approx 1 \tag{4.9}$$

For the optimized MPL-grating solid-state dye laser oscillator, a laser linewidth of $\Delta v \approx 350$ MHz ($\Delta\lambda \approx 0.00041$ nm at $\lambda = 590$ nm) was measured at a pulse duration of $\Delta t \approx 3$ ns [37]. This means that the measured linewidth was close to the limit allowed by the uncertainty principle for that pulse duration. Also, the spectral power density delivered by this narrow-linewidth oscillator is $\rho \approx 95$ W/MHz at $\lambda \approx 590$ nm.

Besides the multiple-prism grating oscillators described here, researchers have also successfully introduced solid-state distributed-feedback dye lasers [42–44]. Oki et al. [45,46] have also investigated waveguide configurations. The DDP matrices, including functional silica nanoparticle distributions, described here are applicable to all the oscillator architectures mentioned in this section as well as simple broadband resonators.

Finally, it should also be mentioned that the excitation methods of the dye-doped solid-state gain media should not be limited to traditional laser, or flashlamp, pumping. Recently, a waveguide method of excitation, designed for an array of pulsed high-brightness light-emitting diodes (LEDs), was disclosed in the literature [47]. One particular waveguide is made of polished aluminum, with an input aperture, for the diode array, having dimensions of 260×9 mm while the output aperture, designed for transverse excitation of the solid-state laser dye medium, has dimensions of 10 mm $\times 250$ μm. The two apertures are separated by 270 mm. The wide dimension of the excitation aperture is parallel to the plane of incidence.

4.3 SYNTHESIS OF DDPN LASER GAIN MEDIA

The new gain media consist of dye-doped, high-purity polymethyl methacrylate (PMMA) including dispersed silica nanoparticles. One example of such laser DDPN gain media is a rhodamine 6G–doped PMMA matrix containing 30% w/w silica in which the silica content is composed of ~ 12 nm SiO_2 particles. This particular DDPN gain medium shows conservation of TEM_{00} spatial beam characteristics approaching that observed in DDP gain media.

Synthesis and methods of fabrication of the DDPN gain media have been described in the recent literature [17,48–51]; however, we shall provide a comprehensive review here. Several variations of gain media preparation are possible, but the following is a fairly detailed discussion of materials and processes. The approach taken here to prepare homogeneous gain media was to obtain or prepare separate stable, moderately concentrated solutions or dispersions of (1) optical-grade PMMA polymers [51], (2) nanoparticulate silica organosols [17,50,51], and (3) laser dyes in organic solvents or solvent mixtures. The process involves physically mixing colloidally stable SiO_2 nanoparticle dispersions (organosols) in methyl ethyl ketone (MEK) with solutions of optical-grade PMMA resins in solvents that are compatible with the silica sol over a wide range of concentrations. The laser dye is also added to the mixture as a dissolved component in a suitable, compatible solvent. We use as high concentrations of each separate component as possible, so that when the mixture of component solutions is made, the polymer/sol remains colloidally stable, and the amount of solvent evaporation required to form the solid phase is minimized.

The materials used in DDPN gain media are all commercially available. The PMMA used was optical-grade resin manufactured for use in video laser disks (VLD) or video optical disks (VOD). Silica organosols are available in a range of organic solvents and particle sizes. In the work described here, silica organosol in MEK was the principal component. For specific listings, see [17,48–51]. An Internet search will also yield specific manufacturers.

The nanoparticle–polymer laser dye composite is formed from this dispersion mixture by slow solvent evaporation from a partially covered mold or container using a solvent-stripping method that provides a saturated vapor over the sample for a period often exceeding 1 week. All proportions of the component solutions are calculated using a spreadsheet to provide the desired concentrations of silica and laser dye in the polymer matrix. The mechanics of the synthesis–manufacturing process is outlined in Figure 4.4.

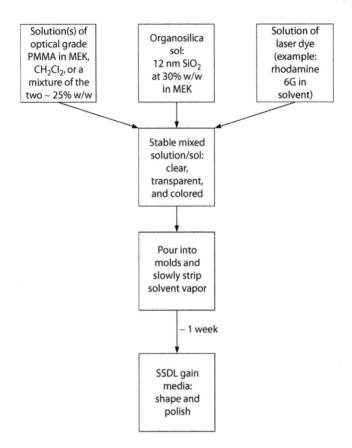

FIGURE 4.4 Synthesis–manufacturing process for DDPN gain media.

An example preparation involves weighing and mixing the following:

1. 54.83 g of silica organosol, composed of 12 nm diameter particles, 30.5% w/w SiO$_2$ in MEK
2. 97.57 g of PMMA solution at 20.0% w/w solids in MEK
3. 65.05 g PMMA solution at 30.0% w/w in methylene chloride
4. 37.17 g of 0.1% w/w solution of rhodamine 6G in methylene chloride

This dispersion example contains 21.92% solids, and the solids are composed of 29.98% SiO$_2$, 69.95% PMMA, and 0.069% rhodamine 6G. The solvent blend is 41.55% MeCl$_2$ and 54.45% MEK. The mass balance of solids and solvents for components and final gain media is shown in Table 4.2. After thorough mixing at room temperature, the clear, colored sol samples are placed in covered containers, and the solvents are slowly stripped away to form a gel. Eventually, this results in a colored, transparent, solid, rigid body.

It is possible to vary the solvent mixture ratios and the SiO$_2$ particle content up to approximately 50% w/w to provide a range of nanoparticle-filled laser DDP gain media.

TABLE 4.2

Mass Balances for Starting Components in Solid-State DDPN Gain Media[a]

Components Dispersions	Mass (g)	Mass Fraction	% w/w Solids	Solids (g)	% w/w Solids/ sol	Volatiles	Solvents
Silica organosol (12 nm diam.)	54.83	0.305	30.5	16.723	—	38.11	MEK
PMMA	97.57	0.20	20	19.514	—	78.06	MEK
PMMA	65.02	0.30	30	19.506	—	45.51	MeCl$_2$
Rhodamine 6G	37.10	0.001	0.1	0.037	—	37.06	MeCl$_2$
Totals	254.52	—	—	55.780	21.92	198.74	—

[a] SiO$_2$: 29.980%, PMMA: 69.953%, rhodamine 6G: 0.067%.
[b] Solvent blend: MeCl$_2$: 41.55%, MEK: 58.45%.

Silica organosols are available with a 9 and 5 nm particle diameter. Laser gain media have also been made with these smaller particles; however, it has proved more difficult to provide stable laser gain media using the 5 nm silica organosols. The magnitude of the thermo-optic coefficient, $\partial n/\partial T$, of the PMMA–silica composite media decreases in a linear fashion with the concentration of silica. However, it is difficult to prepare samples with greater than 50% w/w silica. Consequently, the negative sign of $\partial n/\partial T$ for PMMA cannot be completely nullified by silica addition alone.

Gain media with trapezoidal cross sections, at a plane parallel to the plane of propagation, are optically polished using a slow polishing technique. Since polymer properties are temperature dependent, care should be exercised not to overheat the sample during polishing. The rhodamine 6G DDP medium, used as a comparison, is the same as that used in previous experiments [7,35–37], and has been characterized in detail by Maslyukov et al. [8] and Popov [52].

4.4 EXPERIMENTAL RESULTS AND LASER EMISSION

In their 1995 paper, Duarte and Pope [16] presented clear interferometric evidence that illustrated a comparison of the internal structure of DDP gain media with the internal structure of hybrid dye-doped organic–inorganic gain media. In their paper, it was suggested that the high degree of internal homogeneity in the case of DDP, such as dye-doped MPMMA, matrices resulted in the absence of internal interference, which manifested itself in the homogeneous emission and propagation of laser beams. In other words, laser emission using these matrices as gain media did not present evidence of laser beam *breakup*. However, at the time, this was not the case for hybrid dye-doped organic–inorganic gain media, in which beam breakup was evident. The result of the propagation of laser beams in a dye-doped hybrid organic–inorganic matrix is shown in Figure 4.5 to illustrate the concepts just outlined.

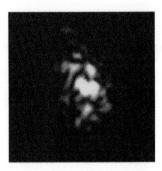

FIGURE 4.5 Interferometrically distorted beam profile following propagation through an inhomogeneous dye-doped organic–inorganic gain medium. Originally the beam, from a He–Ne laser emitting at $\lambda \approx 632.8$ nm, had a TEM_{00} profile. (Reproduced from Duarte, F. J. and R. O. James, Tunable solid-state lasers incorporating dye-doped, polymer-nanoparticle gain media, *Opt. Lett.* 28: 2088–2090, 2003. With permission from Optical Society of America.)

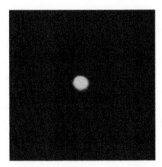

FIGURE 4.6 Preservation of laser beam profile following propagation through a homogeneous DDP gain medium. The preserved TEM_{00} beam profile is from a He–Ne laser emitting at $\lambda \approx 632.8$ nm. (Reproduced from Duarte, F. J. and R. O. James, Tunable solid-state lasers incorporating dye-doped, polymer-nanoparticle gain media, *Opt. Lett.* 28: 2088–2090, 2003. With permission from Optical Society of America.)

The same experiment using a rhodamine 6G-doped MPPMA gain matrix, as used in narrow-linewidth tunable laser oscillators, results in the preservation of the TEM_{00} beam profile, as illustrated in Figure 4.6.

4.4.1 TUNABLE LASER EMISSION

The laser experiments were performed using a prismatic tunable coumarin 152 laser as the excitation laser, delivering approximately 2 mJ in the 520–552 nm region. This laser was pumped transversely by a nitrogen laser at 337 nm. The emission from the green tunable laser was used to excite longitudinally a simple mirror-grating resonator. The cavity was comprised of a 2400 lines/mm grating, deployed in Littrow configuration, and an output-coupler mirror with a reflectivity of ~20%. The overall length of the cavity, illustrated in Figure 4.7, was about 75 mm, and it was configured

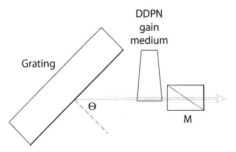

FIGURE 4.7 Mirror-grating cavity used in the DDPN gain media experiments.

to allow the interchange of trapezoidal solid-state gain media without altering the alignment of the resonator. In fact, it was possible to switch easily from one medium to another without disturbing the alignment of the cavity. Effort was devoted to this feature to ensure a fair comparison among media. The trapezoidal configuration of the gain medium enabled us to maintain a gain length of ~ 10 mm for all gain media used in these experiments. Lasing was also achieved, under direct nitrogen laser excitation, in a simple mirror–mirror cavity using a coumarin 500 DDPN at 30% w/w SiO_2 gain medium [17].

Beam profiles were recorded using black-and-white silver halide film, and energetic and temporal measurements were performed using the usual instrumentation [17]. Given previous experience with single-transverse-mode single-longitudinal-mode tunable laser oscillators in the solid state [7,35–37], it was decided to characterize and compare the new DDPN gain media by measuring the beam emission profiles of the new lasers. This was done because single-transverse-mode emission is a crucial precondition to achieving narrow-linewidth emission [35]. In other words, it is not possible to achieve single-longitudinal-mode lasing in the presence of more than one single transverse mode. Further, one of our main hypotheses was that a more favorable $\partial n / \partial T$ for the gain medium would possibly yield improved beam divergences and open the door for higher prfs. A simple preliminary experiment is to observe the beam profile of a propagating TEM_{00} beam through the DDPN gain medium. The result of this observation is shown in Figure 4.8, where it is clearly observed that for a DDPN at 30% w/w SiO_2, the TEM_{00} beam profile of a He–Ne laser, at $\lambda = 593.93$ nm, is nicely preserved.

Besides the demonstration of lasing in these new DDPN gain media, a primary objective of the measurements became the characterization of the laser emission beam. A typical profile of a laser beam from these new organic–inorganic media is shown in Figure 4.9. This beam profile has the usual homogeneous characteristics associated with broadband liquid, or DDP, tunable dye lasers. Albeit a tenuous secondary ring structure is observed, the profile can be fairly characterized as near TEM_{00}. This beam was measured to have a divergence of $\Delta\theta \approx 1.9$ (mrad), which is ~ 1.3 times the diffraction limit [17].

A summary of the laser emission results for DDP and DDPN matrices is presented in Table 4.3. In addition to the homogeneous beam profile, the feature that

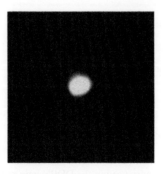

FIGURE 4.8 Conservation of TEM_{00} beam profile following propagation through a DDPN gain medium at 30% w/w SiO_2. The beam was generated by a He–Ne laser at $\lambda = 593.93$ nm.

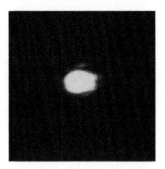

FIGURE 4.9 Laser beam profile generated with a mirror-grating resonator incorporating a rhodamine 6G DPN gain medium. The beam is similar to those obtained with liquid media and is primarily distributed in a central mode while displaying some weak secondary ring structure.

TABLE 4.3

Performance of Solid-State Lasers Incorporating DDP and DDPN Gain Matrices Using Rhodamine 6G Dye

Gain Medium	C (mM)	λ_p (nm)	Tuning Range (nm)	$\Delta\theta$ (mrad)	Eff. (%)[a]
DDP (%)	0.50^b	~525	563–610	2.3	49
DDPN 30 w/w SiO_2	$0.31^{b,c}$	~525	567–603	1.9	63
DDPN 50 w/w SiO_2	$0.31^{b,c}$	~550	575–600	1.6	9

Source: Adapted from Duarte, F. J. and R. O. James, *Opt Lett.* 28: 2088–2090, 2003.

[a] Overall optical efficiency.

[b] Initial dye concentration.

[c] The dye concentration in the solid gain volume increases to ~1.9 mM.

TABLE 4.4
$\partial n / \partial T$ in DDP and PN Matrices[a]

Matrix[a] (%)	λ (nm)	$\partial n / \partial T$ (×10⁻⁴)	References
DDP	593.93	1.4 ± 0.2	[54][b]
PN 0 w/w SiO₂	632.82	−1.0317	[17][c]
PN 30 w/w SiO₂	632.82	−0.8840	[17][c]
PN 50 w/w SiO₂	632.82	−0.6484	[17][c]

Source: Adapted from Duarte, F. J. and R. O. James, *Opt Lett.* 28: 2088–2090, 2003.

[a] P stands for the PMMA polymer and N stands for nanoparticle.

[b] Refractive measurement at minimum deviation.

[c] The polymer was not dye doped, and the measurement was performed in a thin-film configuration using a prism-coupling device.

immediately becomes of interest is the lower beam divergences observed in the emission from the DDPN lasers relative to the DDP laser. In fact, the beam divergence from the DDPN (30% w/w SiO₂) $\Delta\theta \approx 1.9$ mrad is found to be ~ 1.3 times the diffraction limit, which is slightly lower than the beam divergence reported for a single-transverse-mode single-longitudinal-mode narrow-linewidth DDP laser exhibiting ~ 1.5 times the diffraction limit [7]. It should be noted that the laser efficiencies observed in these experiments are in line with previously reported laser efficiencies for DDP lasers, which are in the 40%–64% range [7,8].

The lower beam divergence observed with these DDPN lasers is a direct consequence of the improved $\partial n / \partial T$ values (see Table 4.4), which enable faster dissipation of heat introduced by the pump laser and the thermal losses inherent in the excitation process [34,53].

Note: Occasionally in the literature, some confusion is expressed in regard to the optical homogeneity of solid-state dye gain media. To summarize: This was a problem in early dye-doped organic–inorganic gain media, as identified in [7,16]. However, it was clearly established that DDP gain media, in the form of MPMMA, were perfectly homogeneous, thus enabling the generation of single-transverse-mode beams and narrow-linewidth emission [7]. It was further established that DDPN gain media were also optically homogeneous, thus enabling the emission of single-transverse-mode beams [17].

4.4.2 NARROW-LINEWIDTH LASER EMISSION

Further experiments with the rhodamine DDPN (30% w/w SiO₂) gain media consisted of the excitation of a double-prism grating oscillator comprising a 3000 lines/mm grating deployed in Littrow configuration. These experiments were performed using a frequency-doubled Nd:YAG laser at $\lambda \approx 532$nm, and yielded single-transverse-mode emission with fairly good beam quality while using a pump energy density of more than 1 J/cm² [54]. In a nonoptimized cavity configuration, lasing was restricted to double-longitudinal-mode oscillation at linewidths in the $1.5 \leq \Delta v \leq 2.0$ GHz range at $\lambda \approx 580$ nm, while illuminating about 80% of the available diffractive width at the Littrow grating.

4.4.3 Optical Ruggedness of Dye-Doped Polymer Gain Media

An important and attractive characteristic of both DDP and DDPN gain media is their optical ruggedness. This means that following irradiation at energy densities above bleaching levels, at $\rho \approx 0.7$ J/cm², "the gain media tends to heal itself in a few days" [55]. More specifically, while using a particular dye-doped MPMMA matrix, at a dye concentration of 0.5 mM, in 1994, photobleaching was induced, and the resulting dye-bleaching energy threshold density measured just below $\rho \approx 1.0$ J/cm² [56]. The very same matrix was used in high-coherence single-longitudinal-mode oscillator experiments yielding laser linewidths in the $350 \leq \Delta v \leq 375$ MHz range 3–5 years later [35,57], with the gain medium exhibiting a total absence of any signs of photobleaching. Indeed, in one of these papers, it is stated that "we have used the same gain media in various experiments for a period in excess of three years without signs of degradation" [57]. The one caveat here is that these experiments were performed at low prfs, that is, ~1 Hz.

This "self-healing" phenomenon at the gain matrix caused by the apparent migration of active laser dye species into bleached, or vacated, polymer volumes has also been observed in dye-doped fibers, and has attracted the attention of researchers interested in what has become known as *reversible photodegradation* [58].

4.5 INTERFEROMETRIC INTERPRETATION

Besides the improvement in thermal characteristics resulting in a decrease in the magnitude of $\partial n / \partial T$, which leads to lower observed laser beam divergences, the most remarkable effect observed in these DDPN matrices is the absence of beam inhomogeneities. As explained earlier, this is observed in both the passive transmission of laser beams and active laser emission.

In 1995, Duarte and Pope [16] had suggested that the origin of beam inhomogeneities in organic–inorganic gain media was the presence of internal interference created by randomized diffraction grating structures formed by minute refractive index differentials. The same effect could be present in DDPN gain media. For instance, the measured refractive index for rhodamine 6G dye-doped MPMMA is $n(\lambda) = 1.4953$, while the refractive index for fused silica is $n(\lambda) = 1.4582$, thus giving $\Delta n \approx 0.0371$. Both these measurements were performed at $\lambda = 593.93$ nm and $T = 297$ K [59].

To study the internal structure of the DDPN gain media, it was decided to obtain electron microscope nanographs of the matrices. To this effect, a JEOL electron microscope (JEM 100CX II), with a resolution of approximately 0.3 nm, was used [50]. The gain media studied were rhodamine 6G DDPN and coumarin 500 DDPN, both at 30% w/w SiO_2. The nanographs from these gain media are shown in Figures 4.10 and 4.11.

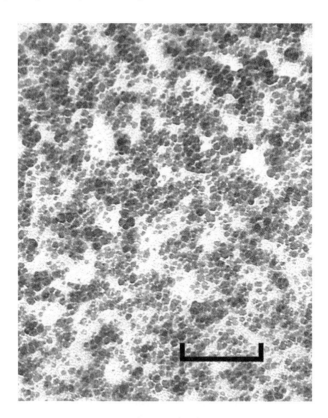

FIGURE 4.10 Nanograph of the rhodamine 6G DDPN solid-state laser matrix. The indicated distance represents 200 nm. (Reproduced from Duarte, F. J. and R. O. James, Spatial structure of dye-doped polymer nanoparticle laser media, *Appl. Opt.* 43: 4088–4090, 2004. With permission from Optical Society of America.)

In the nanographs, it became clearly evident that there are areas of higher concentration of nanoparticles and areas that show a near-total absence of nanoparticles. These are the areas corresponding to the DDP. This morphology may be related to a nondeterministic volumetric transmission grating, as previously suggested [16]. By looking at a cross section of the two-dimensional planes observed in the nanographs, it is possible to estimate the average dimensions of slits and isles for DDPN matrices. These results are summarized in Table 4.5.

The effect of a diffractive morphology on the propagation of coherent emission, either deterministic or randomized, can be analyzed via three-dimensional, two-dimensional, or one-dimensional generalized N-slit interference equations [60,61]. For a detailed description of the interferometric approach, the reader is referred to Chapter 10. In essence, the generalized one-dimensional interferometric equation is given by [60,61]

$$|\langle x|s\rangle|^2 = \sum_{j=1}^{N} \Psi(r_j)^2 + 2\sum_{j=1}^{N} \Psi(r_j) \left(\sum_{m=j+1}^{N} \Psi(r_m)\cos(\Omega_m - \Omega_j) \right) \qquad (4.10)$$

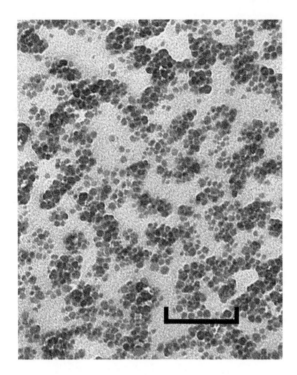

FIGURE 4.11   Nanograph of the coumarin 500 DDPN solid-state laser medium. The indicated distance represents 200 nm. (Reproduced from Duarte, F. J. and R. O. James, Spatial structure of dye-doped polymer nanoparticle laser media, *Appl. Opt.* 43: 4088–4090, 2004. With permission from Optical Society of America.)

TABLE 4.5

Dimensions of the Silicate Structure in the DDPN Matrices

Matrix	Slit Dimensions (nm)	Island Dimensions (nm)
Rhodamine 6G DDPN	49 ± 29	42 ± 31
Coumarin 500 DDPN	55 ± 32	57 ± 41

Source: From Duarte, F. J. and R. O. James, *Appl Opt.* 43: 4088–4090, 2004.

---

where the cosine term is the origin of the well-known diffraction equation [62,63]:

$$d_j(\sin\Theta_j \pm \sin\Phi_j) = m\lambda \qquad (4.11)$$

where:

- λ is the wavelength
- m the diffraction order
- d_j the sum of the dimensions of the slits plus the islands
- Θ_j the angle of incidence
- Φ_j the angle of diffraction.

Using the results from Table 4.4, it can be established that for the rhodamine 6G DDPN matrix, $d_j \approx 91$ nm, which, for $\lambda \approx 580$ nm and $m = 1$, yields

$$\frac{m\lambda}{d_j} \approx 6.37 \tag{4.12}$$

For the coumarin 500 DDPN matrix, $d_j \approx 99$ nm, $\lambda \approx 510$ nm, and $m = 1$, we have

$$\frac{m\lambda}{d_j} \approx 5.15 \tag{4.13}$$

Now, from Equation 4.2, the condition for diffraction is satisfied only with

$$\frac{m\lambda}{d_j} < 2 \tag{4.14}$$

which for the rhodamine 6G DPN matrix, at $\lambda \approx 580$ nm, imposes $d_j > 290$ nm. For the coumarin 500 DDPN matrix, $\lambda \approx 510$ nm, the imposition for diffraction becomes $d_j > 255$ nm.

Clearly, the size of the nanoparticles, coupled with their relatively uniform distribution in the DDP space, does not meet the conditions for diffraction, resulting in the absence of internal interference and the spatial homogeneity of the laser emission beam.

4.6 INVISIBILITY OF NANOPARTICLE DISTRIBUTIONS IN THE VISIBLE ELECTROMAGNETIC SPECTRUM

The subject of invisibility has evoked interest in the scientific literature for a long time [64–66]. In this particular section, we are interested in invisibility qualities in the microscopic domain that may lead to new and useful optics materials and devices. Here, invisibility is simply defined as the ability to avoid detection when illuminated in the visible portion of the electromagnetic spectrum. In particular, we are interested in transparency and in the ability to conserve the spatial characteristics of the electromagnetic field on transmission in an optical gain medium.

Two of the prominent tools to accomplish the invisibility of the internal structure of a gain medium are index of refraction matching and the use of extraordinarily small optical features. Organic–inorganic gain matrices exhibiting a very slight mismatch of refractive indices can produce inhomogeneities in a propagating beam of coherent electromagnetic radiation in the visible spectrum. This is certainly true for the refractive index difference of $\Delta n \approx 0.04$ between DDP and silica.

Given the existing mismatch in refractive indices, the improvement of $\partial n / \partial T$ characteristics, using silica, in a dye-doped solid-state organic–inorganic gain matrix requires a secondary approach. In our experience, this secondary approach can be provided by silica nanoparticles, provided they are uniformly distributed.

In the previous section, it was shown that albeit the nanoparticles do form clusters, these clusters are sufficiently small and assume a spatial distribution that is not favorable to the attainment of the conditions necessary for internal diffraction. Hence, no diffraction means no distortion of the propagating electromagnetic field, thus no detection, and therefore *invisibility*. This was accomplished for distributions of SiO_2 nanoparticles in laser DDP matrices, as clearly shown in Figures 4.8 and 4.9 [17].

Albeit these experiments successfully demonstrated invisible distributions of nanoparticles, with a different refractive index from the host matrix, there is one further avenue to enhance the effect if necessary. This approach consists of augmenting the invisibility of the nanoparticles themselves. As explained by Duarte and James [51] and James et al. [67], using the teachings of Kerker [64–66], the conditions for invisibility can be improved if core–shell nanoparticles are used rather than traditional nanoparticles.

For a composite core–shell nanoparticle, it can be shown that for the condition

$$n_{shell} < n_{polymer} < n_{core} \tag{4.15}$$

there is a particular ratio of shell core radius (a) to the coated composite radius (b) (see Figure 4.11) at which the scattering produced by the coated nanoparticle will be at a minimum, so that the haze will be very low and hence transparency will be very high [67]. This condition of particle invisibility is found at the ratio [64–67]:

$$\frac{b}{a} = \left(\frac{(2f_2^2 + 1)(f_2^2 - f_1^2)}{(f_2^2 - 1)(f_1^2 + 2f_2^2)} \right)^{1/3} \tag{4.17}$$

where $f_1 = n_{core}/n_{polymer}$ and $f_2 = n_{shell}/n_{polymer}$.

In [51,67], an example is described using composite nanoparticles with a shell of silica and a core of ZnS dispersed in a polymer such as PMMA. This type of composite particle has a positive, higher value of $\partial n/\partial T$ than pure silica, to offset the

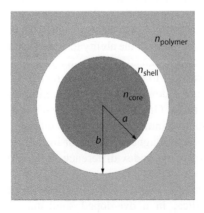

FIGURE 4.12 Simple diagram of a core–shell particle depicting the various parameters included in Equation 4.17.

negative $\partial n / \partial T$ of the (PMMA) polymer matrix. This *core–shell* or *cloaked* particle in, say, PMMA provides an inorganic–organic hybrid with a lower-magnitude $\partial n / \partial T$ than would be possible with silica particles alone in PMMA. For detailed discussions of the electromagnetic theory applicable to core–shell particles dispersed in a polymeric matrix, readers are referred to additional papers published over the past two decades [68–70].

4.7 APPLICATIONS FOR DDPN GAIN MEDIA

Tunable dye lasers, in the liquid state, created a renaissance and golden age for a plethora of scientific applications [71]. Prominent among these applications were laser spectroscopy [72] and laser medicine [73]. For an updated review of tunable dye laser applications in medicine, please see Chapter 8 [74]. Some of these applications have also become applications for solid-state dye lasers and solid-state dye laser gain media. Here, a brief survey of these application fields is provided, and a number of areas are suggested in which tunable solid-state dye lasers using DDPN gain media could be useful.

4.7.1 LASER SPECTROSCOPY

Laser spectroscopy is a vast and diverse field. Among the numerous books and reviews on laser spectroscopy, the following are particularly informative: Demtröder [75], Radziemski et al. [74], and Orr et al. [76]. In particular, here we refer to pulse laser spectroscopy using narrow-linewidth tunable lasers. This class of solid-state tunable narrow-linewidth lasers is described in Section 4.2. These lasers yield tunable radiation in low divergence single-transverse-mode beams, in the spatial domain, and single-longitudinal-mode emission, in the spectral domain. In particular, these organic solid-state lasers are capable of delivering linewidths in the $350 \leq \Delta v \leq 650$ MHz range. Laser linewidths in this range are ideally suited for the excitation of single vibrational–rotational levels in small molecules, such as I_2, and for selective excitation in a wide range of atomic species, as explained further in Chapter 11 [77,78].

Albeit narrow-linewidth multiple-prism grating laser oscillators incorporating DDPN gain media have yet to be demonstrated, knowing what we already know about the spatial homogeneity of the emission with these media in the broadband domain, it is likely that the performance achieved with DDP media will be matched. The added advantage will be reduced beam divergence and the opportunity to operate at slightly higher prfs. In summary, narrow-linewidth tunable laser oscillators using solid-state DDP, or DDPN, gain media offer researchers involved in exploratory studies an attractive, optically rugged, and inexpensive alternative for performing laser spectroscopy.

4.7.2 LASER MEDICINE

Dye lasers have an ample and rich history of applications in medicine. Relevant reviews and collective works include Goldman [73,79] and Costela et al. [74]. Here, we provide a very brief overview of the main applications of dye lasers to medicine, and then mention more specific areas applicable to solid-state dye lasers that could also be applicable to solid-state dye lasers incorporating DDPN gain media.

Some of the more emblematic applications of tunable dye lasers in medicine include photodynamic therapy (PDT) [73,79], dermatology [73,79], urology [80], lithotripsy [80], and treatment of vascular lesions [81,82]. A dual tunable laser system for PDT, in which the excitation laser is also used as a diagnostic tool, was described by Duarte [83]. This concept is directly applicable to solid-state dye laser systems and other solid-state systems [84].

Solid-state pulsed dye lasers are applicable to many of the applications in which liquid dye lasers have been put to use. These applications include dermatology, lithotripsy, and urolithiasis. Further, solid-state dye lasers have already been applied in thrombolysis [85]. DDPN gain media offer improved thermal characteristics, good beam quality, and reduced beam divergence. Hence, it is reasonable to expect good performance, in these medical applications, using tunable lasers incorporating DDPN gain media.

As indicated previously, the continuous tuning range demonstrated with narrow-linewidth solid-state dye lasers, powered by rhodamine 6G DDP gain media, is 565–610 nm [36]. The continuous tuning range demonstrated by dye lasers powered by rhodamine 6G DDPN gain media, is 567–603 nm [17]. These tuning ranges overlap and cover wavelength regions of interest for ophthalmology, dermatology, and biomedical diagnostics, for which all-solid-state lasers are also being developed [86,87]. The particular cited wavelength regions are $573 \le \lambda \le 580$ nm [86] and $\lambda \approx 588$ nm [87], which are positioned near the maximum efficiency of the solid-state dye laser tuning ranges [17,36].

For the abovementioned medical applications, the wavelength coverage available from dye-doped solid-state gain media is optimal. The excellent performance of tunable narrow-linewidth laser oscillators based on DDP gain media has been amply documented [36–38]. Also, for applications needing relatively large pulse energies at low prfs, these lasers are quite viable since they can be engineered to deliver tens to hundreds of millijoules per pulse. The limitations in the area of average power can be partly minimized using DDPN gain media and other physical approaches. These physical approaches include rotation of the gain medium [88], which would have to be performed on a gain medium previously dimensioned using high-precision automated machinery, using high-precision turning techniques to minimize measurable frequency jitter and microvariations in the beam profile. An extensive review of the nanobiophotonic properties of hybrid organic–inorganic materials is given by Escribano et al. [89].

4.7.3 LASER DEVELOPMENT AND NONLINEAR OPTICS

In addition to the laser development outlined in this chapter, mainly focused on laser efficiency and tunable narrow-linewidth emission, organic DDPN gain media are also compatible with the technology of organic solid-state integrated laser devices [90]. An additional area of research interest in DDPN gain media can be found in the development and engineering of microcavity solid-state organic lasers [30,31]. Furthermore, these particular composite nanostructured organic–inorganic materials have also become important to researchers studying fundamental local field effects in nonlinear optics [91, 92].

REFERENCES

1. Sorokin, P. P. and J. R. Lankard, Stimulated emission observed from an organic dye, chloroaluminum phthalocyanine, *IBM J. Res. Dev.* 10: 162–163, 1966.
2. Schäfer, F. P., W. Schmidt, and J. Volze, Organic dye solution laser, *Appl. Phys. Lett.* 9: 306–309, 1966.
3. Soffer, B. H. and B. B. McFarland, Continuously tunable narrow-band organic dye lasers, *Appl. Phys. Lett.* 10: 266, 1967.
4. Peterson, O. G. and B. B. Snavely, Stimulated emission from flashlamp-excited organic dyes in polymethyl methacrylate, *Appl. Phys. Lett.* 12: 238–240, 1968.
5. Pacheco, D. P., H. R. Aldag, I. Itzkan, and P. S. Rostler, A solid-state flashlamp-pumped dye laser employing polymer hosts. In F. J. Duarte (Ed.), *Proceedings of the International Conference on Lasers '87*, pp. 330–337, STS, McLean, VA, 1988.
6. Dunn, B., J. D. Mackenzie, J. I. Zink, and O. M. Stafsudd, Solid-state tunable lasers based on dye-doped sol-gel materials, *Proc. SPIE* 1328: 174–182, 1990.
7. Duarte, F. J., Solid-state multiple-prism grating dye-laser oscillators, *Appl. Opt.* 33: 3857–3860, 1994.
8. Maslyukov, A., S. Solokov, M. Kaivola, K. Nyholm, and S. Popov, Solid-state dye laser with modified poly(methyl methacrylate)-doped active elements, *Appl. Opt.* 34: 1516–1518, 1995.
9. Duarte, F. J., J. J. Ehrlich, W. E. Davenport, T. S. Taylor, and J. C. McDonald, A new tunable dye laser oscillator: Preliminary report. In C. P. Wang (Ed.), *Proceedings of the International Conference on Lasers '92*, pp. 293–296, STS, McLean, VA, 1993.
10. Hermes, R. E., T. H. Allik, S. Chandra, and J. A. Hutchinson, High-efficiency pyrromethene doped solid-state dye lasers, *Appl. Phys. Lett.* 63: 877–879, 1993.
11. Rahn, M. D. and T. A. King, Comparison of laser performance of dye molecules in sol-gel, polycom, ormosil, and poly(methyl methacrylate) host media, *Appl. Opt.* 34: 8260–8271, 1995.
12. Costela, A., I. García-Moreno, and R. Sastre, Handbook of advanced electronic and photonic materials. In H. S. Nalwa (Ed.), *Liquid Crystals, Display and Laser Materials*, pp. 161–208, Academic, New York, 2001.
13. Costela, A., I. García-Moreno, and R. Sastre, Polymeric solid-state dye lasers: Recent developments, *Phys. Chem. Chem. Phys.* 5: 4745–4763, 2003.
14. Duarte, F. J. and A. Costela, Dye lasers. In B. D. Guenther (Ed.), *Encyclopedia of Modern Optics*, pp. 400–414, Elsevier, New York, 2004.
15. Costela, A., I. García-Moreno, and R. Sastre, Solid-state dye lasers. In F. J. Duarte (Ed.), *Tunable Laser Applications*, 2nd edn, Chapter 3, Taylor & Francis, New York, 2008.
16. Duarte, F. J. and E. J. A. Pope, Optical inhomogeneities in sol-gel derived ORMOSILS and nanocomposites, *Ceram. Transac.* 55: 267–273, 1995.
17. Duarte, F. J. and R. O. James, Tunable solid-state lasers incorporating dye-doped, polymer-nanoparticle gain media, *Opt. Lett.* 28: 2088–2090, 2003.
18. Costela, A., I. García-Moreno, D. del Agua, O. García, and R. Sastre, Silicon-containing organic matrices as host for highly photostable solid-state dye lasers, *Appl. Phys. Lett.* 85: 2160–2162, 2004.
19. Costela, A., I. García-Moreno, D. del Agua, O. García, and R. Sastre, Highly photostable solid-state dye lasers based on silicon-modified organic matrices, *J. Appl. Phys.* 101: 073110, 2007.

20. Costela, A., I. García-Moreno, D. del Agua, O. García, and R. Sastre, Solid-state dye lasers: New materials based on silicon, *Opt. J.* 1: 1–6, 2007.

21. Yang, Y., C. Ye, W. H. Ni, K. Y. Wong, M. Q. Wang, D. Lo, and G. D. Qian, Amplified spontaneous emission from infrared dye-doped zirconia-organically modified silicate thin film waveguides, *J. Sol-Gel Sci. Tech.* 44: 53–57, 2007.

22. Yang, Y., J. Zou, H. Rong, G. D. Qian, Z. Y. Wang, and M. Q. Wand, Influence of various coumarin dyes on the laser performance of laser dyes co-doped into ORMOSILs, *Appl. Phys. B* 86: 309–313, 2007.

23. Yang, Y., G. Lin, J. Zou, Z. Wang, M. Wang, and G. Qian, Enhanced laser performances based on energy transfer of multi-dyes co-doped solid media, *Opt. Commun.* 277: 138–142, 2007.

24. Sathiyamoorthy, K., C. Vijayan, and M. P. Kothiyal, Design of a low power optical limiter based on a new nanocomposite material incorporating silica-encapsulated phthalocyanine in nafion, *J. Phys. D: Appl. Phys.* 40: 6121–6128, 2007.

25. Nedumpara, R. J., K. Geetha, V. J. Dann, C. P. G. Vallabham, V. P. N. Nampoori, and P. Rhadakrishnan, Light amplification in dye-doped polymer films, *J. Opt. A: Pure Appl. Opt.* 9: 174–179, 2007.

26. Ray, A. K., S. Kumar, N. V. Mayekar, S. Sinha, S. Kundu, S. Chattopadhyay, and K. Dasgupta, Role of the stimulated-emission rate in the photostability of solid-state dye lasers, *Appl. Opt.* 44: 7814–7822, 2005.

27. Bañuelos Prieto, J., F. López Arbeloa, O. García, and I. López Arbeloa, Photophysics and lasing correlation of pyrromethene 567 dye in crosslinked polymeric networks, *J. Lumines.* 126: 833–837, 2007.

28. Maier, G. V., T. N. Kopilova, V. A. Svetlichnyi, V. M. Podgaetskii, S. M. Dolotov, O. V. Ponomareva, A. E. Monich, et al., Active polymer fibres doped with organic dyes: Generation and amplification of coherent radiation, *Quantum Electron.* 37: 53–59, 2007.

29. Zhu, J., Y. Zhang, G. Dong, Y. Guo, and L. Guo, Single-layer dichromated gelatin material for Lippmann color holography, *Opt. Commun.* 241: 17–21, 2004.

30. Popov, S., S. Ricciardi, A. T. Friberg, and S. Sergeyev, Mode suppression in a microcavity solid-state dye laser, *J. Euro. Opt. Soc.* 2: 07023, 2007.

31. Ricciardi, S., S. Popov, A. Friberg, and S. Sergeyev, Thermally induced wavelength tunability of microcavity solid-state dye lasers, *Opt. Express* 15: 12971–12978, 2007.

32. López Arbeloa, F., J. Bañuelos, V. Martínez, T. Arbeloa, and T. López Arbeloa, Structural, photophysical and lasing properties of pyrromethene dyes, *Int. Rev. Phys. Chem.* 24: 339–371, 2005.

33. Duarte, F. J., Narrow-linewidth pulsed dye laser oscillators. In F. J. Duarte and L. W. Hillman (Eds), *Dye Laser Principles*, Chapter 4, Academic, New York, 1990.

34. Duarte, F. J., *Tunable Laser Optics*, Elsevier Academic, New York, 2003.

35. Duarte, F. J., Solid-state dispersive dye laser oscillator: Very compact cavity, *Opt. Commun.* 117: 480–484, 1995.

36. Duarte, F. J., Multiple-prism near-grazing-incidence grating solid-state dye laser oscillator, *Opt. Laser Technol.* 29: 513–516, 1997.

37. Duarte, F. J., Multiple-prism grating solid-state dye laser oscillator: Optimized architecture, *Appl. Opt.* 38: 6347–6349, 1999.

38. Duarte, F. J., T. S. Taylor, A. Costela, I. García-Moreno, and R. Sastre, Long-pulse narrow-linewidth dispersive solid-state dye laser oscillator, *Appl. Opt.* 37: 3987–3989, 1998.

39. Duarte, F. J., Technology of pulsed dye lasers. In F. J. Duarte and L. W. Hillman (Eds), *Dye Laser Principles*, Chapter 5, Academic, New York, 1990.

40. Duarte, F. J., Multiple-return-pass beam divergence and the linewidth equation, *Appl. Opt.* 40: 3038–3041, 2001.

41. Dirac, P. A. M., *The Principles of Quantum Mechanics*, 4th edn, Oxford University, London, 1978.
42. Wadsworth, W. J., I. T. McKinnie, A. D. Woolhous, and T. G. Haskell, Efficient distributed feedback solid state dye laser with a dynamic grating, *Appl. Phys. B* 69: 163–165, 1999.
43. Zhu, X-L., S-K. Lam, and D. Lo, Distributed-feedback dye-doped solgel silicate lasers, *Appl. Opt.* 39: 3104–3107, 2000.
44. Oki, Y., S. Miyamoto, M. Tanaka, D. Zuo, and M. Maeda, Long lifetime and high repetition rate operation from distributed feedback plastic waveguided dye lasers, *Opt. Commun.* 214: 277–283, 2002.
45. Oki., Y., K. Aso, D. Zuo, N. J. Vasa, and M. Maeda, Wide-wavelength range operation of a distributed-feedback dye laser with a plastic waveguide, *Jpn. J. Appl. Phys.* 41: 6370–6374, 2002.
46. Oki, Y., M. Tanaka, Y. Ogawa, H. Watanabe, and M. Maeda, Development of quasi-end-fired waveguide plastic dye laser, *IEEE J. Quantum Elect.* 42: 389–396, 2006.
47. Duarte, F. J., Light emitting diode-pumped laser and method of excitation, U.S. Patent 2005/0083986A1, 2005.
48. Duarte, F. J., R. O. James, and L. A. Rowley, Dye-doped polymer nanoparticle gain medium for use in a laser, U.S. Patent 2004/0120373 A1, 2004.
49. Duarte, F. J. and R. O. James, Dye-doped polymer-nanoparticle gain media for tunable solid-state lasers, *Mat. Res. Soc. Symp. Proc.* 817: 201–206, 2004.
50. Duarte, F. J. and R. O. James, Spatial structure of dye-doped polymer nanoparticle laser media, *Appl. Opt.* 43: 4088–4090, 2004.
51. Duarte, F. J. and R. O. James, Dye-doped polymer nanoparticle gain medium, U.S. Patent 688862 B2, 2005.
52. Popov, S., Influence of pump repetition rate on dye photostability in a solid-state dye laser with a polymeric gain medium, *Pure Appl. Opt.* 7: 1379–1388, 1998.
53. Hillman, L. W., Laser dynamics. In F. J. Duarte and L. W. Hillman (Eds), *Dye Laser Principles*, Chapter 2, Academic, New York, 1990.
54. Duarte, F. J., Tunable organic dye lasers: Physics and technology of high-performance liquid and solid-state narrow-linewidth oscillators, *Prog. Quant. Electron.* 36: 29–50, 2012.
55. Duarte, F. J. and R. O. James, Tunable lasers based on dye-doped polymer gain media incorporating homogeneous distributions of functional nanoparticles. In F. J. Duarte (Ed.), *Tunable Laser Applications*, 2nd edn, Chapter 4, CRC Press, New York, 2009.
56. Duarte, F. J., Solid-state multiple-prism grating dye-laser oscillators, *Appl. Opt.* 33: 3857–3860, 1994.
57. Duarte, F. J., Multiple-prism near-grazing-incidence grating solid-state dye laser oscillator, *Opt. Laser Technol.* 29: 513–516, 1997.
58. Anderson, B. and M. G. Kusyk, Generalizing the correlated chromophore domain model of reversible photodegradation to include the effects of an applied electric field, *Phys. Rev. E* 89: 032601, 2014.
59. Duarte, F. J, A. Costela, I. García-Moreno, and R. Sastre, Measurements of $\partial n/\partial T$ in solid-state dye-laser gain media, *Appl. Opt.* 39: 6522–6523, 2000.
60. Duarte, F. J., Dispersive dye lasers. In F. J. Duarte (Ed.), *High Power Dye Lasers*, Chapter 2, Springer, Berlin, 1991.
61. Duarte, F. J., On a generalized interference equation and interferometric measurements, *Opt. Commun.* 103: 8–14, 1993.
62. Duarte, F. J., *Tunable Laser Optics*, Chapter 2, Elsevier Academic, New York, 2003.
63. Duarte, F. J., Interference, diffraction, and refraction, via Dirac's notation, *Am. J. Phys.* 65: 637–640, 1997.
64. Kerker, M., *The Scattering of Light and Other Electromagnetic Radiation*, Academic, New York, 1969.

65. Kerker, M., Invisible bodies, *J. Opt. Soc. Am.* 65: 376–379, 1975.
66. Kerker, M., Elastic scattering, absorption, and surface-enhanced raman scattering by concentric spheres comprised of a metallic and a dielectric region, *Phys. Rev. B* 26: 4052–4063, 1982.
67. James, R. O., L. A. Rowley, D. F. Hurley, and J. Border, Core shell nanocomposite optical plastic article, U.S. Patent 7091271 B2, 2006.
68. Salib, S. K., Interaction of monochromatic waves and bodies of nonhomogeneous morphology. In F. J. Duarte (Ed.), *Proceedings of the International Conference on Lasers '87*, pp. 810–825, STS, McLean, VA, 1988.
69. Alu, A. and N. Engheta, Achieving transparency with plasmonic and metamaterials coatings, *Phys. Rev. E.* 72: 016623, 2005.
70. Small, A., S. Hong, and D. Pine, Scattering properties of core-shell particles in plastic matrices, *J. Poly. Sci. B: Poly. Phys.* 43: 3534–3548, 2005.
71. F. J. Duarte, J. A. Paisner, and A. Penzkofer, Dye lasers: Introduction by the feature editors, *Appl. Opt.* 31: 6977–6978, 1992.
72. Demtröder, W., *Laser Spectroscopy*, 3rd edn, Springer, Berlin, 2003.
73. Goldman, L., Dye lasers in medicine. In F. J. Duarte and L. W. Hillman (Eds), *Dye Laser Principles*, Chapter 10, Academic, New York, 1990.
74. Costela, A., I. García-Moreno, and R. Sastre, Medical applications of dye lasers. In F. J. Duarte (Ed.), *Tunable Laser Applications*, 2nd edn, Chapter 7, CRC Press, New York, 2008.
75. Demtröder, W., *Laser Spectroscopy*, Springer, Berlin, 2003.
76. Orr, B. J, R. T. White, and Y. He, Spectroscopic applications of tunable optical parametric oscillators. In F. J. Duarte (Ed.), *Tunable Laser Applications*, 3rd edn, Chapter 2, CRC Press, New York, 2015.
77. Radziemski, L. J., R. W. Solarz, and J. A. Paisner (Eds), *Laser Spectroscopy and Its Applications*, Marcel Dekker, New York, 1987.
78. Duarte, F. J. and D. R. Foster, Lasers, dye. In T. G. Brown et al. (Eds), *The Optics Encyclopedia*, Volume 2, pp. 1065–1096, Wiley-VCH, Weinheim, 2004.
79. Goldman, L. (Ed.), *Laser Non-Surgical Medicine*, Technomic, Lancaster, PA, 1991.
80. Floratos, D. L. and J. J. M. C. H. de la Rosette, Lasers in urology, *BJU Int.* 84: 204–211, 1999.
81. Clement, R. M., M. N. Kiernan, and K. Donne, Treatment of vascular lesions, U.S. Patent 6398801 B1, 2002.
82. Clement, R. M. and M. N. Kiernan, Reduction of vascular blemishes by selective thermolysis, U.S. Patent 6605083 B2, 2003.
83. Duarte, F. J., Two-laser therapy and diagnosis device, Patent EP 0284330 A1, 1988.
84. Duarte, F. J., Liquid and solid-state tunable organic dye lasers for medical applications. In H. Jelinkova (Ed.), *Lasers for Medical Applications*, Chapter 7, Woodhead, Oxford, 2013.
85. Aldag, H. R., Solid-state dye laser for medical applications, *Proc. SPIE* 2115: 184–189, 1994.
86. Sinha, S., C. Langrock, M. J. F. Digonnet, M. F. Fejer, and R. L. Byer, Efficient yellow-light generation by frequency doubling a narrow-linewidth 1150 nm ytterbium fiber oscillator, *Opt. Lett.* 31: 347–349, 2006.
87. Dekker. P., H. M. Pask, and J. A. Piper, All-solid-state 704 mW continuous-wave yellow source based on an intracavity, frequency doubled crystalline Raman laser, *Opt. Lett.* 32: 1114–1116, 2007.
88. Abedin, K. M., M. Alvarez, A. Costela, I. García-Moreno, O. García, R. Sastre, D. W. Coutts, et al., 10 kHz repetition rate solid-state dye laser pumped by diode-pumped solid-state laser, *Opt. Commun.* 218: 359–363, 2003.

89. Escribano, P., B. Julian-Lopez, J. Planelles-Aragó, E. Cordoncillo, B. Viana, and C. Sanchez, Photonic and nanobiophotonic properties of luminescent lanthanide-doped hybrid organic–inorganic materials, *J. Mater. Chem.* 18: 23–40, 2008.
90. Grivas, C. and Pollnau, M., Organic solid-state integrated amplifiers and lasers, *Lasers Photon. Rev.* 6: 419–462, 2012.
91. Dolgaleva, K., R. W. Boyd, and P. W. Milonni, The effects of local fields on laser gain for layered and Maxwell Garnett composite materials, *J. Opt. A: Pure Appl. Opt.* 11: 024002, 2009.
92. Dolgaleva, K. and R. W. Boyd, Local field effects in nanostructured photonic materials, *Adv. Opt. Photon.* 4: 1–77, 2012.

5 Broadly Tunable External-Cavity Semiconductor Lasers

F. J. Duarte

CONTENTS

5.1   INTRODUCTION

Tunable semiconductor lasers have become widely used in a plethora of applications, including communications, imaging, interferometry, medicine, metrology, remote sensing, and spectroscopy. The advantages of tunable semiconductor lasers include direct electrical excitation, compactness, low cost, and simplicity.

The approximate spectral coverage available from tunable semiconductor lasers is outlined in Table 5.1. The most widely used tunable external-cavity semiconductor (ECS) lasers belong to the III–V classification and employ GaAlInP, GaAlAs, and InGaAsP semiconductors. The single-device continuous-wave (CW) power levels offered by these lasers, at room temperature, can range from a few milliwatts to hundreds of milliwatts. Continuous-wave powers in the multiwatt regime are available from diode arrays. In general, these lasers are of the index-guided class with buried heterostructures.

TABLE 5.1

Approximate Wavelength Ranges
Covered by Broadly Tunable
Semiconductor Lasers

Semiconductor Type	Spectral Range (nm)
II–VI and III–V	$395 \leq \lambda \leq 410$
AlGaInP/GaAs	$660 \leq \lambda \leq 680$
GaAlAs	$815 \leq \lambda \leq 825$
InGaAsP/InP	$1255 \leq \lambda \leq 1335$
InGaAsP/InP	$1530 \leq \lambda \leq 1570$

Semiconductor lasers are intrinsically tunable, and the extent of their tunability depends on the characteristics of the energy bandgap, operating temperature, and current density. The basic physics and technological features are explained and discussed in several books and review articles [1–9].

In this chapter, attention is focused on semiconductor tunable lasers operating at room temperature. Further, the scope of this coverage is limited to tunable semiconductor lasers using external dispersive or frequency-selective optics. This approach is justified because the use of external cavities has been shown to be a very effective avenue to frequency tuning in semiconductor lasers. In addition, the use of external cavities provides access to a variety of optical architectures and well-proven, frequency-selective techniques previously developed for other tunable lasers, such as dye lasers, crystalline solid-state lasers, and gas lasers [10–13].

The discussion on frequency selectivity and tuning in this chapter is applicable in general to any emission wavelength, type of semiconductor, and physical dimensions of the active medium. Albeit most of the open literature information concerning tunable ECS lasers refers to III–V semiconductors, the event of II–VI type lasers [14–16] has also led to the introduction of ECS lasers powered by II–VI gain media, which will be mentioned in Section 5.6.

5.2   DISPERSIVE OSCILLATOR CAVITIES

In general, tunable ECS lasers employ cavity configurations developed for earlier tunable lasers, such as the dye laser. A detailed survey and classification of dispersive cavity configurations for organic dye lasers, both in liquid and in solid state, are given in [10–13]. In this regard, it should also be mentioned that cavity configurations developed for dye lasers have been specifically adopted to provide narrow-linewidth tunable emission in various other types of lasers, including high-power gas lasers [12,17] and semiconductor lasers [18].

Although, in principle, the concepts and configurations can be easily adopted from the domain of the dye laser for application to ECS lasers, it must be observed that there are some intrinsic differences to be considered. First, dye lasers are high-gain pulsed lasers, and the boundary between the gain medium and the cavity can easily be made to yield low reflectivity by the use of antireflection (AR) coating or the use of windows at an angle relative to the plane of propagation. On the other hand, semiconductor and diode lasers of interest emit in the cw regime, and the high refractive indices available naturally yield high reflectivity at the gain boundaries. Because the achievement of extended-wavelength tuning ranges, in ECS lasers, depends on the availability of facets with low reflectivities, the use of AR coatings becomes very important. In this regard, AR coatings are particularly relevant to the semiconductor facet adjacent to the tuning optics.

Given the existence of facets with intrinsic high reflectivity, the concepts of *open* and *closed* cavities assume a heightened degree of importance. This can be further emphasized by the need to protect the cavity from unwanted external optical feedback.

An *open* cavity is configured to couple the output beam via the reflection losses of one of its optical or dispersive components [12,13]. In a *closed* cavity, the output beam exits the cavity through an output-coupler mirror. The advantage of closed-cavity over open-cavity laser configurations was highlighted by Duarte and Piper [19,20]. In those works, it was demonstrated that in the case of high-gain tunable laser oscillators, closed-cavity configurations yielded considerable reductions in optical noise emission, or amplified spontaneous emission (ASE), and prevented unwanted optical feedback with optical elements external to the cavity.

Here, a survey is given of open and closed dispersive cavities. In the case of open cavities, it is assumed that one of the facets of the semiconductor is AR coated, whereas in the case of the closed-cavity configuration, both output facets are required to be AR coated.

Open cavities are illustrated in Figure 5.1 and include a simple mirror-grating cavity with intracavity étalon(s), where the output is coupled via an intracavity beam splitter [21]. Additional open-cavity configurations include the single-prism grating cavity [22] and the pure grazing-incidence cavity [23], illustrated in Figure 5.1b and c. In the case of the single-prism cavity, the output is coupled via the reflection losses of the prism, and in the case of the grazing-incidence cavity, the output emission exits the cavity via the reflection losses at the grating. This latter cavity can also be used in a closed configuration [24]. Grazing-incidence grating cavities are also known in the literature as Littman cavities.

Closed cavities are depicted in Figure 5.2. These include simple mirror-grating cavities in which the output emission is coupled via the output mirror [25]. These cavities can also incorporate one or more étalons, as shown in Figure 5.2b.

Additional closed-cavity configurations include the multiple-prism grating cavities [12,13,26], as illustrated in Figure 5.3. The multiple-prism Littrow (MPL) grating laser cavities use multiple-prism beam expanders in a variety of configurations [13] deployed to either augment or neutralize the intracavity multiple-prism dispersion (see Figure 5.3a and b). The basic principle of these cavities is to expand the intracavity beam to totally illuminate the dispersion grating deployed in a Littrow configuration. An alternative design that yields higher dispersions but lower efficiencies is the hybrid multiple-prism near grazing-incidence (HMPGI) grating laser cavity, depicted in Figure 5.4. However, HMPGI grating cavities can be more compact than MPL grating resonators and more efficient than pure grazing-incidence

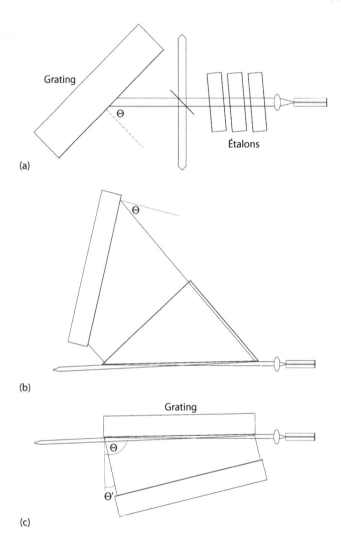

FIGURE 5.1 Open-cavity configurations. (a) Mirror-grating cavity incorporating intracavity étalons, (b) single-prism grating cavity, and (c) grazing-incidence grating cavity.

configurations used in a closed-cavity mode. Extensive discussions on the performance and design of these cavities are provided in [12,13]. It should be noted that an alternative abbreviation for MPL grating cavities is MPLG cavities. Also, HMPGI grating cavities can be abbreviated to MPNGIG cavities. The early use of the word *hybrid* was meant to convey the dual use of prismatic beam expansion with gratings deployed in a near grazing-incidence configuration. Here, we continue using MPL and HMPGI to maintain consistency with early literature on the subject. In general, both configurations can be referred to as multiple-prism grating cavities.

Closed cavities in tunable semiconductor lasers were introduced early by Fleming and Mooradian [25] in a simple mirror-grating configuration. Also, the emission

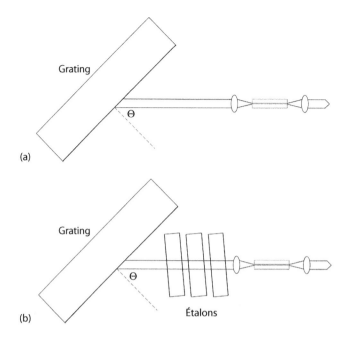

FIGURE 5.2 Closed-cavity configurations. (a) Mirror-grating cavity and (b) mirror-grating cavity incorporating intracavity étalons. Note that the use of an independent output-coupler mirror is not a common practice because most designs use a high-reflectivity coating at the external facet of the semiconductor.

characteristic advantages of these configurations have been clearly highlighted in cavities comprising generalized multiple-prism grating tuning configurations [18,26–28] since the early 1990s. However, for a long time they were the exception rather than the rule. Slowly, they have become more prevalent, and today they take center stage in tunable cavity configurations controlled by microelectromechanical systems (MEMS) [29].

In the following discussion, tunable ECS lasers using dispersive optics for frequency selectivity are referred to as dispersive ECS lasers or, more appropriately, as dispersive ECS laser oscillators.

5.2.1 OPTIMIZED DISPERSIVE OSCILLATOR CAVITIES

In addition to the open-cavity noise and vulnerability to external coupling, designers of tunable semiconductor lasers have to deal with the asymmetry of the emission beam, which is often not circular but ellipsoidal. These problems can be eliminated in an integrated approach to dispersive cavity configurations applicable to ESC lasers. Prior to further details, the reader might wish to consult the literature on optimized solid-state organic tunable lasers, where the basics are discussed [13,30].

A variant of a closed cavity was introduced by Laurila et al. [31]. These authors coupled the output from a transmission grating deployed in a Littrow configuration. An improvement on this approach can also solve the problem of beam asymmetry.

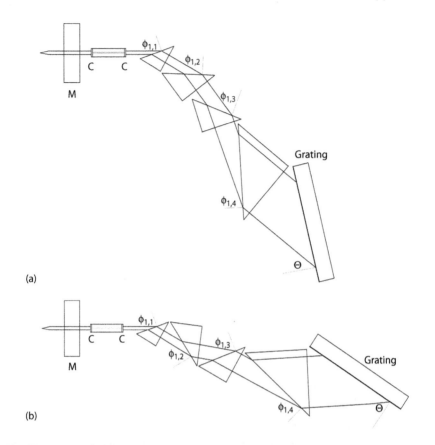

(a)

(b)

FIGURE 5.3 Multiple-prism Littrow (MPL) grating oscillator configurations. (a) The multiple-prism expander can be deployed in a (+, +, +, −) configuration or (b) a (+, −, +, −) configuration. (Adapted from Duarte, F. J., *Laser Focus World* 29(2), 103–109, 1993. With permission from PennWell.)

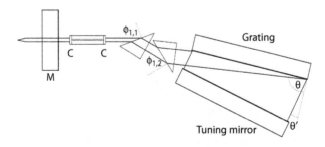

FIGURE 5.4 Hybrid multiple-prism near grazing-incidence (HMPGI) grating laser oscillator. (Adapted from Duarte, F. J., *Laser Focus World* 29(2), 103–109, 1993. With permission from PennWell.)

This is caused by the fact that the cross-sectional area of the gain region, perpendicular to the plane of propagation, is often asymmetrical, with dimensions such as 4×1 μm [32]. In this regard, deployment of the gain region to yield a vertically elongated ellipsoidal beam can be compensated by using prismatic, or multiple-prism, beam expansion parallel to the plane of propagation to yield a circular beam. Such cavity architecture was disclosed in [13].

A disadvantage with this concept, however, is that tuning performed by the angular rotation of the grating might lead to minor deviation of the output beam due to refraction induced at the substrate of the transmission diffraction grating. A better solution is to use beam expansion at both ends of the cavity, that is, beam expansion as previously disclosed to illuminate the tuning grating and reduced beam expansion at the output coupler end to correct for beam asymmetry. The architecture of such an oscillator is shown in Figure 5.5.

A reflection diffraction grating, in a Littrow configuration, is illuminated by an expanded intracavity beam to induce narrow-linewidth oscillation. At the output end of the cavity, moderate beam expansion is used to produce a near-circular beam profile. Albeit more elaborate, this double multiple-prism architecture eliminates the possible beam deviations induced by substrate refraction while coupling the beam via a transmission grating. It should also be noted that in this configuration, the beam expansion illuminating the grating can be as large as necessary to illuminate the whole useful diffractive length of the grating. This circular-beam concept also applies to HMPGI grating configurations. Collimators, adjacent to the gain media, are identified by the letter C, while the output-coupler mirrors are labeled M.

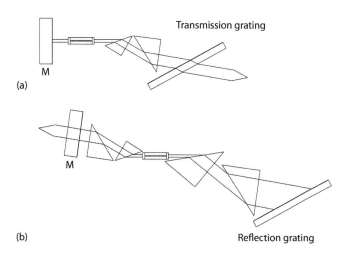

FIGURE 5.5 Circular-beam close-cavity MPL grating laser oscillators. (a) Moderate beam expansion corrects the asymmetry of the vertically elongated beam and enhances the dispersion of the cavity via the expanded illumination of a transmission diffraction grating. (b) Beam expansion at both ends of the cavity.

5.3 OPTICAL THEORY

In this section, theoretical elements applicable to the characterization of intracavity beam propagation are summarized. In this regard, the topics considered are interference and diffraction, intracavity dispersion, and beam propagation matrices.

5.3.1 INTERFERENCE AND DIFFRACTION

Application of the Dirac method [33] to describe the interaction of electromagnetic radiation and a generalized grating leads to the probability equation [11,34]:

$$|\langle x \mid s \rangle|^2 = \sum_{j=1}^{N} \Psi(r_j)^2 + 2 \sum_{j=1}^{N} \Psi(r_j) \left(\sum_{m=j+1}^{N} \Psi(r_m) \cos(\Omega_m - \Omega_j) \right) \qquad (5.1)$$

In this generalized, one-dimensional, interferometric equation, $\langle x \mid s \rangle$ represents the probability amplitude for propagation from a source (s) to a screen (x) via a grating (j) comprised of N slits. The wave functions $\Psi(r_j)$ and $\Psi(r_m)$ are "ordinary wave functions of classical optics" as described by Dirac [33], and $\cos(\Omega_m - \Omega_j)$ is the interference term. The interference term, in conjunction with the geometry of the N-slit interferometer, gives origin to the diffraction grating equation [34,35]:

$$m\lambda = d(\sin\Theta \pm \sin\Theta') \qquad (5.2)$$

where:
   λ is the wavelength
   m is the order of diffraction
   d is the number of slits (or grooves) per meter
   Θ is the angle of incidence
   Θ' is the angle of diffraction

For further details, see Chapter 10.

Equation 5.1 can be used to describe diffraction by a single wide slit, or aperture, which can be represented by a large number of small slits [34,35]. Hence, the transverse-mode structure characteristic of the given physical dimensions of a gain region can also be established.

As the cross-sectional areas (transverse to the optical axis) of the gain regions in semiconductor lasers are very small, the corresponding Fresnel numbers are also small. An example where these calculations can be useful concerns relatively wide cross-sectional areas. For instance, Voumard [36] discusses the use of a GaAlAs laser in an external cavity at $\lambda \approx 874$ nm. The dimensions of the gain region are given as 285 μm long and 20 μm wide [36]. Hence, the Fresnel number along the 20 μm width becomes $N \approx 0.4$, and the beam profile along this dimension can be calculated using Equation 5.1. At this stage, it should be emphasized that for a true external cavity, where the facets of the diode are AR coated, the beam profile will be determined by the emission wavelength, the dimensions of the aperture, and the *overall length* of the cavity.

5.3.2   INTRACAVITY DISPERSION

Dispersive cavities incorporate prisms, gratings, or combinations of these optical elements. Indeed, multiple-prism grating assemblies are widely used in narrow-linewidth tunable dye, gas, and solid-state lasers [10,13]. Here, the basic dispersion formulas of gratings, multiple prisms, and multiple-prism grating assemblies are given.

By differentiating Equation 5.2, the dispersion of a grating mirror combination (see Figure 5.4) can be shown [37] to be given by

$$\nabla_\lambda \Theta_G = \frac{2(\sin\Theta \pm \sin\Theta')}{\lambda \cos\Theta} \tag{5.3}$$

or in its equivalent form,

$$\nabla_\lambda \Theta_G = \frac{2m}{d\cos\Theta} \tag{5.4}$$

where:
$\nabla_\lambda = (\partial/\partial\lambda)$
   m is the diffraction order
   d is the groove spacing

For a grating in a Littrow configuration (Figure 5.3), the dispersion is given [38] by

$$\nabla_\lambda \Theta_G = \frac{2\tan\Theta}{\lambda} \tag{5.5}$$

Note that in the Littrow configuration, the angle of incidence Θ equals the angle of diffraction Θ', that is, $\Theta = \Theta'$.

For a multiple-prism grating assembly, the double-pass dispersion is given by [10,11]

$$\nabla_\lambda \Theta = M \nabla_\lambda \Theta_G + \nabla_\lambda \Phi_P \tag{5.6}$$

where the generalized multiple-prism dispersion for a prismatic assembly composed of r prisms (see Figure 5.7) is given, for a single pass, by [10,11,13,39]

$$\nabla_\lambda \phi_{2,m} = \mathcal{H}_{2,m} \nabla_\lambda n_m \pm (k_{1,m} k_{2,m})^{-1} \left(\mathcal{H}_{1,m} \nabla_\lambda n_m \pm \nabla_\lambda \phi_{2,m-1} \right) \tag{5.7}$$

the double-pass version of which, in a more explicit notation, becomes [10,40]

$$\nabla_\lambda \Phi_P = 2M \sum_{m=1}^{r} (\pm 1) \mathcal{H}_{1,m} \left(\prod_{j=m}^{r} k_{1,j} \prod_{j=m}^{r} k_{2,j} \right)^{-1} \nabla_\lambda n_m$$
$$+ 2 \sum_{m=1}^{r} (\pm 1) \mathcal{H}_{2,m} \left(\prod_{j=1}^{m} k_{1,j} \prod_{j=1}^{m} k_{2,j} \right) \nabla_\lambda n_m \tag{5.8}$$

where

$$\mathcal{H}_{1,m} = \frac{\tan \phi_{1,m}}{n_m} \tag{5.9}$$

$$\mathcal{H}_{2,m} = \frac{\tan \phi_{2,m}}{n_m} \tag{5.10}$$

and

$$M = \prod_{j=1}^{r} k_{1,j} \prod_{j=1}^{r} k_{2,j} \tag{5.11}$$

is the total beam expansion. Also,

$$k_{1,j} = \frac{\cos \psi_{1,j}}{\cos \phi_{1,j}} \tag{5.12}$$

$$k_{2,j} = \frac{\cos \phi_{2,j}}{\cos \psi_{2,j}} \tag{5.13}$$

where $\phi_{1,j}$ and $\phi_{2,j}$ are the incidence and exit angles, respectively, at each individual prism. The angles of incidence and refraction are related by the positive law of refraction, also known as Snell's law:

$$\sin \phi_{1,j} = n(\lambda) \sin \psi_{1,j} \tag{5.14}$$

As a matter of generality, the reader should be aware that the diffraction grating equation (Equation 5.2), Snell's law, and the reflection law can be derived, in sequence, from the generalized interference equation (Equation 5.1) (Figure 5.6) [13,35].

Here, it should be noted that the single-pass dispersion provided by the multiple-prism beam expander can be obtained by multiplying $\nabla_\lambda \Phi_P$ by $1/2\ M$ (this is given in Chapter 10).

For the case of a multiple-prism expander composed of right-angled prisms (see Figure 5.3) designed for orthogonal beam exit, that is, $\phi_{2,m} = \psi_{2,m} = 0$, Equation 5.8 reduces to

$$\nabla_\lambda \Phi_P = 2M \sum_{m=1}^{r} (\pm 1) \mathcal{H}_{1,m} \left(\prod_{j=m}^{r} k_{1,j} \right)^{-1} \nabla_\lambda n_m \tag{5.15}$$

where the beam-expansion factor now assumes the simpler form:

$$M = \prod_{j=1}^{r} k_{1,j} \tag{5.16}$$

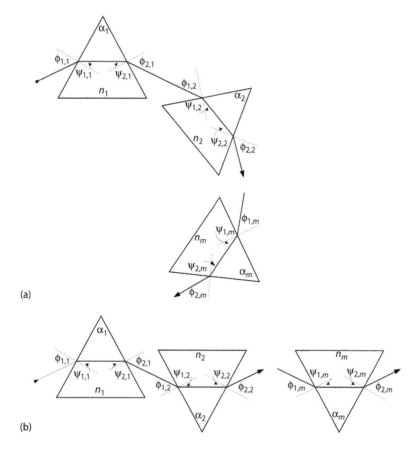

(a)

(b)

FIGURE 5.6 Generalized multiple-prism array deployed in (a) an additive configurational and (b) a compensating configuration. (Adapted with permission from Duarte, F. J. and J. A. Piper, *Am. J. Phys.* 51: 1132–1134, 1983. Copyright 1983, American Association of Physics Teachers.)

Further, if the angle of incidence at each prism is the Brewster angle, and all prisms are made of the same material, then Equation 5.15 can be succinctly expressed as [10]

$$\nabla_\lambda \Phi_P = 2 \sum_{m=1}^{r} (\pm 1) n^{m-1} \nabla_\lambda n \tag{5.17}$$

and the beam-expansion coefficient becomes

$$M = n^r \tag{5.18}$$

In Equations 5.8, 5.15, and 5.17, the (± 1) factor designates whether the prism is being deployed in a positive (+) or a compensating (−) configuration. Explicit examples of the closed-form analytical design of dispersionless, that is, $\nabla_\lambda \Theta_P = 0$, multiple-prism beam expanders are given in [11] and [40].

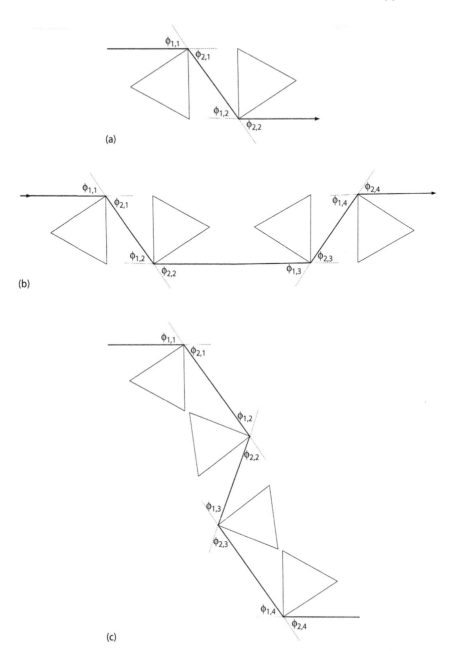

FIGURE 5.7 Multiple-prism pulse compressors configured by (a) two compensating prisms; (b) two compensating pairs of prisms; and (c) two groups of prisms deployed in an additive configuration, with each group deployed in a compensating configuration relative to the other.

Dispersionless multiple-prism beam expanders are useful for relinquishing control of the tuning characteristics of the oscillator exclusively to the grating. Further, as discussed by Duarte [10], the design of a multiple-prism beam expander with $\nabla_\lambda \Theta_P = 0$ reduces intracavity beam deviations due to thermal changes, because [10]

$$\nabla_T \phi_{2,r} = \nabla_\lambda \phi_{2,r} \left(\nabla_\lambda n \right)^{-1} \nabla_T n \qquad (5.19)$$

where

$$\nabla_\lambda \phi_{2,r} = (2M)^{-1} \nabla_\lambda \Phi_P \qquad (5.20)$$

This can be quite important in the design and construction of stabilized dispersive oscillators.

5.3.3 Dispersion Theory of Multiple-Prism Pulse Compression

For pulse-compression calculations in lasers incorporating multiple-prism compressors, using

$$\nabla_n \phi_{2,m} = \nabla_\lambda \phi_{2,m} (\nabla_\lambda n_m)^{-1} \qquad (5.21)$$

the single-pass dispersion, that is, Equation 5.7, can be restated as [39,41–43]

$$\nabla_n \phi_{2,m} = \mathcal{H}_{2,m} + (\mathcal{M})^{-1} \left(\mathcal{H}_{1,m} \pm \nabla_n \phi_{2,(m-1)} \right) \qquad (5.22)$$

where the identity

$$k_{1,m}^{-1} k_{2,m}^{-1} = (\mathcal{M})^{-1} \qquad (5.23)$$

applies. Hence, the complete second derivative of the refraction angle, or first derivative of the dispersion $\nabla_\lambda \phi_{2,m}$, is given by [41]

$$\nabla_n^2 \phi_{2,m} = \nabla_n \mathcal{H}_{2,m}$$
$$+ (\nabla_n \mathcal{M}^{-1})(\mathcal{H}_{1,m} \pm \nabla_n \phi_{2,(m-1)}) \qquad (5.24)$$
$$+ (\mathcal{M}^{-1})(\nabla_n \mathcal{H}_{1,m} \pm \nabla_n^2 \phi_{2,(m-1)})$$

The second derivative of the dispersion $\nabla\lambda \phi_{2,m}$ is given by [43]

$$\nabla_n^3 \phi_{2,m} = \nabla_n^2 \mathcal{H}_{2,m}$$
$$+ (\nabla_n^2 \mathcal{M}^{-1})(\mathcal{H}_{1,m} \pm \nabla_n \phi_{2,(m-1)})$$
$$+ 2(\nabla_n \mathcal{M}^{-1})(\nabla_n \mathcal{H}_{1,m} \pm \nabla_n^2 \phi_{2,(m-1)}) \qquad (5.25)$$
$$+ (\mathcal{M}^{-1})(\nabla_n^2 \mathcal{H}_{1,m} \pm \nabla_n^3 \phi_{2,(m-1)})$$

and the third derivative of the dispersion $\nabla_\lambda \phi_{2,m}$ is given by [43]

$$\nabla_n^4 \phi_{2,m} = \nabla_n^3 \mathcal{H}_{2,m}$$

$$+ (\nabla_n^3 \mathcal{M}^{-1})(\mathcal{H}_{1,m} \pm \nabla_n \phi_{2,(m-1)})$$

$$+ 3(\nabla_n^2 \mathcal{M}^{-1})(\nabla_n \mathcal{H}_{1,m} \pm \nabla_n^2 \phi_{2,(m-1)}) \qquad (5.26)$$

$$+ 3(\nabla_n \mathcal{M}^{-1})(\nabla_n^2 \mathcal{H}_{1,m} \pm \nabla_n^3 \phi_{2,(m-1)})$$

$$+ (\mathcal{M}^{-1})(\nabla_n^3 \mathcal{H}_{1,m} \pm \nabla_n^4 \phi_{2,(m-1)})$$

Higher-phase derivatives are given explicitly by Duarte [43–45]. A generalized equation allowing the computation of Nth order derivatives is also available [44,45].

For the case of a multiple-prism compressor designed for collinear beam transmission and composed of two balanced compensating pairs [46], as illustrated in Figure 5.7b, the derivatives reduce to [39,41]

$$\nabla_n \phi_{2,1} = \nabla_n \phi_{2,3} = 2 \qquad (5.27)$$

$$\nabla_n \phi_{2,2} = \nabla_n \phi_{2,2} = 0 \qquad (5.28)$$

$$\nabla_n^2 \phi_{2,1} = \nabla_n^2 \phi_{2,3} = 4n - \frac{2}{n^3} \qquad (5.29)$$

$$\nabla_n^2 \phi_{2,2} = \nabla_n^2 \phi_{2,4} = 0 \qquad (5.30)$$

for minimum deviation and incidence of the Brewster angle. Certainly, for incidence at angles other than the Brewster angle, Equations 5.22 and 5.24 must be used. Duarte [42] has calculated the $\nabla_n \phi_{2,m}$ and $\nabla_n^2 \phi_{2,m}$ values for incidence at angles other than the Brewster angle.

The $\nabla_n \phi_{2,m}$ and $\nabla_n^2 \phi_{2,m}$ values are used in calculating the second derivative of the optical path length $\nabla_\lambda^2 P$ through the prisms. In turn, $\nabla_\lambda^2 P$ is used to determine the value of the group-velocity-dispersion (GVD) constant [46].

Recent progress in prismatic, and multiple-prism, pulse compression includes the detailed experimental measurements of Osvay et al. [47,48], where the effect of beam deviations was studied. These researchers studied, using an 18 fs Ti:sapphire laser, the effect of slight beam deviations on a double-prism pulse compressor [47]. They obtained excellent agreement between theoretical predictions, using Equations 5.22 and 5.24, and measurements. These studies were extended to include the effect of noncompensated angular dispersion on the temporal lengthening of femtosecond pulses [48]. A more recent study of pulse compression with prism pairs was reported by Arissian and Diels [49]. An excellent review on the subject of prismatic pulse compression is given by Diels and Rudolph [50].

The transmission efficiency of intracavity multiple prisms can be estimated using expressions for the cumulative reflection losses at the incidence face of the *m*th prism [11]:

$$L_{1,m} = L_{2,m-1} + (1 - L_{2,m-1})R_{1,m} \tag{5.31}$$

and the cumulative reflection losses at the exit face:

$$L_{2,m} = L_{1,m} + (1 - L_{1,m})R_{2,m} \tag{5.32}$$

Here, $R_{1,m}$ and $R_{2,m}$ are the individual losses occurring at the *m*th prism and are given by the well-known Fresnel equations [13,37] for *s*- and *p*-polarization. At this stage, it should be mentioned that the oscillators incorporating multiple-prism grating assemblies emit radiation that is strongly polarized parallel to the plane of incidence (or propagation) [10,45]. The issue of polarization in multiple-prism grating oscillators is discussed in [10].

5.3.4 RAY TRANSFER MATRICES

Ray transfer matrices of interest include the well-known *ABCD* matrices and the more complete 3×3 and 4×4 matrix systems. For an introduction to ray transfer matrix systems, the reader should consult [11,51–54]. Ray transfer matrices of interest to ECS lasers include those incorporating parameters to describe intracavity space, lenses, grating, mirrors, and prisms. In this regard, ray transfer matrices describing the overall optical system can be derived and used in describing the profile of the intracavity beam [55] via

$$w(x) = w_0 \left[A^2 + \left(\frac{B}{L_\mathcal{R}} \right)^2 \right]^{1/2} \tag{5.33}$$

where w_0 is the beam waist at the output facet of the gain region and

$$L_\mathcal{R} = \frac{\pi w^2}{\lambda} \tag{5.34}$$

is the Rayleigh length.

The *ABCD* ray transfer matrix for a length of space L with a refractive index n is given by [52]

$$\begin{pmatrix} A & B \\ C & D \end{pmatrix} = \begin{pmatrix} 1 & L/n \\ 0 & 1 \end{pmatrix} \tag{5.35}$$

For a lens, the ray transfer matrix is given by

$$\begin{pmatrix} A & B \\ C & D \end{pmatrix} = \begin{pmatrix} 1 & 0 \\ C & 1 \end{pmatrix} \tag{5.36}$$

where $C=-1/f$ for a convex lens and $C=1/|f|$ for a concave lens. Here, f is the focal length of the lens. For a flat grating, the corresponding matrix is given by [56]

$$\begin{pmatrix} A & B \\ C & D \end{pmatrix} = \begin{pmatrix} \dfrac{\cos\Theta'}{\cos\Theta} & 0 \\ 0 & \dfrac{\cos\Theta}{\cos\Theta'} \end{pmatrix} \tag{5.37}$$

where Θ and Θ' are the corresponding angles of incidence and diffraction, respectively. For a grating deployed in the Littrow configuration, the A and D components in Equation 5.37 become unity; that is, $A=D=1$ and $C=B=0$, which also applies to a mirror used at normal incidence [11].

For a generalized multiple-prism beam expander array, the ray transfer matrix is [11,57]

$$\begin{pmatrix} A & B \\ C & D \end{pmatrix} = \begin{pmatrix} M & B \\ 0 & 1/M \end{pmatrix} \tag{5.38}$$

where:
  M is defined by Equation 5.11
  B term is given in Chapter 13

For an étalon, the ray transfer matrix can be written as [11]

$$\begin{pmatrix} A & B \\ C & D \end{pmatrix} = \begin{pmatrix} 1 & (l_e/n)(\cos\phi_e/\cos\psi_e)^2 \\ 0 & 1 \end{pmatrix} \tag{5.39}$$

where l_e is the thickness of the étalon. Here, $A=D=1$, ϕ_e is the angle of incidence, and ψ_e is the corresponding angle of refraction. At normal incidence, Equation 5.39 takes the form of Equation 5.35.

A more elaborate system of matrices is the 4×4 matrices, which can take the form of [54]

$$\begin{pmatrix} A & B & D & E \\ C & D & 0 & F \\ G & H & 1 & I \\ 0 & 0 & 0 & 1 \end{pmatrix} \tag{5.40}$$

In these matrices, the four upper-left components are the usual $ABCD$ terms. Other components are related to quantities representing well-known optical phenomena. This has been particularly well established for the F term of the 4×4 matrix system describing a generalized multiple-prism array, where the single-pass dispersion can be written as [57]

$$\frac{1}{2M}\nabla_\lambda \Phi_P = F \nabla_\lambda v \tag{5.41}$$

For further discussions on matrices applicable to pulse compression and intracavity dispersion, the reader should consult [57,58].

The usefulness of the matrix approach, via terms such as A and B, becomes self-evident when determining the beam profile, using Equation 5.33, and the beam divergence through equations such as [11]

$$\Delta\theta = \frac{\lambda}{\pi w}\left[1+\left(\frac{L_R}{B}\right)^2+\left(\frac{L_R A}{B}\right)^2\right]^{1/2} \tag{5.42}$$

Here, it should be mentioned that in well-designed cavities, the terms in parentheses become very small, so that the laser beam divergence tends to its *diffraction limit*, whose origin can be traced to the uncertainty principle [13,45,59]:

$$\Delta\theta \approx \frac{\lambda}{\pi w} \tag{5.43}$$

5.3.5 LASER LINEWIDTH

The dispersive linewidth of a multiple-prism grating oscillator is given by [60]

$$\Delta\lambda_D = \Delta\theta\left(RM\nabla_\lambda \Theta_G + R\nabla_\lambda \Phi_P\right)^{-1} \tag{5.44}$$

where:
   $\Delta\theta$ is the beam divergence
   R is the number of intracavity return passes
   $\nabla_\lambda \Theta_G$ is the grating dispersion in either Littrow or near grazing-incidence configuration
   $\nabla_\lambda \Phi_P$ is the single return-pass, or double-pass, dispersion of the multiple-prism expander

In practice,

$$M\nabla_\lambda \Theta_G \gg \left|\nabla_\lambda \Phi_P\right| \tag{5.45}$$

Furthermore, the design of dispersionless multiple-prism beam expanders $\nabla_\lambda \Phi_P \approx 0$ [45,61], so that the intracavity dispersion is completely dominated by the diffraction grating characteristics and

$$\Delta\lambda_D \approx \Delta\theta\left(RM\nabla_\lambda \Theta_G\right)^{-1} \tag{5.46}$$

In high-gain pulsed lasers, such as laser-pumped dispersive dye laser oscillators, Equation 5.44 provides an upper limit for the observed linewidth [10]. For high-performance narrow-linewidth high-gain dispersive laser oscillators yielding pulses $\Delta t \leq 5$ ns [30], it has been found that $R \approx 3$ [61]. Furthermore, for long-pulse dispersive dye laser oscillators, the measured linewidth can be significantly narrower than the estimate provided by Equation 5.44 [10,62]. For instance, for a laser yielding pulses $\Delta t \approx 200$ ns in duration, the estimated double-pass dispersive linewidth is $\Delta v \approx 2.16$ GHz, whereas the measured linewidth is $\Delta v \leq 360$ MHz [63]. This measured laser linewidth corresponds to double-longitudinal-mode oscillation, that is, $\Delta v \leq c/2 L_c$, where L_c is the length of the cavity. Indeed, if oscillation is restricted to a single longitudinal mode by reducing the cavity length, for example, the measured Δv can be even narrower. In this regard, Equation 5.44 can be used to estimate the dispersion necessary to restrict oscillation to a single longitudinal mode. Further insight into the multiple-pass linewidth-narrowing mechanism is given in [60,61].

Since ECS lasers are used mainly in the cw regime, the measured linewidth will always be much narrower than the calculated dispersive linewidth. In this regard, the main objective is to design a dispersive cavity that would be characterized by $\Delta v_D \leq c/2L_c$. The linewidth of a single longitudinal mode in an ECS laser can be characterized using the expression given by Harrison and Mooradian [64]. In this equation, the modified Schalow–Townes linewidth is multiplied by a factor having the length of the external cavity at the denominator. The equation is [64]

$$\Delta v = \Delta v_m \left(\frac{n_g L}{n_g L + L_c} \right)^2 \left(\frac{g_c}{g} \right)^2 \tag{5.47}$$

where:
Δv_m is the modified Schawlow–Townes linewidth
n_g is the ratio of c to the group velocity
L is the length of the semiconductor active region

The g factors are related to the gains at threshold with (g_c) and without (g) the external cavity [64]. From Equation 5.47, it is apparent that single-longitudinal-mode linewidths can be reduced substantially by the use of external cavities with appropriate lengths in the centimeter range.

Gavrilovic et al. [65], using external dispersive cavities, have noted that at higher power levels, the emission changes from single-longitudinal-mode oscillation to multimode oscillation. Under these conditions, the linewidth of the emission is limited to the dispersive linewidth at 4 GHz [65]. Duarte [27] has estimated the single-return pass dispersive linewidths ($R = 1$) for MPL and HMPGI oscillators to be $\Delta v \approx 2.37$ GHz and $\Delta v \approx 1.2$ GHz, respectively. These calculations were made for an index-guided diode laser emitting at 670 nm for fully illuminated 2400 lines/mm diffraction gratings. In both cases, the cavity lengths are about 10 cm, yielding a free spectral range of $FSR \approx 1.5$ GHz [27]. An additional example is described and discussed in Chapter 10.

An important point to make here is that given the narrow dimensions of the gain waveguide in semiconductor lasers (usually a few micrometers), the emission tends to be a single transverse mode with very large divergence. Therefore, for very compact cavity designs, the diffraction grating can be illuminated directly once the intracavity beam is collimated, in the absence of further beam expansion. This explains the proliferation of very simple open cavities with gratings in a Littrow configuration illuminated with "expanded beams" from an intracavity collimating lens system. A generic system of this class is illustrated in Figure 5.8.

In Figure 5.9, a compact, closed-cavity, multiple-prism grating oscillator is illustrated. The double-prism expander is composed of two identical prisms providing identical beam expansion, so that the overall beam expansion is $M \approx 3.43$. In this type of design, the beam exits the prisms at a near-orthogonal angle, thus reducing the likelihood of backreflections.

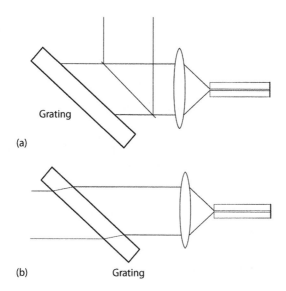

FIGURE 5.8 Compact open-cavity tunable narrow-linewidth diode laser configured with a Littrow grating cavity. The cavity length in this type of cavity is often less than 10 mm, which corresponds to a free spectral range greater than 15 GHz. (a) Here, the output is coupled via a beam splitter. (b) Alternative closed-cavity configuration employing a transmission Littrow grating as the output coupler.

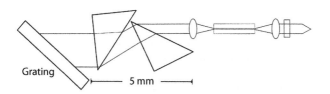

FIGURE 5.9 Compact closed-cavity tunable narrow-linewidth diode laser configured with a double-prism expander and a Littrow grating cavity. The cavity length in this type of cavity is often less than 10 mm, which corresponds to a free spectral range greater than 15 GHz.

5.3.6 Wavelength Tuning

Semiconductor lasers are inherently tunable devices, whose tuning characteristics depend on the energy gap of the semiconductor. Additional parameters affecting the emission wavelength are current density and temperature. Cassidy et al. [66] provide a good survey of temperature-dependent wavelength tuning in semiconductor lasers emitting in a single longitudinal mode. The widest tuning ranges quoted are 1485–1527 nm in an InGaAsP laser for $\Delta v = 120°C$, and 752–781 nm in a GaAlAs laser for $\Delta v = 135°C$ [66].

Here, optical means of wavelength tuning are considered, and the temperature is assumed to remain constant to maintain the fixed optical path length of the semiconductor. Using grating tuning, one of the largest wavelength tuning ranges reported has been 80 nm in InGaAsP/InP by Zorabedian [26].

Tuning in a grating is straightforward and follows the diffraction grating equation

$$m\lambda = d(\sin\Theta \pm \sin\Theta')$$

For a grating in a Littrow configuration, this reduces to

$$m\lambda = 2d\sin\Theta \tag{5.48}$$

Thus, the simple angular rotation of the grating relative to the optical axis of the cavity yields a change in the resonant wavelength. Note that for multiple-prism grating cavities incorporating multiple-prism expanders in the compensating mode, the wavelength characteristics of the cavity depend exclusively on the grating.

In the case of a prismatic cavity with prisms deployed in an additive configuration (see Figure 5.6), the exit angle of the mth prism as a function of wavelength is given by [10]

$$\phi_{2,m} = \arcsin\left\{ n(\lambda)\sin\left[\alpha_m - \arcsin\left(\frac{\sin\phi_{1,m}}{n(\lambda)} \right) \right] \right\} \tag{5.49}$$

where α_m is the apex angle of the mth prism, and the incidence angle of this prism $(\phi_{1,m})$ is related geometrically to the exit angles of the previous prism $\phi_{2,m-1}$.

For an étalon, the tuning properties can be characterized by the simple equation [37]:

$$m_e\lambda = 2n(\lambda)d_e\cos\psi_e \tag{5.50}$$

where:

m_e is an integer
d_e is the distance between the reflective surfaces
ψ_e is related to the angle of incidence by $\sin\phi_e = n(\lambda)\sin\psi_e$

The dispersion of an étalon is given by [10]

$$\nabla_\lambda\phi_e = \left(\frac{\sin\psi_e}{\cos\phi_e} \right)\nabla_\lambda n + n\left(\frac{\cos\psi_e}{\cos\phi_e} \right)\nabla_\lambda\psi_e \tag{5.51}$$

where

$$\nabla_\lambda \psi_e = \frac{1}{\tan \psi_e} \left(\frac{1}{n} \nabla_\lambda n - \frac{1}{\lambda} \right) \tag{5.52}$$

Wavelength tuning by rotating the grating, by rotating a mirror at the end of a prismatic array, or by rotating an étalon does not guarantee smooth wavelength tuning over an extensive wavelength range. This is due to the change in the optical cavity length as λ is varied.

To achieve synchronous wavelength tuning, a number of schemes have been implemented [67–69]. Synchronous wavelength tuning in semiconductor lasers is described by Favre et al. [70], who report a 15 nm tuning range at 1260 nm, and by Trutna and Stokes [71], who achieved a 17 nm tuning range at 1310 nm. Synchronous tuning in MEMS-driven cavities is described in the next section.

5.3.7 TUNING MINIATURE MEMS-DRIVEN CAVITIES

Miniature semiconductor laser cavities tuned by MEMS are of intense interest for various applications, including telecommunications. Here, three wavelength tuning approaches compatible with MEMS techniques are described, albeit the techniques are applicable in general. These are the basic grating tuning technique, the synchronous tuning technique, and the longitudinal tuning technique based on changing the cavity length of the resonator.

From Heisenberg's uncertainty principle [33]:

$$\Delta x \Delta p \approx h \tag{5.53}$$

it follows that [13]

$$\Delta \lambda \approx \frac{\lambda^2}{\Delta x} \tag{5.54}$$

which can also be expressed as

$$\delta \lambda \approx \frac{\lambda^2}{\Delta x} \tag{5.55}$$

where $\delta \lambda$ can be related to the separation, in the wavelength domain, between two longitudinal modes, and Δx can be related to twice the cavity optical length ($\Delta x = 2L$) of the resonator, or oscillator, generating the emission. This version of Heisenberg's uncertainty principle indicates that whenever the wavelength changes, that is, whenever the oscillator is tuned, the *FSR* or the spacing between modes ($\delta \lambda$) also changes. This phenomenon can lead to abrupt jumps in the wavelength domain as a cavity is tuned, and is known in the literature as *mode-hopping*. The solution to this phenomenon is given by Equation 5.53, which shows that to maintain $\delta \lambda$ fixed, as λ changes, Δx must vary accordingly. To be consistent with the terminology of the literature, it is useful to also write Equation 5.55 as the familiar identity:

$$FSR \approx \frac{\lambda^2}{2L} \tag{5.56}$$

To maintain $\delta\lambda$, or the *FSR*, constant, we need to define a central value for this quantity $(\delta\lambda)_c$, which is then maintained constant as determined from the initial central wavelength λ_i of the scan, so that

$$(\delta\lambda)_c \approx \frac{\lambda_i^2}{\Delta x} \tag{5.57}$$

Then, using

$$m\lambda = d(\sin\Theta \pm \sin\Theta')$$

the cavity optical length should be maintained according to

$$\Delta x \approx (\delta\lambda)_c^{-1}\left(\frac{d}{m}\right)^2 (\sin\Theta \pm \sin\Theta')^2 \tag{5.58}$$

as the wavelength is scanned. This equation is applicable to a grazing-incidence grating cavity being tuned by rotating its tuning mirror around its central axis, thus changing Θ', which is perpendicular to the plane of incidence. For a cavity using a grating in a Littrow configuration, this expression reduces to

$$\Delta x \approx 4(\delta\lambda)_c^{-1}\left(\frac{d}{m}\right)^2 \sin^2\Theta \tag{5.59}$$

This time, the tuning is performed by changing Θ by rotating the grating about its central axis, which is centered at the optical axis of the cavity and perpendicular to the plane of incidence. Thus, maintaining Δx according to Equation 5.58 or 5.59 ensures the condition of a constant *FSR* or $(\delta\lambda)_c$. It should be noted that these equations also apply to multiple-prism grating cavities, since for either a Littrow or a grazing-incidence configuration, the dispersive contribution of the multiple-prism expander in

$$\Delta\lambda_D = \Delta\theta\left(M\nabla_\lambda\Theta_G + \nabla_\lambda\Phi_P\right)^{-1}$$

can be reduced, by design, to

$$\nabla_\lambda\Phi_P \approx 0 \tag{5.60}$$

In all these $(\delta\lambda)_c$ approaches, it is necessary to precision change Δx as either Θ or Θ' is changed. This requires careful control, and calibration, of the angular and longitudinal parameters mentioned.

An approach that simultaneously changes Δx as Θ' is varied was introduced by Liu and Littman [67] for grazing-incidence grating cavities in dye lasers. This type of tuning is geometrically accomplished by establishing a common rotational point, also referred to as the *pivot point*, defined by the intersection of the projections from the diffraction grating surface, the tuning mirror surface, and the reflective surface of the output coupler. In this setup, L_f is the distance from the center of the diffraction grating surface to the reflective surface of the output coupler, while L_p is the distance from the center of the diffraction grating to the rotational point. Thus, in this approach, the overall cavity length is made a function of Θ' and is given by [67]

$$L = (L_f + L_p \sin \Theta')\qquad(5.61)$$

This type of synchronous tuning was first demonstrated in a miniature grazing-incidence grating cavity, driven by MEMS, by Berger et al. [72].

An additional type of fine tuning applicable to MEMS-driven miniature laser cavities is one of the most basic types of tuning and consists simply in changing the cavity length as outlined in Figure 5.10. In this regard, this approach exploits the very fact that the *FSR* of the cavity is a function of Δx. Going back to

$$\delta \lambda \approx \frac{\lambda^2}{\Delta x}$$

one can write for an initial wavelength λ_1:

$$\delta \lambda_1 \approx \frac{\lambda_1^2}{2L}\qquad(5.62)$$

and for a subsequent wavelength λ_2:

$$\delta \lambda_2 \approx \frac{\lambda_2^2}{2(L \pm \Delta L)}\qquad(5.63)$$

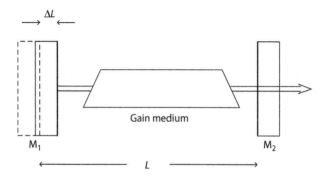

FIGURE 5.10 Wavelength tuning using the displacement of one of the mirrors of the resonator, thus effectively changing the length of the cavity L.

In addition, it is useful to define the number of longitudinal modes in each case as

$$N_1 = \frac{\Delta\lambda_1}{\delta\lambda_1} \tag{5.64}$$

$$N_2 = \frac{\Delta\lambda_2}{\delta\lambda_2} \tag{5.65}$$

where $\Delta\lambda_1$ and $\Delta\lambda_2$ are the corresponding laser linewidths. Now, if the laser linewidth, during this ΔL change is maintained so that $\Delta\lambda_1 \approx \Delta\lambda_2$, then taking the ratio of Equations 5.60 and 5.61 leads to [13]

$$\lambda_2 \approx \lambda_1 \left(\frac{N_1}{N_2}\right)^{1/2} \left(1 \pm \frac{\Delta L}{L}\right)^{1/2} \tag{5.66}$$

Further, for $N_1 \approx N_2$, or single-longitudinal-mode oscillation, this equation reduces to [13]

$$\lambda_2 \approx \lambda_1 \left(1 \pm \frac{\Delta L}{L}\right)^{1/2} \tag{5.67}$$

Uenishi et al. [73] report on experiments using the $\Delta L/L$ method to perform wavelength tuning in an MEMS-driven semiconductor laser cavity. In their experiment, Uenishi et al. [73] observed wavelength tuning in the absence of mode-hopping as long as the change in wavelength did not exceed $\lambda_2 - \lambda_1 \approx 1$ nm. Using their graphical data for the scan initiated at $\lambda_1 \approx 1547$ nm, it is established that $\Delta L \approx 0.4$ μm, and using $L \approx 305$ μm, Equation 5.65 yields $\lambda_2 \approx 1548$ nm, which approximately agrees with the author's observations [73]. In this regard, it should be mentioned that Equation 5.65 was implicitly derived with the assumption of a wavelength scan obeying the condition $\delta\lambda_1 \approx \delta\lambda_2$.

The MEMS tuning technique considered here is for the fine-tuning of a narrow-linewidth emission over a limited wavelength range. Other MEMS-tunable semiconductor lasers providing wide tuning ranges, and broader linewidths, are considered in Section 5.6.

5.3.8 TUNING USING BRAGG GRATINGS

One further method of wavelength tuning, applicable to ECS lasers, that has gained renewed interest recently involves the use of Bragg gratings [74]. A Bragg grating can be visualized as a wavelength-selective mirror satisfying the Bragg condition:

$$\lambda = 2n\Lambda \tag{5.68}$$

where:
  n is the refractive index
  Λ is the grating period

The linewidth selectivity can be estimated using Equation 5.48, with $\Delta x = 2nd$, for propagation in a bulk material of refractive index n:

$$\Delta\lambda \approx \frac{\lambda^2}{2nd} \qquad (5.69)$$

where d is the thickness of the grating. The grating period can also be defined as $\Lambda = d/N$, where N is the number of planes in the grating. Thus, in terms of explicit grating parameters, the wavelength can expressed as

$$\lambda \approx \frac{2nd}{N} \qquad (5.70)$$

and the linewidth as

$$\Delta\lambda \approx \frac{2nd}{N^2} \qquad (5.71)$$

For assessment and comparison purposes, it is useful to restate this identity in frequency units

$$\Delta\nu \approx \frac{c}{2nd} \qquad (5.72)$$

Further aspects of Bragg grating tuning as applied to fiber lasers are discussed in Chapter 6.

5.4 PERFORMANCE OF TUNABLE EXTERNAL-CAVITY SEMICONDUCTOR LASERS

A common feature in most tunable ECS lasers considered here is the use of AR coatings in the internal facet of the semiconductor leading to the intracavity frequency-selective optics. As discussed previously, this is an important requirement to achieve oscillation with characteristics that are totally dependent on the intracavity frequency-selective optics. In this regard, excessive amounts of reflectivity at the facet adjacent to the frequency-selective optics can lead to uncontrolled emission, or noise, and lack of control of the frequency characteristics by the tuning optics. This problem is analogous to the competition between narrow-linewidth emission and ASE observed in dispersive dye laser oscillators [10,11]. Evidence of background superluminescence in narrow-linewidth tunable ECS lasers is provided by Gavrilovic et al. [65]. These authors used a semiconductor with an internal facet, adjacent to the dispersive optics, AR coated to 2%. The design adopted by these authors was a grazing-incidence grating cavity in an open configuration [65].

One traditional feature in tunable laser oscillators is the use of an independent output-coupler mirror (e.g., see [10,11]). In the realm of the ECS laser, very few designs have implemented that feature [25,27]. Although the use of an independent output-coupler mirror can add to the cost, complexity, and physical dimensions, it can provide a further degree of alignment control and the means to collimate the output beam intracavity [27] (see Figures 5.4 and 5.5). The reflectivity of the output-coupler mirror can vary from 40% to 95% [25,65]. So far, however, most authors using closed-cavity configurations have opted for the use of high-reflectivity coatings at the external, or output, facet of the semiconductor.

The performance of ECS laser oscillators using dispersive intracavity optic elements is listed in Table 5.2. The reported linewidths vary from 10 kHz to 32 MHz and the output powers from 1 to 70 mW. It should be noted that the tuning range reported by Favre et al. [70] corresponds to synchronous wavelength tuning.

The performance of ECS lasers using alternative frequency-selective methods such as Bragg gratings, liquid crystals, and acousto-optic filters is given in Table 5.3. Again, AR coatings are used at the internal facet of the semiconductor adjacent to the frequency-selective optics. One method that appears particularly promising is the use of external volumetric Bragg gratings. This method has been demonstrated in ECS lasers [81,82], optically pumped solid-state lasers [81], and fiber lasers [82]. In the case of the ECS lasers, the Bragg grating configuration has been successful in providing frequency selectivity to diode laser arrays [81,82]. In one particular experiment, a total cw power of 13.5 W is reported at a laser linewidth of 7 GHz [82].

Another important area of activity in tunable semiconductor lasers is frequency stabilization [88–93]. A subtle distinction here is that many of these lasers can be classified, according to Weiman and Hollberg [94], as *pseudo*-ECS lasers. As discussed previously, in true ECS lasers, the semiconductor facet adjacent to the frequency-selective optics is AR coated. Under these conditions, oscillation is achieved with the feedback from the frequency-selective optics. In the case of pseudo-ECS lasers, oscillation can proceed in the absence of external optics, although lasing can also be established in a regime where the dispersive optics provides the frequency information of the emission [94].

A widely applied method of frequency stabilization is the use of external reference cavities such as confocal Fabry–Perot resonators [88–91]. In this regard, Laurent et al. [88] report on a 50–60 dB frequency noise reduction and linewidths of less than 4 kHz [88]. Hollberg and colleagues [32] provide an excellent review of various methods of frequency stabilization applicable to tunable diode lasers. The techniques discussed by these authors include optical controlling techniques, electronic controlling techniques, and a combination of optical and electronic techniques [32].

The performance of external-cavity quantum cascade lasers is outlined in Table 5.4, while the performance of external-cavity quantum dot lasers is tabulated in Table 5.5.

5.5 PERFORMANCE OF ULTRASHORT-PULSE EXTERNAL-CAVITY SEMICONDUCTOR LASERS

External-cavity semiconductor lasers have been demonstrated to oscillate using passive [101], active [102,103], and hybrid [104] mode-locking techniques. The saturable absorber demonstrated in the passively mode-locked ECS laser is a multiple-quantum

TABLE 5.2
Performance of External-Cavity Semiconductor Lasers

Laser Semiconductor	Cavity	$\Delta\nu$	Tuning Range	Power	AR Coating[a] (%)	References
InGaAsP/InP	Littrow grating	10 kHz	55 nm @ 1500 nm	—	3–4	[77]
InGaAsP/InP	Littrow grating[b]	31 kHz	1285–1320 nm	≥1 mW	—	[78]
InGaAsP/InP	Littrow grating	20 kHz	15 nm @ 1260 nm	—	<0.01 (SiO)	[70]
InGaAsP/InP	MPL grating[b]	100 kHz	1255–1335 nm	—	<0.01 (SiO)	[26]
GaAlAs	Littrow grating[b,c]	<1.5 MHz	815–825 nm	5 mW	<0.2 (SiO)	[25]
GaAlAs	Littrow grating[b]	~200 kHz	32 nm @ 850 nm	1 mW	<0.5	[79]
GaAlAs	Double étalon[b]	32 MHz	10 nm @ 875 nm	—	Yes	[36]
GaAlAs	Étalon[b]	4 kHz	—	—	<0.4 (SiO–Si_2O_3)	[64]
GaAlAs	GI grating[d]	10 kHz	~20 nm @ 780 nm	—	>2	[80]
GaAlAs	GI grating[d]	≤15 MHz	~30 nm @ 820 nm	30 mW	2 (Al_2O_3)	[65]
InGaAsP/InP	GI grating[d,e]	2 MHz	42 nm @ 1550 nm	70 mW	—	[72]
Index guided	Littrow grating plus étalon[d]	—	20 nm @ ~670 nm	6 mW	~1 (SiO)	[21]
	Mirror[e]	—	20 nm @ 1540 nm	—	—	[73]
	Mirror[e]	12.7 GHz	16 nm @ 1536 nm	~17 nW	—	[75]
InGaAsP/InP	Littrow grating[e]	~1.3 GHz	30 nm @ 1525 nm	~1 mW	0.19	[76]

[a] AR coating of the internal facet adjacent to the frequency-selective optics.
[b] Closed-cavity configuration.
[c] Employs an independent output-coupler mirror.
[d] Open-cavity configuration.
[e] Tuned using MEMS.

TABLE 5.3
Performance of External-Cavity Semiconductor Lasers Using Alternative Tuning Methods

Laser Semiconductor	Tuning Method	$\Delta\nu$	Tuning Range	AR Coating[a] (%)	References
	Bragg grating	7 GHz	750–758 nm	0.5	[82]
GaInAsP	Fiber grating	—	45 nm @ 1500 nm	~1(Pb–SiO$_2$)	[85]
GaInAsP/InP	Liquid crystal filter[b]	~350 MHz	6 nm @ 1500 nm	0.02	[86]
GaAs	Acousto-optic filter[b]	—	35 nm @ 850 nm	1.5	[87]

[a] AR coating of the internal facet next to the frequency-selective optics.
[b] Closed-cavity configuration.

TABLE 5.4
Performance of Tunable External-Cavity Quantum Cascade Lasers

Stages in Cascade	Cavity	Tuning Range (µm)	$\Delta\nu$	Output Power	References
20	Littrow	8.2–10.4	SM[a]	15 mW	[95]
74	Littrow	7.6–11.4	~3.59 GHz	65 µW	[96]
	DFB[b]	—	5 GHz[b]	—	[97]

Source: Duarte, F. J., *Quantum Optics for Engineers*, CRC Press, New York, 2014.
[a] Single mode.
[b] Distributed feedback: primary emissions around 9 and 10.22 µm.

TABLE 5.5
Performance of Quantum Dot Lasers

QD[a]	Cavity	Tuning Range (nm)	$\Delta\nu$	Output Power (mW)	References
InAs	Littrow	1033–1234	—	—	[98]
InAs	Littrow	1125–1288	200 kHz	200	[99]
InAs/GaAs	Littrow	1122–1324	—	480	[100]

Source: Duarte, F. J., *Tunable Laser Optics*, 2nd edn, CRC Press, New York, 2015. With permission.
[a] Quantum dot.

well (MQW) section adjacent to the gain MQW region [101]. Delfyett et al. [104] also use an MQW region as a saturable absorber. In this latter case, however, the saturable absorber is removed from its substrate and placed in contact with the end mirror of the cavity [104]. In addition to MQW semiconductors, saturable absorbers can also result from damaged semiconductor materials that develop saturable absorbing regions [102].

The hybrid mode-locked ECS laser of Delfyett et al. [104] employs a four-prism sequence configured for collinear transmission in a compensating mode [46]. To this prism sequence, the first- and second-derivative values given in Equations 5.27 through 5.30 apply directly.

An alternative pulse-compression multiple-prism array is a six-prism array in which the first three prisms are deployed in an additive configuration, with the second group of three prisms also deployed in a positive configuration [103]. However, the two groups of prisms are deployed in a compensating configuration relative to each other (see Figure 5.7). By adjusting the prism separation, these authors were able to continuously vary the GVD from positive to negative [103]. It should be emphasized that for this more general class of prismatic configuration, the special case considered by Equations 5.27 through 5.30 does not apply. Instead, the generalized equations given by [39,41,42], namely, Equations 5.22 through 5.26, are used. The generality of this approach was elegantly demonstrated in the experiments by Osvay et al. [47,48].

Another interesting cavity design is that of Salvatore et al. [101]. These authors use a 5% AR coating on the facet of the gain section of their four quantum well laser. This AR facet leads to a Littrow-mounted grating, which is used for tuning. The second section is the MQW saturable absorber, whose output facet leads to a double-grating pulse compressor. This facet is coated for 90% reflectivity.

The performance of the short-pulse ECS lasers outlined in this section is listed in Table 5.6. At this stage, it is clear that this is a field that offers ample opportunities

TABLE 5.6

Performance of Ultrashort-Pulse External-Cavity Semiconductor Lasers

Laser Semiconductor	Cavity	Mode-Locking Technique	Δt	Tuning Range or Emission λ	AR Coating[a] (%)	References
InGaAsP	Étalon[b]	Active	580 fs	1300 nm	<1	[102]
InGaAsP	Littrow grating[c]	Internal SA[d]	2.5 ps	40 nm @ 1300 nm	No	[105]
AlGaAs	Four prisms[c]	Hybrid, MQW SA[d]	200 fs	~838 nm	—	[104]
AlGaAs	Six prisms[b]	Active, uses intracavity SA[d]	650 fs	805 nm	Yes	[103]
MQW	Littrow grating and grating pair compressor[c]	Passive	260 fs	16 nm @ 846 nm	<5	[101]

[a] AR coating of the internal facet next to the frequency-selective optics.
[b] Closed-cavity configuration.
[c] Open-cavity configuration.
[d] Saturable absorber.

for further developments in the areas of spectral coverage and attaining shorter emission pulses.

5.6 APPLICATIONS

ECS lasers have been shown to yield narrow-linewidth widely tunable emission in a variety of configurations (see Tables 5.2 through 5.5). Since the publication of the first edition of this book in 1995 [28], these lasers have become the laser of choice for a wide spectrum of applications. ECS lasers have also made significant and crucial contributions in areas such as laser cooling and Bose–Einstein condensation [106]. ECS lasers have also become workhorses in the optical communications industry, which requires narrow-linewidth tunable radiation in their C-band (~ 1530–1565 nm) and L-band (~ 1570–1610 nm) [72,107]. Additional applications that have benefited directly from the availability of tunable ECS lasers include imaging, interferometry, remote sensing, and spectroscopy. Applications to imaging and interferometry are described in Chapter 13.

Given its wavelength agility, direct electrical excitation, light weight, and compactness, an application that is quite suitable for ECS lasers is that of remote sensing and light detection and ranging (LIDAR). An informative review on the various categories of LIDAR applications is given by Grant [108]. A description on the application of ECS lasers to LIDAR can be obtained from Diekmann [109] (and references therein). This author employed an electronically tuned diode laser in conjunction with a fiber Mach–Zehnder interferometer and a Michelson interferometer to perform distance measurements [109]. In addition to the advantages already mentioned, ECS lasers also offer LIDAR applications the alternative of fairly narrow emission linewidths and attractive tuning ranges.

A particular application that has made significant use of tunable semiconductor lasers is spectroscopy [94,110]. Wieman and Hollberg [94] provide an excellent listing of the different areas of spectroscopy employing semiconductor lasers. These areas include optical pumping, fast frequency modulation, high-resolution spectroscopy, high-sensitivity spectroscopy, and trapping and cooling of atoms [94]. Here, it should be noted that high-resolution and high-sensitivity spectroscopy are applications that benefit from the availability of frequency-stabilized diode lasers. Also, stabilized narrow-linewidth ($\Delta v \leq 1$ MHz) semiconductor lasers are very useful in the trapping and cooling of atoms [94]. As mentioned earlier, tunable ECS lasers have been central to laser cooling and Bose–Einstein condensation experiments [94,110]. For an interesting description of the use of tunable semiconductor lasers in the cooling of atoms, the reader should refer to Weidemuller et al. [111]. This experiment uses two excitation lasers, a repumping laser, a probing laser, and a counterpropagating cooling laser. This last laser is a Littrow grating-tuned semiconductor laser with $\Delta v \leq 1$ MHz and a 6 GHz continuous tuning range at ~ 670 nm [111]. All five lasers are semiconductor lasers.

One application mentioned in detail in Chapters 11 and 12 is that of laser isotope separation (LIS) in Li atoms using a tunable ECS laser emitting at the visible red end of the spectrum [112]. In these experiments, ^{7}Li was separated from ^{6}Li using sequential laser excitation. This required smooth wavelength tuning of the ECS laser in the 670.77–670.81 nm region capable of resolving the hyperfine spectrum of lithium involving the ^{6}Li D_1, ^{6}Li D_2, ^{7}Li D_1, and ^{7}Li D_2 lines [112]. Note that for spectroscopy and laser cooling applications, in addition to narrow-linewidth oscillation (e.g., $\Delta v \leq 1$ MHz [110]), the availability of continuous and smooth wavelength tuning, without mode-hopping, is important. A comparison of ECS lasers, based on Littrow grating and grazing-incidence grating configurations, for applications to Raman spectroscopy has been provided by Cooney et al. [113].

Spectroscopic applications of blue GaN ECS lasers emitting in the 373–472 nm portion of the spectrum have been reported by Scheibner et al. [114] and Olejnicek et al. [115]. These authors used open-cavity Littrow grating configurations to study the $^2S_{1/2} - ^2P_{1/2}$ and $^2S_{1/2} - ^2P_{3/2}$ transitions of Al in hollow cathode and magnetron discharges, respectively.

Finally, tunable ECS lasers, at shorter wavelengths, might be suitable for cancer diagnostics using molecules such as hematoporphyrin derivative (HpD) that absorb in the blue and fluoresce in the red [116,117]. In this regard, the availability of higher average power diode laser systems, emitting at the red end of the spectrum, has created the alternative for compact and reliable systems for laser photodynamic therapy (PDT). A diode laser–based system, analogous to that described by Duarte [118] for tunable dye lasers, using dual wavelength emission, was briefly outlined for both diagnosis and PDT for suitable cancers [119]. For a description of PDT using tunable lasers, the reader is referred to Goldman [116].

An additional and significant application of external-cavity tunable diode lasers is in optical coherence tomography (OCT) in medicine. Specific applications of OCT are found in cardiology, dentistry, dermatology, and ophthalmology. Briefly, tunable diode laser systems operating in this field use MEMS tuning techniques to achieve high tuning sweeping rates, from tens to hundreds of kilohertz, while attaining tuning ranges of 100 nm or more, at laser linewidths in the gigahertz range [120,121].

A brief overview summary of tunable narrow-linewidth diode laser applications, including communications, isotope separation, laser cooling, OCT, and spectroscopy, is given in Table 5.7.

5.7 CONCLUSIONS

In this chapter, the architecture, optical elements, and performance characteristics of tunable ECS lasers have been outlined. Particular attention was given to dispersive optical oscillator configurations relevant to the design of tunable ECS lasers. The oscillator configuration and the elements of optical theory considered apply, in general, to any class of semiconductor material irrespective of its physical dimensions and emission wavelength region.

The difference between open- and closed-cavity configurations has been highlighted, and the importance of AR coatings at the semiconductor facet adjacent to the frequency-selective optics has been discussed.

In general, it is found that dispersive ECS laser oscillators offer very narrow-linewidth emission and excellent wavelength tuning ranges. Further, it should be indicated that, as disclosed in the literature, dispersive optical oscillators using

TABLE 5.7
Brief Survey of ECS Laser Applications

Laser Semiconductor	Cavity	Tuning Range	Application	References
GaN	Littrow grating[a]	394.40–396.15 nm[b]	Spectroscopy of Al in hollow-cathode discharges ($^2S_{1/2} - ^2P_{1/2}$ and $^2S_{1/2} - ^2P_{3/2}$ transitions)	[114]
GaN	Littrow grating[a] $\Delta \approx 1$ MHz	394.40–396.15 nm[b,c]	Absorption spectroscopy of Al in a magnetron discharge	[115]
AlGaAs	Littrow grating	~5 GHz @ 780 nm[e]	Measurement of the hyperfine structure of the $^5S_2$ state of ^{17}O	[122]
Index guided	Littrow grating plus étalon[d]	20 nm @ 670 nm	Fluorescence spectrum of ^{6}Li ($2S_{1/2} - 2P_{1/2}$ transition)	[21]
	Littrow grating[e] $\Delta \leq 100$ kHz	6 GHz @ 670.8 nm	Cooling of Li atoms ($2\,^2S_{1/2} - 2\,^2P_{3/2}$ transition)	[111]
	Littrow grating[f]	18 GHz @ 670 nm	Absorption spectrum of ^{7}Li (D_1 and D_2 transitions)	[123]
	GI grating[a] $\Delta \approx 100$ kHz	25 nm @ 672 nm	Laser isotope separation in Li	[112]
InGaAsP/InP	GI grating[g] $\Delta \approx 2$ MHz	42 nm @ 1550 nm	Optical communications	[72]
	Non-Littrow grating plus mirror[g] $\Delta \approx 30$ GHz	100 nm @ 1310 nm	Optical coherence tomography	[120]
VCSEL[h]	$\Delta \approx 3$ GHz[g]	110 nm @ 1310 nm	Optical coherence tomography	[121]

a Commercial ECS laser.

b The overall tuning range of these lasers is approximately 373 nm ≤ λ ≤ 472 nm including several gaps.

c Quoted tuning range includes several gaps.

d AR coating of the semiconductor facet adjacent to the frequency-selective optics. Laser output is coupled via an intracavity beam splitter.

e This is a coarse tuning range. A 1.2 GHz range is quoted for continuous fine tuning.

f The semiconductor facet adjacent to the grating is not AR coated.

g Tuned using MEMS.

h Optically pumped vertical-cavity surface emitting laser (VCSEL). A microcavity is configured between a Bragg reflector and a MEMS-driven mirror [121].

closed-cavity configurations offer enhanced reduction of background emission noise and greater protection against unwanted external optical feedback.

By the time of publication of the first edition of *Tunable Laser Applications* (1995), dispersive ECS laser oscillators had been demonstrated to cover spectral regions in the red and near-infrared using III–V semiconductors to power the various dispersive laser oscillator architectures described here. Since then, however, the development of commercially available II–VI and III–V blue-green laser semiconductors [124,125] has opened a new spectral region for tunable ECS lasers. This remains a research and development area of opportunity.

The stable, narrow-linewidth emission characteristics of dispersive ECS laser oscillators make them attractive for many spectroscopic applications. One disadvantage, however, is the relatively low peak powers available. Hence, the use of these optical oscillators in hybrid tunable laser systems in which amplification is provided by a complementary class of laser remains an attractive alternative. For instance, the use of dispersive ECS laser oscillators in conjunction with existing tunable solid-state laser technology should open doors for further applications in need of high peak powers. In this regard, advances in solid-state dye lasers [126,127] suggest the realization of low-cost hybrid systems incorporating dispersive ECS laser oscillators and solid-state dye laser media at the amplification stages. Indeed, as blue dispersive ECS lasers become more widely available, the injection of high-power lasers in that region of the spectrum is only a matter of time.

On a more futuristic note: the demonstration of spatial coherence, characterized in the form of nearly diffraction-limited beams, and emission linewidths comparable to broadband dye laser emission from electrically excited organic semiconductors [128–130] could lead to a new generation of miniature tunable sources emitting the visible spectrum.

For OCT applications: new improved miniature MEMS-driven ECS lasers yielding single-longitudinal-mode laser linewidths in the megahertz or kilohertz regime at improved sweeping rates and tuning ranges should be possible.

REFERENCES

1. Yariv, A., *Quantum Electronics*, Wiley, New York, 1975.
2. Yariv, A., *Optical Electronics*, Holt, Rinehart and Winston, New York, 1985.
3. Murata, S. and I. Mito, Frequency-tunable semiconductor lasers, *Opt. Quantum Electron.* 22: 1–15, 1990.
4. Ohtsu, M., *Highly Coherent Semiconductor Lasers*, Artech House, Boston, 1992.
5. Zory, P. S. (Ed.), *Quantum Well Lasers*, Academic, New York, 1993.
6. Coleman, J. J., Semiconductor lasers. In R. Waynant and M. Ediger (Eds), *Electro-Optics Handbook*, Chapter 6, McGraw-Hill, New York, 1994.
7. Chow, W. W. and S. W. Koch, *Semiconductor Laser Fundamentals*, Springer, Berlin, 1999.
8. Kapon, E., *Semiconductor Lasers II*, Academic, New York, 1999.
9. Ye, C., *Tunable External Cavity Diode Lasers*, World Scientific, Singapore, 2004.
10. Duarte, F. J., Narrow linewidth pulsed dye laser oscillators. In F. J. Duarte and L. W. Hillman (Eds), *Dye Laser Principles*, Chapter 4, Academic, New York, 1990.
11. Duarte, F. J., Dispersive dye lasers. In F. J. Duarte (Ed.), *High Power Dye Lasers*, Chapter 2, Springer, Berlin, 1991.

12. Duarte, F. J., *Tunable Lasers Handbook*, Academic, New York, 1995.
13. Duarte, F. J., *Tunable Laser Optics*, 1st edn, Elsevier-Academic, New York, 2003.
14. Zmudzinski, C. A., Y. Guan, and P. S. Zory, Room temperature photopumped ZnSe lasers, *IEEE Photon. Tech. Lett.* 2: 685–687, 1991.
15. Jeon, H., M. Hagerott, J. Ding, A. V. Nurmikko, D. C. Grillo, W. Xie, M. Kobayashi, et al., Pulsed room-temperature operation of a blue-green ZnSe quantum-well diode laser, *Opt. Lett.* 18: 125–127, 1993.
16. Nakamura, S. and G. Fasol, *The Blue Laser Diode*, Springer, Berlin, 1998.
17. Duarte, F. J., Multiple-prism Littrow and grazing-incidence pulsed CO_2 lasers, *Appl. Opt.* 24: 1244–1245, 1985.
18. Zorabedian, P., Tunable external cavity semiconductor lasers. In F. J. Duarte (Ed.), *Tunable Lasers Handbook*, Chapter 8, Academic, New York, 1995.
19. Duarte, F. J. and J. A. Piper, A double-prism beam expander for pulsed dye lasers, *Opt. Commun.* 35: 100–104, 1980.
20. Duarte, F. J. and J. A. Piper, Prism preexpanded grazing-incidence grating cavity for pulsed dye lasers, *Appl. Opt.* 20: 2113–2116, 1981.
21. Boshier, M. G., D. Berkeland, E. A. Hinds, and V. Sandoghdar, External-cavity frequency-stabilization of visible and infrared semiconductor lasers for high resolution spectroscopy, *Opt. Commun.* 85: 355–359, 1991.
22. Hanna, D. C., P. A. Karkkainen, and R. Wyatt, A simple beam expander for frequency narrowing of dye lasers, *Opt. Quantum Electron.* 7: 115–119, 1975.
23. Shoshan, I., N. N. Danon, and U. P. Oppenheim, Narrowband operation of a pulsed dye laser without intracavity beam expansion, *J. Appl. Phys.* 48: 4495–4497, 1977.
24. Littman, M. G. and H. J. Metcalf, Spectrally narrow pulsed dye laser without beam expander, *Appl. Opt.* 17: 2224–2227, 1978.
25. Fleming, M. W. and A. Mooradian, Spectral characteristics of external-cavity controlled semiconductor lasers, *IEEE J. Quantum Elect.* QE-17: 44–59, 1981.
26. Zorabedian, P., Characteristics of a grating-external-cavity semiconductor laser containing intracavity prism beam expanders, *J. Lightwave Technol.* 10: 330–335, 1992.
27. Duarte, F. J., Multiple-prism grating designs tune diode lasers, *Laser Focus World* 29(2): 103–109, 1993.
28. Duarte, F. J., Dispersive external cavity semiconductor lasers. In F. J. Duarte (Ed.), *Tunable Laser Applications*, 1st edn, Chapter 3, Marcel-Dekker, New York, 1995.
29. Liu, A. Q. and X. M. Zhang, A review of MEMS external-cavity tunable lasers, *J. Micromech. Microeng.* 17: R1–R13, 2007.
30. Duarte, F. J., Multiple-prism grating solid-state dye laser oscillator: Optimized architecture, *Appl. Opt.* 38: 6347–6349, 1999.
31. Laurila, T., T. Joutsenoja, R. Hernberg, and M. Kuittinen, Tunable external-cavity laser at 650 nm based on a transmission diffraction grating, *Appl. Opt.* 27: 5632–5637, 2000.
32. Fox, R. W., L. Hollberg, and A. S. Zibrov, Semiconductor diode lasers. In F. B. Dunning and R. G. Hulet (Eds), *Atomic, Molecular, and Optical Physics: Electromagnetic Radiation*, Chapter 4, Academic, New York, 1997.
33. Dirac, P. A. M., *The Principles of Quantum Mechanics*, 4th edn, Oxford University, London, 1978.
34. Duarte, F. J., On a generalized interference equation and interferometric measurements, *Opt. Commun.* 103: 8–14, 1993.
35. Duarte, F. J., Interference, diffraction, and refraction, via Dirac's notation, *Am. J. Phys.* 65: 637–640, 1997.
36. Voumard, C., External-cavity-controlled 32-MHz narrow-band CW GaAlAs-diode lasers, *Opt. Lett.* 1: 61–63, 1977.
37. Born, M. and E. Wolf, *Principles of Optics*, 7th edn, Cambridge University Press, Cambridge, 1999.

38. Hänsch, T. W., Repetitively pulsed tunable dye laser for high resolution spectroscopy, *Appl. Opt.* 11: 895–898, 1972.
39. Duarte, F. J. and J. A. Piper, Dispersion theory of multiple-prism beam expanders for pulsed dye lasers, *Opt. Commun.* 43: 303–307, 1982.
40. Duarte, F. J., Transmission efficiency in achromatic nonorthogonal multiple-prism laser beam expanders, *Opt. Commun.* 71: 1–5, 1989.
41. Duarte, F. J., Generalized multiple-prism dispersion theory for pulse compression in ultrafast dye lasers, *Opt. Quantum Electron.* 19: 223–229, 1987.
42. Duarte, F. J., Prismatic pulse compression: Beam deviations and geometrical perturbations, *Opt. Quantum Electron.* 22: 467–471, 1990.
43. Duarte, F. J., Generalized multiple-prism dispersion theory for laser pulse compression: Higher order phase derivatives, *Appl. Phys. B* 96: 809–814, 2009.
44. Duarte, F. J., Tunable laser optics: Applications to optics and quantum optics, *Prog. Quant. Electron.* 37: 326–347, 2013.
45. Duarte, F. J., *Tunable Laser Optics*, 2nd edn, CRC Press, New York, 2015.
46. Fork, R. L., O. E. Martínez, and J. P. Gordon, Negative dispersion using pairs of prisms, *Opt. Lett.* 9: 150–152, 1984.
47. Osvay, K., A. P. Kovács, Z. Heiner, G. Kurdi, J. Klebniczki, and M. Csatári, Angular dispersion and temporal change of femtosecond pulses from misaligned pulse compressors, *IEEE J. Sel. Top. Quant.* 10: 213–220, 2004.
48. Osvay, K., A. P. Kovács, G. Kurdi, Z. Heiner, M. Divall, J. Klebniczki, and I. E. Ferincz, Measurements of non-compensated angular dispersion and the subsequent temporal lengthening of femtosecond pulses in a CPA laser, *Opt. Commun.* 248: 201–209, 2005.
49. Arissian, L. and J. C. Diels, Carrier to envelope and dispersion control in a cavity with prism pairs, *Phys. Rev. A* 75: 013814, 2007.
50. Diels, J. C. and W. Rudolph, *Ultrashort Laser Pulse Phenomena*, 2nd edn, Academic, New York, 2006.
51. Brouwer, W., *Matrix Methods in Optical Instrument Design*, W. A. Benjamin, New York, 1964.
52. Siegman, A. E., *Lasers*, University Science Books, Mill Valley, CA, 1986.
53. Wollnik, H., *Optics of Charged Particles*, Academic, New York, 1987.
54. Kostenbauder, A. G. Ray-pulse matrices: A rational treatment for dispersive optical systems, *IEEE J. Quantum Elect.* 26: 1148–1157, 1990.
55. Turunen, J., Astigmatism in laser beam optical systems, *Appl. Opt.* 25: 2905–2911, 1986.
56. Siegman, A. E., *ABCD*-matrix elements for a curved diffraction grating, *J. Opt. Soc. Am. A* 2: 1793, 1985.
57. Duarte, F. J., Multiple-prism dispersion and 4×4 ray transfer matrices, *Opt. Quantum Electron.* 24: 49–53, 1992.
58. Martinez, O. E., Matrix formalism for pulse compressors, *IEEE J. Quantum Elect.* 24: 2530–2536, 1988.
59. Duarte, F. J., *Quantum Optics for Engineers*, CRC Press, New York, 2014.
60. Duarte, F. J. and J. A. Piper, Multi-pass dispersion theory of prismatic pulsed dye lasers, *Opt. Acta* 31: 331–335, 1984.
61. Duarte, F. J., Multiple-return-pass beam divergence and the linewidth equation, *Appl. Opt.* 40: 3038–3041, 2001.
62. Schäfer, F. P., Principles of dye laser operation. In F. P. Schäfer (Ed.), *Dye Lasers*, Chapter 1, Springer, Berlin, 1990.
63. Duarte, F. J., J. J. Ehrlich, W. E. Davenport, and T. S. Taylor, Flashlamp pumped narrow-linewidth dispersive dye laser oscillators: Very low amplified spontaneous emission levels and reduction of linewidth instabilities, *Appl. Opt.* 29: 3176–3179, 1990.

64. Harrison, J. and A. Mooradian, Linewidth and offset frequency locking of external cavity GaAlAs lasers, *IEEE J. Quantum Elect.* QE-25: 1152–1155, 1989.

65. Gavrilovic, P., A. V. Chelnokov, M. S. O'Neill, and D. M. Beyea, Narrow-linewidth operation of broad-stripe single quantum well laser diodes in a grazing incidence external cavity, *Appl. Phys. Lett.* 60: 2977–2979, 1992.

66. Cassidy, D. T., D. M. Bruce, and B. F. Ventrudo, Short-external-cavity module for enhanced single-mode tuning of InGaAsP and AlGaAs semiconductor diode lasers, *Rev. Sci. Instrum.* 62: 2385–2388, 1991.

67. Liu, K. and M. G. Littman, Novel geometry for single-mode scanning of tunable lasers, *Opt. Lett.* 6: 117–118, 1981.

68. Littman, M. G., Single-mode pulsed tunable dye laser, *Appl. Opt.* 23: 4465–4468, 1984.

69. McNicholl, P. and H. J. Metcalf, Synchronous cavity mode and feedback wavelength scanning in dye laser oscillators with gratings, *Appl. Opt.* 24: 2757–2761, 1985.

70. Favre, F., D. LeGuen, J. C. Simon, and B. Landousies, External-cavity semiconductor laser with 15 nm continued tuning range, *Electron. Lett.* 22: 795–796, 1986.

71. Trutna, W. R. and L. F. Stokes, Continuously tuned external cavity semiconductor laser, *J. Lightwave Technol.* 11: 1279–1286, 1993.

72. Berger, J. D. and D. Anthon, Tunable MEMS devices for optical networks, *Opt. Photonics News* 14(3): 43–49, 2003.

73. Uenishi, Y., K. Honna, and S. Nagaoka, Tunable laser diode using a nickel micromachined external mirror, *Electron. Lett.* 32: 1207–1208, 1996.

74. Kogelnik, H. and C. V. Shank, Coupled-wave theory of distributed feedback lasers, *J. Appl. Phys.* 43: 2327–2335, 1972.

75. Liu, A. Q., X. M. Zhang, V. M. Murukeshan, and Y. Lam, A novel integrated micromachined tunable laser using polysilicon 3-D mirror, *IEEE Photon. Tech. Lett.* 13: 427–429, 2001.

76. Zhang, X. M., A. Q. Liu, C. Lu, and D. Y. Tang, Continuous wavelength tuning in micromachined Littrow external-cavity lasers, *IEEE J. Quantum Elect.* 41: 187–197, 2005.

77. Wyatt, R. and W. J. Devlin, 10 kHz linewidth 1.5 μm InGaAsP external cavity laser with 55 nm tuning range, *Electron. Lett.* 19: 110–112, 1983.

78. Shan, X., A. S. Siddiqui, D. Simeonidou, and M. Ferreira, Rebroadening of spectral linewidth with shorter wavelength detuning away from the gain curve peak in external cavity semiconductor laser sources. In *Conference on Lasers and Electro-Optics, 1991,* pp. 258–259, Optical Society of America, Washington, DC, 1991.

79. DeLabachelerie, M. and P. Cerez, An 850 nm semiconductor laser tunable over a 30 nm range, *Opt. Commun.* 55: 174–178, 1985.

80. Harvey, K. C. and C. J. Myatt, External-cavity diode laser using a grazing-incidence diffraction grating, *Opt. Lett.* 16: 910–912, 1991.

81. Volodin, B. L., S. V. Dolgy, E. D. Melnik, E. Downs, J. Shaw, and S. V. Bans, Wavelength stabilization and spectrum narrowing of high-power multimode laser diodes and arrays by use of volume Bragg gratings, *Opt. Lett.* 29: 1891–1893, 2004.

82. Meng, L. S., B. Nizamov, P. Nadasami, J. K. Brasseur, T. Henshaw, and D. K. Newmann, High-power 7-GHz bandwidth external-cavity diode laser array and its use in optically pumping singlet delta oxygen, *Opt. Express* 14: 10469–10474, 2006.

83. Chung, T-Y, A. Rapaport, V. Smirnov, L. B. Glebov, M. C. Richardson, and M. Bass, Solid-state laser spectral narrowing using a volumetric photothermal refractive Bragg grating cavity mirror, *Opt. Lett.* 31: 329–331, 2006.

84. Jelder, P. and F. Laurell, Efficient narrow-linewidth volume-Bragg grating-locked Nd:fiber laser, *Opt. Express* 15: 11336–11340, 2007.

85. Whalen, M. S., K. L. Hall, D. M. Tennant, U. Koren, and G. Raybon, Tunable fibre-extended-cavity laser, *Electron. Lett.* 23: 313–314, 1987.

86. Wacogne, B., J. P. Goedgebuer, A. P. Onokhov, and M. Tomilin, Wavelength tuning of a semiconductor laser using nematic liquid crystals, *IEEE J. Quantum Elect.* 29: 1015–1017, 1993.

87. Coquin, G. A. and K. W. Cheung, Electronically tunable external-cavity semiconductor laser, *Electron. Lett.* 24: 599–600, 1988.

88. Laurent, P., A. Clairon, and C. Breant, Frequency noise analysis of optically self-locked diode lasers, *IEEE J. Quantum Elect.* 25: 1131–1142, 1989.

89. Hemmerich, A., D. H. McIntyre, D. Schropp, D. Meschede, and T. W. Hänsch, Optically stabilized narrow linewidth semiconductor laser for high resolution spectroscopy, *Opt. Commun.* 75: 118–122, 1990.

90. Fox, R. W., A. S. Zibrov, H. G. Robinson, L. Hollberg, N. Mackie, and R. Ellingsen, Diode lasers stabilization. In F. J. Duarte and D. G. Harris (Eds), *Proceedings of the International Conference on Lasers'91*, pp. 601–607, STS, McLean, VA, 1992.

91. Celikov, A., F. Riehle, V. L. Velichansky, and J. Helmcke, Diode laser spectroscopy in a Ca atomic beam, *Opt. Commun.* 107: 54–60, 1994.

92. Maki, J. J., N. S. Campbell, C. M. Grande, R. P. Knorpp, and D. H. McIntyre, Stabilized diode-laser system with grating feedback and frequency-offset locking, *Opt. Commun.* 102: 251–256, 1993.

93. Lee, S. and L. W. Hillman, Frequency stabilization of diode lasers. In F. J. Duarte and D. G. Harris (Eds), *Proceedings of the International Conference on Lasers'91*, pp. 608–612, STS, McLean, VA, 1992.

94. Weiman, C. E. and L. Hollberg, Using diode lasers for atomic physics, *Rev. Sci. Instrum.* 62: 1–20, 1991.

95. Maulini, R., A. Mohan, M. Giovannini, J. Faist, and E. Gini, External cavity quantum-cascade laser tunable from 8.2 to 10.4 µm using a gain element with a heterogeneous cascade, *Appl. Phys. Lett.* 88: 201113, 2006.

96. Hugi, A., R. Terazzi, Y. Bonetti, A. Wittmann, M. Fischer, M. Beck, J. Faist, et al., External cavity quantum cascade laser tunable from 7.6 to 11.4 µm, *Appl. Phys. Lett.* 95: 061103, 2009.

97. Lu, Q. Y., N. Bandyopadhyay, S. Slivken, Y. Bai, and M. Razeghi, High performance terahertz quantum cascade laser sources based on intracavity difference frequency generation, *Opt. Express.* 21: 968–973, 2013.

98. Varangis, P. M., H. Li, G. T. Liu, T. C. Newell, A. Stintz, B. Fuchs, K. J. Malloy, et al., Low-threshold quantum dot lasers with 201 nm tuning range, *Electron. Lett.* 36: 1544–1545, 2000.

99. Nevsky, A. Yu., U. Bressel, I. Ernsting, Ch. Eisele, M. Okhapkin, S. Schiller, A. et al., A narrow-linewidth external cavity quantum dot laser for high-resolution spectroscopy in the near infrared and yellow spectral ranges, *Appl. Phys. B* 92: 501–507, 2008.

100. Fedorova, K. A., M. A. Cataluna, I. Krestnikov, D. Livshits, and E. U. Rafailov, Broadly tunable high-power InAs/GaAs quantum dot external cavity diode lasers, *Opt. Express* 18: 19438–19443, 2010.

101. Salvatore, R. A., T. Schrans, and A. Yariv, Wavelength tunable source of subpicosecond pulses from CW passively mode-locked two-section multiple-quantum-well laser, *IEEE Photon. Tech. Lett.* 5: 756–758, 1993.

102. Corzine, S. W., J. E. Bowers, G. Przybylek, U. Koren, B. I. Miller, and C. E. Soccolich, Actively mode-locked GaInAsP laser with subpicosecond output, *Appl. Phys. Lett.* 52: 348–350, 1988.

103. Pang, L. Y., J. G. Fujimoto, and E. S. Kintzer, Ultrashort-pulse generation from high-power diode arrays by using intracavity optical nonlinearities, *Opt. Lett.* 17: 1599–1601, 1992.

104. Delfyett, P. J., L. Florez, N. Stoffel, T. Gmitter, N. Andreadakis, G. Alphonse, and W. Ceislik, 200 fs optical pulse generation and intracavity pulse evolution in a hybrid mode-locked semiconductor diode-laser/amplifier system, *Opt. Lett.* 17: 670–672, 1992.

105. Bouchoule, S., N. Stelmakh, M. Cavelier, and J. M. Lourtioz, Highly attenuating external cavity for picosecond-tunable pulse generation from gain/Q-switched laser diodes, *IEEE J. Quantum Elect.* 29: 1693–1700, 1993.

106. Myatt, C. J., N. R. Newbury, R. W. Ghrist, S. Loutzenhizer, and C. E. Wieman, Multiply loaded magneto-optical trap, *Opt. Lett.* 21: 290–292, 1996.

107. Berger, J. D., Y. Zhang, J. D. Grade, H. Lee, S. Hrinya, H. Jerman, A. Fennema, et al., External cavity diode lasers tuned with silicon MEMS, *IEEE LEOS Newslett.* 15(5): 9–10, 2001.

108. Grant, W. B., Lidar for atmospheric and hydrospheric studies. In F. J. Duarte (Ed.), *Tunable Laser Applications*, 1st edn, Chapter 7, Marcel-Dekker, New York, 1995.

109. Dieckmann, A., FMCW-LIDAR with tunable twin-guide laser diode, *Electron. Lett.* 30: 308–309, 1994.

110. Camparo, J. C., The diode laser in atomic physics, *Contemp. Phys.* 26: 443–477, 1985.

111. Weidemuller, M., C. Gabbanini, J. Hare, M. Gross, and S. Harcoche, A beam of laser cooled lithium Rydberg atoms for precision microwave spectroscopy, *Opt. Commun.* 101: 342–346, 1993.

112. Olivares, I. E., A. E. Duarte, E. A. Saravia, and F. J. Duarte, Lithium isotope separation with tunable diode lasers, *Appl. Opt.* 41: 2973–2977, 2002.

113. Cooney, T. F., H. T. Skinner, and S. M. Angel, Evaluation of external-cavity diode lasers for Raman spectroscopy, *Appl. Spectrosc.* 49: 1846–1851, 1995.

114. Scheibner, H., St. Franke, S. Solyman, J. F. Behnke, C. Wilke, and A. Dinklage, Laser absorption spectroscopy with a blue diode laser in an aluminum hollow cathode discharge, *Rev. Sci. Instrum.* 73: 378–382, 2002.

115. Olejnicek, J., H. T. Do, Z. Hubicka, R. Hippier, and L. Jastrabik, Blue diode laser absorption spectroscopy of pulse magnetron discharge, *Jpn. J. Appl. Phys.* 45: 8090–8094, 2006.

116. Goldman, L., Dye lasers in medicine. In F. J. Duarte and L. W. Hillman (Eds), *Dye Laser Principles*, Chapter 10, Academic, New York, 1990.

117. Dougherthy, T. J., Tumor detection and treatment: Hematoporphyrin derivative and photofrin II. In L. Goldman (Ed.), *Laser Non-Surgical Medicine*, Technomic, Lancaster, 1991.

118. Duarte, F. J., Two-laser therapy and diagnosis device, EP 0284330 A1, 1988.

119. Duarte, F. J., Broadly tunable external cavity semiconductor lasers. In F. J. Duarte (Ed.), *Tunable Laser Applications*, 2nd edn, Chapter 5, CRC Press, New York, 2009.

120. Gloor, S., A. H. Bachmann, M. Epitaux, T. vonNiederhäusern, P. Vorreau, N. Matuschek, K. Hsu, et al., High-speed miniaturized swept sources based on resonant MEMS mirrors and diffraction gratings, *SPIE Proc.* 8571, 2013.

121. Grulkowski, I., J. J. Liu, B. Potsaid, V. Jayaraman, C. D. Lu, J. Jiang, A. E. Cable, et al., Retinal, anterior segment and full eye imaging using ultrahigh speed swept source OCT with vertical-cavity surface emitting lasers, *Biomed. Opt. Express* 3: 2733–2751, 2012.

122. Tino, G. M., L. Hollberg, A. Sasso, M. Inguscio, and M. Barsanti, Hyperfine structure of the metastable $^5S_2$ state of ^{17}O using a AlGaAs diode laser at 777 nm, *Phys. Rev. Lett.* 64: 2999–3002, 1990.

123. Atutov, S. N., E. Mariotti, M. Meucci, P. Bicchi, C. Marinelli, and L. Moi, A 670 nm external-cavity single mode diode laser continuously tunable over 18 GHz range, *Opt. Commun.* 107: 83–87, 1994.

124. Taniguchi, S., T. Hino, S. Itoh, K. Nakano, N. Nakayama, A. Ishibashi, and M. Ikeda, 100h II-VI blue-green laser diode, *Electron. Lett.* 60: 552–553, 1996.

125. Nakamura, S., The roles of structural imperfections in InGaN-based blue light-emitting diodes and laser diodes, *Science* 281: 956–961, 1998.

126. Duarte, F. J., Multiple-prism grating solid-state dye laser oscillators: Optimized architecture, *Appl. Opt.* 38: 6347–6349, 1999.

127. Duarte, F. J. and R. O. James, Tunable solid-state lasers incorporating dye-doped polymer-nanoparticle gain media, *Opt. Lett.* 28: 3088–3090, 2003.
128. Duarte, F. J., L. S. Liao, and K. M. Vaeth, Coherence characteristics of electrically excited tandem organic light-emitting diodes, *Opt. Lett.* 30: 3072–3074, 2005.
129. Duarte, F. J., Coherent electrically excited organic semiconductors: Visibility of interferograms and emission linewidth, *Opt. Lett.* 32: 412–414, 2007.
130. Duarte, F. J., Coherent electrically excited organic semiconductors: Coherent or laser emission? *Appl. Phys. B* 90: 101–108, 2008.

6 Tunable Fiber Lasers

T. M. Shay and F. J. Duarte

CONTENTS

6.1 INTRODUCTION

Fiber lasers have become ubiquitous with the emergence of the telecommunications industry. Fiber lasers have been demonstrated spanning wavelengths from just below 400 nm to nearly 3 μm. Among fiber lasers, the most widely used rare earth–doped silica fibers are doped with Er^{+3}, Nd^{+3}, Yb^{+3}, and Tm^{+3}. These systems have the advantage of having pump bands that are compatible with highly efficient diode lasers as well as having quantum efficiencies that range from 0.63 to 0.95 depending on the rare earth ion being excited and the pump and emission wavelengths. All-fiber-based systems provide a tunable performance with minimal sensitivity to environmental disturbances as well as high reliability because the all-fiber laser cavity cannot be misaligned and diffraction-limited beams are generally ensured by the use of single-mode optical fibers. As a result of these advantages, fiber lasers are being employed in a steadily increasing number of applications that previously employed conventional solid-state lasers. Finally, the availability of very efficient and very high-power fiber amplifiers offers a simple means of scaling the output power of tunable fiber laser systems.

The three most widely tunable fiber laser media, Er^{+3}, Yb^{+3}, and Tm^{+3}, will be discussed. Tunable Yb-doped fiber lasers (YDFL) and tunable Tm-doped fiber lasers (TDFL) are not as well explored a technology as the tunable Er-doped fiber lasers (EDFL) used for telecommunications applications. In the remaining sections, some of the tuning techniques that have been employed in tunable YDFL, EDFL, and TDFL will be discussed.

6.2 CORE- AND CLADDING-PUMPED FIBER LASERS

Conceptually, the simplest fiber laser configuration is to efficiently launch a high-brightness laser into the single-mode core with reflectors on both ends. This configuration can lead to very short cavities, and hence can provide a laser with fewer cavity modes than are achievable in equivalent lasers with longer cavities. Core-pumped lasers have the disadvantage that the pump must be high brightness for efficient coupling into the single-mode core of the fiber. For an optical fiber to be single mode, the product of the mode field diameter and the numerical aperture must be

$$2a_{\text{laser}}NA \leq \frac{\lambda}{\pi}2.405 \qquad (6.1)$$

where:
  a_{laser} represents the fiber core radius
  NA represents the numerical aperture of the fiber

In a typical $\lambda \approx 1$ μm single-mode fiber laser, the core diameter is 10 μm, and $NA \approx 0.08$. The numerical aperture for an optical fiber is defined as

$$NA = n\sin\theta \qquad (6.2)$$

where:
  n represents the index of refraction for the optical fiber
  θ represents the fiber acceptance angle

The conservation of brightness requires that the product of the numerical aperture and the beam radius at any two points in the beam path be conserved:

$$NA_1 r_1 = NA_2 r_2 \qquad (6.3)$$

where $NA_{1,2}$ and $r_{1,2}$ represent the numerical apertures and radii, respectively, at two points in the beam path. The practical impact of Equation 6.3 for a fiber laser is that it requires that the product of the pump lasers' NA and spot radius be conserved. Therefore, the only sources that can efficiently pump a core-pumped single-mode fiber laser are very nearly diffraction-limited laser diodes, which are only available at relatively low powers. To achieve high efficiency and high powers in fiber lasers, it is necessary to pump the gain medium with low-brightness, very high-power diode lasers. A dual-cladding fiber [1] can be used to efficiently convert the high-power low-brightness light into a high-power diffraction-limited output beam from a single-mode optical fiber. The dual-cladding fiber geometry is illustrated in Figure 6.1.

In a dual-clad fiber design, a single-mode rare earth–doped core is embedded within a multimode pump waveguide. The pump light from a low-brightness fiber laser can be efficiently coupled into the multimode pump waveguide, and the pump light is absorbed only in the single-mode core, since the pump waveguide is undoped silica with insignificant optical losses. The practical advantage of this configuration is that the dual-clad fiber laser acts as an efficient brightness converter, taking the high output power from diode lasers that have between 50% and 75% electrical efficiency and converting that low-brightness light into the diffraction-limited output beam from the single-mode fiber core. In YDFL, the optical diode pump radiation

- Large-diameter pump waveguide
  - Inner cladding surrounded by low-index outer cladding
  - Efficient low-brightness diode can pump single-mode core

- Single-mode doped core embedded within the pump waveguide

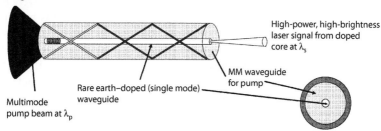

FIGURE 6.1 Dual-clad gain fiber configuration.

has been converted to the single-mode fiber laser output beam with an optical-to-optical conversion efficiency of 85% or more. The dual-clad fiber laser geometry was a key catalyst [2] in the development of high-power, high-efficiency, diffraction-limited lasers.

The increase in brightness available from dual-clad fiber lasers relative to the pump light can be estimated from the following equation:

$$B_{\text{ratio}} = \frac{P_{\text{Laser}}}{\pi\left(NA_{\text{Laser}} \cdot a_{\text{Laser}}\right)^2} \frac{1}{\dfrac{P_{\text{pump}}}{\pi\left(NA_{\text{pump}} \cdot a_{\text{pump}}\right)^2}} = \eta_{\text{optical}} \frac{\left(NA_{\text{pump}} \cdot a_{\text{pump}}\right)^2}{\left(NA_{\text{Laser}} \cdot a_{\text{Laser}}\right)^2} \quad (6.4)$$

where:

P_{Laser} and P_{pump} represent the fiber laser and pump powers, respectively

NA_{Laser} and NA_{pump} represent the single-mode laser core and pump cladding numerical apertures, respectively

a_{Laser} and a_{pump} represent the laser and pump delivery fiber radii, respectively

η_{optical} represents the optical conversion efficiency of pump power into single-mode fiber laser power

For example, a typical single-mode fiber laser operating at $\lambda \approx 1.064$ µm has a 5 µm core radius and a numerical aperture of 0.08. Pump cladding for this single-mode core can have a diameter of between 125 and 400 µm with a numerical aperture of 0.44. Assuming a typical value for η_{optical} of 80% and a pump cladding diameter of 400 µm with a single-mode core at $\lambda \approx 1.064$ µm, the brightness enhancement can be calculated from Equation 6.4 as

$$B_{\text{ratio}} = \eta_{\text{optical}} \frac{\left(NA_{\text{pump}} \cdot a_{\text{pump}}\right)^2}{\left(NA_{\text{Laser}} \cdot a_{\text{Laser}}\right)^2} \cong 38,000 \quad (6.5)$$

The application of dual-clad fibers [2] has been a key enabling technology that has allowed the development of efficient high-power fiber lasers.

Er-, Yb-, and Tm-doped silica fiber lasers all have very wide absorption and emission bands. For example, Yb has absorption from 910 nm, peaking at 977 nm and tailing off rapidly beyond 1060 nm, while emission is relatively low for wavelengths below 970 nm, peaks at 977 nm as absorption does, and remains relatively high for wavelengths as long as 1100 nm. In YDFL, tunable laser action has been demonstrated from 1020 to 1100 nm [3]. Er absorbs between 920 and 1480 nm with an absorption peak at 975 nm, and the emission wavelength for Er extends from 1480 to 1600 nm, with most systems designed to operate at wavelengths in the 1520–1560 nm range. Finally, Tm has absorption bands between 780 and 1880 nm and emission wavelengths between 1800 and 2500 nm. These rare earths are popular laser media for tunable fiber lasers, in part because of the wide tuning ranges, and also because the absorption bands are compatible with highly efficient diode laser systems.

6.3 TUNABLE FIBER LASER CONFIGURATIONS

Fiber laser systems have been tuned using both ring and linear cavity geometries. In addition, the frequency-selective elements encompass external-cavity gratings [4–8], fiber Bragg gratings [9–18], fiber loop mirrors [19], multiple coupled ring cavities [19], fiber Fabry–Perot cavities [19,20], and acousto-optic tunable filters [21,22], and several other tuning methods have also been employed. In many cases, several frequency-selective elements are used in a single tunable laser. As is typical of many widely tunable lasers, the highest-power tunable laser oscillators usually have fairly broad spectral widths, while the narrowest spectral width, or narrowest linewidth, oscillators produce lower output powers. There are a great many tunable fiber laser configurations. In this chapter, a number of the most common and interesting configurations from the literature will be discussed.

The external grating tuned cavities typically are operated in the Littrow or grazing-incidence (GI) grating configurations. These two configurations are illustrated in Figures 6.2 and 6.3, respectively. For both configurations, the laser consists of an optical pump beam, an output coupler, a doped fiber gain medium, an optional cladding mode stripper, a collimating lens, and a diffraction grating. The pump beam

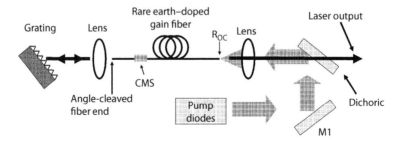

FIGURE 6.2 Littrow diffraction grating tuned rare earth–doped fiber laser. CMS represents a cladding mode stripper, and ROC represents the output-coupler mirror.

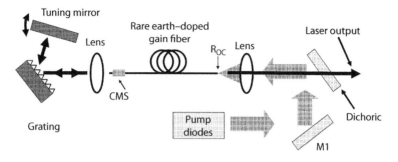

FIGURE 6.3 GI diffraction grating tuned rare earth–doped fiber laser. This type of cavity is also known in the literature as a Littman–Metcalf or Littman cavity. CMS represents a cladding mode stripper, and ROC represents an output coupler.

is generally launched through the output coupler for the laser cavity. The output coupler can be a bulk mirror or a fiber Bragg grating or, in the case of a high-power laser, simply the ~4% reflection from a flat cleaved silica fiber end. The gain medium is a rare earth–doped fiber. The cladding mode strippers shown in Figures 6.2 and 6.3 are sometimes used in high-power cladding pumped fiber lasers to prevent the unabsorbed pump power from damaging the tuning elements. The laser light exits the fiber core and is collimated by a lens, and then the light is directed to the tuning element. A fiber laser tuned directly by a diffraction grating in a Littrow configuration is shown in Figure 6.2, while Figure 6.3 illustrates a fiber laser tuned by the diffraction grating–mirror combination of the GI grating configuration.

The wavelength tuning of a diffraction grating is determined by the diffraction grating equation [23]:

$$m\lambda = d\left(\sin\theta \pm \sin\theta'\right) \tag{6.6}$$

where:

- m represents the diffraction order
- λ represents the wavelength
- d represents the groove spacing
- θ and θ' represent the angles of incidence and diffraction on the grating, respectively

Equation 6.6 is used to calculate the oscillation wavelength for both GI grating and Littrow grating laser cavities (see Chapter 5 for further details).

The spectral resolution of a diffraction grating depends on the number of grooves illuminated by collimated light incident on the grating. The well-known resolution of the diffraction grating is

$$R = \frac{\lambda}{\Delta\lambda} = m \cdot N \tag{6.7}$$

where:
- $\Delta\lambda$ represents the spectral width of the diffraction grating
- N represents the number of grooves illuminated on the grating surface

Substituting for m from Equation 6.6 into Equation 6.7 and solving for the spectral width, or linewidth $\Delta\lambda$, we obtain

$$\Delta\lambda = \frac{\lambda^2}{Nd(\sin\theta \pm \sin\theta')} \tag{6.8}$$

where N times d represents the product of the groove spacing and the number of grooves.

For the Littrow grating tuned laser cavity, the angles of incidence and refraction are the same, so that $\theta = \theta'$, and therefore the lasing wavelength is

$$\lambda = \left(\frac{2d}{m}\right)\sin\theta \tag{6.9}$$

and

$$\Delta\lambda = \frac{\lambda^2}{2Nd\sin\theta} \tag{6.10}$$

These linewidth equations implicitly assume illumination of the whole grating length Nd by a nearly collimated beam with a Gaussian profile. For the GI grating tuned laser cavity, the incident angle is typically $88° \leq \theta \leq 89°$. Therefore, the lasing wavelength of a GI grating tuned laser cavity is, to a very good approximation,

$$\lambda \cong \frac{2d}{m}(1 + \sin\theta') \tag{6.11}$$

In fiber lasers, the GI grating configuration has produced narrower spectral widths than the Littrow configuration, as demonstrated experimentally [4]. The disadvantage of bulk grating tuned fiber lasers is that both the pump and the signal light are free space coupled in and out of the fiber laser. These free-space coupled fiber lasers are less robust than the all-fiber tunable lasers. For a general discussion of the efficiency and linewidth performances of both Littrow and GI grating cavities, the reader should refer to [23].

An all-fiber tunable oscillator is much less sensitive to environmental and mechanical disturbances than a free-space coupled tunable fiber oscillator. The development of fiber Bragg grating tuning elements has allowed the production of all-fiber tunable lasers. The reflection of a fiber Bragg grating is the result of a periodic small permanent index variation along a short length of fiber. The periodic index variation is induced by the irradiation of the fiber with an ultraviolet laser. The fiber Bragg grating reflection wavelength, λ_B, is

$$\lambda_B = 2n\Lambda \tag{6.12}$$

where:

  n represents the average index of the grating
  Λ represents the grating period

The spectral selectivity associated with a Bragg grating can be expressed as (see Chapter 5)

$$\Delta\lambda_B \approx \frac{\lambda^2}{2nd} \tag{6.13}$$

where d is the thickness of the Bragg grating. Commercial fiber Bragg gratings are frequency selective in reflection, and gratings with reflection spectral widths as low as $\Delta\lambda_B \approx 0.1$ nm are readily available. The fiber Bragg grating reflection wavelength depends on the grating period Λ. Therefore, any physical effect that results in a change in the grating period will tune the grating wavelength. Physical processes that change the fiber Bragg grating period, including applying stress, strain, or thermal expansion or contraction, are applied to tune the fiber Bragg grating. Therefore, the fiber Bragg grating reflection wavelengths can be tuned thermally [9,10], by stretching [9,11,12], or by compression [13–15]. Compression of the fiber Bragg grating is most easily induced by bending the fiber. The maximum tuning range for a fiber Bragg grating of 45 nm was demonstrated in an Yb^{+3}-doped fiber laser tuned by bending the grating [15]. The wavelength shift in the Bragg wavelength, $\delta\lambda_B$, as a function of strain and temperature is given by [24]

$$\delta\lambda \approx 2n\Lambda \left\{ \left[1 - \left(\frac{n^2}{2} \right) \left(p_{12} - v_p (p_{11} + p_{12}) \right) \right] \varepsilon + \left(\alpha + \frac{\nabla_T n}{n} \right) \Delta T \right\} \tag{6.14}$$

where:

  p_{ij} represent the Pockels coefficients of the stress-optic tensor
  v_p represents Poisson's ratio
  α represents the coefficient of thermal expansion of the fiber material
  Δ_T represents the temperature change

In a typical silica fiber, the temperature effects account for 95% of the observed wavelength shift [9]. However, temperature tuning is slow, and therefore most fiber Bragg grating tuned lasers are tuned by strain.

   A fiber Bragg grating compression configuration is shown in Figure 6.4. The fiber Bragg grating is glued to a beam, which is then bent to compress the fiber. Under these conditions, the strain in the fiber is given by [15]

$$\varepsilon = -\frac{d}{2R} \tag{6.15}$$

where:

  d represents the thickness of the beam
  R represents the radius of curvature of the beam

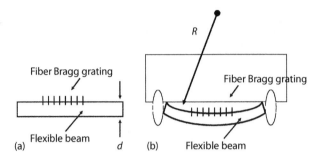

FIGURE 6.4 (a) Flexible beam of thickness d with fiber Bragg grating glued to the beam. (b) Flexible beam bent at the radius of curvature R with compressed fiber Bragg grating.

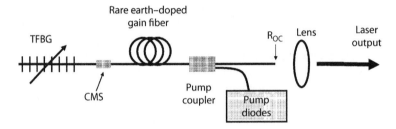

FIGURE 6.5 Generic linear cavity all-fiber tunable rare earth–doped fiber laser. CMS represents a cladding mode stripper, and R_{OC} represents the output-coupler mirror.

Note that care must be taken to keep the strain below the fiber's breaking point strain [16] of approximately 0.07.

The common basic linear and basic ring cavity configurations for all-fiber rare earth–doped fiber lasers are shown in Figures 6.5 and 6.6, respectively.

The basic tunable linear all-fiber cavity consists of a tunable fiber Bragg grating (TFBG) that selects lasing wavelength, a diode pump source, a pump coupler, a rare earth–doped gain fiber, an optional cladding mode stripper, and an output coupler. For a core-pumped single-mode fiber laser, the pump is coupled in by a wavelength division multiplexor that couples the pump light into the doped laser core. The wavelength division multiplexor is designed to be transparent to the fibers' lasing wavelength. In the case of cladding-pumped fiber lasers, either a tapered fiber bundle or side couplers are used to launch the pump light into the pump cladding. The single-mode region of the gain fiber is doped with the rare earth ions that absorb the pump light to create the population inversion. The cladding-pumped configurations are preferred for fiber lasers with output powers exceeding a few watts. In high-power cladding-pumped lasers, a cladding mode stripper is used to prevent the unabsorbed pump power from damaging the pumps or other power-sensitive laser components. A cladding mode stripper consists of a short section of fiber in which the low-index outer cladding that trapped the pump light has been removed and replaced by a high-index coating that allows any unabsorbed pump light to escape from the pump

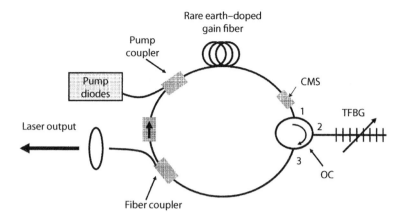

FIGURE 6.6 Generic unidirectional ring cavity all-fiber tunable rare earth–doped fiber laser. CMS represents a cladding mode stripper, OC represents a three-port optical circulator, and the output coupler is a fiber power splitter.

cladding. The output coupler for these systems can be either a partially transmitting fiber Bragg grating or simply a flat cleaved fiber end.

A generic tunable all-fiber ring cavity is illustrated in Figure 6.6. The ring cavity has a few more elements compared with the linear cavity; however, it generally produces a significantly narrower laser linewidth. The ring cavity consists of a TFBG that selects the lasing wavelength, a diode pump source, a pump coupler, a rare earth–doped gain fiber, an optical isolator, an optical circulator, an output coupler, and an optional cladding mode stripper. As was the case for the linear fiber cavity, the pump coupler consists of a wavelength division multiplexor that couples the pump light into the doped core for core-pumped fibers; for cladding-pumped fibers, a tapered fiber bundle or side couplers are used to launch the pump light into the pump cladding. The single-mode region of the gain fiber is doped with the rare earth ions that absorb the pump light to create the population inversion. The optical isolator ensures that the laser light travels only in one direction. Unidirectional oscillation of the ring laser ensures that hole-burning effects will be avoided, and the ring laser cavity oscillates with fewer modes than the comparable linear cavity laser. Because TFBGs are frequency selective only in reflection, the three-port optical circulator allows light from Port 1 to be directed to the TFBG at Port 2. Here, the narrow bandwidth reflection from the TFBG spliced to Port 2 provides frequency selection. The light reflected from the TFBG is then returned to Port 3 of the optical circulator, thus providing frequency selection in each trip around the ring laser cavity. The output coupler for these systems is generally an evanescent coupled fiber power splitter that outcouples some fraction of the power in the laser cavity. In general, the output power from fiber ring cavities is polarized by a polarizing element in the laser cavity. Common polarizing elements include sensitive optical circular or polarization-sensitive optical isolators. These elements, in conjunction with polarization-maintaining coupled fibers or manual polarization-control paddles, will provide stable polarized output from the ring laser. While polarization-control paddles and nonpolarization-maintaining fibers can be used, this system often requires frequent adjustments, and therefore, a much more robust system is obtained if polarization-maintaining gain fibers are used. As with the linear cavity case, the cladding-pumped system is preferred for fiber lasers with output powers exceeding a few watts. In the case of high-power cladding-pumped lasers, a cladding mode stripper is used to prevent the unabsorbed pump power from damaging the pumps, TFBG, or other optical components in the laser.

6.3.1 MULTIPLE-PRISM GRATING CONFIGURATION

Now, we revisit the linewidth issue from a slightly different perspective. The cavity linewidth equation is given by [23]

$$\Delta\lambda \approx \Delta\theta\left(\nabla_\lambda\Theta\right)^{-1} \tag{6.16}$$

where:
  $\Delta\theta$ is the beam divergence of the beam, at the gain region, with a beam waist of w
  $\nabla_\lambda\Theta = (\partial\Theta/\partial\lambda)$ is the overall cavity dispersion

For a single-transverse-mode beam, with a Gaussian profile, experiencing a beam expansion M from the exit of the gain medium to the entrance of the grating, the linewidth is given by

$$\Delta\lambda \approx \Delta\theta\left(M\nabla_\lambda\Theta_G\right)^{-1} \tag{6.17}$$

where $\nabla_\lambda\Theta_G$ is the grating dispersion in either GI, near-GI, or Littrow configuration. Assuming a nearly diffraction-limited beam profile [23]:

$$\Delta\theta = \frac{\lambda}{\pi w} \tag{6.18}$$

and a GI or near-GI grating configuration, the linewidth equation takes the form of

$$\Delta\lambda \approx \frac{\lambda^2}{\pi M w}\left(\frac{\cos\theta}{\sin\theta \pm \sin\theta'}\right) \tag{6.19}$$

Again, this equation assumes that the whole diffractive length of the grating is being illuminated by a Gaussian beam of modified, or expanded, width $2Mw$. The linewidth expression for a Littrow configuration follows by setting the angle of incidence equal to the angle of diffraction, that is, $\theta = \theta'$.

Multiple-prism grating configurations, with the grating deployed in either the Littrow or the near-GI configuration, have been applied and demonstrated with a variety of gain media [23]. Beyond traditional high-gain, homogeneously broadened, broadly tunable laser media, these configurations have also been applied to gas lasers [25–27] and semiconductor lasers [28,29]. In the case of gas lasers, single-longitudinal-mode oscillation has been reported for cavity lengths of approximately 107 cm, with a laser linewidth of $\Delta v \approx 140$ MHz [26]. This result is particularly relevant to contemporary fiber lasers, in which optimized multiple-prism grating configurations should yield tunable single-longitudinal-mode lasing.

For example, let us consider a hypothetical Yb-doped fiber laser oscillator with a core fiber diameter of $2w = 30$ μm and an overall cavity length of 1 m. These types of lasers have been demonstrated to lase in the $1531 \leq \lambda \leq 1568$ nm range [30], so we shall consider a central wavelength $\lambda = 1550$ nm. Following the approach outlined in [23], a five-prism achromatic expander is selected to illuminate a 1200 lines/mm grating deployed in its first diffraction order. For this, a grating with a length of 100 mm is selected (see Figure 6.7). The parameters imposed by the core of the fiber and the dimensions of the grating dictate that the multiple-prism beam expander should provide an overall magnification factor of $M \approx 990$. The multiple-prism dispersion equation, for orthogonal beam exit, is given by [23] (also, see Chapters 5 and 10)

$$\nabla_\lambda \phi_{2,r} = \sum_{m=1}^{r} (\pm 1) \mathcal{H}_{1,m} \left(\prod_{j=m}^{r} k_{1,j} \right)^{-1} \nabla_\lambda n_m \qquad (6.20)$$

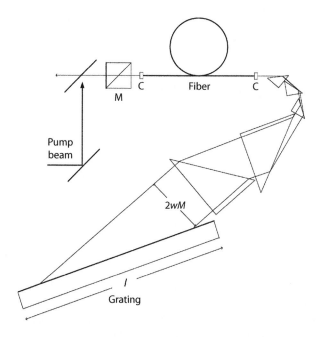

FIGURE 6.7 Multiple-prism Littrow (MPL) grating configuration for narrow-linewidth tunable fiber lasers. This simplified diagram is not drawn to scale. The length of the grating is $l = 100$ mm, and the width of the one-dimensional expanded beam illuminating the grating is calculated to be $2wM \approx 29.61$ mm. The letter C indicates the position of collimators, and the M at the output stands for mirror. This output-coupler mirror is a Glan–Thompson polarizer with its reflective coating at the exit surface (see text).

Setting $\nabla_\lambda \phi_{2,m} \approx 0$, then, for four right-angle prisms, with identical angular dimensions, deployed at the same angle of incidence, and designed for orthogonal beam exit, plus a fifth compensating prism, we arrive at

$$\left(k_{1,1} + k_{1,1}\, k_{1,2} + k_{1,1}\, k_{1,2}\, k_{1,3} + k_{1,1}\, k_{1,2}\, k_{1,3}\, k_{1,4}\right) n \tan \psi_{1,1} = \left(k_{1,1}\, k_{1,2}\, k_{1,3}\, k_{1,4}\right) \tan \phi_{1,5} \quad (6.21)$$

For fused silica at 1550 nm ($n \approx 1.44402$), selecting the beam expansion of the first four prisms as

$$k_{1,1} = k_{1,2} = k_{1,3} = k_{1,4} = 5$$

yields

$$\phi_{1,1} = \phi_{1,2} = \phi_{1,3} = \phi_{1,4} = 81.65°$$

and

$$\psi_{1,1} = \psi_{1,2} = \psi_{1,3} = \psi_{1,4} \approx 43.25°$$

Then, using Equation 6.21, the parameters for the fifth prism, deployed in a compensating mode, become $\phi_{1,5} \approx 59.46°$, $\psi_{1,5} \approx 36.62°$, and $k_{1,5} \approx 1.58$, so that

$$k_{1,1} k_{1,2} k_{1,3} k_{1,4} k_{1,5} \approx 987$$

Thus, assuming a single transverse mode, with nearly diffraction-limited divergence, and using $M \approx 987$, in [23]

$$\Delta\lambda \approx \Delta\Theta \left(M \nabla_\lambda \Theta_G\right)^{-1}$$

the estimated double-pass, or return-pass, linewidth becomes $\Delta\lambda \approx 0.01$ nm or $\Delta v \approx 1.27$ GHz at $\lambda = 1550$ nm. It should be noted that double-pass dispersive linewidth estimates are known to be an *upper limit* of the observed laser linewidth [23,31,32]. This means that for long-pulse or continuous-wave operation, the emission might well approach a *single longitudinal mode* for a cavity length of approximately 1 m where the longitudinal mode spacing is ~150 MHz. In the present configuration, only ~81 mm of the grating is illuminated at 1550 nm, leaving ample diffractive space at the grating for tuning to longer wavelengths. It should be noted that the use of high-density diffraction gratings with diffractive lengths of up to 140 mm is a known and proved feature in long-pulse narrow-linewidth tunable laser oscillators [33]. In practice, the beam expansion needed should be somewhat smaller, given that the emerging beam diameter from the collimators will be greater than the 2w generated at the exit of the gain medium.

Albeit on the surface this design might appear somewhat unusual, it should be remembered that the multiple-prism beam expansion can be accomplished in a fairly compact manner, requiring little extra cavity space. Also, the cavity configuration remains *closed* (see Chapter 5), thus reducing the amount of amplified spontaneous emission (ASE) in the output. As compared with GI grating designs, deployment in a Littrow configuration is known to offer higher efficiencies. Again, the efficiency of GI grating configurations can be improved using prism pre-expansion [23,26,32].

As hinted previously, this should be considered as the first step, in an iterative process, to design an optimized multiple-prism configuration capable of yielding single-longitudinal-mode oscillation at reasonable efficiencies. An alternative design using only a *four-prism expander* with $k_{1,1} k_{1,2} k_{1,3} \approx 8$ and an overall beam expansion of $M \approx 773$ yields a double-pass linewidth estimate of $\Delta\lambda \approx 0.013$ nm or $\Delta v \approx 1.63$ GHz at $\lambda = 1550$ nm. This would also require the use of a 1200 lines/mm grating; however, its length only needs to be ~70 mm.

As far as polarization is concerned, the multiple-prism grating assembly induces a strong polarization parallel to the plane of incidence [23,32–34], which is further reinforced by the Glan–Thompson output-coupler mirror [23,35]. In this polarizer output coupler, the inner surface is antireflection coated, while the exit surface is typically coated at ~20%, depending on the gain conditions. This added polarization feature also reduces the amount of ASE in the output emission [23].

In general, the aim of this multiple-prism grating approach to linewidth narrowing is to illuminate the whole available diffractive length of the grating with a single transverse mode of near-Gaussian profile. The larger the number of grooves that are thus illuminated, the narrower the dispersive linewidth [23].

6.4   TUNABLE FIBER LASER PERFORMANCE

A selected summary of a few specific demonstrations of fiber laser performance are listed in Tables 6.1 and 6.2. The tables list for the most part some recently reported results. Table 6.1 lists tunable fiber laser results reported in the literature for EDFL. Tunable EDFL have received most attention due to their importance in fiber telecommunications. All the techniques described in this chapter, and others, have been employed to tune EDFL. In the case of Yb- and Tm-doped tunable fiber lasers, only bulk diffraction grating tuning and fiber Bragg gratings have been used for wavelength tuning.

TABLE 6.1

Characteristics of Er-Doped Tunable Fiber Lasers

Tuning Technique	Tuning Range (nm)	Linewidth	Power (W)	η_{slope} (%)	References
Diffraction grating	1533–1600	0.25 nm	6.7	38	[6]
Fiber Bragg grating	1532–1567	0.15 nm	43	32	[8]
	1510–1580	100 MHz	5×10^{-4}	—	[17]
Multiple ring cavities	1481–1513	0.02 nm	1×10^{-3}	—	[19]
Acousto-optic tunable	1540–1578	9 GHz	0.1	—	[22]
filter	1533–1581	1.3 kHz	1.2×10^{-4}	—	[21]

TABLE 6.2

Characteristics of Tunable YDFL and TDFL

Tuning Technique	Tuning Range (nm)	Linewidth	Power (W)	η_{slope} (%)	References
Diffraction grating (Yb^{+3})	1027–1100	0.3 nm	2.8	16	[3]
Diffraction grating (Tm^{+3})	1859–2061	<0.5 nm	17.4	65	[7]
	2275–2415	207 MHz	0.006	19	[4]
HTGIG[a] (Yb^{+3})	1032–1124	2.5 GHz	10 W	85	[37]
Fiber Bragg grating (Yb^{+3})	1048–1093	0.15 nm	6	60	[15]
	1040–1100	0.1 nm	0.8	52	[18]

[a] Hybrid telescope grazing-incidence grating configuration in a ring cavity.

Table 6.1 lists a high-power and narrow-linewidth result for most of the tuning techniques. For example, the first entry is the high-power bulk diffraction grating tuned system reported by Nilsson et al. [6]. In their experiments, a Littrow configuration was used for frequency selectivity. They demonstrated a very wide tuning range of 67 nm and moderate power with a linewidth of 0.25 nm at a slope efficiency of 38%.

A fiber Bragg grating tuned EDFL providing 35 nm of tuning, with 43 W of output power, at a linewidth of 0.15 nm and a slope efficiency of 38% was reported by Jeong et al. [8]. In rare earth–doped fiber lasers, the oscillation shifts to longer wavelengths as the fiber length is increased. It is well known that in an Er–Yb-codoped glass, Yb^{+3} ions excited by 975 nm photons will transfer their energy to the upper laser level of Er^{+3}. To ensure that the tunable oscillator remained in the 1550 nm spectral region, the 3.5 m long large-mode area gain fiber was codoped with Yb. The diameter of the large-mode area fiber was 30 μm. The large-mode area fiber is a multimode fiber in which coiling has been used to increase the losses in the higher-order modes, and hence nearly single-mode output can be maintained in a multimode fiber [36]. This laser was a free-space pumped linear cavity in which a dichroic mirror was used at the output of the laser to separate the pump light delivered to the dual-cladding laser and the single-mode tunable laser light. The unabsorbed pump light was prevented from reaching the TFBG by a 1 m long section of single-mode fiber that was taper-spliced to the large-mode Er–Yb-doped gain fiber. To prevent broadband reflections from contributing optical feedback, the end of the TFBG was angle cleaved. The TFBG was tuned by compression.

A fiber ring laser with a 100 MHz linewidth that tuned over 70 nm, with an output power of 0.5 mW, was reported by Chen et al. [17]. The linewidth was narrowed by a tunable fiber Bragg filter and a fiber Fabry–Perot filter, and a saturable absorption section of Er-doped fiber was located at a port of an optical circulator.

A multiple ring cavity fiber laser that was tunable over 32 nm with a linewidth of 0.02 nm, at an output power of 1 mW, was reported by Yeh et al. [19]. The multiple ring cavity is an all-fiber configuration that is a variation of the ring cavity illustrated in Figure 6.8, in which a tunable fiber Fabry–Perot cavity and a main fiber ring with two subrings form coupled cavities with the main ring. In this design, the only wavelengths that can oscillate are the wavelengths that resonate simultaneously in all three ring cavities and the fiber Fabry–Perot cavity. Unidirectional oscillation is guaranteed by optical isolators, and the output-coupling is accomplished by an evanescent outcoupler, as described earlier.

The final two entries in Table 6.1 are the acousto-optically tuned lasers. These both have very narrow linewidths. Tuning over 38 nm was reported with a linewidth of 9 GHz at an output power of 100 mW [22]. This acousto-optically tuned all-fiber laser is another all-fiber configuration, which is a variation of the ring configuration of Figure 6.6, in which an in-line acousto-optic tunable filter replaces the TFBG and optical circulator combination shown in Figure 6.6. One significant advantage of the acousto-optic tuned fiber laser is that the laser wavelength can be shifted on timescales of a few milliseconds [22]. The final laser configuration listed in Table 6.1 is an all-fiber ring laser variation with an in-line acousto-optic tunable filter, again replacing the TFBG and optical circulator configuration, and adding an unpumped Er-doped fiber segment as a saturable absorber at Port 2 of an optical circular. This design was tunable over 48 nm at an output power of ~100 µW but with a linewidth of 1.3 kHz, which implies that this system operated in a single longitudinal mode.

As shown in Table 6.1, EDFL have demonstrated tuning ranges of up to 70 nm, up to 43 W of tuned laser power, and linewidths as low as 1.3 kHz. However, at present, each of those impressive results was obtained using a different laser cavity design. Perhaps in the future, a single system will be available that can simultaneously provide all of these characteristics.

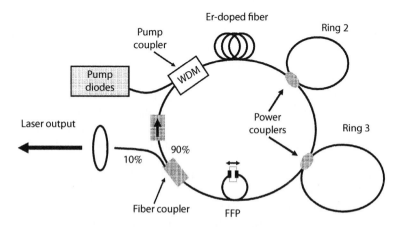

FIGURE 6.8 A multi-ring cavity all-fiber tunable EDFL. FFP represents a fiber Fabry–Perot filter, the pump coupler is a wavelength division multiplexor (WDM), two passive ring cavities are coupled to the laser cavity, and the output coupler is a 90/10 fiber power splitter.

Table 6.2 lists some of the recent tunable laser performance reported for YDFL and TDFL systems. There has been much less research on tunable YDFL and TDFL than on Er-doped tunable fiber lasers.

The bulk diffraction grating systems are listed first in Table 6.2. A bulk diffraction grating tuned Yb-doped fiber laser with a tuning range of 73 nm, at an output power of 2.8 W, with a 0.3 nm linewidth and a slope efficiency of 16% was reported in [3]. This design is a variation of the linear cavity configuration shown in Figure 6.2, in which the light exiting the tuning end of the fiber is reflected off a dichroic mirror that reflects the signal light and transmits the pump light to protect the diffraction grating from damage by the unabsorbed pump light. The signal light is turned 90° by the dichroic mirror so that it is incident on the Littrow grating, and then the frequency-selected light is sent back into the linear laser cavity.

A hybrid telescope GI grating (HTGIG) configuration in a ring cavity is reported to yield a laser linewidth of $\Delta v \approx 2.5$ GHz, tunable over $1032 \leq \lambda \leq 1124$ nm at 10 W power [37]. This class of HTGIG configuration is a variant of the prism-pre-expanded GIG cavities originally introduced for tunable organic lasers [34,38].

The last rows of Table 6.2 list the all-fiber Yb-doped fiber laser systems. Tuning over 45 nm with a linewidth of 0.15 nm, at an output power of 6 W, with 60% slope efficiency was reported in [15]. This all-fiber linear cavity design uses the configuration of Figure 6.5 with a TFBG. The fiber Bragg grating is tuned in compression by gluing the fiber Bragg grating to a flexible beam and bending the beam as shown in Figure 6.4. The authors report that compressing the fiber Bragg grating increases the grating reflection coefficient and in their case, results in increased output power. The next laser is in an all-fiber ring cavity configuration (see Figure 6.6) with a tunable filter in the ring. This system reported 70 nm of tuning with a 0.1 nm linewidth, at an output power of 0.8 W, and a sloped efficiency of 52% [18].

Finally, the Tm-doped tunable fiber lasers selected are both bulk grating tuned devices. The highest-power results listed are 17.4 W, with a tuning range of 202 nm, at 0.5 nm linewidth, and a slope efficiency of 65% [7]. This cladding-pumped design is a variation of the linear cavity configuration shown in Figure 6.2, in which the light exiting the tuning end of the fiber is reflected off a dichroic mirror that reflects the signal light and transmits the pump light to protect the diffraction grating from damage by the unabsorbed pump light. The signal light is turned 90° by the dichroic mirror so that it is incident on the Littrow grating, and then the frequency-selected light is sent back into the linear laser cavity. These authors also report tuning a core-pumped Tm-doped fiber laser from 1723 to 1973 nm. The final Tm-doped tunable fiber laser design is a GI grating design. This bulk grating tuned laser was tunable over 140 nm, at an output power of 6 mW, with a slope efficiency of 19%, and a linewidth of 210 MHz [4].

Table 6.2 indicates that Tm-doped tunable fiber lasers can have tuning ranges of 202 nm, powers of 17 W, and linewidths as low as 210 MHz. However, similarly to the Er-doped tunable fiber laser systems, not all the aforementioned accomplishments can be demonstrated in a single device. Finally, the research on tunable Yb-doped fiber has also shown wide tuning ranges and significant powers.

6.5 SUMMARY

There are a large number of tunable fiber oscillator laser configurations. A few of the most common and some interesting tunable fiber laser systems have been discussed in this chapter. All-fiber tunable lasers with linewidths in the kilohertz range have been demonstrated [21]. All-fiber tunable lasers with tuning ranges of 70 nm have also been reported [17]. Bulk diffraction grating tuned fiber lasers have been demonstrated with a tuning range of 202 nm [7]. Linewidths as low as 210 MHz have also been demonstrated in a GI grating fiber laser cavity [4]. Many of the tunable fiber lasers have demonstrated slope efficiencies of more than 30%. There is a great deal of activity in the development of tunable fiber laser systems, and further improvements are to be expected.

While this chapter has only discussed *tunable laser oscillators*, it is important to note that all-fiber kilohertz-linewidth fiber amplifiers with power levels of 177 W have been reported. A properly designed fiber amplifier seeded by a tunable source is a straightforward method for producing a high-power narrow-linewidth tunable fiber source. There is currently a great deal of effort devoted to developing narrow-linewidth fiber amplifiers. Recently, a narrow-linewidth Yb-doped fiber amplifier has amplified a 1 mW source up to 500 W [39]. It is possible to design a high-power narrow-linewidth tunable optical source by using a narrow-linewidth tunable low-power oscillator as a seed for a chain of high-power fiber amplifiers. As previously shown, in other types of high-power tunable lasers [23], when this master-oscillator power-amplifier approach is used, tunable high power and narrow linewidth are completely compatible.

Note that one area of application for injection-seeded Raman fiber amplifiers, whose output is then frequency doubled into the visible, is the generation of coherent emission at $\lambda \approx 589$ nm [40,41]. This application consists in the generation of *laser guide star* emission for astronomical applications [42]. These lasers are proposed as an alternative to narrow-linewidth dye lasers that generate the emission directly in the visible [34,43].

REFERENCES

1. Maurer, R., Optical waveguide light source, U.S. Patent 3808549, 1974.
2. Zenteno, L., High power double-clad fiber lasers, *IEEE J. Lightwave Tech.* 11: 1435–1446, 1993.
3. Nilsson, J., W. A. Clarkson, R. Selvasa, J. K. Sahu, P. W. Turner, S.-U. Alam, and A. B. Grudinin, High power wavelength-tunable cladding-pumped rare-earth-doped silica fiber lasers, *Opt. Fiber Tech.* 10: 5–30, 2004.
4. McAleavey, F. J., J. O'Gorman, J. F. Donegan, B. D. MacCraith, J. Hegarty, and G. Maze, Narrow linewidth, tunable Tm^{+3}-doped fluoride fiber laser for optical-based hydrocarbon gas sensing, *IEEE J. Selec. Top. Quantum Electron.* 3: 1103–1111, 1997.
5. Soh, D. B. S., S. Yoo, J. Nilsson, J. K. Sahu, K. Oh, S. Baek, Y. Jeong, et al., Neodymium-doped cladding pumped aluminosilicate fiber laser tunable in the 0.9-μm wavelength range, *IEEE J. Quantum Elect.* 40: 1275–1282, 2004.
6. Nilsson, J., S. Alam, J. A. Alvarez-Chavez, P. W. Turner, W. A. Clarkson, and A. B. Grudinin, High-power and tunable operation of erbium-ytterbium co-doped cladding-pumped fiber lasers, *IEEE J. Quantum Elect.* 39: 987–993, 2003.

7. Shen, D. Y., J. K. Sahu, and W. A. Clarkson, High-power widely tunable Tm: Fibre lasers pumped by an Er,Yb co-doped fibre laser at 1.6-μm, *Opt. Express* 14: 6084–6090, 2006.

8. Jeong, Y., C. Alegria, J. K. Sahu, L. Fu, M. Ibsen, C. Codemard, M. R. Mokhtar, et al., A 43-W C-band tunable narrow-linewidth erbium-ytterbium codoped large-core fiber laser, *IEEE Photon. Tech. Lett.* 16: 756–758, 2004.

9. Liaw, S-K., W. Y. Jang, C-J. Wang, and K. L. Hung, Pump efficiency improvement of a C-band tunable fiber laser using an optical circular and tunable fiber gratings, *Appl. Opt.* 46: 2280–2285, 2007.

10. Liaw, S-K., K.-L. Hung, Y.-T. Lin, C.-C. Chinag, and C.-S. Shin, C-Band tunable lasers using tunable fiber Bragg gratings, *Opt. Laser Technol.* 39: 1214–1217, 2007.

11. Hernandez-Cordero, J., J. B. Escalante-Garcia, and F. Nunez-Orozco, Programmable control system for wavelength tuning and stabilization of optical fiber lasers, *Opt. Eng.* 44: 044201, 2005.

12. Zhang, S-M., F.-Y. Lu, and J. Wiang, High-power narrow linewidth tunable cladding pumped Er:Yb co-doped fiber laser, *Microwave Opt. Tech. Lett.* 48: 1736–1739, 2006.

13. Goh, C. S., S. Y. Set, and K. Kikuchi, Widely tunable optical filters based on fiber Bragg gratings, *IEEE Photon. Tech. Lett.* 14: 1306–1308, 2002.

14. Fu, L. B., M. Ibsen, D. J. Richardson, J. Nilsson, D. N. Payne, and A. B. Grudinin, Compact high-power tunable three-level operation of double cladding pumped Nd-doped fiber laser, *IEEE Photon. Tech. Lett.* 17: 306–308, 2005.

15. Akulov, V. A., D. M. Afanasiev, S. A. Babin, D. V. Churkin, S. I. Kablukov, M. A. Rybakov, and A. A. Vlasov, Frequency tuning and doubling in Yb-doped fiber lasers, *Laser Phys.* 17: 124–129, 2007.

16. Mokhtar, M. R., C. S. Goh, S. A. Butler, S. Y. Set, K. Kikuchi, D. J. Richardson, and M. Ibsen, Fiber Bragg grating compression-tuned over 110-nm, *Electron. Lett.* 39: 509–511, 2003.

17. Chen, H., F. Babin, M. Leblanc, and G. W. Schinn, Widely tunable single-frequency erbium-doped fiber lasers, *IEEE Photon. Tech. Lett.* 15: 185–187, 2003.

18. Hideur, A., T. Chartier, and C. Ozkul, All-fiber tunable ytterbium-doped double-clad fiber ring laser, *Opt. Lett.* 26: 1054–1056, 2001.

19. Yeh, C-H., T-T. Huang, H-C. Chien, C-H. Ko, and S. Chi, Tunable S-band erbium-doped triple-ring laser with single-longitudinal-mode operation, *Opt. Express* 15: 382–386, 2007.

20. Zheng, L., J. Vaillancourt, C. Armiento, and X. Lu, Thermo-optically tunable fiber ring laser without any mechanical moving parts, *Opt. Eng.* 45: 070503, 2005.

21. Kang, M. S., M. S. Lee, J. C. Yong, and B. Y. Kim, Characterization of wavelength-tunable single-frequency fiber laser employing acoustooptic tunable filter, *IEEE J. Lightwave Tech.* 24: 1812–1823, 2006.

22. Yun, S. H., D. J. Richardson, D. O. Culverhouse, and B. Y. Kim, Wavelength-swept fiber laser with frequency shifted feedback and resonantly swept intra-cavity acoustooptic tunable filter, *IEEE J. Select. Top. Quantum Electron.* 3: 1087–1096, 1997.

23. Duarte, F. J., *Tunable Laser Optics*, 1st edn, Elsevier-Academic, New York, 2003.

24. Kersey, A. D., M. A. Davis, H. J. Patrick, M. LeBlanc, K. P. Koo, C. G. Akins, M. A. Putnam, et al., Fiber grating sensors, *J. Lightwave Tech.* 15: 1442–1463, 1997.

25. Duarte, F. J., Variable linewidth high-power TEA CO_2 laser, *Appl. Opt.* 24: 34–37, 1985.

26. Duarte, F. J., Multiple-prism Littrow and grazing-incidence pulsed CO_2 lasers, *Appl. Opt.* 24: 1244–1245, 1985.

27. Sze, R. C., and D. G. Harris, Tunable excimer lasers. In F. J. Duarte (Ed.), *Tunable Lasers Handbook*, Chapter 3, Academic, New York, 1995.

28. Duarte, F. J., Dispersive external-cavity semiconductor lasers. In F. J. Duarte (Ed.), *Tunable Laser Applications*, 1st edn, Chapter 3, Marcel-Dekker, New York, 1995.

29. Zorabedian, P., Tunable external-cavity semiconductor lasers. In F. J. Duarte (Ed.), *Tunable Lasers Handbook*, Chapter 8, Academic, New York, 1995.

30. Shen, D. Y., J. K., Sahu, and W. A. Clarkson, Highly efficient Er, Yb-doped fiber laser with 188 W free running and >100 W tunable output power, *Opt. Express* 13: 4916–4921, 2005.

31. Schäfer, F. P. (Ed.), *Dye Lasers*, Springer, Berlin, 1990.

32. Duarte, F. J., Narrow linewidth pulsed dye laser oscillators. In F. J. Duarte and L. W. Hillman (Eds), *Dye Laser Principles*, Chapter 4, Academic, New York, 1990.

33. Duarte, F. J., W. E. Davenport, J. J. Ehrlich, and T. S. Taylor, Ruggedized narrow-linewidth dispersive dye laser oscillator, *Opt. Commun.* 84: 310–316, 1991.

34. Duarte, F. J., and J. A. Piper, Narrow-linewidth, high-prf copper laser-pumped dye-laser oscillators, *Appl. Opt.* 23: 1391–1394, 1984.

35. Duarte, F. J., Solid-state multiple-prism grating dye-laser oscillators, *Appl. Opt.* 33: 3857–3860, 1994.

36. Koplow, P., L. Golberg, R. P. Moeller, and D. A. V. Kliner, Single-mode operation of a coiled multimode fiber amplifier, *Opt. Lett.* 25: 442–444, 2000.

37. Auerbach, M., P. Adel, D. Wandt, C. Fallnich, S. Unger, S. Jetschke, and H-R. Müller, 10 W widely tunable narrow linewidth double-clad fiber ring laser, *Opt. Express* 10: 139–144, 2002.

38. Duarte, F. J., and J. A. Piper, Prism preexpanded grazing-incidence grating cavity for pulsed dye lasers, *Appl. Opt.* 20: 2113–2116, 1981.

39. Jeong, Y., J. Nilsson, J. K. Sahu, D. N. Payne, R. Horley, L. M. B. Hickey, and P. W. Turner, Power scaling of single-frequency Ytterbium-doped fiber master-oscillator power-amplifier sources up to 500-W, *IEEE J. Select. Top. Quantum Electron.* 13: 546–551, 2007.

40. Feng, Y., L. R. Taylor, and D. B. Calia, 25 W Raman-fiber-amplifier-based 589 nm laser for laser guide star, *Opt. Express* 17: 19021–19026, 2009.

41. Henry, L. J., T. M. Shay, G. T. Moore, and G. R. Grosek, Seeded Raman amplifier for applications in the 1100–1500 nm spectral region, U.S. Patent 8472486 B1, 2013.

42. F. J. Duarte, *Tunable Laser Optics*, 2nd edn, CRC Press, New York, 2015.

43. Bass, I. L., R. E. Bonanno, R. H., Hackel, and P. R. Hammond, High-average power dye laser at Lawrence Livermore National Laboratory, *Appl. Opt.* 31: 6993–7006, 1992.

7 Fiber Laser Overview and Medical Applications

S. Popov

CONTENTS

7.1 INTRODUCTION

Fiber lasers began their remarkable history in the early 1960s, when the first working laser of its kind was demonstrated, and very soon after, optical fibers with reasonably small attenuation were developed [1,2]. Initially, optical fibers mainly found application in signal transmission in optical telecom networks. It took about two decades before fully functional fiber-based optical amplifiers and fiber lasers appeared on the scene of research and industrial applications. Optical fibers with different dopants, mainly rare earth metal ions, have opened virtually unlimited opportunities as unique gain materials operating in the near- and mid-infrared (IR) bands of the optical spectrum. Currently, fibers of complicated chemical structure with gain properties in the far IR, over 3 µm, are being actively explored [3–6].

The earliest implementations of fibers in active optical components were realized in fiber lasers and fiber-optical amplifiers (FOAs) almost simultaneously [7,8].

Originally targeted to enhance the performance of fiber-optic networks for telecommunications, erbium-doped fiber amplifiers (EDFAs) have stimulated the development of a large class of fiber lasers with an outstanding performance record. Such lasers have quickly found their own place in various research and industrial areas. Rapidly progressing technology in the development of lasing materials and the sophisticated design of optical fibers have firmly positioned fiber lasers as indispensable leaders in such fields as the automotive and processing industry, machinery, metrology, telecom, the biosciences, and medicine.

Medicine and the biosciences are important fields for implementing fiber lasers. Interest has been significantly driven by the fortunate matching of a wide variety of wavelengths generated by fiber lasers to several absorption spectral bands of organic compounds and water-based (or hydroxyl-based) molecule groups, found in a wide variety of organic tissues and living cells. Various operational regimes—continuous wave (CW), Q-switched, or mode-locked—along with wavelength tunability have opened additional opportunities for fiber lasers in this field. During the infancy period of fiber lasers, before versatile gain materials with rich sets of transition spectra were developed, their medical applications were primarily in laser micromachining and the marking of instruments and tools used in surgery, dentistry, and ophthalmology.

A fair amount of information and discussion about recent achievements, technical performance, and ubiquitous applications of fiber lasers is continually generated in the literature, from scientific journals to commercial booklets and manuals. In this survey, we present key areas of fiber lasers used in medicine-related branches. This chapter focuses on practical applications of fiber lasers and their specific advantages provided by radiation with tunable wavelengths for medical tasks, whereas most physical aspects and design details related to laser tunability itself are discussed in Chapter 6. It is worth mentioning that fiber lasers have not been the first actors in laser history to demonstrate impressive tunability. In this context, dye lasers might be considered direct competitors of fiber lasers due to broadband wavelength tenability accompanied by high-intensity radiation, especially in Q-switched or mode-locked operation regimes. Chapter 8 provides an excellent basis to make a comparative analysis for trade-offs in both types of lasers.

Since fiber lasers are part of a larger laser group, it is reasonable to start with a short overview of common laser usage in medicine, in both clinical and research areas. It is also instructive to recollect the main physical principles of the interaction of laser radiation with organic tissues, as well as the basics of the gain properties and operation principles of fiber lasers.

7.2   LASERS IN MEDICINE AND LIFE SCIENCES

Even before early lasers had left research laboratories for industrial applications, medicine was considered an important "consumer" of laser technologies, first as manufacturing tools for medical instruments, then as working instruments themselves. Practically all types of laser have found their specific niches in important branches of medicine: research, monitoring, imaging, probing, therapy, surgery, and others. Referring to more specific applications, lasers are used literally everywhere: in biomedical investigation, for fluorescent spectroscopy, microscopy, and flow cytometry; in surgery, for "bloodless" operations in cardiology and on abdominal and thoracic organs, and for skull and brain microsurgery; in cosmetics and aesthetic medicine, for smoothing wrinkles, resurfacing the skin, and bleaching tattoos; in therapy, for the treatment of cancer, spider veins, and vascular dysfunction; in diagnostics, for endoscopic investigations and optical coherence tomography (OCT). This list can be extended further by going more deeply into subclassifications and interdisciplinary topics.

Depending on the particular requirements, numerous types of lasers can provide different wavelengths, energy levels, and operation modes. As a short overview, Table 7.1 provides some examples of the most typical and commercially available systems, as well as their particular uses.

Fiber lasers should be considered successors of trends in medical applications rather than "pioneers" discovering untouched fields. However, due to the inherent flexibility of their physical principles and design, as well as their outstanding performance, fiber lasers have enormous potential to bring new opportunities to medicine.

Before specifying the particular applications of fiber lasers in medicine, it is instructive to briefly depict some of the main fields in which lasers are commonly used for health care, monitoring, and research regardless of which particular type of laser is considered. Such a classification is commonly arranged according to how organic tissues react to laser radiation.

TABLE 7.1
Main Laser Types and Fields of Application in Medicine

Laser Type and Operation Mode	Wavelength (µm)	Application
Carbon dioxide (cw, pulsed)	10.6	Surgery: general and eye; dental therapy
Argon (cw)	0.488, 0.514	Sealing blood vessels in retina, eye microsurgery, plastic surgery, photodynamic therapy
Nd:YAG (cw, Q-switched)	1.06	General surgery, dentistry: therapy and surgery
Nd:YAG (Q-switched)	0.532 (double frequency)	Surgery, ophthalmology, dermatology, cosmetic, photodynamic therapy
Ruby (Q-switched)	0.694	Plastic surgery, dermatology, photodynamic therapy
Er:YAG (Q-switched)	2.94	Skin resurfacing (superficial ablation), dental therapy and surgery
Ho:YAG (cw, pulsed)	2.12	Ablation, incision, tissue hemostatic vaporization, cancer tumor treatment
Diode lasers (cw, pulsed)	0.63, 0.82, 0.83, 0.98, 1.45	Photodynamic therapy, endovenous treatment, aesthetic medicine, vascular lesions
Alexandrite lasers (cw, Q-switched)	0.755	Pigmented lesions, tattoo bleaching, vascular lesions, skin treatment, hair removal
Dye lasers (cw, Q-switched, tunable)	0.570–0.650	Treatment of malignant tissues, photodynamic therapy, cosmetic, vascular lesions, hair removal

7.2.1 Optical versus Thermal Response

Using the terminology adopted among medical professionals, the reaction of organic tissues to laser radiation is typically described as either an optical or a thermal response (Figure 7.1) [9,10]. In the optical response, the light energy absorbed does not damage or destroy the tissues. Most effects are achieved either (1) by selective resonance absorption of specific laser wavelengths by fluorophores or photosensitizers with sequentially photoinduced changes of the tissues or (2) by exposure with short light pulses of high peak intensity leading to material ablation. The thermal response is normally produced by cw or long-pulse laser radiation, when higher power delivered to organs is converted to heat and destroys the surrounding tissue. How tissues react to laser radiation depends in particular on the chosen wavelength, mode of operation, pulse duration, and energy, as well as the laser spot size.

The optical response is fundamental to various therapeutic and cosmetic treatments using physical and chemical photoinduced processes, either directly or as side effects. The former are based on the direct absorption of light by organic compounds and cells naturally constituting the tissues, with subsequent conversion of the energy, through nonradiative transitions, into chemical changes or tissue ablation. A second type of photoinduced effect exploits light absorption by specialized photoacceptors (photosensitizers) or separate molecules that are not natural parts of the tissues but are artificially injected into the patient's body for treatment. The molecules transfer the energy to other agents, such as rhodopsin, phytochrome, or chlorophyll, which participate in the activation of chemical reactions in the tissue and its surroundings [10]. For example, these reactions are essential for photodynamic therapy (PDT) of tumors or for treating skin diseases in dermatology (Figure 7.1). The photosensitizers alone are harmless and have no effect on either healthy or abnormal tissues until they are illuminated with light of the necessary wavelength. Typically, treatment and therapy based on the optical response do not require high-power laser radiation.

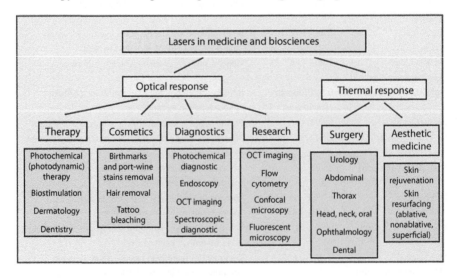

FIGURE 7.1 General applications of lasers in medicine and life sciences.

An example of PDT without using external agents is the removal of port-wine stains, reddish birthmarks typically found on the neck or face. Port-wine stains, which consist of thousands of blood vessels, are exposed to green laser light and are literally burned away. The surrounding skin remains unharmed and unheated, since it does not absorb the green light as efficiently as the red formations. A similar procedure is used to remove tattoos when the colors are bleached with appropriately chosen laser light. For this type of PDT, laser wavelength is a crucial parameter, because the efficiency of the procedure strongly depends on how accurately the wavelength matches the resonance absorption of the treated tissue. Thus, the ability to tune the laser wavelength, as first demonstrated in dye lasers (Table 7.1), is essentially a favorable feature for this application [11].

Another example of the optical response without resonance absorption of laser radiation is the scattering or attenuation of light during its propagation inside a tissue. The physical and chemical properties of the surrounding area remain unchanged during this process, which is extensively used for investigation purposes. One of the best-known uses of such scattering is OCT, introduced in the early 1990s [12,13]. This noninvasive imaging technique is primarily conducted by the low-coherence Michelson interferometer. It requires broadband light sources, such as supercontinuum (SC) or short-pulse lasers, and provides resolution of the order of micrometers, with possible penetration to a depth of millimeters inside the tissue to be investigated. These days, OCT is rapidly developing as a versatile investigation method, in demand in practically all branches of the life sciences [14–18].

Compared with nondestructive optical effects, the thermal response of the laser–tissue interaction involves damage to treated organic matter: cutting, fragmentation, vaporization, or coagulation. Such destructive changes are caused by intensive heating of the tissues by high-power radiation, delivered by either cw or pulsed lasers.

Traditionally, the best-known and most popular medical application for lasers using the light–tissue thermal response is surgery. It can include both open and endoscopic implementations. In the latter case, laser energy is delivered by a fiber to the treated organ without dissecting the patient's body, for example, through large blood vessels in cardiovascular operations, or through urethral channels. Focused to a microscopic dot of high energy density, the laser beam works as the tiniest of cutting and cauterizing instruments [10,19,20].

Resonance absorption of laser radiation by water contained in organic tissues is a main cause of the thermal laser–tissue response. Such absorption is used to produce different results, depending on the mode and power of the laser applied. Operating in the pulse mode, either Q switched or cw modulated, the laser heats water very rapidly to several hundred degrees Celsius. The overheated water expands explosively, and, depending on the hardness of the tissue, either breaks it into fragments (e.g., tiny stones) or vaporizes it into medium–hard substances. The energy absorption in water takes place regardless of the composition, hardness, or color of the tissue, and enables a highly efficient procedure, roughly the same for both hard and soft tissues. Due to this instantaneous impact, heating is restricted to the area in the immediate vicinity, while the surrounding area remains almost unaffected. Such thermal ablation is useful in many surgical treatments. By varying the power and pulse duration of the laser, it is possible to achieve different impacts on various organs and tissues.

Use of high-energy short pulses increases the effect in lithotripsy (stone fragmentation), while operating with longer pulses enhances coagulation. This is another irrefutable advantage of laser "scalpels," an excellent alternative to traditional methods. In such cases, typical pulse repetition rates can vary between 10 and 20 Hz.

Laser surgery is also a well-established technique used in dentistry. With precise tuning of the radiation wavelength, one can selectively adjust absorption of the laser pulses by different parts of the teeth, either enamel or dentin. This can significantly relieve the patient's sensations of pain and irritation during the drilling and burning typical of the work necessary to repair tooth cavities. Lasers also make dental procedures more accurate.

Another branch, ophthalmology, is probably the most "natural" area for noninvasive treatments applying medical lasers. Propagating through the transparent cornea and crystal, laser light can be directly used for restoring detached retinas, removing blood vessels, treating glaucoma, or reshaping the cornea.

It is not an exaggeration to say that the combination of laser and fiber-optic technology has revolutionized noninvasive surgery. For example, cutting prostate or superficial bladder cancer tumors, lithotripsy, and vessel treatment with lasers are hugely beneficial. An optical fiber inserted into a blood vessel through a needle-sized opening can deliver laser light to practically any part of the blood system and enable noninvasive angioplasty, that is, the removal of fatty plaques from arteries, to prevent heart attacks or strokes caused by clogged blood vessels. This approach can also be used to perform endovenous laser treatment to cure spider and varicose veins. A comprehensive review of the laser methods used for health care is given in [9,10].

More examples of the laser applications not included in Figure 7.1 will be discussed in the sections considering particular types of fiber lasers. In comparison with other fields that use fiber lasers, medicine and bioscience do not demand very high-power instruments, say in the kilowatt range that is typical for machinery or the automotive industry. Depending on which of the two main effects of laser radiation on the organic tissues is required—optical or thermal—fiber lasers with an average power of between hundreds of milliwatts and tens of watts are needed.

Although it will be briefly discussed in Section 7.4.7, we omitted from Figure 7.1 one more application marginally related to medicine: the implementation of lasers for making and marking medical instruments, components, and devices. This involves the interaction of radiation with inorganic materials (metals, plastics, ceramics) rather than the treatment of biological tissues. For such tasks, fiber-based systems delivering necessary power at the corresponding wavelengths are becoming widely used.

To elucidate the reasons for their leading role, as well as to comprehend the advantages and potential of fiber lasers in medicine, we should review the basic features of these lasers.

7.3 PRINCIPLES, TYPES, AND PERFORMANCE OF FIBER LASERS

Optical fibers can be used in fiber lasers either as a gain medium, combined with the cavity functionality, or as a passive part of the laser cavity, solely to realize conditions for forming cavity modes. In the latter case, another active component, such as a semiconductor gain material, should be included for amplification and lasing. Here, we consider exclusively "classical" fiber lasers, that is, those using the optical fibers as key components for the gain, building up the modes, and lasing.

7.3.1 HOST FIBERS: SILICA-, PHOSPHATE-, AND FLUORIDE-BASED GLASSES

Amplification in optical fibers is realized by embedding dopants in the form of ions of rare earth metals into host fibers. These dopants provide specific energy transitions available for laser generation. The main host materials used in contemporary optical fibers are silica, silica fluoride, and phosphate-based glasses. Traditional silica-based fibers are employed in lasers based on direct transition, 3- (4-)level schemes. For most rare earth ions, easily allowed lasing transitions are allocated in near- and mid-IR bands. Until recently, this property precluded developing fiber lasers in the visible range, although there exist numerous medical applications demanding lasers with these wavelengths (Table 7.1).

Advances in the development of two novel types of fibers, phosphate- and fluoride-based glasses, have dramatically increased progress with high-power and efficient fiber lasers. Phosphate fibers provide higher internal gain in comparison with silica-based fibers, and enable more efficient and higher-power fiber lasers with very short active fibers [21,22]. Another family member is the ZBLAN fiber, a fluoride-based fiber incorporating additives of heavy metals such as zirconium or lead, and a more complicated composition of barium, lanthanum, aluminum, and sodium. The acronym ZBLAN stands for its components. ZBLAN fibers demonstrate important advantages: they exhibit high transparency in the mid-IR range, whereas silica-based fibers start to absorb around 2 µm; and rare earth dopants in ZBLAN fibers reduce the quenching caused by multiphonon transitions, thus increasing the lifetime of metastable states. Therefore, ZBLAN fibers have encouraged the development of a novel class of fiber lasers exploiting upconversion, or excited-state transitions (ESTs), and radiating in the visible range [23,24]. Although fluoride-based fibers are not free from problems, such as fragility and absorbing ambient moisture (mainly water), the rapid development of glass materials demonstrates considerable progress with ZBLAN fiber lasers [25,26].

Active optical fibers utilizing different host glasses and various active rare earth dopants allow near-IR, mid-IR, and visible parts of the spectrum to be covered. More details, energy-level structures, and corresponding wavelengths for different fiber lasers will be discussed along with particular applications in further sections.

7.3.2 GAIN MEDIA

To build a complete fiber laser, the gain fiber should be equipped with two reflectors playing the roles of back mirror and output coupler/mirror. They can be either traditional external mirrors using free-space optics components to couple the light in and out of fibers, or deposited directly on the fiber facets; or components embedded inside fibers, for example, fiber Bragg gratings (FBGs) [27]. An intermediate variant for the back mirror is a semiconductor saturable absorbing mirror (SESAM) (Figure 7.2), which is an external semiconductor device fiber-coupled to the gain fiber [28].

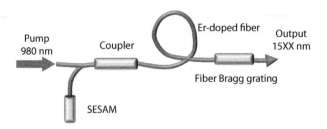

FIGURE 7.2   Classical design of fiber laser using SESAM as a back mirror. Depending on the particular parameters of the SESAM, the laser can operate in Q-switched or mode-locked regime.

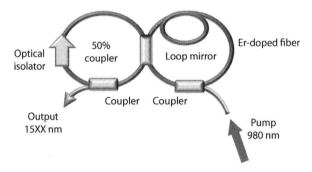

FIGURE 7.3   Mode-locked fiber laser with loop-mirror cavity design with a nonlinear fiber to obtain femtosecond pulse generation.

Some applications, such as nonthermal ablation in dentistry, sophisticated micro-surgery in the human brain, or refractive eye surgery, combined with an endoscopic approach, require fiber lasers generating ultrashort pulses, in the picosecond or femtosecond range [29,30]. To achieve this goal, a fiber loop mirror and a strongly nonlinear fiber in the gain section can be used (Figure 7.3). Strong fiber nonlin-earity is commonly used to manipulate the fiber dispersion properties over a wide wavelength bandwidth, which is in demand to create ultrashort optical pulses [31]. Recent progress with photonics crystal fibers (PCFs), or fibers having a crystal-like structure in their cross section (Figure 7.4), has brought novel opportunities for creat-ing extremely broadband and ultrafast fiber lasers [32]. In certain cases, possessing a very sophisticated design (Figure 7.5), such fibers can provide conditions for zero-dispersion and single-mode operation over a very wide wavelength range, creating high gain, and maintaining high power density inside the core [33,34]. These are important issues for the practical realization of fiber lasers in medicine.

As they do not affect essential operational or performance parameters, we do not specify laser cavity details or the output-coupling design of fiber lasers in this survey. For a discussion on cavities for tunable fiber lasers, please refer to Chapter 6. To focus on medical applications, we discuss the gain material, operating mode (cw or pulsed), wavelength, and energy characteristics, such as average power or pulse energy. All these parameters are relevant to specific applications of interest for fiber lasers in medicine.

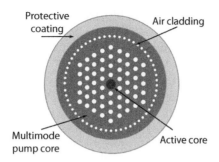

FIGURE 7.4 Schematic overview of most typical PCF cross section.

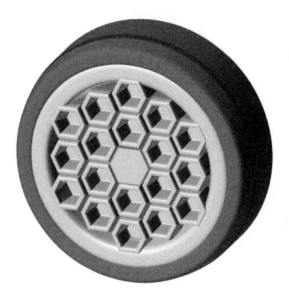

FIGURE 7.5 Examples of crystal fibers designed for double-cladding pumping schemes and supercontinuum fiber laser sources.

7.3.3 LASING WAVELENGTHS

An essential parameter for medical applications is wavelength, which defines how efficiently the laser radiation is transmitted, scattered, or absorbed by the tissue. For example, 2–3 μm wavelengths are suitable for accurate cutting, removing, or coagulation of soft tissues due to the strong absorption of this radiation by water present in the majority of biological objects [35,36]. On the other hand, radiation within the wavelength band of 650–1200 nm can penetrate up to several millimeters into tissue, which is advantageous for imaging and diagnostic procedures [37]. Various fiber lasers are capable of generating a rather large set of wavelengths using various physical phenomena.

The main and most developed approach is doping the fibers with different rare earth ions, such as erbium (Er^{3+}), praseodymium (Pr^{3+}), thulium (Tm^{3+}), neodymium

(Nd^{3+}), holmium (Ho^{3+}), or ytterbium (Yb^{3+}). Direct energy transitions characteristic of these elements cover almost the whole near- and mid-IR range of the spectrum. A complementary method to build fiber lasers operating in the visible spectrum is the use of upconversion transitions. With this technique, also known as *excited-state absorption*, several ladder-like energy levels of rare earth ion are excited sequentially to reach the highest lasing level. Compared with classical laser schemes, the lasing wavelength is shorter than the pumping one in this case.

Figure 7.6 displays one of the typical transition structures for the thulium fiber laser radiating in the blue range [38]. However, such a scheme requires rather high pump intensity and intermediate levels with long lifetimes. Standard silica-based fibers are not capable of providing such features. The problem can be resolved with ZBLAN fibers using fluoride-based materials mentioned in Section 7.3.1. With increased lifetimes of the intermediate levels, it is easier to start upconversion lasing. Recently demonstrated upconversion fiber lasers covering the visible spectrum from blue to red, using erbium, praseodymium, and thulium ions, have been reported [39–42]. Lasers in the visible spectrum are in high demand for numerous therapies and noninvasive treatments for dermatology, aesthetic medicine, cosmetic surgery, and cancer PDT (Table 7.1).

Another effect enabling more lasing frequencies from fiber lasers is stimulated Raman scattering (SRS) producing the Raman gain inside the fiber [43–45]. This strongly nonlinear phenomenon reveals itself under high-intensity pumping, typically provided by another laser, semiconductor, or fiber. The remarkable feature of the Raman gain is its manifestation in practically all fibers and its frequency dependence on the pump wavelength only rather than on a particular fiber material. The lasing wavelength is typically shifted 80–100 nm apart from the pumping source. With several pairs of FBGs nested into each other, one can shift the Raman gain in several steps, thus realizing a cascaded Raman laser with wavelength transfer up to

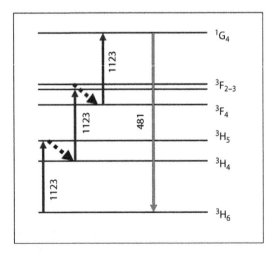

FIGURE 7.6 Energy levels of thulium (Tm^{3+}) ions, showing how multiphoton excitation with 1123 nm wavelength results in blue fluorescence through upconversion (dotted arrows denote relaxation transitions).

hundreds of nanometers [46]. The efficiency and strength of the Raman gain can be manipulated by the appropriate chemical composition of the fiber compounds and the suitable design of the fiber core [47].

7.3.4 PUMPING AND LASER EFFICIENCY

In addition to the generous choice of available wavelengths and tunability, fiber lasers offer attractive conversion efficiencies. More pumping energy is converted into useful radiation than into heating the gain media, which makes it possible to abandon bulky cooling systems. This leads to smaller sizes, simpler construction, and lower costs of reliable turnkey devices. With optimized pumping sources and carefully engineered active fiber cores, pump-lasing optical efficiencies of about 20%–30% are routinely reported for fibers with almost all rare ion dopants [6,21,26]. For some elements with a "lucky" energy structure, such as Yb^{3+} dopants, considered in Section 7.4.2, optical conversion efficiency of 80% and up to 30% wall-plug efficiencies have been reported [48,49].

In addition to high conversion efficiencies, the excellent heat dissipation of fiber lasers is facilitated by a large surface-to-volume ratio of the active medium. Gradual pump absorption and smooth distribution of the amplification within the fiber provide high beam quality of the guided mode, which is defined by the core design rather than pumping or generated power. This is a significant advantage for high-power devices. Near-perfect resistance to power dissipation and heating, as well as to thermal optical problems, makes fiber lasers good candidates for power scaling. Being coupled with negligible losses into amplifying fibers and strictly confined within the core, the pumping wave interacts efficiently with the lasing radiation. This results in a low pump threshold and high gain, which can be an order of magnitude larger than in crystalline solid-state lasers. Really high-power fiber lasers operating in the cw mode (kilowatt-class and more) have been routinely reported and have become commercially available during recent years [50–52].

However, lasers requiring high pump intensity may suffer from nonlinear effects, which can worsen conditions and cause beam quality distortion. Fortunately, there are some techniques and solutions to overcome the nonlinear phenomena induced by high power [31]. On the other hand, nonlinear effects such as SRS or stimulated Brillouin scattering (SBS), can, under proper control, provide additional opportunities for wavelength conversion, as was exemplified in Section 7.3.3 [46,53].

An important factor contributing to the growth in popularity, and applicability, of fiber lasers is pumping solutions. Rapid progress in the development of high-power laser diodes continually leads to the gradual displacement of other pump sources, such as flashlamps and traditional lasers. Until recently, a high-quality beam could be generated by a single-mode fiber laser in which the pumping beam also propagated in the same core. This used to restrict the output power of the laser to only tens of milliwatts. Using multimode fibers to enhance pumping and lasing power would immediately destroy the beam quality. An efficient alternative to increase the fiber laser power, yet maintain the high quality of the beam, is the implementation of double-clad pumping. This breakthrough technology utilizes crystal fibers with inner cladding placed between the main core (which, in turn, has a complicated

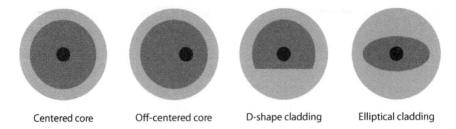

Centered core   Off-centered core   D-shape cladding   Elliptical cladding

FIGURE 7.7 Different shapes of double-clad fibers to improve pump-lasing mode overlapping.

structure, e.g., PCF) and outer cladding, and separated from each other by air holes (Figure 7.4).

The double-clad pumping technique considerably relaxes the requirements for the quality of pump sources. Due to the high numerical aperture (NA) of the PCF, a low-quality beam from a high-power diode laser can be easily launched into the fiber, and can propagate while trapped inside the inner cladding. The simple circular symmetry shown in Figures 7.4 and 7.5 does not ensure the best possible coupling between the pumping and lasing modes, because the light partially propagates as skewed "beams" outside the central core. Avoiding circular symmetry in the PCF mitigates the problem of poor pump/lasing mode overlap. The most commonly used alternatives for the double-clad design (shown in Figure 7.7) can admit low-quality high-power pumping and provide efficient absorption by the active area [54,55].

Employing symmetry-broken double-clad pumping in crystal fibers produces several advantages in one step. First, due to much better pump/lasing overlap and an enlarged core area (50–60 μm in comparison with the traditional 12 μm in standard single-mode fibers), high-power lasing can be obtained in a shorter fiber. This significantly reduces the risk of nonlinear phenomena, such as self-phase modulation, SBS, or undesired SRS. On the other hand, inherent physical properties of the PCF restrict the lasing to a single-mode field across the whole large-mode area (LMA) for broad wavelength bands. Single-mode cw operation of almost diffraction-limited quality (factor M2 < 1.05) was demonstrated with 100–500 W fiber lasers [50,56,57]. Finally, due to the LMA, implementing multidiode pumping is a natural solution to combine a single-mode operation, capability for power scaling, and excellent conditions for heat dissipation, described at the start of this section. Fiber lasers with power-independent beam quality and delivering output power levels in the kilowatt range, in both cw and pulse mode, have been increasingly reported [58–60].

7.3.5 Advantages and Challenges

Summarizing the basic facts about fiber lasers, one can argue that they might gradually replace other types of lasers employed in branches of biomedicine. As discussed at the beginning of the chapter, laser radiation at practically all wavelengths, both visible and IR, is in great demand for medical applications. One of the main obstacles precluding successful "switching" of traditional procedures and methods in medicine to relevant laser technologies is the cost of the equipment.

Considerably lower costs for fiber lasers are mainly based on higher lasing efficiency and excellent heat dissipation performance, which allow cooling systems to be abandoned and many advanced systems to be reduced to A4 footprint size. Rather cheap and simple maintenance is also a considerable contribution to increasing fiber laser competitiveness.

There is no significant price variation for fiber lasers depending on wavelength, operation mode, and power (except a minor scaling factor for the pump diode costs), since they exploit the same physical principles and similar material technologies.

Depending on the particular biomedical application, fiber lasers can operate in all required regimes—cw, pulsed, Q-switched, or mode-locked—producing the necessary power. The additional advantages of fiber lasers are wavelength tunability and power-independent high-quality beams deliverable directly to an application area without coupling losses.

Although only certain types of fiber lasers have been established in the medical market so far, numerous promising results for biomedicine and medical applications are continually being demonstrated in research laboratories and preliminary clinical trials.

7.4 GAIN MATERIAL AND OPERATION MODE— RELATION TO PARTICULAR APPLICATIONS

In the previous sections, we outlined general laser uses in medicine and bioscience, and reviewed some of the basics of fiber lasers. Here, we are going to depict application examples customary for particular types of fiber lasers. Since the diversity of applications exceeds the range of lasers available, it is more instructive to link a certain laser type to relevant applications rather than vice versa. It is also more convenient to discuss fiber lasers in reference to the dopant ions responsible for amplification in the active fibers, because other features, such as wavelength, power, and cw/pulsed operation mode, cannot be attributed uniquely to any laser in particular.

Although almost all rare earth metal ions have been tested and investigated for possible lasing with direct, upconversion, or Raman-shifted transitions, only a limited number have been demonstrated as practical active media in fiber lasers [61]. Thus, our discussion will concern only those rare earth ions that are used in fiber lasers outside research laboratories: erbium, thulium, ytterbium, holmium, neodymium, and praseodymium (Table 7.2). As host materials, both silica- and fluoride-based fibers are used where they can demonstrate particular advantages.

7.4.1 ERBIUM LASERS

Erbium-doped lasers can be considered veterans and founders of the family of fiber lasers. A manifold energy level structure with easily allowed transitions made them a popular object of research and applications. The set of most often used transitions, shown in Figure 7.8, offers numerous opportunities to build erbium fiber lasers [58].

Soon after the pioneering demonstration of broadband amplification and lasing in the near-IR range around 1500–1600 nm [62–64], erbium-doped fiber lasers became widely applied in the fields of medicine and biology. Their use in OCT is well

TABLE 7.2

Rare Earth Metal Ions Commonly Used in Fiber Lasers, and Laser Applications in Medicine

Laser, Host Fiber and Operation Mode	Wavelengths (μm)	Applications
Er^{3+}; silica; ZBLAN; cw, pulsed	0.55, 1.5–1.6, 2.7, 3	Optical coherence tomography; cosmetic surgery and therapy; soft-tissue surgery
Yb^{3+}; silica; ZBLAN; cw, pulsed	0.98–1.1, 0.512–0.532 (SHG)	Optical coherence tomography; dermatology; PDT; soft- and hard-tissue surgery; dentistry, gynecology
Tm^{3+}; silica; ZBLAN; cw, pulsed	0.48, 0.8, 1.45–1.53, 1.7–2.1	Surgery: thorax, otolaryngology, urology, ophthalmology, cardiology, neurosurgery; lithotripsy
Nd^{3+}; silica; cw, pulsed	0.9–0.95, 1.03–1.1, 1.32–1.35	Dentistry; hard-tissue surgery; orthopedic surgery
Ho^{3+}; silica; ZBLAN; cw, pulsed	2.1, 2.8–2.9	Gastroenterology with endoscopic or direct access; surgery on blood-rich tissues; lithotripsy
Pr^{3+}; silica, ZBLAN; cw, pulsed	0.49, 0.52, 0.6, 0.635, 1.3	Cosmetic surgery and therapy; cancer therapy; photodynamic therapy

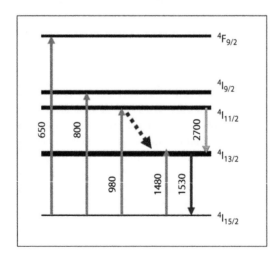

FIGURE 7.8 Energy levels of erbium (Er^{3+}) ions and main transitions (in nanometers) in silica-based fibers used to obtain amplification and lasing.

documented [65,66]. Since promising performance was shown with erbium lasers, other fiber lasers have manifested their potential to replace the complicated and expensive femtosecond-pulsed lasers commonly used in OCT systems [67,68]. Briefly, the OCT method is based on the use of a Michelson interferometer with a broadband light source. Unlike the classical Michelson interferometer, in which the light propagates in free space between a beam splitter and mirrors, a fiber-based four-port optical coupler (typically of 50/50 splitting ratio) plays the role of beam splitter, whereby two output optical fibers form the two-arm interferometric system to deliver the optical signal both to the object under investigation and to the reference mirror (Figure 7.9).

The broadband spectrum of the source results in the low coherence of radiation and considerably limits the area of high visibility of the interference pattern. Thus, high visibility (or a high-intensity peak on an interferogram; see Chapter 12) is achieved when full optical paths of the light in the "probe" and reference arms are equal with high accuracy. If light in the probe arm is scattered by some material, the position of the scanning mirror in the reference arm defines a corresponding tiny area inside the tissue, which scatters most of the light contributing to the interfering signal. By displacing the mirror and processing the scattered signal, one can restore the information about the tissue properties, depending on the depth. By choosing the appropriate broadband light source and suitable central wavelength within the IR range, the tissue structure can be imaged to a depth of several millimeters due to good penetration of this radiation into biological objects. The short coherence length due to the broadband spectrum results in smaller tissue volume, contributing to the main interferometric response and higher spatial resolution. Since the probe light is scattered by all regions in the tissue where it propagates and produces noisy background scattering, a high-brightness source is required to provide a strong response signal. Classical light sources, such as high-intensity tungsten or xenon lamps, cannot compete with fiber lasers or optical amplifiers generating broadband amplified spontaneous emission (ASE). The results reported with Er-doped fiber lasers have stimulated development of other broadband fiber-based light sources for OCT applications, including SC lasers and low-noise ASE amplifiers [69–71].

Cosmetic therapy and surgery is one more field that is being conquered by erbium-doped fiber lasers, mainly with radiation wavelength around 1550 nm. A challenging application of these lasers is treating wrinkles and skin photoaging due to UV exposure, which is unavoidable in everyday life. The final effect of photoaging might be very unpleasant, since sunlight causes thinning of the epidermis and can lead to the growth of skin lesions, such as actinic keratoses and cell carcinomas [72].

Treating wrinkles or photoaging is a procedure of skin resurfacing that can be performed in both ablative and nonablative forms. Traditionally practiced ablative

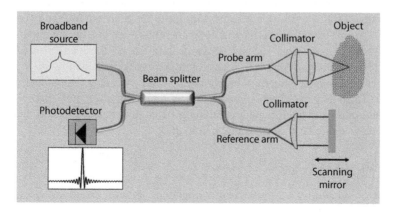

FIGURE 7.9 Simplified scheme of the optical coherence tomography setup.

treatments exploit high-power lasers and can be a rather painful procedure with a long recovery time. The laser removes the overlying epidermal skin surface with the subsequent growth of renewed tissue. With nonablative skin resurfacing, a fiber laser with subablative energy pulses generates heat within dermal connective tissue without necessarily removing the overlying skin surface. Such a method offers higher efficiency, more convenient handling, and lower risks of side effects as compared with the use of traditional lasers in this area. A commercially available 1550 nm system has demonstrated very promising results in the nonablative treatment of atrophic facial acne with 8–16 J/cm^2 pulse energy in modulation mode [73,74].

An intermediate variant of laser therapy efficiently treating wrinkles and photoaging is fractional resurfacing. Here again, an erbium fiber laser is the main working instrument, albeit the operating mode is slightly different. High-intensity short pulses, up to 40 J/cm^2, drill small pinpoint areas of the skin. The light penetrates to the right depth, ~1.3 mm instead of the 300–800 µm attained with nonablative curing, and as it heals, the tissue tightens. This procedure has been shown to result in quick recovery after the treatment [75].

The potential uses of erbium fiber lasers in cosmetology and aesthetic medical applications are practically unlimited. This fact has apparently been recognized by leading players in the market of fiber lasers. Today, they offer a big family of lasers oriented to this branch of medicine: models with wavelengths of 1065, 1075, 1090, and 1550 nm operating in cw and modulated-pulsed modes and delivering between 10 and 100 W average power [76].

Rapid progress in the development of fibers codoped with different rare earth ions and using efficient double-clad diode pumping schemes has opened a path for erbium lasers into other branches of surgery, such as cardiology, dentistry, and ophthalmology. Using ZBLAN fluoride-based fibers doped with Er^{3+}–Yb^{3+} or Er^{3+}–Pr^{3+} combinations has made it possible to realize high-power lasers operating at wavelengths of 2.7 and 3 µm with output power up to 1 W and more [77,78]. For example, using high-intensity diode pumping with 980 nm and Pr^{3+} as a codopant allows increasing depopulation of the lower level and enables efficient lasing at the 2.7 µm transition, which is rather weak in standard silica-based fibers. Operation at 3 µm can be achieved using absorption from excited states (or upconversion) and relaxation through upper states (transition schemes similar to those shown in Figure 7.6) [79]. ZBLAN upconversion fiber lasers will be further discussed in a later section.

The growing popularity in, and active penetration of, the medical market by erbium fiber lasers operating at 2.7 and 3 µm are easily explained by their advantages over alternative counterparts such as Er^{3+}:YAG solid-state lasers operating at 2.94 µm. Since they are cheaper, more efficient, more compact, and easier to operate, the use of erbium fiber lasers is continually expanding in areas such as dentistry, dermatology, angioplasty, and ophthalmology [80].

7.4.2 Ytterbium Lasers

In terms of popularity in biomedical applications, erbium lasers are closely followed by ytterbium fiber lasers. Possessing a rather simple energy-level structure (Figure 7.10), Yb^{3+} ion transitions offer potentially high pumping efficiency due to

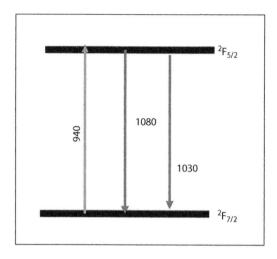

FIGURE 7.10 Two-level transition structure for Yb^{3+} ions.

their small quantum defect, that is, the energy (or frequency) difference between the pumping and lasing photons. The ytterbium laser, operating around 1 µm, offers small nonradiative losses and low heating, and provides conversion efficiencies approaching 80% and approximately 25% wall-plug efficiency.

As a result, high-power cw ytterbium fiber lasers continue to advance in the market due to lower cost, compact design, and simpler maintenance [56,81]. Numerous sublevels exhibit the broadband fluorescence spectrum, which allows tunability of the Yb^{3+} fiber lasers within the 100 nm window [82]. Using high lasing efficiency and broadband tunability, ytterbium-pulsed lasers with high peak power operating in Q-switched and mode-locking regimes have been rapidly advancing [83–85]. With radiation around the wavelength of 1030–1080 nm, Q-switched ytterbium fiber lasers are becoming an attractive alternative to Nd:YAG lasers, which traditionally occupied a large sector of the medical applications industry employing the 1064 nm wavelength. Pulsed Yb lasers delivering more than 80 W of peak power with microsecond pulses are applicable to diverse areas such as gynecology, abdominal surgery, cardiovascular surgery, and dental curing [86]. Yb fiber laser tunability opens additional possibilities. Tunable subnanosecond-pulsed Yb lasers using second harmonic generation (SHG) to achieve lasing in the visible range have found uses in bioscience investigations: DNA sequencing, flow cytometry, and laser microscopy [87,88]. In addition, attaining green emission (515–532 nm) with frequency doubling is very advantageous for applications in dermatology and PDT. The generous tunability of ytterbium lasers is also favorable for high-resolution OCT techniques [89].

7.4.3 THULIUM LASERS

Among other fibers containing rare earth ion dopants, thulium-doped materials occupy a special place due to their specific and efficient properties usable in fiber lasers. What makes thulium lasers attractive for many applications is the manifold and sophisticated structure of Tm^{3+} transitions available for lasing (Figure 7.11) [90,91]. Operating typically around the 2 μm wavelength with silica-based fibers and extending to the 3–4 μm range in codoped (with other rare earth ions) or ZBLAN fibers, Tm^{3+} fiber lasers fill an important mid-IR gap, which enables minimally invasive surgery in various branches: otolaryngology, urology, ophthalmology, and cardiology [35]. Along with lasing in the mid-IR, several almost equidistantly allocated transition levels (shown in a more complete transition scheme in Figure 7.6) offer the opportunity to realize fiber lasers generating several wavelengths in the visible range using multiple excited state absorption (ESA), or upconversion, mechanisms [40]. This unique feature is realized in ZBLAN fibers, thus bringing thulium fiber lasers to the field of dermatology, cosmetic, and cancer treatment.

The growing selection of laser designs with a versatile choice of power and operation modes is continually demonstrated. One of the first widely tunable thulium lasers (1.9–2.1 μm) delivering about 5 W in the cw regime was reported by Jackson and King as long as 16 years ago [92]. This wavelength range has great practical importance for abdominal, thoracic, and neurological surgery in which soft tissues are treated. Practical advantages of the 2 μm thulium fiber lasers over traditionally used CO_2 lasers were demonstrated in comparative clinical research by Verdaasdonk et al. [93]. In these trials, the cw thulium lasers have demonstrated high efficiency for superficial tissue ablation, with minimal coagulation depth both in air and in water, which makes such lasers very useful for the treatment of tissues containing a lot of water, such as the lungs or liver.

The wide tunability of thulium fiber lasers around 2 μm makes them very attractive for other important branches in surgery, including such critical issues in health care as lithotripsy (kidney stone fragmentation) and the treatment of benign hyperplasia of the prostate [94]. The laser tunability in the range of strong water absorption

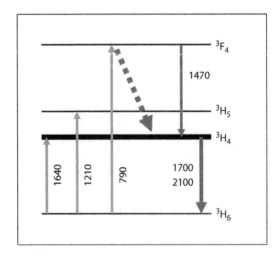

FIGURE 7.11 Selected set of energy levels of thulium (Tm^{3+}) in silica fiber with pumping, absorption, and lasing transitions.

allows the laser radiation to be adjusted on or off the absorption peak, thus carefully manipulating the degree of interaction with specific tissues.

A high-power 110 W thulium laser radiating at the wavelength of 1.91 μm in cw mode was highly efficient in testing for vaporization and coagulation of urinary tissue (prostate) [94,95]. Providing a small coagulation zone, about 500–2000 μm, and rapid tissue vaporization at the rate of 0.83 ± 0.11 g/min, such lasers have proved their potential for practically bloodless surgery of the soft tissues. Successful urinary stone fragmentation was reported with a high-power thulium laser using a slightly different wavelength of 1.94 μm. Operating in cw mode with a modulation of 10 Hz repetition rate, the 100 W laser was capable of breaking both hard and soft urinary stones with a mass of 800 mg into 2 mg pieces at a rate of about 400 and 25 mg/min, respectively [96].

However, to be qualified for full-scale clinical use, high-power thulium fiber lasers operating in short-pulse modes have to be developed to provide sufficiently rapid vaporization of tumor tissues and more precise incision of the urethral/bladder-neck structures [97]. When the necessary performance is achieved, such lasers might replace traditional crystalline solid-state lasers for this application.

7.4.4 HOLMIUM LASERS

Holmium fiber lasers exhibit an interesting example of technology development. As considered in the previous section, thulium fiber lasers have rapidly attracted much interest as a replacement for the Ho:YAG crystal lasers widely used in soft-tissue surgery. After tunable Tm^{3+} fiber lasers achieved maturity and became available on the market as research and industrial instruments, they turned out to be a suitable pumping source for holmium fiber lasers [98]. Being rather expensive instruments, and gradually being replaced by more efficient thulium lasers, Ho:YAG lasers still have a place as a working tool in some specific fields of surgery, such as in the laparoscopic sector or in treating benign prostatic hyperplasia, or noncancerous enlargement of the prostate gland [99]. Holmium-based lasers continue to be used in surgical applications because their radiation wavelength, slightly over 2.1 μm, falls at the very edge of the thulium fiber laser bandwidth, where thulium lasers cannot achieve high power. In [99], a high-power device, about 80–100 W, operating in modulated mode with pulse energy of 2–3 J and a repetition rate of 25–40 Hz, combines the thermal ablation of the soft tissues and coagulation of the operated area. This results in smaller blood loss during treatment.

The energy levels of Ho^{3+}-doped fibers offer additional opportunities for lasing (Figure 7.12). Along with typical generation around 2.1 μm, and reaching a record 83 W with 42% slope efficiency (in a Tm^{3+}-codoped version), holmium fiber lasers emitting at 3 μm have been demonstrated [98,100]. Operation in this mid-IR part of the spectrum, and the possibility of moving farther over the 3 μm boundary, makes holmium fiber lasers almost a unique tool. This mid-IR lasing can be obtained in combination with other rare earth dopants or in ZBLAN-based fibers using upconversion transitions to affect the lifetime of lower levels. More details are given in the next section, devoted to codoped fiber lasers.

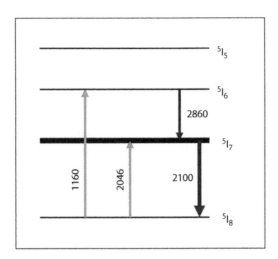

FIGURE 7.12   Simplified energy levels of holmium (Ho^{3+}) in silica fiber.

Confirming their promising results in research projects and clinical tests, holmium fiber lasers are rapidly acquiring the status of reliable and cost-effective commercial systems designed for use in delicate fields of surgery such as urology, orthopedics, lithotripsy, or gastroenterology with endoscopic or direct access.

7.4.5   CODOPED AND **ZBLAN** FIBER LASERS

The main effect of ZBLAN host glasses in fiber-optic technology is their impact on the lifetime of dopants impregnated into fibers. Complicated interactions between the host material and doping ions of rare earth metals typically used in fiber lasers (Er^{3+}, Pr^{3+}, Tm^{3+}, and Ho^{3+}) influence the kinetics of excitation and phonon relaxation of the active levels. The induced changes enable "turning on" lasing transitions, which otherwise are low efficiency or almost prohibited, while using traditional silica-based host glasses [101]. The versatile set of ZBLAN laser wavelengths is typically found at the mid-IR range. This makes these fiber lasers attractive tools for surgery due to strong absorption of the radiation by organic tissues around the 3 μm wavelength range. Using the thermal response in radiation–tissue interactions and operating mainly in the cw regime, ZBLAN lasers are efficient instruments for endoscopic abdominal, thoracic, and brain surgery. Numerous examples and clinical data about the use of ZBLAN lasers in surgery are given in [6,35].

Although ZBLAN lasers were introduced about two decades ago, they possessed a number of drawbacks, which precluded their practical use in medicine. At the beginning of the fiber laser era, when Er-ion doping was the most developed and popular approach, ZBLAN lasers with Er^{3+} ions were actively attempted [102]. Among the most challenging tasks were attempts to improve the resistance of fluoride-based glasses against water absorption and to increase the lasing efficiency [103,104]. Another significant obstacle to using the lasers for medical applications was the modest output power due to the relatively long lifetime of the Er^{3+} ions at the

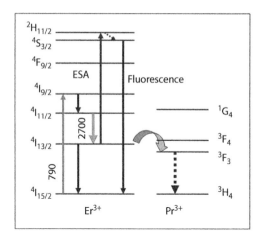

FIGURE 7.13 Energy levels of codoped Er^{3+}:Pr^{3+}:ZBLAN glass fiber.

lower lasing level. Recently, a 10 W Er–ZBLAN laser with a heavily doped double-clad structure was demonstrated to have promising performance, which might solve the problems mentioned [105]. In this particular solution, energy-transfer upconversion was used to reduce the lifetime of the lower level, thus increasing the lasing efficiency dramatically.

In contemporary fiber-optic technology, codoping the fiber host with several different rare earth ions simultaneously has become a popular technique. Along with the advances in developing high-power semiconductor diode lasers for pumping, implementing other dopants has broadened the range of the operating wavelengths of ZBLAN fiber lasers. Codoped Er^{3+}:Pr^{3+} (with low-intensity double-clad diode pumping) and Ho^{3+}:Pr^{3+} (pumped with a Nd:YAG laser) ZBLAN lasers were capable of delivering over 1 W of power in the cw mode at 2.78 and 2.87 μm wavelengths, respectively [35,106]. In this design, a rather sophisticated excitation scheme was used to overcome the bottleneck related to the long lifetime of the Er^{3+} low level (Figure 7.13).

For the cw operation mode, aimed at thermal ablation of soft and hard water-rich tissues, ZBLAN lasers do not need to provide extremely high power: 1–10 W class lasers have proved their efficiency for diverse surgical applications [6,35,107].

7.4.6 SUPERCONTINUUM FIBER LASERS

The stream of breakthrough achievements related to fiber lasers and the intensive research in biomedicine, biophysics, and other sectors of the life sciences would not be complete without highlighting sophisticated monitoring and imaging techniques. We have already mentioned OCT. Fluorescent imaging (including flow cytometry and confocal fluorescence microscopy) and two- and three-dimensional (3-D) live-cell imaging are just selected examples that extensively use advanced spectroscopic and microscopic instrumentation (see Chapter 9 for a discussion on laser microscopy). To attain the best efficiency, these methods require broadband light sources with high brightness, which is extremely difficult to obtain with classical thermal (black body) radiation sources such as tungsten-based lamps. SC fiber lasers turned out to be excellent tools for solving this problem.

The first fiber SC sources were reported in around 2000. They were capable of covering the spectral band from 400 nm to almost 2 μm and used high nonlinear optical fibers as active media, such as photonic crystal fibers (PCF) or tapered fibers [69,108,109]. To obtain such a broadband spectrum, a short light pulse (in the femtosecond to nanosecond range) from a Q-switched or mode-locked laser, for example a Ti:sapphire or ytterbium fiber, is launched into PCF with a carefully engineered core structure providing close to zero dispersion in the visible range [110,111]. This enables generating a more than 1000 nm spectral band of extremely bright light (Figure 7.14). Although the first systems could offer rather modest total radiation power, SC fiber lasers have rapidly turned into a mature technology, and reliably deliver several watts of high-quality laser beam (M2 < 1.1) with commercially available systems [112].

Immediately after the first demonstrations, the SC fiber lasers were in high demand for OCT imaging to replace relatively narrowband sources (30–40 nm), radiating within the 1.3–1.5 μm range, which mainly comprised ASE from fiber-optic amplifiers or superluminescent light-emitting diodes (SLED). Although these wavelengths are attractive for the investigation of biological species due to good penetration into the tissues, they limit longitudinal resolution, which is inversely proportional to the spectral width of the light source. Using SC radiation with wide bandwidth leads to tremendous improvement of the resolution. In 2001, Hartl et al. reported 2.5 μm longitudinal resolution with a 370 nm wide SC source centered

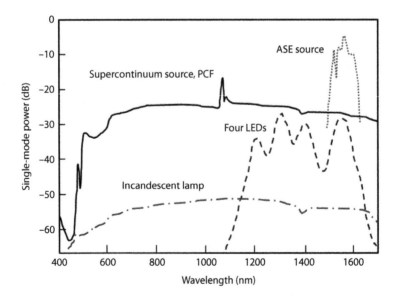

FIGURE 7.14 Comparison of supercontinuum spectra generated by different sources. The spectrum obtained with PCF covers the visible, near-IR, and IR range.

around 1300 nm, which was built using a 100 fs Ti:sapphire mode-locked laser and a nonlinear PCF [113].

Another approach to achieving ultrahigh resolution using SC sources is to implement dual wavelength combination. The results of OCT with resolution around 1.8 μm were demonstrated with sources emitting at 840 and 1230 nm with a 200 nm bandwidth at each wavelength [114]. Using both wavelengths simultaneously also improved the image quality, with reduced speckle pattern.

Fluorescent imaging is one more domain in biology-related applications for which the use of bright white sources is essential. Flow cytometry relies on the laser excitation of fluorophores, which have versatile spectral structure and demand broadband illumination for detailed analysis. Before SC lasers were introduced, sources with discrete numbers of wavelengths were used, thus leaving a rather large spectrum gap uncovered. Many types of fluorophore were unusable due to this limitation [115].

Confocal fluorescent microscopy is another imaging technique that is valuable in the biosciences and definitely gains from the use of SC fiber lasers. A high-power SC fiber laser covering a 450–700 nm spectral range and equipped with acousto-optical tunable filters was recently used to realize a scanning microscope providing 3-D live-cell images [116]. This laser is also a commercially available system incorporating a low-power mode-locked Yb fiber master laser and a high-power fiber amplifier with nonlinear PCF [112].

Despite their rather short history, SC laser sources have drastically progressed during the last 5 years. At the moment, instruments routinely generating up to 6 W with the tremendous range of 460–2500 nm are off-the-shelf turnkey devices operating in cw mode. Figure 7.15 displays a simplified design of such a source, implementing a PCF with specially tailored dispersion properties.

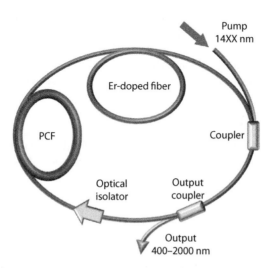

FIGURE 7.15 Schematic design of SC coherent source making use of Er-doped amplifier and nonlinear PCF.

7.4.7 Making and Marking Tools and Instruments for Medical Industry

To complete the survey of fiber laser applications in life sciences and medicine, it is worth mentioning one more domain implicitly related to medicine. This is the industry of making, postprocessing, and marking medical instruments and tools. Regulations in many countries on the market of medical instruments impose strict requirements for the quality and identification of most surgical tools and implants.

Numerous tools used in contemporary medicine, especially in branches such as neurosurgery or ophthalmology, are often manufactured with microscale accuracy from extremely hard materials or alloys containing cobalt, chrome, nitinol, and tantalum. To provide the highest quality for such instruments in a cost-effective way, no ordinary mechanical machining equipment can compete with high-power-pulsed fiber lasers built with ytterbium-doped fibers. Outperforming laser properties, such as high-pulse power up to 40 kW, excellent beam profile (often M < 1.05 for TEM00 mode), and small beam size, satisfy production quality specifications [60]. Very small cutting width and a small heat-affected zone can be achieved by carefully choosing the suitable laser tool and its operational mode.

Furthermore, laser processing such components as burs, narrow and parallel kerfs, scalpels, and tweezers, among others, can drastically improve the working properties of the instruments without thermally induced stresses or distortions, which are hard to avoid with mechanical processing. Making "active" tools for surgery or implants is not the only branch of manufacture that is profiting from the use of fiber lasers as processing instruments. Nonintrusive devices for cardiovascular and neurological applications, such as catheters, medical stems, implants, and biodegradable components, can be efficiently and easily manufactured by the use of fiber lasers [117]. Laser technology also provides diverse opportunities for reliably joining together various materials, such as polymers, metals, and glasses [118].

Strictly speaking, all the applications mentioned here have already been served by machinery exploiting lasers other than fiber lasers. Due to the technical and cost advantages discussed in this chapter, such as higher power and efficiency, smaller size, and easier operation and maintenance routines, fiber lasers are gradually expanding their influence over the biomedical application sector.

ACKNOWLEDGMENTS

The author is greatly thankful to the book editor, Dr. F. J. Duarte, for supportive discussions and enthusiastic guidance during the preparation of the chapter.

REFERENCES

1. Koester, C. J. and E. Snitzer, Amplification in a fiber laser, *Appl. Opt.* 3: 1182–1186, 1964.
2. Snitzer, E., Proposed fiber cavities for optical masers, *J. Appl. Phys.* 32: 36–39, 1961.
3. Moizan, V., V. Nazabal, J. Troles, P. Houizot, J-L. Adam, F. Smektala, J-L. Doualan, et al., Mid-infrared fiber laser application:Er^{3+}-doped chalcogenide glasses, *Proc. SPIE* 6469: 64690E, 2007.

4. Coleman, D., S. Jackson, P. Golding, T. King, H. Se, B. Yong, and H. Jong, Heavy metal oxide and chalcogenide glasses as new hosts for Er^{3+} and Er^{3+}/Pr^{3+} mid-IR fiber lasers. In *OSA Proceedings, Trends in Optics and Photonics: Advanced Solid State Lasers*, 34: 434–439, Optical Society of America, Washington, DC. 2000.

5. Carrig, T., G. Wagner, W. Alford, and A. Zakel, Chromium-doped chalcogenide lasers, *Proc. SPIE* 5460: 74–82, 2004.

6. Tafoya, J., J. Pierce, R. Jain, and B. Wong, Efficient and compact high-power mid-IR (~3 µm) lasers for surgical applications, *Proc. SPIE* 5312: 218–222, 2004.

7. Mears, R., L. Reekie, S. Poole, and D. Payne, Neodymium-doped silica single-mode fibre lasers, *Electron. Lett.* 21: 738–740, 1985.

8. Mears, R., L. Reekie, I. Jauncey, and D. Payne, Low-noise erbium-doped fibre amplifier operating at 1.54 µm, *Electron. Lett.* 23: 1026–1028, 1987.

9. Welch, A. J. and M. J. C. van Gemert (Eds), *Optical-Thermal Response of Laser-Irradiated Tissue*, Springer, Dordrecht, 1995.

10. Waynant, R. W. (Ed.), *Lasers in Medicine*, CRC Press, Boca Raton, 2002.

11. Goldman, L., Dye lasers in medicine. In Duarte, F. J. and L. W. Hillman (Eds), *Dye Laser Principles*, Chapter 10, Academic, New York, 1990.

12. Huang, D., E. Swanson, C. Lin, J. Schuman, W. Stinson, W. Chang, M. Hee, et al., Optical coherence tomography, *Science* 254: 1178–1781, 1991.

13. Swanson, E., J. Izatt, M. Hee, D. Huang, C. Lin, J. Schuman, C. Puliafito, et al., In vivo retinal imaging by optical coherence tomography, *Opt. Lett.* 18: 1864–1866, 1993.

14. Brezinski, M. E. *Optical Coherence Tomography Principles and Applications*, Academic Press, Burlington, MA, 2006.

15. Tearney, G., B. Bouma, S. Boppart, B. Golubovic, E. Swanson, and J. Fujimoto, Rapid acquisition of in vivo biological images by use of optical coherence tomography, *Opt. Lett.* 21: 1408–1410, 1996.

16. Podoleanu, A. Gh., Optical coherence tomography, *Br. J. Radiol.* 78: 976–988, 2014.

17. Calabresi, P. A., L. J. Balcer, and E. M. Frohman (Eds), *Optical Coherence Tomography in Neurologic Diseases*, Cambridge University Press, London, 2015.

18. Vakoc, B. J., D. Fukumura, R. K. Jain, and B. E. Bouma, Cancer imaging by optical coherence tomography: Preclinical progress and clinical potential, *Nat. Rev. Cancer* 12: 363–368, 2012.

19. Chen, W., P. Xue, T. Yun, and D. Chen, Medical application of ultrafast laser, *Proc. SPIE* 3934: 87–92, 2000.

20. Palumbo, G. and R. Pratesi (Eds), *Lasers and Current Optical Techniques in Biology*, European Society for Photobiology, Royal Society of Chemistry, Cambridge, 2004.

21. Wu, R., J. Myers, and M. Myers, New generation high power rare-earth-doped phosphate glass fiber and fiber laser, *Proc. SPIE* 4267: 56–60, 2001.

22. Dianov, E., M. Grekov, I. Bufetov, S. Vasiliev, O. Medvedkov, V. Plotnichenko, V. Koltashev, et al., CW high power 1.24 µm and 1.48 µm Raman lasers based on low loss phosphosilicate fibre, *Electron. Lett.* 33: 1542–1544, 1997.

23. Smart, R., D. Hanna, A. Tropper, S. Davey, S. Carter, and D. Szebesta, CW room temperature upconversion lasing at blue, green and red wavelengths in infrared-pumped Pr^{3+}-doped fluoride fibre, *Electron. Lett.* 27: 1307–1309, 1991.

24. Whitley, T., C. Millar, R. Wyatt, M. Brierley, and D. Szebesta, Upconversion pumped green lasing in erbium doped fluorozirconate fibre, *Electron. Lett.* 27: 1785–1786, 1991.

25. Poulain, M., Fluoride glass fibers: Applications and prospects, *Proc. SPIE* 3416: 2–12, 1998.

26. Xiushan, Z. and R. Jain, Numerical analysis and experimental results of high-power Er/Pr:ZBLAN 2.7 µm fiber lasers with different pumping designs, *Appl. Opt.* 45: 7118–7125, 2006.

27. Kashyap, R., *Fiber Bragg Gratings*, Academic, London, 1999.

28. Gomes, L., L. Orsila, T. Jouhti, and O. Okhotnikov, Picosecond SESAM-based ytterbium mode-locked fiber lasers, *IEEE J. Quantum Elect.* 10: 129–136, 2004.

29. Perry, M., B. Stuart, P. Banks, D. Feit, V. Yanovsky, and A. Rubenchik, Ultrashort-pulse laser machining of dielectric materials, *J. Appl. Phys.* 85: 6803–6810, 1999.

30. Juhasz, T., F. Loesel, R. Kurtz, C. Horvath, J. Bille, and G. Mourou, Corneal refractive surgery with femtosecond lasers, *IEEE J. Quantum Elect.* 5: 902–910, 1999.

31. Dausinger, F., F. Lichtner, and H. Lubatschowski (Eds), *Femtosecond Technology for Technical and Medical Applications* (Topics in Applied Physics, v 96), Springer, London, 2004.

32. Andersen, T., O. Schmidt, C. Bruchmann, J. Limpert, C. Aguergaray, E. Cormier, and A. Tünnermann, High repetition rate tunable femtosecond pulses and broadband amplification from fiber laser pumped parametric amplifier, *Opt. Express* 14: 4765–4773, 2006.

33. De Matos, C. J. S., R. Kennedy, S. Popov, and J. Taylor, 20-kW peak power all-fiber 1.57-μm source based on compression in air-core photonic bandgap fiber, its frequency doubling, and broadband generation from 430 to 1450 nm, *Opt. Lett.* 30: 436–438, 2005.

34. Hansen, K., J. Broeng, A. Petersson, M. Nielsen, P. Skovgaard, C. Jakobsen, and H. Simonsen, High-power photonic crystal fibers, *Proc. SPIE* 6102: 61020B, 2006.

35. Pierce, M., S. Jackson, P. Golding, B. Dickinson, M. Dickinson, T. King, and P. Sloan, Development and application of fiber lasers for medical applications, *Proc. SPIE* 4253: 144–154, 2001.

36. Steiner, R., New laser technology and future applications, *Med. Laser Appl.* 21: 131–140, 2005.

37. Tearney, G., B. Bouma, S. Boppart, B. Golubovic, E. Swanson, and J. Fujimoto, Rapid acquisition of in vivo biological images by use of optical coherence tomography, *Opt. Lett.* 21: 1408–1410, 1996.

38. Paschotta, R., N. Moore, W. Clarkson, A. Tropper, D. Hanna, and G. Maze, 230 mW of blue light from a thulium-doped upconversion fiber laser, *IEEE J. Quantum Elect.* 3: 1100–1102, 1997.

39. Gaebler, V. and H. Eichler, Monolithic blue upconversion fiber laser, *Proc. SPIE* 4629: 94–98, 2002.

40. Qin, G., S. Huang, Y. Feng, A. Shirakawa, M. Musha, and K.-I. Ueda, Power scaling of Tm^{3+} doped ZBLAN blue upconversion fiber lasers: Modeling and experiments, *Appl. Phys. B* 82: 65–70, 2006.

41. Tohmon, G., H. Sato, J. Ohya, and T. Uno, Thulium: ZBLAN blue fiber laser pumped by two wavelengths, *Appl. Opt.* 36: 3381–3386, 1997.

42. Ping, X. and T. Gosnell, Room-temperature upconversion fiber laser tunable in the red, orange, green, and blue spectral regions, *Opt. Lett.* 20: 1014–1016, 1995.

43. Chernikov, S., N. Platonov, D. Gapontsev, D. Chang, M. Guy, and R. Taylor, Raman fibre laser operating at 1.24 μm, *Electron. Lett.* 34: 680–681, 1998.

44. Dianov, E., Advances in Raman fibers, *J. Lightwave Technol.* 20: 1457–1462, 2002.

45. Dianov, E. and A. Prokhorov, Medium-power CW Raman fiber lasers, *IEEE J. Quantum Elect.* 6: 1022–1028, 2000.

46. Rini, M., I. Cristiani, V. Degiorgio, A. Kurkov, and V. Paramonov, Experimental and numerical optimization of a fiber Raman laser, *Opt. Commun.* 203: 139–144, 2002.

47. Xiong, Z., N. Moore, Z. Li, G. Lim, D. Liu, and D. Huang, Experimental optimization of high power Raman fiber lasers at 1495 nm using phosphosilicate fibers, *Opt. Commun.* 239: 137–145, 2004.

48. Goldberg, L., J. Koplow, and D. A. V. Kliner, Highly efficient 4-W Yb-doped fiber amplifier pumped by a broad-stripe laser diode, *Opt. Lett.* 24: 673–675, 1999.

49. Dominic, V., S. MacCormack, R. Waarts, S. Sanders, S. Bicknese, R. Dohle, E. Wolak, et al., 110 W fibre laser, *Electron. Lett.* 35: 1158–1160, 1999.

50. Limpert, J., A. Liem, H. Zellmer, and A. Tunnermann, 500 W continuous-wave fibre laser with excellent beam quality, *Electron. Lett.* 39: 645–647, 2003.

51. Dorsch, F., V. Bluemel, M. Schroeder, D. Lorenzen, P. Hennig, and D. Wolff, Fiber coupled diode laser systems up to 2 kW output power, *Proc. SPIE* 3945: 42–44, 2000.

52. Hecht, J., High-power fiber lasers: Pumping up the power, *Laser Focus World* 8: 66–70, 2005.

53. De Matos, C. J. S., J. Taylor, and K. Hansen, All-fibre Brillouin laser based on holey fibre yielding comb-like spectra, *Opt. Commun.* 238: 185–189, 2004.

54. Bedo, S., W. Luthy, and H. Weber, The effective absorption coefficient in double-clad fibres, *Opt. Commun.* 99: 331–335, 1993.

55. Anping, L. and K. Ueda, The absorption characteristics of circular, offset, and rectangular double-clad fibers, *Opt. Commun.* 132: 511–518, 1996.

56. Gapontsev, V., N. Platonov, O. Shkurihin, and I. Zaitsev, 400 W low-noise single-mode CW ytterbium fiber laser with an integrated fiber delivery. In *Proceedings of Conference on Lasers and Electro-Optics (CLEO'2003)* (Cat. #CH37419-TBR): 3, 2003.

57. Carter, A., K. Tankala, B. Samson, D. Machewirth, V. Khitrov, and U. Manyam, Continued advancements in the design of double clad fibers for use in high output power fiber lasers and amplifiers, *Proc. SPIE* 5662: 470–475, 2004.

58. Limpert, J., F. Roser, S. Klingebiel, T. Schreiber, C. Wirth, T. Peschel, R. Eberhardt, et al., The rising power of fiber lasers and amplifiers, *IEEE J. Quantum Elect.* 13: 537–545, 2007.

59. Tünnermann, A., S. Hofer, A. Liem, J. Limpert, M. Reich, F. Roser, T. Schreiber, et al., Power scaling of high-power fiber lasers and amplifiers, *Laser Phys.* 15: 107–117, 2005.

60. Babushkin, A., N. Platonov, and V. Gapontsev, Multi-kilowatt peak power pulsed fiber laser with precise computer controlled pulse duration for materials processing, *Proc. SPIE*, 5709: 98–102, 2005.

61. Digonnet, M. J. F. (Ed.), *Rare-Earth-Doped Fiber Lasers and Amplifiers*, 2nd edn, CRC Press, Boca Raton, 2001.

62. Reekie, L., R. Mears, S. Poole, and D. Payne, Tunable single-mode fiber lasers, *J. Lightwave Technol.* LT-4: 1985, 1985.

63. Laming, D., M. Farries, P. Morkel, L. Reekie, D. Payne, P. Scrivener, F. Fontana, et al., Efficient pump wavelengths of erbium-doped fibre optical amplifier, *Electron. Lett.* 25: 12–14, 1989.

64. Barnes, W., P. Morkel, L. Reekie, and D. Payne, High-quantum-efficiency Er^{3+} fiber lasers pumped at 980 nm, *Opt. Lett.* 14: 1002–1004, 1989.

65. Bouma, B., L. Nelson, G. Tearney, D. Jones, M. Brezinski, and J. Fujimoto, Optical coherence tomographic imaging of human tissue at 1.55 µm and 1.81 µm using Er and Tm-doped fiber sources, *J. Biomed. Opt.* 3: 76–79, 1998.

66. Fercher, A., W. Drexler, and C. Hitzenberger, Ocular partial coherence tomography, *Proc. SPIE* 2732: 229–241, 1996.

67. Hee, M., J. Izatt, E. Swanson, and J. Fujimoto, Femtosecond transillumination tomography in thick tissues, *Opt. Lett.* 18: 1107–1109, 1993.

68. Povazay, B., B. Hofer, B. Hermann, A. Unterhuber, J. Morgan, C. Glittenberg, S. Binder, et al., Minimum distance mapping using three-dimensional optical coherence tomography for glaucoma diagnosis, *J. Biomed. Opt.* 12: 1–8, 2007.

69. Wadsworth, W., A. Ortigosa-Blanch, J. Knight, T. Birks, T.-P Man, and P. Russell, Supercontinuum generation in photonic crystal fibers and optical fiber tapers: A novel light source, *J. Opt. Soc. Am. B* 19: 2148–2155, 2002.

70. Rulkov, A., A. Ferin, J. Travers, S. Popov, and J. Taylor, Broadband, low intensity noise CW source for OCT at 1800 nm, *Opt. Commun.* 281: 154–156, 2008.

71. Rusu, M., A. Grudinin, and O. Okhotnikov, Slicing the supercontinuum radiation generated in photonic crystal fiber using an all-fiber chirped-pulse amplification system, *Opt. Express* 13: 6390–6400, 2005.

72. Oppel, T. and H. Korting, Actinic keratosis: The key event in the evolution from photo-aged skin to squamous cell carcinoma, *Skin Pharmacol. Physiol.* 17: 67–76, 2004.

73. Wanner, M., E. Tanzi, and T. Alster, Fractional photothermolysis: Treatment of facial and nonfacial cutaneous photodamage with a 1550-nm erbium-doped fiber laser, *Dermatol. Surg.* 33: 23–28, 2007.

74. Kincade, K., Biophotonics-fiber lasers find opportunities in medical applications, *Laser Focus World*, 9: 76–80, 2005.

75. Lawrence, S., Rejuvenation of the aging face using Fraxel laser treatment, *Aesthet. Surg. J.* 25: 307–309, 2005.

76. Norman, S. and M. Zervas, Fiber lasers prove attractive for industrial applications, *Laser Focus World* 8: 93–98, 2007.

77. Srinivasan, B., J. Tafoya, and R. Jain, High-power "Watt-level" CW operation of diode-pumped 2.7 μm fiber lasers using efficient cross-relaxation and energy transfer mechanisms, *Opt. Express* 4: 490–495, 1999.

78. Pollnau, M., Ch. Ghisler, M. Bunea, W. Luthy, and H. Weber, Erbium 3-μm fiber laser in the power range for surgery, *Proc. SPIE* 2629: 234–244, 1996.

79. Pollnau, M., Route toward a diode-pumped 1-W erbium 3-μm fiber laser, *IEEE J. Quantum Elect.* 33: 1982–1990, 1997.

80. Serafetinides, A. and D. Papadopoulos, Lasers and new trends in laser-tissue interaction, *Proc. SPIE* 5449: 212–221, 2004.

81. Even, P. and D. Pureur, High power double clad fiber lasers: A review, *Proc. SPIE* 4638: 1–12, 2002.

82. Okhotnikov, O., L. Gomes, N. Xiang, T. Jouhti, and A. Grudinin, Mode-locked ytterbium fiber laser tunable in the 980-1070-nm spectral range, *Opt. Lett.* 28: 1522–1524, 2003.

83. Nickel, D., A. Liem, J. Limpert, H. Zellmer, U. Griebner, S. Unger, G. Korn, et al., Fiber based high repetition rate, high energy laser source applying chirped pulse amplification, *Opt. Commun.* 190: 309–315, 2001.

84. Limpert, J., S. Hofer, A. Liem, H. Zellmer, A. Tunnermann, S. Knoke, and H. Voelckel, 100-W average-power, high-energy nanosecond fiber amplifier, *Appl. Phys. B.* B75: 477–479, 2002.

85. Limpert, J., A. Liem, T. Gabler, H. Zellmer, A. Tünnermann, S. Unger, S. Jetschke, et al., High-average-power picosecond Yb-doped fiber amplifier, *Opt. Lett.* 26: 1849–1851, 2001.

86. Engelbrecht, M., D. Wandt, and D. Kracht, Microsecond-pulsed ytterbium fiber laser system with a broad tuning range and a small spectral linewidth, *Proc. SPIE* 6453: 645321, 2007.

87. Laroche, M., P. Leproux, V. Couderc, C. Lesvigne, H. Gilles, and S. Girard, Compact sub-nanosecond wideband laser source for biological applications, *Appl. Phys. B* B86: 601–604, 2007.

88. Kang, J., K. Chang-Seok, and J. Khurgin, Fiber laser SHG yields broad bandwidth at high power, *Laser Focus World*, 2: 55–58, 2002.

89. Hyungsik, L., J. Yi, W. Yimin, H. Yu-Chih, C. Zhongping, and F. Wise, Ultrahigh-resolution optical coherence tomography with a fiber laser source at 1 μm, *Opt. Lett.* 30: 1171–1173, 2005.

90. Agger, S., J. Povlsen, and P. Varming, Single-frequency thulium-doped distributed-feedback fiber laser, *Opt. Lett.* 29: 1503–1505, 2004.

91. Jackson, S. and T. King, Theoretical modeling of Tm-doped silica fiber lasers, *J. Lightwave Technol.* 17: 948–956, 1999.

92. Jackson, S. and T. King, High-power diode-cladding-pumped Tm-doped silica fiber laser, *Opt. Lett.* 23: 1462–1464, 1998.

93. Verdaasdonk, R., A. Rem, S. van Thoor, T. de Boorder, J. Klaessens, and H-O. Teichmann, Comparison of the CO_2, cw thulium and diode laser in a thermal imaging model for the optimization of various clinical applications, *Proc. SPIE* 6084: 126–136, 2006.

94. Fried, N. and K. Murray, High-power thulium fiber laser ablation of the canine prostate, *Proc. SPIE* 5686: 176–182, 2005.

95. Fried, N., High-power laser vaporization of the canine prostate using a 110 W Thulium fiber laser at 1.91 μm, *Lasers Surg. Med.* 36: 52–56, 2005.

96. Fried, N., Thulium fiber laser lithotripsy: An in vitro analysis of stone fragmentation using a modulated 110-watt Thulium fiber laser at 1.94 μm, *Lasers Surg. Med.* 37: 53–58, 2005.

97. Fried, N. and K. Murray, High-power thulium fiber laser ablation of urinary tissues at 1.94 μm, *J. Endourol.* 19: 25–31, 2005.

98. Jackson, S., Midinfrared holmium fiber laser, *IEEE J. Quantum Elect.* 42: 187–191, 2006.

99. Kuo, R., S. Kim, J. Lingeman, R. Paterson, S. Watkins, G. Simmons, and R. Steele, Holmium laser enucleation of prostate (HoLEP): The Methodist Hospital experience with greater than 75 gram enucleations, *J. Urol.* 170: 149–152, 2003.

100. Jackson, S., A. Sabella, A. Hemming, S. Bennetts, and D. Lancaster, High-power 83 W holmium-doped silica fiber laser operating with high beam quality, *Opt. Lett.* 32: 241–243, 2007.

101. Allain, J. Y., M. Monerie and H. Poignant, Tunable CW lasing around 0.82, 1.48, 1.88 and 2.35 μm in thulium-doped fluorozirconate fibre, *Electron. Lett.* 25: 1660–1662, 1989.

102. Auzel, F., D. Meichenin and H. Poignant, Laser cross-section and quantum yield of Er^{3+} at 2.7 μm in a ZrF_4-based fluoride glass, *Electron. Lett.* 24: 909–910, 1988.

103. Robinson, M. and G. L. Tangonan, Light scattering in fluoride glass, *Mater. Res. Bull.* 23: 943–951, 1988.

104. Esterowitz, L., R. Allen, G. Kintz, I. Aggarwal, and R. J. Ginther, Laser emission in Tm^{3+} and Er^{3+}-doped fluorozirconate glass at 2.25, 1.88, and 2.70 μm, in *Proc. Conference on Lasers and Electro-Optics (CLEO'1988)*, 7: 318–320, Optical Society of America, Washington, DC. 1988.

105. Zhu, X. and R. Jain, 10-W-level diode-pumped compact 2.78 μm ZBLAN fiber laser, *Opt. Lett.* 32: 26–28, 2007.

106. Qamar, F., T. King, S. Jackson, and Y. Tsang, Holmium, praseodymium-doped fluoride fiber laser operating near 2.87 μm and pumped with a Nd:YAG laser, *J. Lightwave Technol.* 23: 4315–4320, 2005.

107. Sumiyoshi, T., H. Sekita, T. Arai, S. Sato, M. Ishihara, and M. Kikuchi, High-power continuous-wave 3- and 2-μm cascade Ho^{3+}:ZBLAN fiber laser and its medical applications, *IEEE J. Quantum Elect.* 5: 936–943, 1999.

108. Husakou, A. and J. Herrmann, Supercontinuum generation of higher-order solitons by fission in photonic crystal fibers, *Phys. Rev. Lett.* 87: 203901/1–203901/4, 2001.

109. Hundertmark, H., D. Kracht, D. Wandt, C. Fallnich, V. V. Kumar, A. George, J. Knight, et al., Supercontinuum generation with 200 pJ laser pulses in an extruded SF6 fiber at 1560 nms, *Opt. Express* 11: 3196–3201, 2003.

110. Hansen, K., Dispersion flattened hybrid-core nonlinear photonic crystal fiber, *Opt. Express* 11: 1503–1509, 2003.

111. Andersen, T., K. Hilligsoe, C. Nielsen, J. Thogersen, K. Hansen, S. Keiding, and J. Larsen, Continuous-wave wavelength conversion in a photonic crystal fiber with two zero-dispersion wavelengths, *Opt. Express* 12: 4113–4122, 2004.

112. Clowes, J., Next generation light sources for imaging, *Imag. Micros.* 9: 55–57, 2007.

113. Hartl, I., X. Li, C. Chudoba, R. Hganta, T. Ko, J. Fujimoto, J. Ranka, et al., Ultrahigh-resolution optical coherence tomography using continuum generation in an air-silica microstructure optical fiber, *Opt. Lett.* 26: 608–610, 2001.

114. Spoler, F., S. Kray, P. Grychtol, B. Hermes, J. Bornemann, M. Forst, and H. Kurz, Simultaneous dual-band ultra-high resolution optical coherence tomography, *Opt. Express* 15: 10832–10841, 2007.

115. Kapoor, V., F. Subach, V. Kozlov, A. Grudinin, V. Verkhusha, and W. Telford, New lasers for flow cytometry: Filling the gaps, *Nat. Method.* 4: 678–679, 2007.

116. Frank, J., A. Elder, J. Swartling, A. R. Venkitaraman, A. Jeyasekharan, and C. Kaminski, A white light confocal microscope for spectrally resolved multidimensional imaging, *J. Micros.*, 227: 203–215, 2007.

117. Kleine, K., B. Whitney, and K. Watkins, Use of fiber lasers for micro cutting applications in the medical device industry, *Proc. 21st Internat. Cong. Appl. Lasers Elect. Opt. (ICALEO 2002)*, 2: 923–932, 2002.

118. Mian, A., G. Newaz, L. Vendra, N. Rahman, D. Georgiev, G. Auner, R. Witte, et al., Laser bonded microjoints between titanium and polyimide for applications in medical implants, *J. Mater. Sci. Mater. Med.*, 16: 229–237, 2005.

8 Medical Applications of Organic Dye Lasers

A. Costela, I. García-Moreno, and C. Gómez

CONTENTS

8.1 INTRODUCTION

Laser systems have been applied in medicine since they first became available, and today they are employed in diagnostic and therapeutic procedures. Dye lasers, in particular, have potential advantages over other lasers as medical instruments.

A dye laser consists of an organic dye solution optically pumped by a light source (flashlamp, pulsed or continuous-wave [CW] laser). The type of output desired and the absorption properties of the dye determine the choice of the pump source. Dye lasers, in contrast to most other lasers, offer the possibility of shifting the output wavelength. The wavelength range covered by a single dye is about 50–100 nm. Employing presently available dyes, it is possible to cover the wavelength range from 400 to 900 nm. In addition to tunability, an intrinsic feature of dye lasers is their inherent ability to yield high pulse energies and high powers in the visible spectrum. Furthermore, dye lasers can be operated in a wide range of temporal regimes: from femtosecond pulses to CW operation, with optical simplicity and potential reliability.

The usual dye laser uses liquid solutions of dyes in appropriate organic solvents. Thus, despite their great versatility, which favors their use in medicine, interest in the medical applications of dye lasers has been hindered by the complexity and inherent risks that the use of dyes in the liquid phase entails (e.g., large volumes of toxic and flammable solvents and potentially carcinogenic organic dyes, complexity of the system, and need for highly specialized manpower). Areas that require development to improve applications of the dye laser in medicine are decreasing weight and volume of the systems to increase compactness and increasing dye lifetime, beam quality, spatial and temporal coherence, and brightness. To this end, it is important to develop more efficient, longer-lived dyes spanning the near-ultraviolet (UV) to near-infrared (IR) spectrum, as well as potentially low-cost, simple sources of dye laser radiation exploiting proven solid-state technology.

At present, dye lasers are used as excitation light sources for photodynamic therapy (PDT) and as therapeutic agents in dermatology due to their absorption by blood, causing coagulation or vaporization; for this reason, they are able to treat vascular changes selectively. Some of the most important therapeutic applications of dye lasers are presented below. Our aim is not so much to carry out an exhaustive review as to give a general overview of the field.

8.2 DYE LASER SYSTEMS FOR PDT

PDT is a noninvasive or minimally invasive procedure that uses photosensitizing drugs (photosensitizers), which once administered to a patient, may be selectively retained by diseased tissues while normal tissues remain unaltered. These photosensitizers, retained in the diseased tissues, can be activated under intense visible light irradiation to achieve the selective photochemical destruction of the diseased cells and neovasculature [1]. Generally, the photosensitizer is activated by light of the appropriate wavelength and then generates the cytotoxic photodynamic reaction, conventionally mediated by singlet oxygen [2].

Although the healing properties of light have been appreciated for many thousands of years, the more recent use of PDT in oncology dates to the early 1970s, when the group of Dr. Dougherty began research on the mechanism and clinical uses of some hematoporphyrin derivatives [3], despite the 100-year-old concept of cell death induced by the photochemical interaction of light and chemicals. An historical review of this therapy and its evolution, predominantly focused on the treatment of oncologic diseases, can be found in [4,5].

Now, PDT is considered both a curative and a palliative procedure—a treatment of precancerous and cancerous lesions and superficial tumors, using light. Thus, PDT has been an accepted option for the treatment of obstructive esophageal cancer, obstructing endobronchial tumors (non-small-cell lung cancer), early-stage endobronchial tumors, early-stage esophageal cancer, cholangiocarcinoma, head and neck cancer, brain tumors, and mesothelioma. PDT has also found a place in the prevention of restenosis after balloon angioplasty for cardiac artery disease and in the treatment of rheumatoid arthritis (inflammatory cells are particularly prone to photosensitizer uptake), as well as in the medical fields of dermatology, ophthalmology, and gynecology [6]. The increasing interest and importance of PDT are based on the serious inconveniences for the patient's health that often accompany traditional chemotherapy and radiotherapy. It is well known that the toxicity of these well-established therapies limits their therapeutic use, while PDT not only shows a distinct degree of tumor specificity but also can be repeatedly applied without significant damage to patients' health.

The three basic elements involved in the PDT process are photosensitizer, light, and oxygen. The photosensitizer absorbs energy in the form of light of appropriate wavelength, converts it to excitation electronic energy, and transmits or transfers it to oxygen molecules present in the medium, thereby forming highly aggressive forms of singlet oxygen as well as other reactive oxygen-based species, such as ozone, superoxide radicals, and hydroxyl and peroxide radicals. Thus, for the success of PDT, factors such as type and dose of the photosensitizer, location and size of the tumor, irradiation wavelength and intensity, frequency and duration of irradiation, and severity of the disease will have to be considered. Successful clinical PDT is a complex interplay of light and photosensitizers interacting in time and space to create the oxygen-dependent, tumor-ablative photodynamic reaction [5,7]. The involvement of both organic chemistry (design and synthesis of new photosensitizers) and optical physics (appropriate laser light irradiation) is needed to design photosensitizers for PDT. The outcome of this fusion will be clear only on carrying out molecular, oncological, and subsequently, clinical studies.

The first light sources used in PDT were the traditional "gaz" lamps, light from which was filtered to select the photoactivating wavelength and to eliminate IR components that can cause significant heating of tissue. The practical use of these lamps was limited by the way in which light was delivered and the low intensity they produce. Moreover, they cannot be used for internal treatment.

The introduction of a combination of laser light and optical fibers improved the potential of PDT. Lasers have the advantage of a narrow emission spectrum and high output power in the required spectral range (matching the absorption wavelengths of the photosensitizer used). The optical fiber allows the light to be delivered, either interstitially or endoscopically, to practically any site in the human body.

Depending on the location of the tumor, an appropriate light delivery system is selected. A simple lens that produces a uniform illumination may be used for the treatment of skin or oral cavity tumors. To reach tumors in body cavities, laser light is passed through endoscopically placed optical diffusers. An optical fiber placed interstitially into the tumor through a biopsy needle is usually used for the treatment of solid or deep-seated cancers. Intraluminal or intracavity illumination can be carried out by using a flexible fiber that can be placed within the instrument channel or a standard endoscope. By modifying the fiber end or placing the fiber in a light-diffusing medium, the spatial distribution of the light can be controlled [4].

Some laser systems used in PDT based on dye laser technology are described in the following sections.

8.2.1 Argon-Pumped Dye Laser

The most widely used laser for PDT has been the CW argon-pumped dye laser, which has been considered the original PDT "workhorse," capable of delivering powerful monochromatic light that can effectively be coupled into an optical fiber for delivery to the tissue. The wavelength of the dye laser is adjusted to match the optimum absorption of the photosensitizer by simply adjusting the internal filters of the laser system, thus providing the capability to be used with different photosensitizers (such as, for example, 630 nm for Photofrin, 635 nm for aminolevulinic acid [ALA], and 652 nm to activate m-tetrahydroxyphenylchlorin [mTHPC]).

These lasers use a dye jet as active medium. The alignment of the pump laser with the dye module is critical and tends to require regular readjustments and a high level of technical support due to the argon laser beam having a narrow cross section. The output of the dye laser pumped by the main argon lines is in the range 10–500 mW/cm^2 despite the intrinsic losses of the dye laser, which is sufficient to develop effective PDT by either direct or fiber-mediated irradiation at wavelengths between 500 and 750 nm with a bandwidth of 5–10 nm. These argon-pumped dye lasers are especially indicated for endoscopic PDT, because the output beam has a very small cross section (<1 mm) and can readily be coupled to optical fibers. Contrariwise, they are not the most convenient choice in typically large superficial lesions (e.g., in the skin or buccal cavity) involving the addition of a beam expander, which can become cumbersome and reduce the fluence rate [8].

A clinical argon-pumped dye laser, specifically designed for PDT with Photofrin, consisting of a CW argon laser producing up to 12 W, which optically pumps an organic dye laser capable of delivering as much as 2.7 W of 630 nm light, is commercially available [9].

8.2.2 METAL-VAPOR-PUMPED DYE LASER

Metal-vapor-pumped dye lasers have been (and still are) a somewhat popular choice for PDT of human cancer in Europe and Australia. Unlike truly CW argon lasers, metal-vapor lasers are normally pulsed, with pulse widths ranging from 10 to 50 ns and pulse rates of 1 KHz (making the source quasi-continuous for clinical purposes). The pump beam provides high primary output power that can be used to pump tunable dye lasers. The output characteristics are similar to those of the argon-pumped systems: fluences in the range 10–500 mW/cm^2 with a bandwidth of 5–10 nm at wavelengths between 500 and 750 nm. One advantage over the argon-pumped systems is that the metal-vapor-pumped dye lasers can be applied without the need to use a beam expander for PDT of large lesions because of their large beam cross section (typically 1–3 cm^2). Alternatively, they can be used for endoscopic PDT by coupling the output to optical fibers. Although the large cross section of the pump-laser beam means that alignment with the dye module is not as critical as for argon lasers, these lasers still require a good level of technical support [8,10].

8.2.3 KTP-PUMPED DYE LASER

The so-called KTP-pumped dye laser is a modular system consisting of an Nd:YAG laser emitting radiation at 1064 nm with a KTP (potassium-titanyl-phosphate) doubling crystal to generate the second harmonic of the fundamental beam at 532 nm, which pumps the dye unit. A company based in California manufactures lasers of this kind for PDT applications working at a repetition rate of 25 kHz and incorporating a specially designed dye laser head via an optical fiber connection. The dye module is designed to deliver effective PDT at the same range of wavelengths and with the same bandwidth as the laser-pumped dye lasers described in Sections 8.2.1 and 8.2.2. The laser energy from the KTP laser is delivered to the dye module using a fiber that allows independent movement of the dye module and the KTP laser. The dye module can be purchased as an accessory to the KTP laser, simplifying the setup of the system. Different dye modules provide 3.2 and 7 W of power when operated at 630 nm for photoactivation of Photofrin. They are portable and can be tuned to other wavelengths when necessary. The advantages of these systems are low cost, portability, durability, and ease of use and handling [10,11].

Both metal-vapor and KTP dye lasers provide pulsed light instead of the CW output of the argon-pumped dye laser, which led initially to some controversy regarding the possible different effects in the laser–tissue interaction between pulsed and CW radiation [12]. Nevertheless, the high pulse repetition rate and low peak power of these systems produced results not markedly different from CW irradiation, with equivalent photobiological effects. Undesirable side effects such as nonlinear absorption or photosensitizer saturation were found to be negligible.

8.2.4 FUTURE PERSPECTIVES

The availability of a wide number of commercial laser dyes with emission covering the visible spectrum, from the blue to the IR region, allows the appropriate dye emission wavelength to be chosen to overlap with the photosensitizer absorption band. As described in Chapter 3, adequate modifications in the structure of commercial dyes have allowed their efficiency and photostability, in both liquid and solid state, to be significantly increased. When incorporated into solid matrices, the careful choice of matrix composition (linear or cross-linked copolymers, incorporation of fluorine or silicon atoms in the matrix structure, hybrid materials or aerogels, dispersion of silica nanoparticles in the matrix) allows further improvements of laser performance, resulting in solid-state dye lasers competitive with their liquid counterparts. Although most of these improvements have been obtained with dyes emitting in the yellow-orange region, recent efforts have enabled the tuning range of solid-state dye lasers to extend to the red-edge spectral regions (see Chapter 3), appropriate for use in PDT applications. In this way, low-cost, simple sources of dye laser radiation may be obtained, which will greatly facilitate the use of dye lasers in PDT and will provide much-desired flexibility for selecting between different emission wavelengths.

On the other hand, current research is also focused on improving and obtaining new photosensitizers, as well as developing more efficient light delivery systems and obtaining an increased understanding of the optical properties of tissues and the photophysical and photochemical behavior and effects of the interaction between drug and light. Once all these challenges have been overcome, PDT will fully show its great potential as a major treatment in minimally invasive cancer therapy.

8.3   DYE LASERS IN DERMATOLOGY

Although over the last 20 years, not so many new wavelengths have been adopted for treating different dermatological diseases, the incorporation of new software into laser equipment has allowed laser technique to be refined. In practice, the irradiation wavelengths that can be effectively used in dermatology treatments are restricted because of the limited number of useful target chromophores in the skin (melanin, hemoglobin, and different kinds of deposited external pigments, e.g., tattoo colors). In addition, the irradiation wavelength should be in the optical window that combines selective absorption by the chromophore with adequate penetration depth into the skin. Thus, dye lasers, with their great versatility, stand out for therapeutic applications in this field.

8.3.1   DYE LASERS FOR VASCULAR LESIONS

There are a number of congenital vascular anomalies consisting of lesions that vary according to signs, symptoms, and clinical behavior. Vascular malformations are lesions present at birth that grow commensurately with the child and fail to regress. Thus, it is advantageous to treat these malformations at an early age to avoid complications and progression of the lesions.

Most vascular abnormalities can be successfully treated with lasers, and there has been a great deal of careful research on diagnosis and indications for laser treatment over the last decades. This is a rapidly evolving field, and new and improved laser systems are appearing on a regular basis, as it is important to use a laser with the appropriate specifications for a given application. At present, selective photothermolysis is the basis for low-risk treatment of microvascular lesions. Laser wavelengths absorbed by hemoglobin are used to treat cutaneous vascular lesions such as portwine stains (PWSs), hemangioma, spider angioma, cherry angioma, venous lake, and telangiectasia of the face and legs. Selective destruction of blood vessels is possible by matching the wavelength of light absorbed by hemoglobin in the vessels and by using an exposure time less than the calculated thermal relaxation time, defined as the time required for the target tissue to lose 50% of its heat. The theoretical formulation of selective photothermolysis in the early 1980s [13] led to the development of flashlamp-pumped pulsed dye lasers (FPDL) especially designed for use in the treatment of cutaneous vascular lesions. The first studies were carried out with a dye laser containing rhodamine dye and excited by a xenon flashlamp, which produced 1 μs pulses at 577 nm of at least 2 J/cm^2. This laser was used to treat pediatric PWSs, and the initial studies showed histologically selective injury with extensive hemorrhage to dermal vessels [14]. The short pulse duration of this laser produced transient purpura because of hemorrhage and delayed vasculitis. In an attempt to minimize vaporization injury and maximize the thermal coagulation of vessels, the pulse duration was lengthened. A 400 μs, 577 nm FPDL was constructed, tested clinically on PWSs, and noted to work well with a low risk of scarring, even in children [15].

Subsequently, in the early 1990s, the wavelength was adjusted to 585 nm because this somewhat longer wavelength allowed deeper penetration into the vascular injury. With this change, the intravascular hemoglobin release may be greater because of the larger blood vessels and concentration of oxyhemoglobin found in the deep vascular plexus of the dermis. Even so, some important limitations of this laser system remained, such as its inability to penetrate to the level of the deeper vessels. Thus, the treatment was not successful for vessels lying beyond the 1.5 mm penetration depth of the 585 nm laser beam, and lesions at this depth were incompletely cleared.

To determine the depth of effective treatment, spot size plays a significant role. The intensity of a narrow beam (small spot size) tends to suffer greater loss with depth, as light is scattered outside the beam diameter. Thus, when target vessels are deep in the skin, larger exposure spots are desirable. Another significant issue is the number of pulses delivered to a single skin site. Multiple lower-fluence pulses that do not cause hemorrhage might be used to accumulate selective, gentler, and more complete damage to microvessels. For these reasons, newer FPDL versions emit tunable 585–600 nm wavelengths with either fixed pulse duration of 1.5 ms or tunable pulse duration in the range 0.4–20 ms in a stuttered-pulse mode, with an integrated cryogen-spray skin-cooling apparatus. These systems are less painful and allow treatment in pigmented skin at somewhat higher fluences without epidermal damage. The pulses in the millisecond domain are produced either as a true millisecond pulse or as a millisecond "macropulse" composed of a burst of shorter "micropulses." In practice, the experience and skill of the laser operator determine to a large extent the clinical outcome, regardless of the type of laser used. Recently, two laser system platforms that avoid many of the aforementioned drawbacks have been introduced by two companies based in Massachusetts. One of these systems combines a pulsed dye laser with a 1064 nm Nd:YAG laser to be sequentially emitted from the same handpiece, and could become the new gold standard for treating vascular lesions.

8.3.1.1   Dye Lasers for PWSs

PWSs are capillary malformations of the slow-flow vascular malformation type. They are congenital malformations consisting of superficial and deep dilated capillaries in the skin. Their incidence is 0.3%–0.6% in newborn infants; the lesions persist throughout life and can appear in any part of the body, although they occur more often in the face. PWSs are characterized clinically by a sharply demarcated macular erythema, which in infants often appears pinker. The PWSs gradually darken to a deep red or deep purple tinge during life, sometimes becoming raised and irregularly thickened depending on flow changes, pressure associated with trauma, and hormonal changes during puberty. Typically, the diameter of the blood vessels in PWSs varies between 10 and 50 µm. Very few are >100 µm, and most are <20 µm.

Treatments of PWSs have included skin grafting, use of ionizing radiation, cryosurgery, tattooing, or dermabrasion, as well as laser treatments. With the advent of the FPDL, PWSs could be treated in infancy and early childhood, and nowadays FPDL is generally accepted as the standard choice in the treatment of these and related malformations [16]. FPDL treatments achieve lightening of PWSs by reducing the number, size, and erythrocyte content of the vessels, with hemoglobin as the target chromophore [17]. The current FPDL treatment of PWSs uses wavelengths ranging from 585 to 600 nm, with pulses of 0.4–1.5 ms duration, and fluences in the range from 3 to 10 J/cm². Typically, exposure spots with diameters from 3 to 12 mm are used, delivered with a maximum spot overlap of 20%. The shorter pulses are ideal for pediatric PWSs, in which the vessel diameters are relatively small, while long-pulsed FPDLs may be more suitable for resistant or adult PWSs. Fluence range is varied according to the age of the patient, the anatomic location, and the color of the lesion: 5.0–5.6 J/cm² in children less than 12 months of age, 5.6–6.4 J/cm² in children 12 months to 4 years of age, and approximately 7 J/cm² in children over 4 years of age. Treatments are usually repeated at 6 week intervals until the desired degree of lightening is achieved. The high pulse peak power of the FPDL disrupts the vessels. Immediately after treatment, the area characteristically becomes blue-gray and turns purple in a few hours, with surrounding erythematous flare; this takes 7–14 days to resolve.

Several prognostic criteria have been used in predicting the outcome of PWS treatments, including age of patient and site, size, color, and microvascular pattern of the lesion. The major determinants of treatment response have been found to be, in order of decreasing importance, PWS location, PWS size, and patient's age [18]. Some studies have reported "recurrence" of PWSs after treatment with FPDL [19]. As children less than 10 years of age did not show any PWS recurrence, the age at which the treatment begins may have an influence on the recurrence rate. Factors that contribute to a better response to treatment in younger patients and newborns are that lesions in children are smaller overall and that vessels are more superficial and of smaller diameter [20].

The laser pulses produce a mild to moderate degree of discomfort. Topical anesthesia is usually satisfactory for the treatment of PWS lesions in adults, but local or regional anesthesia may be required. General anesthesia should be considered in children less than 12 years of age to minimize the risk of eye injury and pain associated with the multiple treatments. Lanigan [21] and Kautz [22] have successfully applied pneumatic skin flattening, which is a procedure that generates a vacuum over the skin and reduces pain while creating contact between the skin and an upper window. The same technology can be used to increase skin blood fraction while operated in a noncontact mode [21,22] (Figure 8.1).

Side effects from FPDL treatment of PWSs occur infrequently, although hyper-pigmentation, atrophic scar, hypopigmentation, crusting, and hypertrophic scar in patients with skin types II–V have been reported after laser treatment [23]. Early treatment prevents the evolution that makes the lesion dark purple, raised, and nodular in many adults [20], and can mitigate the hypertrophy of affected areas, which is a common complication of extensive PWS, and permanent deformity associated with the lesions.

8.3.1.2 Dye Lasers for Hemangiomas

Hemangiomas are common benign vascular tumors caused by an overgrowth of endothelial cells—the cells that line blood vessels. These lesions occur mainly on the head and neck area (more than 80% of them), but a minor proportion of them can appear anywhere on the body. They are present at birth in approximately 3% of newborns and about 10% by the end of the first year of life [24,25], and are more common in girls. Although the majority of these lesions are benign and exhibit self-limiting conditions, some of them can be associated with complications or may be signs of systemic disorders. Most of the uncomplicated hemangiomas eventually involute and

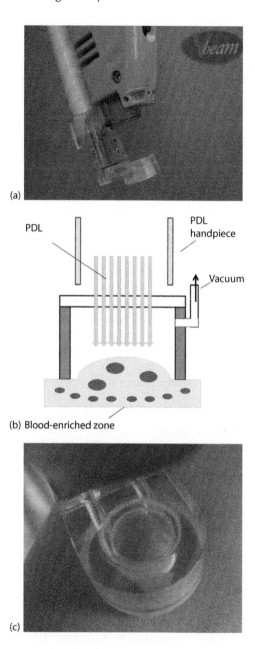

FIGURE 8.1 (a) Vacuum chamber used in the clinical study, connected to the VBeam One Handpiece. (b) Operating principles of the noncontact Serenity Pro vacuum chamber. (c) Blood enrichment can be seen through the vacuum chamber window on contact with the skin (healthy individual). It is evident that even in healthy patients there is a strong skin reaction. (With kind permission from Springer Science+Business Media: *Lasers Med. Sci.*, Treatment of resistant port wine stains (PWS) with pulsed dye laser and non-contact vacuum: A pilot study, 25, 2010, 525–529, Kautz, G., I. Kautz, J. Segal, and S. Zehren, Copyright 2009).

disappear without treatment; thus, allowing spontaneous regression remains a viable therapeutic option. However, some hemangiomas can be disfiguring and psychologically distressing, so early medical intervention is sometimes necessary.

Attempted therapy may cause adverse systemic or cutaneous side effects, particularly scarring, and consequently, intervention is reserved for patients with significant complications. Superficial hemangiomas are generally treated with local corticosteroids (potent topical or intralesional), FPDL, or both. However, alarming hemangiomas or larger lesions with a deeper component usually require the administration of systemic corticosteroids. The treatment of hemangioma must be individualized according to location, rate of growth or involution, age of the patient, and potential risk for complications [26]. Even in carefully selected patients with relatively superficial lesions, the effectiveness of FPDL treatment varies, presumably because of the continued growth of a deeper component not reached by the laser radiation [27].

FDPL treatment may successfully prevent enlargement and promote involution of cutaneous hemangiomas with minimal adverse effects [28]. Therapy should be initiated when the hemangioma is flat or superficial (as early as possible, even in the first weeks of life), and thus, before the lesions have reached an exponential growth phase. The spot size and overlap used are the same as in the treatment of PWSs, with energy fluences in the range from 5 to 7 J/cm^2, although they should be reduced for irradiation over the eyelids, hands, scrotum, and gluteal region. Generally, patients are evaluated at 2–4 weeks after FDPL treatment, and, depending on the degree of response, the entire lesion is then treated again, usually 4 weeks after the first session. Also, cutaneous hemangiomas benefit from FDLP treatment even during the involution phase.

The efficacy of FDPL treatment is limited to 1–2 mm depth of vascular injury. Thus, subcutaneous or mixed hemangiomas, which extend far beyond this depth into the subcutaneous tissue, do not benefit from FDPL during either the growth phase or the involution phase. For these types of hemangiomas, prior treatment with IR Nd:YAG laser radiation with continuous ice-cube cooling is required. The superficial component may respond much better to treatment with the pulsed dye laser once the underlying subcutaneous vessels have been treated with the IR radiation.

8.3.1.3 Dye Lasers for Telangiectases

Telangiectasia and angiokeratoma are classified in the same category as PWSs [29]. Telangiectases, also known as spider veins, are small dilated blood vessels near the surface of the skin measuring between 0.5 and 1 mm in diameter. Although they can develop anywhere on the body, they are most commonly seen on the face around the nose, cheeks, and chin. Angiokeratoma is a benign cutaneous lesion of capillaries, resulting in small marks of red to blue color, and characterized by thickening of the stratum corneum.

Photoaging-induced and rosacea-associated facial redness and telangiectases do not respond to topical or systemic medications. Although electrocoagulation can be used for local or individual vessels, this is an impractical option for extensive vessels seen in telangiectatic photodamage and in patients with rosacea or diffuse facial redness. FPDL has been shown to be a useful alternative. In particular, treating telangiectases in acne rosacea patients with FPDLs can also diminish the papule–pustule load as well as redness and flushing [30]. Use of stacked pulses and multiple passes with

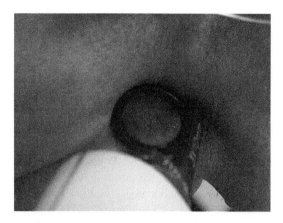

FIGURE 8.2 Vessel tracking with elliptical spot on the Vbeam® pulsed dye laser. (With kind permission from Springer Science+Business Media: *Lasers Med.Sci.*, Using the ultra-long pulse width pulsed dye laser and elliptical spot to treat resistant nasal Telangiectasia, 25, 2010, 151–154, Madan, V. and J. Ferguson, Copyright 2009).

the 10 ms, 595 nm FPDL at subpurpuric settings has been considered to be the best option for the treatment of diffuse facial telangiectases [31]. An image of a vessel tracking with the radiation from a pulsed dye laser system is shown in Figure 8.2 [32].

8.3.1.4 Dye Lasers for Human Papilloma Virus-Induced and Other Warts

Warts (verrucae) are common benign epidermal proliferations caused by human papillomavirus (HPV) infection. The treatment of warts (verrucae vulgaris, verrucae plana) includes surgical excision, cryotherapy, curettage, topical cytotoxic medications (5-fluorouracil, dinitrochlorobenzene), intralesional bleomycin, IR coagulation, PDT, electrosurgery, and laser therapy. FPDL destroys the capillary supply of the wart, causing wart necrosis. At high fluences, FPDL also causes thermal damage to the infected cells. Thus, FPDL treatment has been recommended as an option in HPV-induced warts. By FPDL-induced photocoagulation of the vessels at fluences in the range of 8–10 J/cm², applied repetitively in several sessions, the viability of the cells is compromised. It is recommended to use high fluences without cooling, which causes nonspecific injury to the treated warts and tissue. This treatment is quite painful, although the pain could be somewhat relieved by blowing cold air on the area for a couple of minutes afterwards [33].

8.3.1.5 Dye Lasers for Hypertrophic Scars and Keloids

A keloid is a benign fibrous growth that develops in scar tissue because of altered wound healing, with overproduction of extracellular matrix and dermal fibroblasts that have a high mitotic rate. After the skin is injured, the healing process usually leaves a flat scar. Sometimes the scar is hypertrophic, or thickened, but confined to the margins of the wound. A keloid, by contrast, is a tough heaped-up scar that rises abruptly over the rest of the skin. It may start some time after the injury and extend beyond the wound site. This tendency to migrate into surrounding areas that were not injured to begin with distinguishes keloids from hypertrophic scars. Keloids typically appear following surgery or injury, but they can also appear spontaneously or as a result of some slight inflammation. They develop most often on the chest, back, shoulders, and earlobes, but rarely on the face (with the exception of the jawline). Although keloids are benign and noncontagious, they not only represent a cosmetic problem but also are usually accompanied by severe itchiness, sharp pains, and changes in texture. In severe cases, the movement of skin can be affected.

Despite increasing knowledge of wound healing and collagen metabolism, so far no universally accepted and completely satisfying method in the treatment of hypertrophic scars and keloids has been established. Some of the methods tried are excisional surgery and cryotherapy, adjunctive intralesional corticosteroid application, pressure therapy, and covering with silicone gel sheets. Radiation therapy following surgical removal has also been used, although it was soon abandoned due to possible long-term carcinogenicity. Treatment strategies are similar for both types of lesions, but hypertrophic scars are far less likely to recur once treated [34].

Laser treatment has been tried for both keloids and hypertrophic scars as an alternative to traditional therapies. To choose the best type of laser or technique with specific effects, a previous assessment of the clinical appearance of these lesions, with their individual color, shape, size, or vascularization, is necessary. The skin type of patient and the localization of the lesion should also be considered.

Erythematous hypertrophic scars and keloids (especially erythematous burn scars and keloids) have been treated with promising results in well-controlled studies with FPDL. The laser irradiation induces selective photothermolysis with irreversible destruction of microvessels, which reduces scar microcirculation and leads to a reduction of erythema, with lightening of scars and keloids [35]. Typically, an FPDL emitting at 585 nm (hemoglobin absorption band) with fluences of 6–8 J/cm^2 is utilized, although fluences as high as 18 J/cm^2 have been used in some cases, with pulse duration of 300 µs, spot size of 5 mm, and spatial overlap between pulses of 10%–20% [36–42]. In the case of intense erythema, continuous cooling of the skin surface with a cooling chamber is advisable to reduce pain and thermal side effects at the epidermis. Multiple treatments can be necessary, with 6–8 weeks between sessions. A purpuric tissue response develops immediately after FPDL treatment, which disappears within 10–15 days. Side effects such as small bubbles or crusting can also develop in the treated area, which heal in some days without intervention. Other rare side effects can include hyperpigmentation or infection. The recurrence rate is very low.

In general, the best results are obtained with erythematous hypertrophic scars, especially hypertrophic burn scars, keloids with small elevations, and newer lesions. The results are less satisfactory in the treatment of prominent and fibrotic keloids, proliferate keloids, dermal contractures within the scars, or lesions older than 2 years [40,41,43]. In these cases, it is advisable to use primary transcutaneous or interstitial Nd:YAG laser treatment.

8.3.2 DYE LASERS FOR PIGMENTED LESIONS

Usually, the removal of pigmented lesions is requested for cosmetic reasons. Since these lesions are easily accessible, a large array of therapeutic options has evolved for their management (curettage, dermashaving, cryotherapy, scalped surgery, electrosurgery, topical chemotherapy, and photonic treatment). However, in many of the epithelial lesions, more selective destruction can be achieved by laser techniques.

Melanin is the main natural cutaneous pigment to be considered when dealing with pigmented lesions. Melanocytes at the base of the epidermis synthesize melanin in the form of 0.5 µm intracellular organelles called melanosomes. Melanin absorbs in a broad spectral range across the UV, visible, and near-IR (NIR) spectrum, with decreasing absorption at longer wavelengths, and consequently is a good target for laser treatment. Target specificity of laser pulses depends on wavelength and pulse width. Lasers with emission lines that are absorbed by melanin preferentially over other cutaneous chromophores can be used to eliminate cutaneous melanin selectively. Lasers that emit shorter wavelengths (green light) penetrate optically very little into skin layers and require relatively less energy to produce irreversible thermal damage to melanosomes; therefore, they should be selected to treat epidermal lesions. Lasers that emit longer wavelengths (red light) should be selected to treat deeper dermal melanosomes (dermal lesions). The appropriate pulse width depends primarily on the size of the target and its thermal relaxation time. The calculated thermal relaxation time for melanosomes is about 250–1000 ns. Therefore, 504 and 510 nm FPDLs with pulse duration of 300 ns can destroy pigment-containing organelles or cells of the epidermal lesions by selective photothermolysis, allowing the melanin chromophore target to dissipate its heat without burning normal adjacent structures [44].

Epidermal pigmented lesions such as ephelides, benign lentigo, café-au-lait macules (CALMs) and seborrheic keratoses, can also be treated with the aforementioned FPDL laser, although purpura formation may occur following laser irradiation because the green wavelength of the laser is also well absorbed by oxyhemoglobin. Occasionally, purpura leads to postinflammatory hyperpigmentation. Treatments are usually initiated at 2.0–3.0 J/cm^2 using nonoverlapping 5 mm laser spots. An immediate ash-white discoloration occurs, followed by purpura, which last for 4–7 days before fading [45]. Repeated treatments are delivered at 6–8 week intervals. Eradication of CALMs may require as many as 8–12 treatment sessions, whereas just one or two laser treatments eradicate lentigines. Some studies have shown that FPDL with compression is superior to cryotherapy in the treatment of solar lentigines in darker skin types [46]. In addition, 595 nm FPDL is effective and safe in the treatment of facial lentigines in the darker skin phototypes [47].

As a note of caution, it should be noted that the aforementioned lasers produce a variable response in dermoepidermal pigmented lesions such as Becker's nevi and melasma. Because of the variability in clinical response, testing the treatment areas of the respective lesion may be prudent prior to engaging in a full treatment [48].

8.3.3 DYE LASERS FOR TATTOO REMOVAL

The practice of tattooing is an old one, and evidence of tattoos has been found in ancient Egyptian mummies. Tattooing is accomplished by injecting colored pigment into small deep holes made in the skin, resulting in marks or designs that are relatively permanent. Although over the last decade tattoos have experienced increased popularity all over the world, there are still negative associations with tattoos, and improved self-image or social stigmatization leads people to turn to physicians to remove tattoos.

Many different methods for tattoo removal have been explored over the centuries. Older techniques involve destruction or removal of the outer skin layers by either mechanical (dermabrasion, salabrasion, excision), chemical, or thermal (direct heat, cautery, IR coagulator) means. In the early 1980s, the principle of selective photo-thermolysis, established by Anderson and Parrish [13,49], revolutionized the treat-ment of tattoos. They proposed that the heat generated by incident laser radiation would be confined to the target if the wavelength was well absorbed by the tattoo inks and the pulse width was equal to or shorter than the thermal relaxation time of the target. To specifically target tattoos, laser wavelength and pulse duration must be appropriately chosen. To target tattoo ink, the best laser wavelength should be that which achieves selective absorption for each ink color while minimizing absorption by the primary endogenous chromophores, hemoglobin and melanin.

There are different types of tattoos, such as professional, amateur, and trau-matic tattoos. In general, amateur and traumatic tattoos require fewer treatments for removal than professional multicolored tattoos. Usually, neither the tattooist nor the tattooed knows the content of the pigment used, which is a concern when choosing the correct laser wavelength. In this regard, reflectance spectrum data for tattoo ink colors may assist in selecting the best available wavelength.

The absorption of laser pulses breaks up the tattoo pigments into smaller par-ticles, which are quickly and readily absorbed by the natural defense system by an inflammatory reaction. The pigment can also be eliminated via a scale or a crust that is shed off. Another result of the treatment is an optical alteration of the pigment to make it less apparent. Absorption by different tattoo colors has been studied and measured in vivo by skin reflectance to establish optical laser wave-lengths for treating different tattoo colors. High efficiency can be reached with lasers operating in the nanosecond range and using an irradiation wavelength at which the percentage of reflection from the pigment is minimal [50,51]. Under this condition, laser pulses can be used with a low fluence, minimizing adverse effects and clinical time [50].

Black pigment is absorptive at all wavelengths (having minimal reflectance), and competition with melanin absorption in the epidermis decreases gradually as wave-length increases. Absorption for blue and green is greatest for wavelengths of 600–800 nm, whereas red absorbs best below 575 nm, tan below 560 nm, flesh-colored pigment below 535 nm, and yellow below 520 nm [52].

The FPDL (510 nm, 300 ns with a 3 mm spot size) is well absorbed by red pig-ments, and the pulse width is short enough to fragment the ink granules. Successful cleaning without scarring usually occurred in three to seven treatments developed at intervals of 1 month using a fluence of 3–3.75 J/cm² [53]. Purple, orange, and yel-low pigments require an average of five treatments to achieve complete removal. No hypopigmentation, textural changes, or marks are observed during treatment. Histologically, fragmentation of red pigment particles is observed, followed by mac-rophage engulfment [54]. In addition, because of the epidermal absorption of this laser, transepidermal ink loss occurs.

It is in this application that the solid-state dye lasers (SSDLs) considered in Chapter 3 are probably going to find immediate application. As described in Chapter 3, it is precisely in the yellow-red region of the spectrum that efficient and stable SSDL lasers have already been developed, exhibiting performances comparable to those of the liquid dye lasers emitting in the same region. The recent promising developments of SSDLs extending the tuning range to the 600–750 nm spectral region (Chapter 3) will enable this technology to be extended to the efficient removal of blue and green tattoo inks.

8.3.4 Dye Lasers for Inflammatory Skin Diseases

Nowadays, the position of the FPDL in the treatment of inflammatory skin diseases is still unclear. While published results are certainly promising enough to be followed up by independent research, they are insufficient to justify the abandonment of traditional methods with proven efficacy. The utilization of FPDL in the treatment of inflammatory skin diseases has recently been examined examined by Erceg and collaborators [55].

8.3.4.1 Plaque Psoriasis

Psoriasis is a prevalent inflammatory skin condition that is characterized by chronic T-cell stimulation, abnormal proliferation of dermal vasculature, and parakeratotic epidermal hyperplasia. Common manifestations of psoriasis involve well-demarcated plaques with overlying scales affecting the extremities, intertriginous regions, and nails. Psoriasis can elicit notable patient discomfort. Many treatment modalities (topical: cortisone, retinoids, vitamin D; systemic: methotrexate, cyclosporine, immunomodulatory drugs; phototherapy) continue to be pursued in an effort to adequately address the effects of this disease.

In 1992, Hacker and Rasmussen described for the first time the treatment of psoriasis with the FPDL [56]. A positive correlation between microvessel number (microvascular density) and plaque severity score has been observed; thus, the extensive destruction of dermal papillary microvessels obtained after FPDL treatment could result in clinical improvement [57,58]. Normalization of the vasculature of psoriatic lesions is correlated with the duration of remission induced by the treatment [57]. In addition, a direct cutaneous immunologic activation has also been reported as a mode of action of the FPDL [59]. Treatment with FPDL should therefore be recommended as an alternative therapy to control psoriasis.

The FPDL has also been investigated in the treatment of some variants of psoriasis. In this regard, several studies indicate that FPDL offers an effective treatment for resistant plaque-type psoriasis or recalcitrant psoriasis lesions such as nail psoriasis [60,61], and the device has been cleared by the U.S. Food and Drug Administration (FDA) for this purpose [62,63].

8.3.4.2 Acne

Acne is not a life-threatening disease, but if it is not treated adequately, it can result in permanent scarring of the affected area, causing substantial and persistent social, psychological, or emotional harm, which renders treatment a necessity. Acne initiates as a result of sebaceous gland hyperactivity and hyperseborrhea, altered keratinization of ductal keratinocytes and resultant follicular plugging, hyperproliferation of *Propionibacterium acnes*, and inflammatory signaling. Various laser and light therapies have been increasingly used for the treatment of acne vulgaris. Absorption of the light of specific wavelengths of FPDL systems by endogenous porphyrins produced by *P. acnes* during its metabolic and reproductive processes is believed to produce phototoxic effects that kill the bacteria. FPDL also reduces vascularity by altering the inflammatory response of active acne as well as decreasing postinflammatory erythema; thus, the use of FPDL for the treatment of inflammatory acne vulgaris has shown sustained improvement in inflammatory lesions such as papules, pustules, and nodules [64,65]. Recently, FPDLs were also proposed to have an immunomodulatory effect on the resolution of inflammatory acne. Amelioration reactions and an increase in transforming growth factor (TGF)-β expression was observed by histopathological examinations of inflammatory acne lesions treated by FPDL [66]. TGF-β1 is known to be a potent stimulator of neocollagenesis, playing a central role in the initiation of wound healing. This immunosuppressive cytokine promotes the resolution of inflammation process and is the most potent inhibitor of keratinocyte proliferation [66]. At present, results on the benefit of FPDL in acne are still questionable. Maintenance treatments are recommended, because the improvement seems to be a short term [67].

8.4 SAFETY DURING OPERATION AND MAINTENANCE OF DYE LASERS

When working with a laser, one should always be aware of the potential risks, not only for the patients but also for the physicians and the surgical staff. Safety issues that should be especially considered when using lasers in medical applications are eye protection, plumes of vaporized tissue, and potential fire hazards [68].

The area of potential hazard is not limited to the immediate surgical site, because unlike other light sources, the laser beam is collimated and propagates over long distances. The laser light itself can, directly or by reflection, be dangerous to unprotected skin or eyes. Laser beams are reflected to some extent from any surface they contact, and reflected light can still cause serious injuries if it reaches the eye, because of the eye's focusing capability. In fact, an examination of laser accident records indicates that the source of accidental ocular exposure is most frequently a reflected beam. Ocular damage may result from the absorption of laser light by the structures in the eye, and therefore the laser surgeon and staff must, whenever the laser is in operation, wear protective eyewear with an optical density (OD) specific for the laser wavelength used. Each pair of goggles should be marked with the appropriate wavelength of protection and OD for the specific lasers in use. Dye lasers in the visible and NIR range of the spectrum have the greatest potential for retinal injury, as the cornea and the lens are transparent to those wavelengths, and the lens can focus the laser energy onto the retina. The maximum absorption of laser energy onto the retina occurs in the range from 400 to 550 nm. Wavelengths of less than 550 nm can cause a photochemical injury similar to sunburn. Photochemical effects are cumulative and result from long exposures (over 10 s) to diffuse or scattered light.

Patient safety is assured by limiting needless exposure to the laser radiation of tissues adjacent to those treated, by using noncombustible materials adjacent to the beam, and by protecting the patient's eyes. Skin damage from laser radiation can occur due to uncontrolled movements of the laser by the surgeon, reflected laser light, or inattentiveness of staff, which may lead to induction of burns, pigment darkening, or photosensitive reactions in the skin during laser therapy. The severity of the injury depends on the length of exposure and the penetration depth of the laser radiation.

For usual liquid dye lasers, another hazardous aspect that must be taken into account is the mixing of chemicals that make up the active lasing medium. Thus, strict controls are necessary for the handling of the chemicals: dye and solvent mixing should be done inside a chemistry fume hood. Gloves, lab coats, and eye protection should be worn. Avoid skin contact. During dye laser disassembly, use proper personal protective equipment and be alert to contaminated parts, for example, dye filters. For waste disposal and spills, emphasis should be placed on solvent characteristics, since dye concentrations are low. In this regard, the SSDLs considered in Chapters 3 and 4 avoid the problems of toxicity and provide a low-cost gain medium; they are also compact and easy to operate and maintain. Thus, they would be much more appropriate for use in a medical environment than the usual liquid dye lasers. The technology of the SSDL lasers is maturing fast, and it is expected that their appearance on the market as competitive products in the near future will avoid hazards of this kind.

Many laser systems require a high-voltage power supply. The most serious accidents with lasers have been electrocutions. Changed condensers can be dangerous even if the laser is disconnected from the electrical supply. Users of this equipment must be familiar with safe procedures and electrical safety controls. Pulsed lasers may additionally interfere electromagnetically with other electronic medical equipment.

We cannot end without insisting on the fact that medical lasers represent complex systems whose effective service depends on different factors such as wavelength, pulse duration, fluences, and so on. To be able to use this service purposefully and safely, it is necessary to have not only theoretical knowledge of optical physics, but also appropriate training. Thus, participation in specific courses of training programs is strongly recommended. Accidents can only be prevented by well-trained staff and an administrative policy that encourages a sustained effort toward safe laser use.

REFERENCES

1. Allison, R., T. S. Mang, G. Hewson, W. Snider, and D. Dougherty, Photodynamic therapy for chest wall progression from breast carcinoma is an underutilized treatment modality, *Cancer* 91: 1–8, 2001.
2. Dougherty, T. J., Photodynamic therapy, *Photochem. Photobiol.* 58: 895–900, 1993.
3. Dougherty, T. J., J. E. Kaufman, A. Goldfarb, K. R. Weishaupt, D. Boyle, and A. Mittleman, Photoradiation therapy for the treatment of malignant tumours, *Cancer Res.* 38: 2628–2635, 1978.
4. Mang, T. S., Lasers and light sources for PDT: Past, present and future, *Photodiagnosis Photodyn. Ther.* 1: 43–48, 2004.

5. Allison, R. R., H. C. Mota, and C. H. Sibata, Clinical PD/PDT in North America: An historical review, *Photodiagnosis Photodyn. Ther.* 1: 263–277, 2004.

6. Berlien, H. P. and G. J. Müller, *Applied Laser Medicine*, Springer, Berlin, 2003.

7. Allison, R. R. and C. H. Sibata, Oncologic photodynamic therapy photosensitizers: A clinical review, *Photodiagnosis Photodyn. Ther* 7: 61–75, 2010.

8. Brancaleon, L. and H. Moseley, Laser and non-laser light sources for photodynamic therapy, *Lasers Med. Sci.* 17: 173–186, 2002.

9. Lambert, R., Esophageal cancer: Photodynamic therapy. In R. Fujita, J. R. Jass, M. Kaminishi, and R. J. Schlemper (Eds), *Early Cancer of the Gastrointestinal Tract: Endoscopy, Pathology and Treatment*, pp. 207–212, Springer, Berlin, 2006.

10. Panjehpour, M. and B. F. Overholt, Therapeutic applications of laser gastroenterology. In T. Vo-Dinh (Ed.), *Biomedical Photonics Handbook*, Chapter 46, pp. 1207–1218, CRC Press, Boca Raton, FL, 2003.

11. Sidoroff, A., Topical sensitization-oncologic indications-actinic keratosis. In P. G. Calzavara-Pinton, R. M. Szeimies, and B. Ortel (Eds), *Photodynamic Therapy and Fluorescence Diagnosis in Dermatology*, Chapter 12, pp. 199–216, Elsevier Science, Amsterdam, 2001.

12. Wilson, B. C., Photodynamic therapy: Light delivery and dosage for second generation photosensitizers. In *Photosensitizing Compounds: Their Chemistry, Biology and Clinical Use*, pp. 60–73, John Wiley, Chichester, 1989.

13. Anderson, R. R. and J. A. Parrish, The optics of human skin, *J. Invest. Dermatol.* 77: 13–19, 1981.

14. Nakagawa, H., O. T. Tan, and J. A. Parrish, Ultrastructural changes in human skin after exposure to a pulsed laser, *J. Invest. Dermatol.* 84: 396–400, 1985.

15. Morelli, J. G., O. T. Tan, J. Garden, R. Margolis, Y. Seki, J. Boll, J. M. Carney, et al. Tunable dye laser (577 nm) treatment of port wine stains, *Lasers Surg. Med.* 6: 94–99, 1986.

16. Mahendran, R. and R. A. Sheehan-Dare, Survey of the practices of laser users in the UK in the treatment of port wine stains, *J. Dermatol. Treat.* 15: 112–117, 2004.

17. Lanigan, S. W. and S. M. Taibjee, Recent advances in laser treatment of port-wine stains, *Br. J. Dermatol.* 151: 527–533, 2004.

18. Adamic, M., A. Troilius, M. Adatto, M. Drosner, and R. Dahmane, Vascular lasers and IPLs: Guidelines for care from the European Society for Laser Dermatology (ESLD), *J. Cosmet. Laser Ther.* 9: 113–124, 2007.

19. Michel, S., M. Landthaler, and U. Hohenleutner, Recurrence of port-wine stains after treatment with the flashlamp-pumped pulsed dye laser, *Br. J. Dermatol.* 143: 1230–1234, 2000.

20. Chapas, A. M., K. Eickhorst, and R. G. Geronemus, Efficacy of early treatment of facial port wine stains in newborns: A review of 49 cases, *Lasers Surg. Med.* 39: 563–568, 2007.

21. Lanigan, S., Reduction of pain in the treatment of vascular lesions with a pulsed dye laser and pneumatic skin flattening, *Lasers Med. Sci.* 24: 617–620, 2009.

22. Kautz, G., I. Kautz, J. Segal, and S. Zehren, Treatment of resistant port wine stains (PWS) with pulsed dye laser and non-contact vacuum: A pilot study, *Lasers Med. Sci.* 25: 525–529, 2010.

23. Wareham, W. J., R. P. Cole, S. L. Royston, and P. A. Wright, Adverse effects reported in pulsed dye laser treatment for port wine stains, *Lasers Med. Sci.* 24: 241–246, 2009.

24. Jacobs, A. H. and R. G. Walton, The incidence of birth-marks in the neonate, *Pediatrics* 58: 218–222, 1976.

25. Urban, P. and B. Algermissen, Stadieneinteilung kindlicher hämangiome nach FKDS-kriterien, *Ultraschall. Med.* 20: 36–40, 1999.

26. Chang, L. C., A. N. Haggstrom, B. A. Drolet, E. Baselga, S. L. Chamlin, M. C. Garzon, K. A. Horii, et al., Growth characteristics of infantile hemangiomas: Implications for management, *Pediatrics* 122: 360–367, 2008.

27. Witman, P. M., A. M. Wagner, K. Scherer, M. Waner, and I.J. Frieden, Complications following pulsed dye laser treatment of superficial hemangiomas, *Lasers Surg. Med.* 38: 116–123, 2006.

28. Kono, T., H. Sakurai, W. F. Groff, H. H. Chan, M. Takeuchi, T. Yamaki, K. Soejima, et al., Comparison study of a traditional pulsed dye laser versus a long-pulsed dye laser in the treatment of early childhood hemangiomas, *Lasers Surg. Med.* 38: 112–115, 2006.

29. Enjolras, O. and J. B. Mulliken, Vascular tumors and vascular malformations (new issues), *Adv. Dermatol.* 13: 375–423, 1997.

30. Tan, S. R. and W. D. Tope, Pulsed dye laser treatment of rosacea improves erythema, symptomatology, and quality of life, *J. Am. Acad. Dermatol.* 51: 592–599, 2004.

31. Rohrer, T. E., V. Chatrath, and V. Iyengar, Does pulse stacking improve the results of treatment with variable-pulse pulsed-dye lasers? *Dermatol. Surg.* 30: 163–167, 2004.

32. Madan, V. and J. Ferguson, Using the ultra-long pulse width pulsed dye laser and elliptical spot to treat resistant nasal Telangiectasia, *Lasers Med. Sci.* 25: 151–154, 2010

33. Komericki, P. and M. Akkilic, Treatment of an intrameatal wart with short pulse dye laser: A case report, *J. Eur. Acad. Dermatol. Venereol.* 21: 1422–1423, 2007.

34. Wolfram, D., A. Tzankov, P. Pülzi, and H. Piza-Katzer, Hypertrophic scars and keloids: A review of their pathophysiology, risk factors, and therapeutic management, *Dermatol. Surg.* 35: 171–181, 2009.

35. Karsai, S., S. Roos, S. Hammes, and C. Raulin, Pulsed dye laser: What new in non-vascular lesions? *J. Eur. Acad. Dermatol. Venereol.* 21: 877–890, 2007.

36. Alster, T. S., Improvement of erythematous and hypertrophic scars by the 585-nm flashlamp-pumped pulsed dye laser, *Ann. Plast. Surg.* 32: 186–190, 1994.

37. Alster, T. S. and C. M. Williams, Treatment of keloid sternotomy scars with 585 nm flashlamp-pumped pulsed dye laser, *Lancet* 345: 1198–1200, 1995.

38. Dierickx, C., M. P. Goldmann, and R. E. Fitzpatrick, Laser treatment of erythematous/hypertrophic and pigmental scars in 26 patients, *Plast. Reconstr. Surg.* 95: 84–89, 1995.

39. Alster, T. S. and C. Handrick, Laser treatment of hypertrophic scars, keloids, and striae, *Semin. Cutan. Med. Surg.* 19: 287–292, 2000.

40. Scharschmidt, D., B. Algermissen, C. Philipp, and H. P. Berlien, Prinzipien der Laserbehandlung von Narben and Keloiden, *J. DGPW* 16: 7–9, 1998.

41. Paquet, P., J. F. Hermanns, and G. E. Piérard, Effect of the 585 nm flashlamp-pumped pulsed dye laser for the treatment of keloids, *Dermatol. Surg.* 27: 171–174, 2001.

42. Kuo, Y. R., W. S. Wu, and F. S. Wang, Flashlamp pulsed-dye laser suppressed TGF-β1 expression and proliferation in cultured keloid fibroblasts is mediated by MAPK pathway, *Lasers Surg. Med.* 39: 358–364, 2007.

43. McCraw, J. B., J. A. McCraw, and N. Bettencourt, Prevention of unfavourable scars using early pulse dye lasers treatments: A preliminary report, *Ann. Plast. Surg.* 42: 7–14, 1999.

44. Fitzpatrick, R. E., M. P. Goldman, and J. Ruiz-Esparza, Laser treatment of benign pigmented lesions using a 300 nanosecond pulse and 510 nm wavelength, *J. Dermatol. Surg. Oncol.* 19: 341–347, 1993.

45. Al-Dujaili, Z. and C. C. Dierickx, Laser treatment of pigmented lesions. In D. J. Goldberg (Ed.), *Laser Dermatology*, 2nd edn, pp. 41–64, Springer, Berlin, 2013.

46. Seirafi, H., S. Fateh, F. Farnaghi, A. H. Ehsani, and P. Noormohammadpour, Efficacy and safety of long-pulsed dye laser delivered with compression versus cryotherapy for treatment of solar lentigines, *Indian J. Dermatol.* 56: 48–51, 2011.

47. Pootonqkam, S. and P. Asawanonda, Purpura-free treatment of lentigines using a long-pulsed 595 nm pulsed dye laser with compression handpiece: A randomized, controlled study, *J. Drugs Dermatol.* 8(11 Suppl): 18–24, 2009.

48. Bukvić Mokos, Z., J. Lipozenčić, R. Ceović, D. Stulhofer Buzina, and K. Kostović, Laser therapy of pigmented lesions: Pro and contra, *Acta Dermatovenerol. Croat.* 18: 185–189, 2010.

49. Anderson, R. R. and J. A. Parrish, Selective photothermolysis: Precise microsurgery by selective absorption of pulsed radiation, *Science* 220: 524–527, 1983.

50. Gómez, C., V. Martín, R. Sastre, A. Costela, and I. García-Moreno, In vitro and in vivo laser treatment of tattoos: High efficiency and low fluences, *Arch. Dermatol.* 146: 39–45, 2010.

51. Kossida, T., D. Rigopoulos, A. Katsambas, and R. R. Anderson, Optimal tattoo removal in a single laser session based on the method of repeated exposures, *J. Am. Acad. Dermatol.* 66: 271–277, 2012.

52. Bäumler, W., E. T. Eibler, U. Hohenleutner, B. Sens, J. Sauer, and M. Landthaler, Q-switch laser and tattoo pigments: First results of chemical and photophysical analysis of 41 compounds, *Lasers Surg. Med.* 26: 13–21, 2000.

53. Grekin, R. C., R. M. Shelton, J. K. Geisse, and I. Frieden, 510-nm pigmented lesion dye laser. Its characteristics and clinical uses, *J. Dermatol. Surg. Oncol.* 19: 380–387, 1993.

54. Tan, O. T., J. G. Morelli, and A. K. Kurban, Pulsed dye laser treatment of benign cutaneous pigmented lesions, *Lasers Surg. Med.* 12: 538–542, 1992.

55. Erceg, A., E. M. de Jong, P. C. van de Kerkhof, and M. M. Seyger, The efficacy of pulsed dye laser treatment for inflammatory skin diseases: A systematic review, *J. Am. Acad. Dermatol.* 69: 609–615, 2013.

56. Hacker, S. M. and J. E. Rasmussen, The effect of flash lamp-pulsed dye laser on psoriasis, *Arch. Dermatol.* 128: 853–855, 1992.

57. Noborio, R., M. Kurokawa, K. Kobayashi, and A. Morita, Evaluation of the clinical and immunohistological efficacy of the 585-nm pulsed dye laser in the treatment of psoriasis, *J. Eur. Acad. Dermatol. Venereol.* 23: 420–424, 2009.

58. Hern, S., A. W. Stanton, R. H. Mellor, C. C. Hardland, J. R. Levick, and P. S. Mortimer, In vivo quantification of the structural abnormalities in psoriatic microvessels before and after pulsed dye laser treatment, *Br. J. Dermatol.* 152: 505–511, 2005.

59. Omi, T., S. Kawana, S. Sato, S. Takezaki, M. Honda, T. Igarashi, R. W. Hankins, et al., Cutaneous immunological activation elicited by a low-fluence pulsed dye laser, *Br. J. Dermatol.* 153(Suppl s2): 57–62, 2005.

60. Fernández-Guarino, M., A. Harto, M. Sánchez-Ronco, I. García-Morales, and P. Jaén, Pulsed dye laser vs photodynamic therapy in the treatment of refractory nail psoriasis: A comparative pilot study, *J. Eur. Acad. Dermatol. Venereol.* 23(8): 891–895, 2009.

61. Oram, Y., Y. Karincaoğlu, E. Koyuncu, and F. Kaharaman, Pulsed dye laser in the treatment of nail psoriasis, *Dermatol. Surg.* 36: 377–381, 2010.

62. Goldust, M. and R. Raghifar, Clinical trial study in the treatment of nail psoriasis with pulsed dye laser, *J. Cosmet. Laser Ther.* Epub ahead of print October 16, 2013. DOI: 10.3109/14764172.2013.854627.

63. Yin, N., S. Choudhary, and K. Nouri, Pulsed dye laser for the treatment of nail psoriasis, *Cutis* 92: 129–135, 2013.

64. Seaton, E. D., A. Charakida, P. E. Mouser, I. Grace, R. M. Clement, and A. C. Chu, Pulsed-dye laser treatment for inflammatory acne vulgaris: Randomized controlled trial, *Lancet* 362: 1347–1352, 2003.

65. Seaton, E. D., P. E. Mouser, A. Charakida, S. Alam, P. M. Seldon, and A. C. Chu, Investigation of the mechanism of action of nonablative pulsed-dye laser therapy in photorejuvenation and inflammatory acne vulgaris, *Br. J. Dermatol.* 155: 748–755, 2006.

66. Choi, Y. S., H. S. Suh, M. Y. Yoon, S. U. Min, D. H. Lee, and D. H. Suh, Intense pulsed light vs. pulsed-dye laser in the treatment of facial acne: A randomized split-face trial, *J. Eur. Acad. Dermatol. Venereol.* 24: 773–780, 2010.

67. Karsai, S., L. Schmitt, and C. Raulin, The pulsed-dye laser as an adjuvant treatment modality in acne vulgaris: A randomized controlled single-blinded trial, *Br. J. Dermatol.* 163: 395–401, 2010.

68. Sliney, D. H. and S. L. Trokel, Laser injury and potential hazards. In D. H. Sliney and S. L. Trokel (Eds), *Medical Lasers and Their Safe Use*, pp. 72–86, Springer, New York, 1993.

9 Tunable Laser Microscopy

F. J. Duarte

CONTENTS

9.1 INTRODUCTION

A laser microscope is a microscope optical system that uses a laser as the illumination source. Very briefly, lasers were introduced to the field of microscopy in the mid-1960s [1], and confocal scanning laser microscopes were disclosed in the late 1960s [2,3]. The concept of scanning meant the displacement of the laser beam cross section over the specimen to be observed [4]. An additional illumination approach in scanning laser microscopy is near-field laser illumination [5,6].

Static, or instantaneous, scanning using extremely elongated Gaussian beams, yielding illumination very wide in one optical axis while very thin in the orthogonal axis, produced via beam expander optics, was introduced to laser microscopy in the late 1980s [7–10]. Analogous laser illumination, produced via cylindrical lenses, was introduced subsequently [11–13].

Coherent illumination sources used in microscopy can either be continuous-wave (CW) lasers or femtosecond pulse lasers, depending on the particular application. Here, a brief survey of various tunable laser microscopy techniques is provided.

9.2 BASIC ILLUMINATION GEOMETRIES FOR MICROSCOPY

Basic illumination geometries used in microscopy are illustrated in Figures 9.1 through 9.3, from a laser perspective. That is, the illuminating beam of light is assumed to be a single-transverse-mode beam with a Gaussian profile and spectrally coherent, or narrow, linewidth, at a wavelength $\lambda \pm \Delta\lambda$, where $\Delta\lambda$ is very small. Relative to the basic focusing system illustrated in Figure 9.1, the widely used parameter in microscopy, known as the *numerical aperture*, or *NA*, is defined as [14]

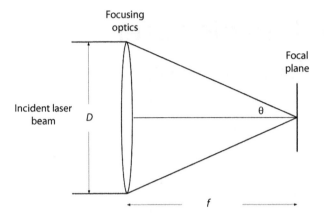

FIGURE 9.1   Basic focusing illumination used in microscopy.

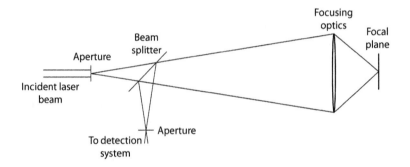

FIGURE 9.2   Confocal illumination geometry.

$$NA \approx n \sin \theta \tag{9.1}$$

where:
  θ is the angle sustained between the optical axis and the outer edge of the focusing beam
  n is the refractive index of the propagating medium

From the geometry of Figure 9.1,

$$NA \approx n \sin \theta \approx n \sin \left(\arctan \frac{D}{2f} \right) \tag{9.2}$$

The same approximation applies to the confocal configuration described in Figure 9.2. In the case of near-field illumination via an optical fiber, as illustrated in Figure 9.3, the numerical aperture is defined as [15]

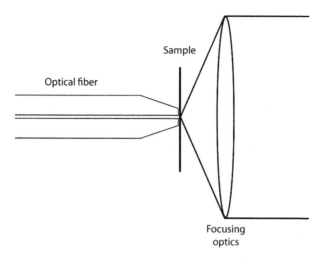

FIGURE 9.3   Fiber illumination for near-field optical microscopy.

$$NA \approx n\sin\theta' \approx \left(n_1^2 - n_2^2\right)^{1/2} \tag{9.3}$$

where:

θ' is the maximum acceptance angle
n_1 is the refractive index of the core
n_2 is the refractive index of the cladding of the fiber [15]

In the case of laser illumination with single-transverse-mode beams with a Gaussian profile, the numerical aperture is sometimes associated with the beam divergence of the laser. This practice is mainly prevalent with single-transverse-mode highly divergent semiconductor waveguides. As such, the numerical aperture for external-cavity semiconductor lasers can be expressed as [16]

$$NA \approx \Delta\theta \approx \frac{\lambda}{\pi w}\left[1+\left(\frac{L_\mathcal{R}}{B}\right)^2+\left(\frac{L_\mathcal{R}A}{B}\right)^2\right]^{1/2} \tag{9.4}$$

where:

λ is the wavelength of emission
w is the beam waist
A and B are propagation matrix terms

and

$$L_\mathcal{R} = \frac{\pi w^2}{\lambda} \tag{9.5}$$

is the Rayleigh (see Chapter 5 for further details).

For well-designed cavities, the terms in the squared brackets approach unity, and

$$NA \approx \frac{\lambda}{\pi w} \tag{9.6}$$

A possible scanning technique is outlined in Figure 9.4. This approach involves the displacing of the focused beam in a direction transverse to the direction of the optical axis of the incident beam. Often, the scanning involves displacement of the focused beam by increments of a fraction of the diameter of the beam. Certainly, an alternative is to move the sample at the focal plane and leave the illuminating beam in a fixed position.

If the optical axis of the illuminating beam is defined as z, then the displacement of the scan shown in Figure 9.4 is in the x direction. Moving the beam in the x direction and the y direction yields information in two dimensions. Again, the same effect can be achieved by moving the sample at the focal plane in the x and y directions. The same observations apply to the near-field technique using fiber illumination.

The description given here applies to the illumination geometries while using either CW or femtosecond lasers. Furthermore, as far as raster scanning is concerned, it should be noted that this can be done either at a low beam velocity or at very high

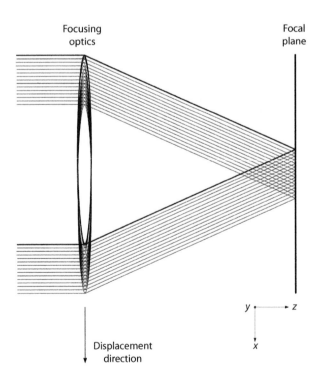

FIGURE 9.4   Point-by-point beam scanning.

linear velocities. In this regard, linear beam-scanning velocities of up to 4000 m/s have been demonstrated using special double-pass rotating polygon systems [17].

Point-by-point beam scanning, as illustrated in Figure 9.4, can be avoided by using extremely elongated Gaussian beam illumination or light sheet illumination (LSI), as explained in Section 9.4.

9.3 MICROSCOPY VIA ULTRASHORT LASER PULSES

Femtosecond pulse lasers, also known as ultrashort pulse lasers or ultrafast lasers, are central to microscopy techniques relying on multiphoton excitation. In the literature, some of those techniques are referred to as multiphoton excited fluorescence microscopy, multiphoton excitation microscopy, or simply multiphoton microscopy. An extensive review on this subject is given by Thomas and Rudolph [18]. These authors consider nonlinear microscopy, via multiphoton fluorescence microscopy, harmonic microscopies, and four-wave mixing microscopy [18]. All these microscopy approaches use femtosecond laser emission as a source of illumination, which by definition is configured by tunable lasers [16]. Here, a brief survey of femtosecond laser sources applicable to microscopy is given, followed by a succinct survey of the various microscopic geometries and their applications.

9.3.1 SURVEY OF FEMTOSECOND LASER SOURCES

For authoritative reviews on ultrashort pulse lasers, the reader should refer to Diels [19] and Diels and Rudolph [20]. Femtosecond semiconductor lasers and prismatic pulse compression are reviewed in Chapter 5. One feature of ultrashort pulse, or femtosecond pulse, lasers is that ideally, their emission linewidth and pulse duration are related by [16]

$$\Delta v \, \Delta t \approx 1 \tag{9.7}$$

so that laser sources yielding very short pulses are associated with a broad emission spectrum. In Table 9.1, the temporal performances of several ultrashort pulse lasers are listed, thus providing a perspective on the class of performance that may be expected from various well-known types of femtosecond-class lasers.

9.3.2 FEMTOSECOND LASER NEAR-FIELD MICROSCOPY

In their review, Thomas and Rudolph [18] focus their attention on nonlinear microscopy, multiphoton fluorescence microscopy, harmonic microscopy, and four-wave mixing microscopy. All these microscopies use femtosecond-type lasers and are configured using the illumination geometries already described. Here, attention is given to near-field scanning optical microscopy (NSOM) [28] using optical fiber illumination [5,6] as described in Figure 9.3.

A laser microscopic technique providing temporal and spatial resolution is known as femtosecond pump-probe near-field optical microscopy [29–31]. A configurational alternative for this scheme is outlined in Figure 9.5. Following [29–31], a femtosecond

TABLE 9.1

Ultrashort Pulse Emission Characteristics of Broadly Tunable Coherent Sources

Emission Source	Central λ[a]	Δt (fs)	References
Dye laser[b]	—	50	[21]
Dye laser[c]	620	6	[22]
$Ti^{3+}:Al_2O_3$ laser[b]	900	5	[23]
ECS[d] laser (AlGaAs)	805	650	[24]
Fiber laser[e]	1200	24	[25]
OPO[f] (BBO[f])	600	4	[26]
Free electron laser	32	25	[27]

[a] Approximate center of the emission spectrum.
[b] Uses a double-prism intracavity pulse compressor.
[c] Uses a four-prism and four-grating pulse compressor.
[d] External-cavity semiconductor laser uses a six-prism pulse compressor.
[e] Includes two double-prism pulse compressors.
[f] Includes a double-prism pulse compressor. BBO, β-barium borate; OPO, optical parametric oscillator.

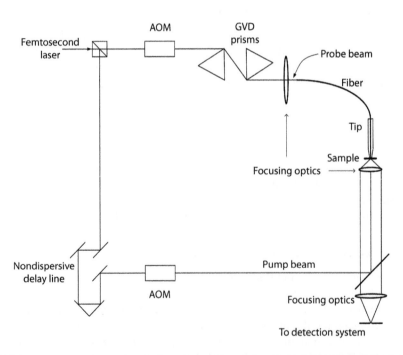

FIGURE 9.5 Approximate description of generic pump-probe near-field laser microscopic configuration. Following prismatic GVD compensation, the probe beam is focused into a fiber connected to the NSOM tip. The pump beam illuminates the sample from the opposite end. Diagram not to scale.

laser beam is divided into a probe and a pump component. Both components are propagated via acousto-optic modulators (AOM). The probe beam then propagates via a double-prism group-velocity-dispersion [32] precompensation stage. The prismatic array yields a negatively chirped pulse that then proceeds to propagate to the entrance of the NSOM fiber and subsequently emerges at the exit of the NSOM tip. The emerging pulse from the NSOM tip is reported to have a duration of ~100 fs or better [29]. The aperture of the fiber NSOM tip is reported to be ~100 nm [29]. The delayed pump femtosecond pulse illuminates the sample from the opposite end.

This pump-probe technique allows a specimen, or sample, to be excited by the femtosecond pump pulse and then to be probed with submicrometer spatial precision by the femtosecond probe pulse. This scheme has been used to observe temporal characteristics as a function of spatial displacement of semiconductor materials such as GaAs/AlGaAs quantum wells [29,30]. Two-dimensional images of quantum wires have also been obtained [31].

9.4 LIGHT SHEET ILLUMINATION

Here, an illumination format for microscopy and nanoscopy applications based on a particular laser beam geometry is described. Over the years, this type of very thin plane laser illumination has become known by several different names, including extremely elongated Gaussian beam illumination [7–9], orthogonal plane illumination [11], selective plane illumination [12], and LSI [13]. This class of illumination obviates the need for point-by-point laser beam scanning. The illumination sources used in this class of microscopy tend to be CW lasers yielding high-quality single-transverse-mode laser beams.

The extremely elongated Gaussian beam illumination (E^2GBI) geometry consists of irradiating the sample, or specimen, of interest with a laser beam, propagating in the z direction, that is very wide in the x direction and very thin in the y direction, as illustrated in Figure 9.6. This class of illumination, extremely wide in the incident plane and very thin in the orthogonal direction to the incident plane, was first disclosed as intracavity illumination of diffraction gratings in tunable lasers [33]. In those experiments, the beam magnification was reported to be $M \approx 60$, albeit further designs describe beam magnifications of $M \approx 200$ [16] or higher (see Chapters 5 and 6). This form of beam expansion is sometimes referred to as *one-dimensional beam expansion*. An illumination optical system consisting of the combination of a conventional two-dimensional transmission telescope, a one-dimensional multiple-prism beam expander, and a focusing lens was reported to yield near-Gaussian beams measuring $20 \times 60,000$ μm, that is, a height to width ratio of 1:3,000 [7]. A detailed description of this class of optical system, including propagation beam matrices, is given in Chapter 10. Several points should be mentioned at this stage: (1) as far as the published literature goes, the focusing optics in these systems has not been optimized to produce thinner beams (i.e., with smaller Δy dimensions); (2) nevertheless, these remain the most elongated near-Gaussian beams (1:3000) so far reported; and (3) the Gaussian profile of the elongated beam can be transformed into a rectangular geometry via diffraction by passing the beam through a wide single slit [9]. When that is done, the intensity profile becomes as illustrated in Figure 9.7 [34]. In practice,

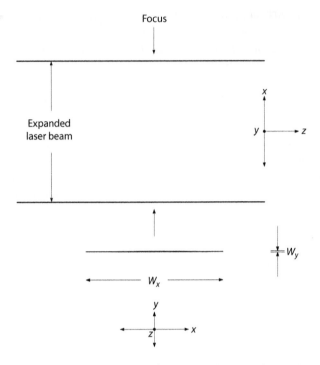

FIGURE 9.6 Beam profile achieved with E²GBI. Note that scanning the beam, or sample, in the *y* direction allows three-dimensional characterization.

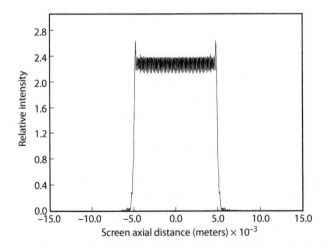

FIGURE 9.7 Diffractive intensity profile of E²GBI, along the *x*-axis, after propagation via a wide slit.

TABLE 9.2

Beam Dimensions at the Focal Plane for Various Laser Illumination Techniques

Illumination	$w_y \times w_x$ (µm)	Wavelength (nm)	References
E²GBI	20×60,000	632.82	[7]
LSI	23×6,500	487.99	[12]
SPI	5.8×660	487.99	[13]
SPI	1.7×5.3	543.30	[35]
	2×8.3	632.82	—

the beams obtained are smoother than the calculated profiles, and there is more than sufficient width to ignore the "batman ears" toward the edges.

SPI and LSI appear to be terminology used to describe equivalent methods of cylindrical lens illumination. An approximate beam geometry description for SPI and LSI is shown in Figure 9.8. From the literature, it appears that the cross section of the beam is uniform or nearly uniform. Also, the ratios of beam height to beam width at the focal plane appear to be more moderate than those reported for extremely elongated Gaussian beams, albeit the beam height, or thickness, is narrower. Beam dimensions for the various illumination techniques at the focal plane are listed in Table 9.2.

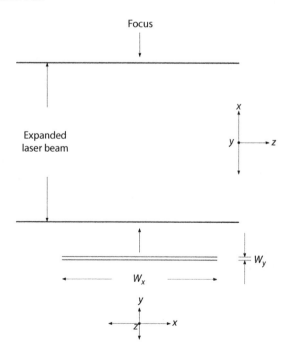

FIGURE 9.8 Approximate beam profile obtained via cylindrical lens focusing assuming a uniform profile, as reported in LSI and SPI.

In Figure 9.9, the optical components and configurations related to E²GBI, LSI, and SPI are outlined. Figure 9.9a outlines the top view of the E²GBI beam profile, which is illustrated in more detail in Figure 9.6. Observation is carried out with a charge-coupled device (CCD) or a complementary metal-oxide semiconductor (CMOS) digital detector deployed along the x-axis, perpendicular to the z-axis. However, the detector could equally be deployed perpendicular to the y-axis. Figure 9.9b outlines the side view of the LSI approach [12]. Observation is carried out perpendicular to the y-axis.

Figure 9.9c and d provide approximate depictions of optical configurations used in SPI microscopy configurations [13,35]. In both cases, as with SPI microscopy, detection is performed along the y-axis. Here, it should be mentioned that LSI microscopy and SPI microscopy have been applied to observe specimens in aqueous solutions [12,35], while SPI microscopy has also been successful in fully characterizing the morphology of biological specimens hundreds of micrometers in length [13].

9.5 INTERFEROMETRIC MICROSCOPY

The principle of N-slit interferometry (see Chapter 10) via the E²GBI optical configuration shown in Figure 9.9a was originally developed for microscopic imaging applications related to silver halide films [10,36]. In particular, it was developed to characterize instantaneously a wide segment of a transmission surface in either the near field or the far field. Figure 9.10 shows the measured interferometric transmission profile in the near field of a grating comprised of $N = 23$ slits, each 100 μm wide and separated by 100 μm. The distance between the grating and the digital detector is 1.5 cm. In essence, this is a classical modulation pattern. Figure 9.11 illustrates the measured interferometric profile created by the illumination of $N = 25$ slits, each 100 μm wide and separated by 100 μm. However, the distance from the N-slit array to the digital detector is now 25 cm.

The beauty of this approach is that these measurements can be fully characterized by the N-slit interferometric equation [8,9]:

$$\left| \langle x | s \rangle \right|^2 = \sum_{j=1}^{N} \Psi(r_j)^2 + 2 \sum_{j=1}^{N} \Psi(r_j) \left(\sum_{j=m+1}^{N} \Psi(r_m) \cos(\Omega_m - \Omega_j) \right) \tag{9.8}$$

which is fully explained in Chapter 10. The main implication of this dual play between theory and experiment is that transmission surfaces can be fully characterized even if the digital detector being used (CCD or CMOS) lacks the pixel resolution to resolve the finer features of the film or transmission surface. That is done by measuring the interferometric profile in the far field and then using the interferometric equation (Equation 9.8) to display the transmission signal in the immediate near field. Thus, by making interferometric measurements in the microscopic domain, the theory allows characterization in the nanoscopic domain.

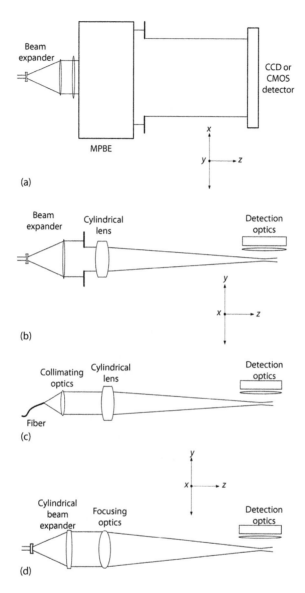

FIGURE 9.9 Approximate depictions of beam profiles available to microscopy via illumination techniques providing very thin sheets of light, also referred as SPI or E²GBI. (a) Top view of optics and beam profile achieved with E²GBI. Observation of the interferometric image is done on the beam itself, along the x-axis, which is perpendicular to the propagation z-axis. The interferometric pattern is incident directly on the CCD or CMOS line array detector in the absence of further imaging optics. Alternatively, for biological applications, the detector could also be deployed perpendicular to the z-axis, off-beam, along the y-axis. The side view of this profile should be similar to the other side profiles described next. (b) Side beam profile of SLI. Detection is done off-beam along the y-axis. (c) and (d) Side beam profiles of SPI. Detection is done off-beam along the y-axis.

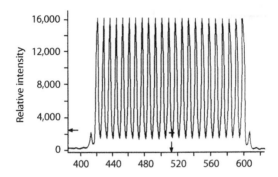

FIGURE 9.10 Measured interferogram originating from a grating with 23 slits each 100 μm wide separated by 100 μm (center-to-center distance of 200 μm). The grating-to screen distance is 1.5 cm. Each pixel is 25 μm wide. (Reprinted from *Opt. Commun.*, 103, Duarte, F. J., On a generalized interference equation and interferometric measurements, 8–14, Copyright (1993), with permission from Elsevier.)

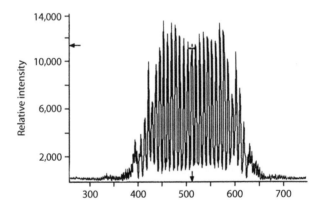

FIGURE 9.11 Measured interferogram originating from a grating with 25 slits each 100 μm wide separated by 100 μm (center-to-center distance of 200 μm). The grating-to screen distance is 25 cm. Each pixel is 25 μm wide. (Reprinted from *Opt. Commun.*, 103, Duarte, F. J., On a generalized interference equation and interferometric measurements, 8–14, Copyright (1993), with permission from Elsevier.)

REFERENCES

1. Peppers, N. A., A laser microscope, *Appl. Opt.* 4: 555–558, 1965.
2. Davidovits, P. and M. D. Eggers, Scanning laser microscope, *Nature* 223: 831, 1969.
3. Davidovits, P. and M. D. Eggers, Scanning laser microscope for biological investigations, *Appl. Opt.* 10: 1615–1619, 1971.
4. Cremer, T. and C. Cremer, Considerations on a laser-scanning-microscope with high resolution and depth of field, *Microsc. Acta* 81: 31–44, 1987.
5. Pohl, D. W., W. Denk, and M. Lanz, Optical stethoscopy: Image recording with resolution lambda/20, *Appl Phys. Lett.* 44: 651–653, 1984.

6. Betzig, E. and J. K. Trautman, Near-field optics: Microscopy, spectroscopy, and surface modification beyond the diffraction limit, *Science* 257: 189–195, 1992.

7. Duarte, F. J., Beam shaping with telescopes and multiple-prism beam expanders, *J. Opt. Soc. Am. A* 4: P30, 1987.

8. Duarte, F. J., Dispersive dye lasers. In F. J. Duarte (Ed.), *High Power Dye Lasers*, Chapter 2, Springer, Berlin, 1991.

9. Duarte, F. J., On a generalized interference equation and interferometric measurements, *Opt. Commun.* 103: 8–14, 1993.

10. Duarte, F. J., Electro-optical interferometric microdensitometer system, U.S. Patent 5255069, 1993.

11. Voie, A. H., D. H. Burns, and F. A. Spelman, Orthogonal-plane fluorescence optical sectioning: Three-dimensional imaging of macroscopic biological specimens, *J. Microsc.* 170: 229–236, 1993.

12. Fuchs, E., J. S. Jaffe, R. A. Long, and F. Azam, Thin laser light sheet microscope for microbial oceanography, *Opt. Express* 10: 147–154, 2002.

13. Huisken, J., J. Swoger, F. Del Bene, J. Wittbrodt, and E. H. K. Stelzer, Optical sectioning deep inside live embryos by selective plane illumination microscopy, *Science* 305: 1007–1009, 2004.

14. Jenkins, F. A. and H. E. White, *Fundamentals of Optics*, McGraw-Hill, New York, 1957.

15. Smith, W. J., *Modern Optical Engineering*, McGraw-Hill, New York, 2000.

16. Duarte, F. J., *Tunable Laser Optics*, 2nd edn, CRC Press, New York, 2015.

17. Duarte, F. J., B. A. Reed, and C. J. Burak, Laser sensitometer, U.S. Patent 6903824 B2, 2005.

18. Thomas, J. L. and Rudolph, W., Biological microscopy with ultrashort laser pulses. In F. J. Duarte (Ed.), *Tunable Laser Applications*, 2nd edn, Chapter 9, CRC Press, New York, 2009.

19. Diels, J-C., Femtosecond dye lasers. In F. J. Duarte and L. W. Hillman (Eds), *Dye Laser Principles*, Chapter 3, Academic, New York, 1990.

20. Diels, J-C. and W. Rudolph, *Ultrafast Laser Pulse Phenomena*, 2nd edn, Academic, New York, 2006.

21. Kafka, J. D. and Baer, T., Prism-pair dispersive delay lines in optical pulse compression, *Opt. Lett.* 12: 401–403, 1987.

22. Fork, R. L., C. H. Brito-Cruz, P. C. Becker, and C. V. Shank, Compression of optical pulses to six femtoseconds by using cubic phase compensation, *Opt. Lett.* 12: 483–485, 1987.

23. Ell, R., U. Morgner, F. X. Kärtner, J. G. Fujimoto, E. P. Ippen, V. Scheuer, G. Angelow, et al., Generation of 5-fs pulses and octave-spanning spectra directly from a Ti:sapphire laser, *Opt. Lett.* 26: 373–375, 2001.

24. Pang, L. Y., J. G. Fujimoto, and E. S. Kintzer, Ultrashort-pulse generation from high-power diode arrays by using intracavity optical nonlinearities, *Opt. Lett.* 17: 1599–1601, 1992.

25. Tauser, F., F. Adler, and A. Leitenstorfer, Widely tunable sub-30-fs pulses from a compact erbium-doped fiber source, *Opt. Lett.* 29: 516–518, 2004.

26. Baltuska, A., T. Fuji, and T. Kobayashi, Visible pulse compression to 4 fs by optical parametric amplification and programmable dispersion control, *Opt. Lett.* 27: 306–308, 2002.

27. Chalupsky, J., L. Juha, J. Kuba, J. Cihelka, V. Hájková, S. Koptyaev, J. Krása, et al., Characteristics of focused soft X-ray free-electron laser beam determined by ablation of organic molecular solids, *Opt. Express* 15: 6036–6043, 2007.

28. Betzig, E. and R. J. Chichester, Single molecules observed by near-field scanning optical microscopy, *Science* 262: 1422–1425, 1993.

29. Nechay, B. A., U. Siegner, M. Achermann, H. Bielefeldt, and U. Keller, Femtosecond pump-probe near-field optical microscopy, *Rev. Sci. Instrum.* 70: 2758–2764, 1999.
30. Nechay, B. A., U. Siegner, M. A. Achermann, F. Morier-Genaud, A. Schertel, and U. Keller, Femtosecond near-field scanning optical microscopy, *J. Microsc.* 194: 329–334, 1999.
31. Siegner, U., M. Achermann, and U. Keller, Spatially resolved femtosecond spectroscopy beyond the diffraction limit, *Meas. Sci. Technol.* 12: 1847–1857, 2001.
32. Duarte, F. J. and J. A. Piper, Dispersion theory of multiple-prism beam expanders for pulsed dye lasers, *Opt. Commun.* 43: 303–307, 1982.
33. Duarte, F. J. and J. A. Piper, A double-prism beam expander for pulsed dye lasers, *Opt. Commun.* 35: 100–104, 1980.
34. Duarte, F. J., *Tunable Laser Optics*, 1st edn, Elsevier Academic, New York, 2003.
35. Ritter, J. G., R. Veith, J-P. Siebrasse, and U. Kubitscheck, High-contrast single-particle tracking by selective focal plane illumination microscopy, *Opt. Express* 16: 7142–7152, 2008.
36. Duarte, F. J., Interferometric imaging. In F. J. Duarte (Ed.), *Tunable Laser Applications*, 1st edn, Chapter 5, Marcel Dekker, New York, 1995.

10 Interferometric Imaging

F. J. Duarte

CONTENTS

10.1 INTRODUCTION

Traditional measurements in imaging science include densitometry, spectropho-tometry, and image structure. In densitometry, macroscopic optical densities are measured as a function of wavelength in either the transmission or the reflection domain. In image structure, measurements include microdensitometry, also known as granularity measurements, and determination of the modulation transfer function (MTF). Microdensitometry provides statistical information on the distributions of microscopic crystal structures in photographic film. MTF measurements determine modulation as a function of spatial frequency in transmission gratings manufactured with either atomic or molecular films. All these imaging measurements, as related to molecular structures, are described in detail by Dainty and Shaw [1].

Traditionally, these measurements have been performed using instrumentation based on incoherent sources of illumination. This is due to the strong and historical link of imaging science and photography. Nevertheless, the use of coherent sources of illumination, in conjunction with digital detectors, was demonstrated in photographic imaging measurements in 1986 [2]. In particular, the use of lasers and photodiode-detector arrays, and charge-coupled devices (CCDs), was investigated in detail [2].

In this chapter, the use of a laser-based interferometer capable of performing a plethora of imaging measurements is described. This N-slit laser interferometer (NSLI) introduced digital detection technology, in the form of photodiode-detector arrays, to molecular imaging diagnostics [2–7]. For instance, it can be used as a straightforward optical densitometer or as a microdensitometer. The use of a laser source, or tunable laser source, provides a long depth of focus and enhances its dynamic range considerably, thus enabling the characterization of high-optical-density surfaces. Further, the photodiode-detector array introduces a feature of spatial discrimination that enables the same instrument to be used as a microdensitometer collecting hundreds, or even thousands, of data points simultaneously. Transmission characteristics from metallic or photographic gratings, as a function of spatial frequency, can also be measured. Further applications not possible with conventional instruments include the assessment of surface structure characteristics in clear film substrates and the detection of microdefects in thin metallic films. Here, in addition to imaging, applications in secure optical communications, textiles, and biomedical areas are discussed.

An important and distinct characteristic of the interferometer detailed here is that the measurements can be described using the Dirac formalism [8]. As such, in typical quantum fashion, the researcher is allowed to predict an output intensity distribution only with knowledge of the input distribution, and the geometry of the interferometer, but without access to the intermediate propagation of the radiation. This approach enables the use of a powerful computer analysis to quantify and predict measurements [2–7]. It is this dual approach that enhances the applicability of the NSIL and the method.

10.2 TUNABLE LASERS

The illumination in the NSLI is provided by a laser. Although a fixed-frequency laser provides the most basic version of the instrument, its applicability is greatly enhanced by a tunable laser. The most important requirement for the tunable laser being used as an illumination source in these measurements is a TEM_{00} transverse-mode beam structure with a Gaussian or near-Gaussian beam profile.

Tunable lasers can be categorized into two subclasses: line-tunable, or discretely tunable, lasers and broadly tunable lasers. Line-tunable lasers include the argon ion (Ar^+), krypton ion (Kr^+), helium cadmium (He–Cd), and helium neon (He–Ne) lasers. In this application, all these lasers are mostly used in the continuous-wave (CW) mode of operation, albeit the interferometer could also use pulsed lasers as a source of illumination. Broadly tunable sources of coherent radiation include optical parametric oscillators (Chapter 2), dye lasers (Chapters 3 and 4), diode lasers (Chapter 5), titanium sapphire lasers, and fiber lasers (Chapters 6 and 7).

Table 10.1 lists the transitions and wavelengths available from Ar^+, Kr^+, He–Cd, and He–Ne lasers. An advantage of the emission from these gas lasers is their low divergence, exquisite TEM_{00} beam profiles, and long-term spectral stability. For details on gas lasers, the reader should refer to [9]. Table 1.4 indicates the approximate wavelength coverage available from various broadly tunable CW lasers.

Table 10.2 includes the tuning range for CW dye lasers, and narrow-linewidth pulsed dye lasers, emitting in the yellow-orange-red region of the spectrum. For a detailed description of CW dye lasers, the reader should refer to [10,11]. Tunable narrow-linewidth pulsed dye lasers are described in [12–14]. Solid-state dye lasers are described in detail in Chapters 3 and 4.

Table 10.3 includes some of the wavelength characteristics of broadly tunable external-cavity semiconductor (ECS) lasers, also known as tunable diode lasers. These lasers are described in detail in Chapter 5.

10.3 THE *N*-SLIT LASER INTERFEROMETER

The *N*SLI is shown schematically in Figure 10.1. The TEM_{00} tunable laser is followed by a variable neutral-density filter. The Gaussian beam is then expanded in two dimensions by a Galilean telescope. Following the telescope, there is an *optional* convex lens whose function is to focus the expanded beam from the telescope. As will be explained later, this lens is optional, and its use depends on the mode of application of the interferometer. The propagating TEM_{00} beam is then expanded again, in one dimension only, by an achromatic multiple-prism beam expander (MPBE) [4,5,18].

10.3.1 EXTREMELY ELONGATED GAUSSIAN BEAMS

In the first mode of operation, the convex lens is part of the optical system and hence yields a well-focused beam at the focal plane. However, because the beam undergoes an additional one-dimensional expansion, the beam thus produced is very focused in the vertical plane and very wide in the horizontal plane (or plane of propagation). As a result, extremely elongated Gaussian beams are produced [4–7,18]. In Figure 10.2, a photograph of a cross section of a highly expanded Gaussian beam, at its focal plane, is shown. In Figure 10.3, an extremely expanded Gaussian beam near its focal plane is approximately depicted. In practice, these beams have been measured to be 10–30 μm in the vertical plane (height) and 35–50 mm in the plane of propagation (width) [4–7]. More specifically, a near-Gaussian beam measuring $20 \times 60{,}000$ μm, that is, a height to width ratio of 1:3000, was reported in 1987 by Duarte [18].

At this stage, it should be mentioned that this class of illumination, via extremely elongated Gaussian beams, can also be described as *light sheet illumination* (LSI) or *selective plane illumination* (SPI) (see Chapter 9). The main difference is that the latter methods use cylindrical lens optics, while here a system comprised of a telescope plus an MPBE is applied. As described next, this optical

TABLE 10.1
Line-Tunable CW Lasers[a]

Laser	Transition[b,c]	Wavelength (nm)
Ar+	$4p\ ^4D^0_{3/2}-4s\ ^2P_{1/2}$	528.69
	$4p\ ^4D^0_{5/2}-4s\ ^2P_{3/2}$	514.53
	$4p'\ ^4D^0_{5/2}-3d\ ^2D_{3/2}$	510.72
	$4p\ ^2D^0_{3/2}-4s\ ^2P_{1/2}$	496.51
	$4p\ ^2D^0_{5/2}-4s\ ^2P_{3/2}$	487.99
	$4p\ ^2P^0_{3/2}-4s\ ^2P_{1/2}$	476.49
	$4p\ ^2D^0_{3/2}-4s\ ^2P_{3/2}$	472.69
	$4p\ ^2P^0_{1/2}-4s\ ^2P_{3/2}$	465.79
	$4p\ ^2S^0_{1/2}-4s\ ^2P_{1/2}$	457.93
	$4p\ ^2P^0_{3/2}-4s\ ^2P_{3/2}$	454.50
Kr+	$5p\ ^4P^0_{3/3}-4d\ ^4D_{1/2}$	799.32
	$5p\ ^4P^0_{3/2}-5s\ ^2P_{1/2}$	752.55
	$5p\ ^4P^0_{5/2}-5s\ ^2P_{3/2}$	647.09
	$5p\ ^4D^0_{5/2}-5s\ ^2P_{3/2}$	568.19
	$5p\ ^4P^0_{5/2}-5s\ ^4P_{3/2}$	530.87
	$5p\ ^4P^0_{3/2}-5s\ ^4P_{3/2}$	520.83
He–Ne	$3s_2-2p_4$	632.82
	$3s_2-2p_6$	611.80
	$3s_2-2p_7$	604.61
	$3s_2-2p_8$	593.93
	$3s_2-2p_{10}$	543.30
He–Cd	$5s\ ^{22}D_{3/2}-5p\ ^2P^0_{3/2}$	441.56
	$6p\ ^2P_{3/2}-5s\ ^{22}D_{3/2}$	488.20
	$4f\ ^2F-5d\ ^2D$	502.50
	$4f\ ^2F^0_{5/2}-5d\ ^2D_{3/2}$	533.75
	$4f\ ^2F_{7/2}-5d\ ^2D_{5/2}$	537.80
	$6g\ ^2G_{7/2}-4f\ ^2F^0_{5/2}$	635.48
	$6g\ ^2G_{9/2}-4f\ ^2F^0_{7/2}$	636.00

[a] Further transitions are available from these lasers. Here, emphasis is given to transitions in the visible spectrum.

[b] Transition assignment has been done following Willett [9].

[c] The laser linewidths of these transitions, in gas lasers, are usually below the few gigahertz range in the absence of intracavity line-narrowing optics.

TABLE 10.2
Broadly Tunable Dye Lasers in the Yellow-Orange-Red Region of the Spectrum

Laser	Laser Linewidth	Tuning Range (nm)	References
Continuous-wave dye laser[a]	$\Delta\nu \approx 1$ MHz	$575 \leq \lambda \leq 639$[b]	[11]
SSDL[c]	$\Delta\nu \approx 350$ MHz[d]	$550 \leq \lambda \leq 603$	[13]

[a] Gain medium is rhodamine 6 G in a water-based solvent [10].
[b] Boundary wavelength values are approximate.
[c] SSDL: Solid-state dye laser. Gain medium is rhodamine 6 G-doped MPMMA [13].
[d] Single-longitudinal-mode emission. Pulse duration is $\Delta t \approx 3$ ns.

TABLE 10.3
Broadly Tunable External-Cavity Semiconductor Lasers[a]

Laser	Laser Linewidth	Tuning Range (nm)	References
GaN	$\Delta\nu \approx 1$ MHz	$394.40 \leq \lambda \leq 396.15$[b,c]	[15]
Index guided	$\Delta\nu \approx 100$ kHz	$660 \leq \lambda \leq 684$[b]	[16]
InGaAsP/InP	$\Delta\nu \approx 100$ kHz	$1255 \leq \lambda \leq 1335$	[17]

[a] These lasers emit in the CW regime.
[b] Obtained with a commercial ECS laser.
[c] The overall tuning range of these lasers is approximately $373 \leq \lambda \leq 472$ nm, which includes several gaps.

system is highly versatile and can be completely described in closed-form analytical expressions.

The second mode of operation of the telescope–MPBE illumination system does not require the presence of the convex lens, and the beam thus produced can be ~10 mm in the vertical plane and 35–60 mm in the plane of propagation. Of course, in both modes of propagation, the resulting beam has a Gaussian beam profile. The extremely elongated Gaussian beam is generally used for microscopic applications, while the unfocused beam is used for straightforward interferometric applications [5–7].

The surface to be examined is deployed on the vertical plane orthogonal to the plane of propagation between the MPBE and the photodiode–detector array. When the convex lens is used, the surface to be examined is positioned at the focal plane.

The ray transfer matrix for an MPBE composed of r prisms is given by [5,7,14,19]

$$\begin{pmatrix} A & B \\ C & D \end{pmatrix} = \begin{pmatrix} M_1 M_2 & B \\ 0 & (M_1 M_2)^{-1} \end{pmatrix} \tag{10.1}$$

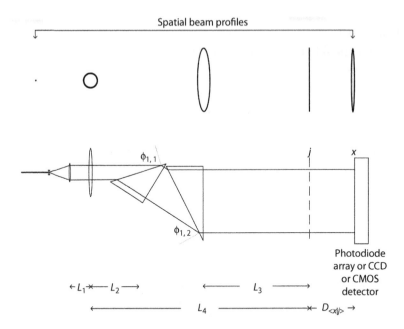

FIGURE 10.1 Schematics of the *N*SLI. The TEM$_{00}$ beam from the tunable laser source is attenuated by a variable neutral-density filter prior to two-dimensional expansion in a Galilean telescope. Following the telescope, there is a convex lens that is followed by an MPBE that provides one-dimensional expansion in the plane of propagation. The surface or transmission grating to be characterized, which gives origin to the interference, is located, at the focal plane, between the multiple-prism array and the photodiode-detector array. The use of the convex lens is optional and depends on whether an extremely elongated Gaussian beam is required. Approximate spatial beam profiles are outlined on top of the diagram. (Reproduced from Duarte, F. J., *Tunable Laser Optics*, 2nd edn, CRC Press, New York, 2015. With permission from Taylor & Francis Group.)

where

$$B = M_1 M_2 \sum_{m=1}^{r-1} L_m \left(\prod_{j=1}^{m} k_{1,j} \prod_{j=1}^{m} k_{2,j} \right)^{-2}$$

$$+ \left(\frac{M_1}{M_2} \right) \sum_{m=1}^{r} (l_m / n_m) \left(\prod_{j=1}^{m} k_{1,j} \right)^{-2} \left(\prod_{j=m}^{r} k_{2,j} \right)^{2} \tag{10.2}$$

$$M_1 = \prod_{m=1}^{r} k_{1,m} \tag{10.3}$$

$$M_2 = \prod_{m=1}^{r} k_{2,m} \tag{10.4}$$

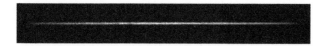

FIGURE 10.2 Photograph of a TEM$_{00}$ beam, from a He–Ne laser, transformed into an extremely elongated near-Gaussian beam following propagation via the optics depicted in Figure 10.1. The width of this beam is approximately 50 mm, and its height appears significantly larger than reality due to intensity saturation in the detection system.

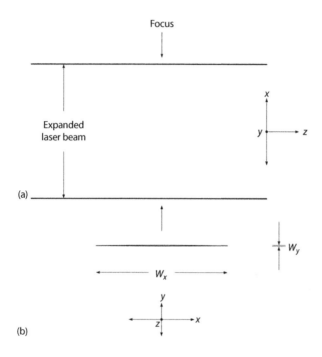

FIGURE 10.3 Approximate propagation outline, left to right, of an extremely elongated Gaussian beam near its focal plane. (a) Top view of the extremely expanded laser beam. (b) Cross section of the propagating extremely elongated near Gaussian. The view shown in (b) corresponds to the expanded profile depicted in Figure 10.2. Drawing is not to scale.

Here, the individual beam-expansion terms for the mth prism are

$$k_{1,m} = \frac{\cos \psi_{1,m}}{\cos \phi_{1,m}} \tag{10.5}$$

$$k_{2,m} = \frac{\cos \phi_{2,m}}{\cos \psi_{2,m}} \tag{10.6}$$

where $\phi_{1,m}$ and $\phi_{2,m}$ are the angles of incidence and emergence, $\phi_{1,m}$ and $\phi_{2,m}$ are related to $\psi_{1,m}$ and $\psi_{2,m}$ via n_m and Snell's law. In Equation 10.2, L_m is the distance separating the prisms, and l_m is the path length at the mth prism.

The overall ray transfer matrix at the plane of propagation is given by [5,7]

$$\begin{pmatrix} M_t\left[M - \left(\dfrac{\zeta}{f}\right)\right] & B_t\left[M - \left(\dfrac{\zeta}{f}\right)\right] + L_1\left(\dfrac{M}{M_t}\right) + \left(\dfrac{\zeta}{M_t}\right)\left[1 - \left(\dfrac{L_1}{f}\right)\right] \\ -\left(\dfrac{M_t}{Mf}\right) & (MM_t)^{-1}\left[1 - \left(\dfrac{L_1}{f}\right) - \left(\dfrac{B_t}{Mf}\right)\right] \end{pmatrix} \tag{10.7}$$

where:

$M = M_1 M_2$

M_t and B_t refer to the A and B terms of the transfer matrix for the Galilean telescope

Also,

$$\zeta = ML_2 + B + \frac{L_3}{M} \tag{10.8}$$

For the vertical component, the corresponding ray transfer matrix becomes

$$\begin{pmatrix} M_t\left[1 - \left(\dfrac{L_2'}{f}\right)\right] & \left[1 - \left(\dfrac{L_2'}{f}\right)\right]\left[B_t + \left(\dfrac{L_1}{M_t}\right)\right] + \left(\dfrac{L_2'}{M_t}\right) \\ -\dfrac{M_t}{f} & M_t^{-1}\left[1 - \left(\dfrac{L_1}{f}\right)\right] - \left(\dfrac{B_t}{f}\right) \end{pmatrix} \tag{10.9}$$

where L_2' is the distance between the convex lens and the N-slit array. Note that in the absence of the convex lens, Equations 10.7 and 10.9 simplify to

$$\begin{pmatrix} (M_t M) & B_t M + L_1\left(\dfrac{M}{M_t}\right) + \dfrac{\zeta}{M_t} \\ 0 & (M_t M)^{-1} \end{pmatrix} \tag{10.10}$$

and

$$\begin{pmatrix} M_t & B_t + \left(\dfrac{L_1}{M_t}\right) + \left(\dfrac{L_2'}{M_t}\right) \\ 0 & M_t^{-1} \end{pmatrix} \tag{10.11}$$

To calculate the width of a Gaussian beam, the following expression is used [20]:

$$w(B') = w_0\left[(A')^2 + \left(\frac{B'}{L_R}\right)^2\right]^{1/2}$$ (10.12)

where A' and B' are given by Equations 10.7 and 10.9, or Equations 10.10 and 10.11. Here,

$$L_R = \frac{\pi w_0^2}{\lambda}$$ (10.13)

is known as the Rayleigh length. For a description of relevant 2×2 and 4×4 propagation matrices, the reader is referred to [4]. Duarte [19] gives the generalized 4×4 matrix for multiple-prism arrays.

Using Equations 10.7 through 10.9 and 10.12, it can be shown that for an optical system illuminated by a $2w_0 = 500$ μm TEM_{00} beam from a He–Ne laser (at $\lambda = 632.8$ nm), and incorporating a convex lens with $f=30$ cm, a telescope with $M_t = 20$, and an MPBE with $M = 5.75$, the resulting laser beam at the focal plane becomes approximately 32.26 μm high and 52.7 mm wide, or approximately $32\times52{,}700$ μm. In the absence of the convex lens, the dimensions of the beam become 10 mm high by 52.7 mm wide.

It should also be mentioned that the depth of focus of this Gaussian beam is better than 2 mm. For microscopy applications, this enormous depth of focus is one of the advantages that this coherent NSLI offers over traditional instrumentation. The ray matrix approach outlined here can also be applied to consider the question of astigmatism [20].

10.3.2 MINIMIZING THE VERTICAL DIMENSIONS OF THE EXTREMELY ELONGATED GAUSSIAN

To minimize the vertical dimension, or thickness, of the beam, the propagation parameters are chosen so that $L_2' \approx f$. This is facilitated if the surface quality and curvature of the convex lens are sufficiently high to ensure focusing at the specified distance. For instance, in the example given above, if L_2' is brought within 100 μm of f, then the vertical dimension of the beam is reduced to 24.5 μm.

In the system described in the previous section, the telescope is introduced to reduce beam divergence; to decrease the need for beam expansion at the multiple beam expander, thus improving the transmission efficiency; and more importantly, to reduce the magnitude of the B' term in Equation 10.12. To illustrate this point, consider the optical system without the telescope, comprised only of the convex lens and the MPBE designed for higher magnification. Under those circumstances, the propagation matrix, given in Equation 10.7, reduces to

$$\begin{pmatrix} \left[M - \left(\dfrac{\zeta}{f}\right)\right] & L_1 M + \zeta\left[1 - \left(\dfrac{L_1}{f}\right)\right] \\ -\left(\dfrac{1}{Mf}\right) & (M)^{-1}\left[1 - \left(\dfrac{L_1}{f}\right)\right] \end{pmatrix}$$ (10.14)

and the matrix given in Equation 10.9 reduces to

$$
\begin{pmatrix}
1-\left(\dfrac{L_2'}{f}\right) & L_1\left[1-\left(\dfrac{L_2'}{f}\right)\right]+L_2' \\[4mm]
-\dfrac{1}{f} & 1-\left(\dfrac{L_1}{f}\right)
\end{pmatrix}
\tag{10.15}
$$

A comparison of Equations 10.9 and 10.15 indicates that the B' term in Equation 10.15 is larger than the B' term in Equation 10.9, or more specifically,

$$
L_1\left[1-\left(\frac{L_2'}{f}\right)\right]+L_2' > \left[1-\left(\frac{L_2'}{f}\right)\right]\left[B_t+\left(\frac{L_1}{M_t}\right)\right]+\left(\frac{L_2'}{M_t}\right)
\tag{10.16}
$$

This is because $[1-(L_2'/f)]$ is a very small number, and L_1 can also be made, by design, into a very small number. Then, in the absence of the telescope, L_2' becomes a significant parameter. Thus, in the search for a minimum beam thickness, there is an optimum M_t for which $[(A')^2+(B'/L_{\mathcal{R}})^2]$, in Equation 10.12, is a minimum. Certainly, a shorter wavelength leading to a larger $L_{\mathcal{R}}$ also helps.

10.3.3 MULTIPLE-PRISM DISPERSION

The overall dispersion of the system is determined by characterizing the MPBE. Here, the overall generalized dispersion equation is given by [4,12,14]

$$
\nabla_\lambda\phi_{2,r} = (M_1M_2)^{-1}\sum_{m=1}^{r}(\pm1)\mathcal{H}_{2,m}\left(\prod_{j=1}^{m}k_{1,j}\prod_{j=1}^{m}k_{2,j}\right)\nabla_\lambda n_m
$$

$$
+\sum_{m=1}^{r}(\pm1)\mathcal{H}_{1,m}\left(\prod_{j=m}^{r}k_{1,j}\prod_{j=m}^{r}k_{2,j}\right)^{-1}\nabla_\lambda n_m
\tag{10.17}
$$

where $\nabla_\lambda = \partial/\partial\lambda$, and

$$
\mathcal{H}_{1,m} = \frac{\tan\phi_{1,m}}{n_m}
\tag{10.18}
$$

$$
\mathcal{H}_{2,m} = \frac{\tan\phi_{2,m}}{n_m}
\tag{10.19}
$$

Note that by making $\nabla_\lambda\phi_{2,r}=0$, a zero-dispersion beam expander can be designed at a given wavelength [4,12]. This enables a significant reduction in thermal deviations because [12]

$$
\nabla_T\phi_{2,r} = \nabla_\lambda\phi_{2,r}(\nabla_\lambda n_m)^{-1}\nabla_T n_m
\tag{10.20}
$$

For a detailed discussion on the design of MPBEs, the reader should consult [4,12,14].

10.4 INTERFEROMETRIC THEORY

In the interferometer schematics shown in Figure 10.4, there is a source (s), an intermediate surface (j), and a detection plane (x). A generalized one-dimensional representation of this optical system is given in Figure 10.4a, where the intermediate surface is represented by a generalized grating (j). Hence, using the Dirac formalism [8], the probability amplitude for photon propagation from the source (s) via the grating (j) to the screen (x) is given by

$$\langle x|s \rangle = \sum_{j=1}^{N} \langle x|j \rangle \langle j|s \rangle \qquad (10.21)$$

Using

$$\langle j|s \rangle = \Psi(r_{s,j})e^{-i\theta_j} \qquad (10.22)$$

$$\langle x|j \rangle = \Psi(r_{j,x})e^{-i\varphi_j} \qquad (10.23)$$

we can write

$$\langle x|s \rangle = \sum_{j=1}^{N} \Psi(r_j)e^{-i\Omega_j} \qquad (10.24)$$

where

$$\Psi(r_j) = \Psi(r_{s,j})\Psi(r_{j,x}) \qquad (10.25)$$

and

$$\Omega_j = \theta_j + \phi_j \qquad (10.26)$$

Here, $\Psi(r_j)$, $\Psi(r_{s,j})$, and $\Psi(r_{j,x})$ are, according to Dirac, the amplitudes of "wave functions of ordinary wave optics" [8]. Thus, the probability distribution at the detector screen is given by [4,6,12]

$$|\langle x|s \rangle|^2 = \sum_{j=1}^{N} \Psi(r_j)^2 + 2\sum_{j=1}^{N} \Psi(r_j)\left(\sum_{j=m+1}^{N} \Psi(r_m)\cos(\Omega_m - \Omega_j) \right) \qquad (10.27)$$

In this equation, the interference term is evaluated using

$$\cos(\phi_m - \phi_j) = \cos\left(\frac{2\pi}{\lambda} \right)|L_m - L_{m-1}| \qquad (10.28)$$

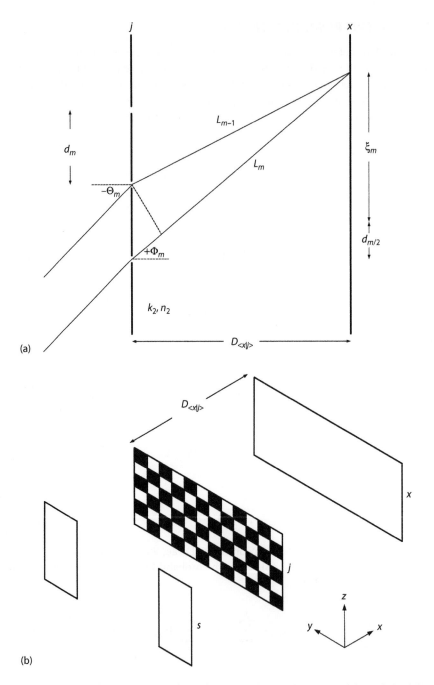

FIGURE 10.4 (a) Generalized one-dimensional geometrical representation of the interferometric measurement. A source (*s*) is generated at the aperture and propagates toward the detection screen (*x*) via the grating (*j*). (b) Three-dimensional representation showing the *zy* plane, which is orthogonal to the plane of propagation.

where the path differences are expressed in terms of the geometry [6]:

$$\left|L_m - L_{m-1}\right| = \frac{2\xi_m d_m}{\left|L_m + L_{m-1}\right|} \tag{10.29}$$

$$L_m^2 = a^2 + \left[\xi_m + \left(\frac{d_m}{2}\right)\right]^2 \tag{10.30}$$

$$L_{m-1}^2 = a^2 + \left[\xi_m - \left(\frac{d_m}{2}\right)\right]^2 \tag{10.31}$$

where:

  a is the j-to-x distance (see Figure 10.4a)
  d_m is the center-to-center distance of the slits
  ξ_m is the displacement on x from the projected medium of d_m to the point of calculation

The approach just described for the generalized N-slit one-dimensional grating can be extended to the case of the two-dimensional grating, as illustrated in Figure 10.4b. Propagation occurs from s to x via a two-dimensional grating j_{zy}. The plane z–y is orthogonal to the plane of propagation. Under these conditions, the probability amplitude for photon propagation from s to x, via j_{zy}, is given by [7]

$$\langle x|s\rangle = \sum_{z=1}^{N}\sum_{y=1}^{N}\langle x|j_{zy}\rangle\langle j_{zy}|s\rangle \tag{10.32}$$

which can be written as

$$\langle x|s\rangle = \sum_{z=1}^{N}\sum_{y=1}^{N}\Psi(r_{j_{zy}})e^{-i\Omega_{zy}} \tag{10.33}$$

Hence, the corresponding probability equation can be expressed as [7]

$$\left|\langle x|s\rangle\right|^2 = \sum_{z=1}^{N}\sum_{y=1}^{N}\Psi(r_{j_{zy}})\sum_{q=1}^{N}\sum_{p=1}^{N}\Psi(r_{j_{qp}})e^{i(\Omega_{qp}-\Omega_{zy})} \tag{10.34}$$

For one dimension,

$$\Psi(r_{j_{zy}}) = \Psi(r_j) \tag{10.35}$$

and

$$\Psi(r_{j_{qp}}) = \Psi(r_m) \tag{10.36}$$

so that Equation 10.34 reduces to

$$\left|\langle x|s\rangle\right|^2 = \sum_{j=1}^{N} \Psi(r_j) \sum_{m=1}^{N} \Psi(r_m) e^{i(\Omega_m - \Omega_j)} \tag{10.37}$$

This equation can be expanded and rearranged to yield the generalized one-dimensional Equation 10.27.

At this stage, it should be mentioned that, in the past, physicists have applied quantum mechanics to describe interference and diffraction. For instance, the contribution of Feynman in this area is well known [21,22]. However, it is interesting to note that Feynman used the path integral method to describe single-slit diffraction [21] and the Dirac formalism to describe the famous two-slit interference experiment *for electrons* [22]. The method described here, which is based on the Dirac formalism, is a unified approach to describe interference and diffraction phenomena. Further, in the interference domain, the description is general and applies to any N number of slits. Explicitly, from the interference term of Equation 10.23 and the geometry of Figure 10.4, a generalized diffraction equation follows [23]:

$$L\pi = d_m(n_1 \sin\Theta_m \pm n_2 \sin\Phi_m)\frac{2\pi}{\lambda} \tag{10.38}$$

where $L = 0, 2, 4...$. For $n_1 = n_2$, this equation reduces to the well-known diffraction grating equation [23]:

$$m\lambda = d_m(\sin\Theta_m \pm \sin\Phi_m) \tag{10.39}$$

where:
   Θ_m is the angle of incidence
   Φ_m is the angle of diffraction [14,23]

Note that the m in $m\lambda$ is the order of diffraction ($m = 1, 2, 3,...$) and is unrelated to the subscript in d_m and the angular quantities. For a grating coated over an optical glass substrate, as the dimensions of the slits, and the distance separating them, decrease well below the wavelength λ, then diffraction ceases to occur [23]. Under those circumstances, Equation 10.34 can only be solved for $L = 0$, thus giving rise to the law of refraction, also known as Snell's law:

$$n_1 \sin\Theta_m = n_2 \sin\Phi_m \tag{10.40}$$

where:

Θ_m is the angle of incidence

Φ_m becomes the angle of refraction [14,23]

Hence, the Dirac description of N-slit interference leads to a succinct unified hierarchical description of optics in the sequential order of interference, diffraction, refraction, and reflection [14,23]. Other alternative descriptions of optics have been recently discussed in the literature [24].

One further aspect of the approach leading to the derivation of Equations 10.27, 10.34, and 10.37 is that they are derived using a particle probabilistic approach applicable to *single-photon propagation*. However, as explained in [25], the resulting interferometric equations are also applicable to describe the interference of a distribution of indistinguishable photons as available from narrow-linewidth lasers. Indeed, in a relevant statement while discussing the exposure of a photographic plate, W. E. Lamb writes: "the wave function … is applied in a probabilistic way for a single electron, and the blacketing of the plate by a beam of many electrons is worked out by plausible non quantum mechanical considerations" [26]. More explicitly, and using the terminology introduced here, as pointed out by Duarte [27], the propagation of a single quanta, at wavelength λ, can be characterized by a more explicit version of Equation 10.27:

$$\left| \langle x | s \rangle \right|_\lambda^2 = \sum_{j=1}^{N} \Psi(r_j)_\lambda^2 + 2 \sum_{j=1}^{N} \Psi(r_j)_\lambda \left(\sum_{m=j+1}^{N} \Psi(r_m)_\lambda \cos(\Omega_m - \Omega_j) \right) \qquad (10.41)$$

while the propagation of an ensemble of quantum, within a wavelength distribution $\lambda \pm \Delta\lambda$, can be described by

$$\sum_{\lambda=\lambda_1}^{\lambda_n} \left| \langle x | s \rangle \right|_\lambda^2 = \sum_{\lambda=\lambda_1}^{\lambda_n} \left(\sum_{j=1}^{N} \Psi(r_j)_\lambda^2 + 2 \sum_{j=1}^{N} \Psi(r_j)_\lambda \left(\sum_{m=j+1}^{N} \Psi(r_m)_\lambda \cos(\Omega_m - \Omega_j) \right) \right) \qquad (10.42)$$

For an ideal very narrow-linewidth laser, $\Delta\lambda \to 0$, so that $(\lambda \pm \Delta\lambda) \to \lambda$, and subsequently

$$\sum_{\lambda=\lambda_1} \left| \langle x | s \rangle \right|_\lambda^2 \to \left| \langle x | s \rangle \right|_\lambda^2 \qquad (10.43)$$

In other words, the measured interferograms generated with narrow-linewidth lasers are nicely described using Equation 10.27 or its equivalent Equation 10.41. The use of quantum mechanical methods with the description of "macroscopic phenomena, which are not disturbed by observation," has previously been eloquently discussed by van Kampen [28].

10.5 INTERFEROMETRIC CALCULATIONS

To illustrate the application of the theory, a number of dual measurements/calculations are considered using a variety of transmission gratings. The gratings used in these measurements are made of metallic coatings on high-quality glass substrates. The dimensions of the slits are uniform within 2%. In these measurements, the detection screen (x) is a photodiode array of 1024 pixels, each 25 μm in width [6,7].

The first case is that of the classical double-slit experiment. Here, each slit is 50 μm wide separated by 50 μm; that is, the center-to-center distance is 100 μm, and the grating-to-screen distance is 10 cm. The measured and calculated interference signal, using Equation 10.27, are shown in Figure 10.5.

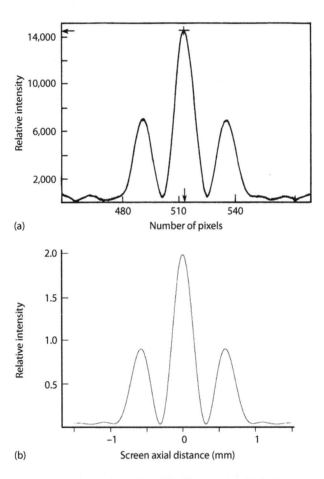

FIGURE 10.5   (a) Measurement of classical double-slit interference. Each slit is 50 μm separated by 50 μm. Each pixel is 25 μm wide. (b) Predicted interference pattern for the double-slit experiment using 50 μm-wide slits separated by 50 μm. (Reproduced from Duarte, F. J., *Quantum Optics for Engineers*, CRC Press, New York, 2014. With permission from Taylor & Francis Group.)

For transmission gratings with a large number of slits, the comparison between measurement and theory is performed using gratings with center-to-center distances of 200 and 60 μm [7]. In the first case, 23 slits of a grating with 100 μm-wide slits, separated by 100 μm, is illuminated for a grating-to-screen distance of 1.5 cm. The resulting near-field interferograms are shown in Figure 10.6. Next, for the grating with 30 μm wide slits, separated by 30 μm, the grating-to-screen distance is 75 cm. The measured and predicted interferograms are shown in Figure 10.7.

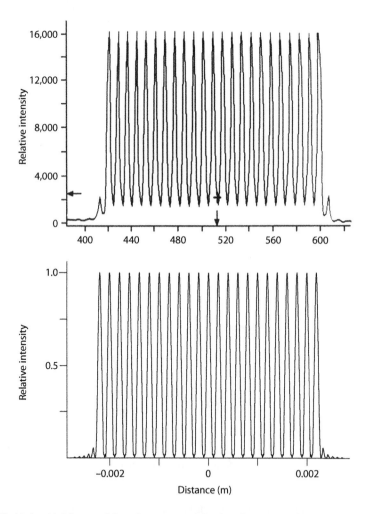

FIGURE 10.6 (a) Measured interferogram originating from a grating with 23 slits each 100 μm wide separated by 100 μm (center-to-center distance of 200 μm). The grating-to-screen distance is 1.5 cm. Each pixel is 25 μm wide. (b) Theoretical reconstruction using the generalized interference equation. (Reprinted from *Opt. Commun.*, 103, Duarte, F. J., On a generalized interference equation and interferometric measurements, 8–14, Copyright (1993), with permission from Elsevier.)

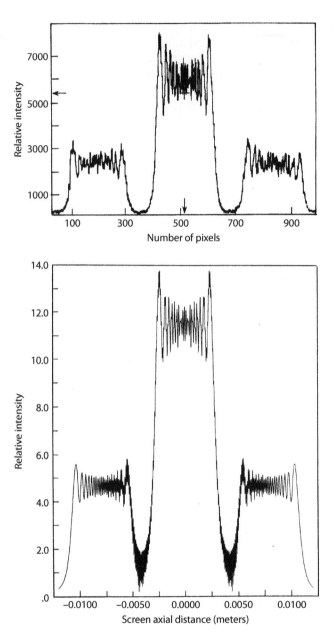

FIGURE 10.7 (a) Measured interferogram originating from a grating with 100 slits 30 μm wide separated by 30 μm (center-to-center distance of 60 μm). The grating-to-screen distance is 75 cm. (b) Corresponding theoretical reconstruction using the generalized interference equation. (Reprinted from *Opt. Commun.*, 103, Duarte, F. J., On a generalized interference equation and interferometric measurements, 8–14, Copyright (1993), with permission from Elsevier.)

At this stage, it should be observed that the calculations have been performed using Equation 10.23, assuming plane-wave illumination of the grating. Under these idealized circumstances, there is excellent agreement between theory and experiment in the spatial frequency domain. Criteria for agreement involve the number of ripples (or peaks) predicted by Equation 10.27 and the number of ripples measured. Also, predicted and measured distances agree to within 1%.

Note that the theory has not been modified to accommodate the background noise of the instrument or the spatial resolution limitations of the detector. Further, beam propagation distortions are not included in the interferometric theory [7].

As mentioned earlier, the gratings used in these experiments have an intrinsic uncertainty in the dimensions of the slits of ~2%. Incorporating a ≤2% uncertainty in the dimensions of the grating yields a calculated interferogram as illustrated in Figure 10.8 for the 30 µm grating at a grating-to-screen distance of 75 cm. Note that the symmetry of the calculation without uncertainty (shown in Figure 10.7)

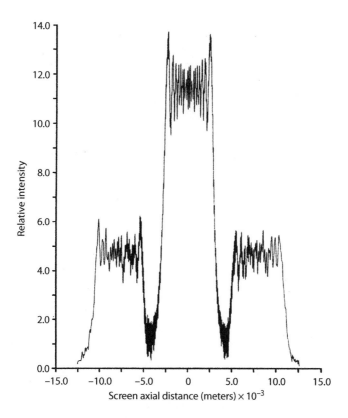

FIGURE 10.8   Theoretical interferogram for the grating composed of 100 slits 30 µm wide separated by 30 µm (center-to-center distance of 60 µm) and assuming a ≤2% uncertainty in the width of the slits. Note a deterioration of the symmetry relative to the calculation shown in the previous figure. (Reprinted from *Opt. Commun.*, 103, Duarte, F. J., On a generalized interference equation and interferometric measurements, 8–14, Copyright (1993), with permission from Elsevier.)

has now deteriorated, and the predicted signal yields a closer resemblance to the measurement.

A further refinement can be achieved by considering the edge effects of illumination on the grating. This occurs because a set of wide slits is used to determine the width of the beam illuminating the grating. In essence, this is a near-field diffraction phenomenon, which can also be calculated using Equation 10.27. This time, the wide slit or aperture is represented by hundreds of subslits. For the case of a 4 mm wide aperture, the diffraction illumination pattern for a distance of 10 cm is shown in Figure 10.9. Here, the 4 mm aperture was represented by 800 slits, 4 μm wide, separated by a 1 μm interslit distance [7]. For this case, the Fresnel number

$$N = \frac{w^2}{L\lambda}$$

(10.44)

is 63.21.

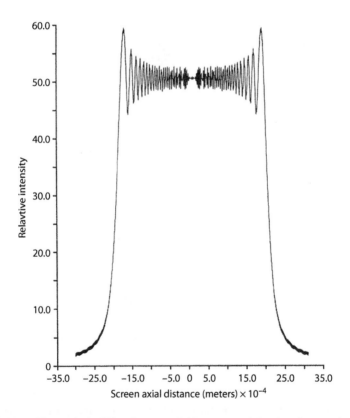

FIGURE 10.9 Theoretical diffraction near-field pattern originating from a 4 mm wide aperture. The calculation distance is 10 cm, and the corresponding Fresnel number is 63.21. (Reprinted from *Opt. Commun.*, 103, Duarte, F. J., On a generalized interference equation and interferometric measurements, 8–14, Copyright (1993), with permission from Elsevier.)

The incorporation of the diffraction pattern, in the incidence wave, modifies the calculated interferograms from those predicted for the plane-wave idealization. For the case of the 100 and 30 µm gratings at a grating-to-screen distance of 75 cm, the predicted interferograms are shown in Figure 10.10. Here, there is a deterioration of the symmetry and a small increase in the magnitude of the oscillation at the central order [7].

The prediction of diffraction patterns resulting from single wide slits, or apertures, enables the application of Equation 10.27 to the calculation of transverse-mode structures in stable laser resonators [7].

The examples illustrated here indicate that the application of the Dirac formalism to beam propagation, via a generalized grating, in classical optics has yielded a unified approach to interference and diffraction. This is achieved by the use of a single and elegant equation.

Initially, the numerical cases considered here were analyzed using a program written in Fortran 77, in an IBM 3090 mainframe computer. Subsequently, Visual

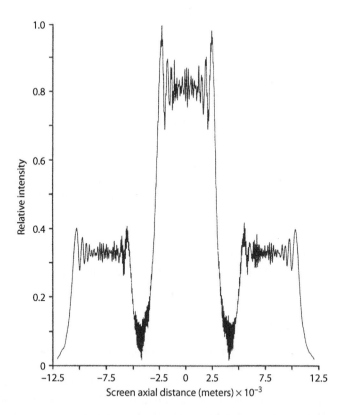

FIGURE 10.10 Theoretical interference patterns for the grating with 100 slits 30 µm wide (at a grating-to-slit distance of 75 cm). This time the diffraction edge effects from the wide illumination slit are incorporated into the calculation. The aperture grating distance is 10 cm. (Reprinted from *Opt. Commun.*, 103, Duarte, F. J., On a generalized interference equation and interferometric measurements, 8–14, Copyright (1993), with permission from Elsevier.)

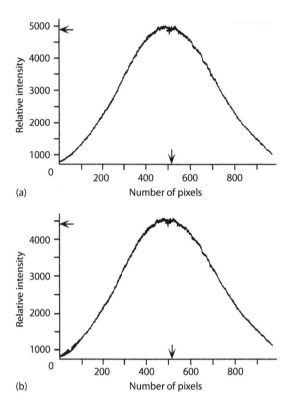

(a)

(b)

FIGURE 10.11 (a) Intensity profile, as a function of radial distance along the expanded axis, of the elongated Gaussian beam following propagation in air. (b) Intensity profile of the elongated Gaussian beam following propagation via a thin microscope slide. Note that the expanded axis is parallel to the plane of incidence. Each pixel is 25 μm wide.

Fortran was used in a PC environment. More recently, programs have been written using MATLAB® [29]. A variety of gratings have been analyzed in the $2 \leq N \leq 2000$ slit range.

10.6 APPLICATIONS

The NSLI described here has found various applications in imaging, has been proposed for uses in secure interferometric communications, and has further uses in textiles and biomedicine. The electro-optical interferometer described here can be used in two different modes, depending on the application. The first mode of application is the straightforward measurement of optical densities in the macroscopic domain for smooth surfaces. Also, transmission modulations can be determined in a classical noninterferometric domain where the detector screen is at a very close distance from the surface being examined, and the slit dimensions are sufficiently wide. The second mode of application is in the interferometric domain.

10.6.1 DENSITOMETRY IN THE MACROSCOPIC DOMAIN

Using the linear photodiode array, the elongated Gaussian beam-intensity profile, following propagation exclusively in air, is shown in Figure 10.11a. Insertion of an optically smooth surface, such as a thin microscope slide, yields little if any alteration to the beam profile, as illustrated in Figure 10.11b. As expected, the only difference is observed in the intensity domain.

This simple exercise illustrates that for optically smooth surfaces, such as neutral-density filters, the instrument can be used as a straightforward densitometer. This is accomplished by integrating the area under the intensity curve due to the substrate alone, denoted by $I_S(\lambda,x)$, and then repeating the measurement with a coated substrate. The simple expression:

$$D(\lambda,x) \approx \log_{10} \frac{\int I_S(\lambda,x)dx}{\int I_{S+C}(\lambda,x)dx} \tag{10.45}$$

yields the optical density D of the coating at a given wavelength. Here, $I_{S+C}(\lambda,x)$ is the spatial intensity distribution measured at the wavelength λ. The advantage of this measurement over traditional density measurements is that any spatially dependent nonuniformity becomes immediately apparent. The spectral distribution of the optical density for a given surface can be obtained by tuning the laser to different wavelengths and evaluating $D(\lambda,x)$. Note that the use of the neutral-density filter prior to the telescope indicates that there is a significant intensity surplus for most measurements. This abundance of intensity enables the instrument to be applied to characterize surfaces with high optical densities. The dynamic range of the instrument can be as high as 10^9.

10.6.2 DETECTION OF SURFACE MICRODEFECTS

The interferometer described here is ideally suited for the detection of surface microdefects. This is illustrated in Figure 10.12a, where dust particles deposited on the microscope slide are easily detected. On the other hand, for a high-optical-density thin metallic film, a microhole causes a strong diffraction signal. Again, spatial information is easily available from the measurement displayed in Figure 10.12b.

As illustrated previously, a simple and inexpensive thin microscope slide yields high-fidelity transmission of the intrinsic elongated Gaussian beam-intensity profile. Replacement of the glass substrate by a polymeric photographic film substrate yields an interferometric response, as illustrated in a sequence of measurements recorded and displayed in the next figure. In Figure 10.13a, the expanded beam-intensity profile following propagation through a smooth glass substrate is displayed with no indication of interference. Replacement of the glass substrate by a high-quality polymeric photographic film substrate yields an interferometric signature, as illustrated in Figure 10.13b. By contrast, a far more pronounced interferometric profile, following propagation via a lower-quality polymeric film substrate, is shown in Figure 10.13c.

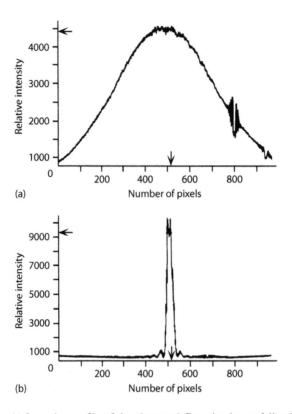

(a)

(b)

FIGURE 10.12 (a) Intensity profile of the elongated Gaussian beam following propagation via a thin microscope slide with some dust particles deposited on it. (b) Intensity profile of a neutral-density filter with an optical density of 4. The diffraction pattern is caused by a micro-hole on the metallic film. Note that, due to Heisenberg's uncertainty principle, the smaller the dimensions of the orifice, the wider the diffraction pattern (see Chapter 5). Each pixel is 25 μm wide. (From Duarte, F. J., *Quantum Optics for Engineers*, CRC Press, New York, 2014.)

It should be noted that the instrument described here provides a fast and unique avenue to quantify defects in clear polymeric film substrates that is not otherwise available. This is due to the fact that at these low optical densities, traditional micro-densitometers, using incoherent illumination sources, encounter serious noise limitations. To quantify the information provided in Figure 10.13, the log ratio of the signal is taken, relative to the intensity transmitted in air, and the standard of deviation calculated. For the spatial profiles shown in Figure 10.13b and c, the standard of deviation is $\sigma = 0.009$ and $\sigma = 0.024$, respectively.

10.6.3 Photographic Film Grain Structure

A further application in the interferometric domain is the characterization of film grain structure in molecular imaging, as described in detail in [5]. For example, the grain structures of black-and-white silver halide photographic film, and various other color films, have been characterized in detail. At this stage, it should

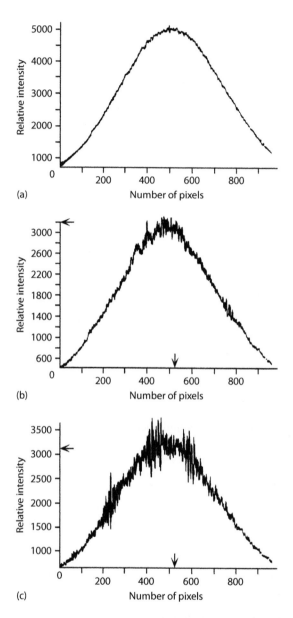

(a)

(b)

(c)

FIGURE 10.13 (a) Elongated Gaussian beam profile transmitted via a smooth thin glass substrate. (b) Interferometric profile of a high-quality clear polymeric film substrate. (c) Interferometric profile of a lower-quality clear polymeric film substrate showing the effect of surface irregularities.

be mentioned that the granularity measurement is performed by recording the microspatial intensity distribution, which is the result of the interaction of the expanded laser beam with the nanodimensioned silver halide crystals of the film and using this distribution to calculate an average microdensity and its standard of deviation according to [14]

$$D(x,\lambda) = \left(\sum_{x=1}^{N} \frac{I_i(x,\lambda)}{I_t(x,\lambda)} \right) N^{-1} \tag{10.46}$$

where:

$I_i(x,\lambda)$ is the incidence intensity
$I_t(x,\lambda)$ is the transmission intensity
N is the total number of micromeasurements

The standard of deviation of this quantity is a measure of the granularity σ of the molecular film or imaging surface.

Using an automated version of the NSLI, in which the surface being illuminated is translated perpendicularly to the plane of propagation, extensive crossover measurements with conventional microdensitometers have been performed. Agreement is excellent in regard to macrodensities, and similar behavior of σ as a function of D was established [14]. However, the absolute values of σ derived from the NSLI are higher than those from traditional microdensitometers, given the enhanced sensitivity of the interferometric measurement. These measurements were performed at various wavelengths of interest throughout the visible. Other advantages of the NSLI include a dynamic range of 10^9, a signal-to-noise ratio of 10^7, a depth of focus greater than 1 mm, and the simultaneous collection of a large number of data points [14].

Finally, from a mathematical perspective, it should be mentioned that the form of Equation 10.37 is similar to the equation for power spectrum widely applied in traditional studies of microdensitometry [14].

The NSLI has also been used in the reflection domain, in a 45° configuration, to assess and quantify surface roughness in photographic, and digital imaging, papers [14].

10.6.4   ASSESSMENT OF TRANSMISSION GRATINGS AND MTF

In addition to the calculations and comparisons presented in the section on interferometric calculations, a straightforward application of the present interferometer, and the theoretical approach previously illustrated, is the assessment of transmission grating characteristics. For instance, one of the features observed in that section is that uncertainty in the dimensions of the slits causes a loss of symmetry in the interferometric/diffraction signal.

An important application is the assessment of transmission interferometric and diffractive properties of gratings coated, on transparent flexible substrates, with silver halide crystals. These gratings are compared with gratings of equal spatial specifications coated with metallic thin films. The interferometric and diffraction characteristics are measured as a function of the spatial frequency of the grating. The modulation is assessed using the usual definition due to Michelson [30]:

$$\mathcal{V} = \frac{I_1 - I_2}{I_1 + I_2} \tag{10.47}$$

In the imaging community, the visibility $\mathcal{V}$ is referred to as the modulation $\mathcal{M}$, while I_1 corresponds to the maximum intensity and I_2 to the minimum intensity. At the same time, the overall measured modulation patterns are compared with the corresponding theoretical prediction. Here, it should be clarified that in the very near field, for an array of sufficiently wide slits, the measured patterns correspond to straightforward classical modulations similar to the distributions shown in Figure 10.6. These modulation or MTF measurements are important, since the higher the modulation, the higher the spatial resolution, or image sharpness, offered by the imaging medium under examination.

These modulation comparisons between photographic and metallic gratings, at the same spatial frequency, are particularly useful to assist in the engineering of crystal-based imaging materials. For example, at a spatial frequency of $f = 20$ lines/mm, the modulation of a particular set of photographic gratings is measured to be in the $0.6 \leq \mathcal{M} \leq 0.8$ range. This compares with $\mathcal{M} \approx 1$ registered from a metallic grating at the same frequency. Also, as the spatial frequency approaches 80 lines/mm and beyond, the spatial definition of the silver halide coatings is adversely affected due to the crystalline grain structure of the photographic film. The dual theoretical/measurement approach described in the fourth and fifth sections is particularly suitable to quantify the deterioration in spatial characteristics of photographic gratings at higher spatial frequencies.

More recently, this technique was extended to assess and compare the spatial resolution, via modulation measurements, of inkjet images using grating patterns of frequencies in the $0.25 \leq f \leq 5$ lines/mm range. For a range of printers, at $f = 5$ lines/mm, the modulations were measured to be in the $0.71 \leq \mathcal{M} \leq 0.87$ range. All these measurements were made at $\lambda = 632.8$ nm.

It should be noted that the applicability of the NSLI extends to any grating-like array and is not just limited to imaging applications. For instance, for micromachining, microdrilling, and similar applications, one can rapidly examine and quantify the uniformity of an array of microscopic orifices or an array of microscopic nozzles.

10.6.5 Theoretical Enhancement of the Resolution of Digital Detectors

The interferometric theory presented in the fourth section, in conjunction with interferometric measurements, can be applied to enhance the resolution of photodiode arrays, CCD detectors, complementary metal-oxide semiconductor (CMOS) detectors, and digital detectors in general.

At present, individual diodes or pixels in a detector array have dimensions in the micrometer range. This size limitation, plus the need to use several diodes or pixels to resolve a given feature, introduces a serious physical limitation to the resolution of these optoelectronic detectors. A solution to this problem is outlined in [5] and rests on the use of the interferometric equations described here.

Assume that a grating with micrometer or nanometer features needs to be characterized. For instance, this characterization may require the determination of the width of the slits of a uniform grating. For this case, positioning of the photodiode array right next to the grating provides no useful information, as the features are beyond the spatial resolution of the detector. Fortunately, as a consequence of the uncertainty principle, the narrow slits, with dimensions in the micrometer or nanometer region, induce significant spatial spread in the far field, so that the light emergent from a single slit can illuminate several individual diodes or pixels. For a large number of slits, the photodiode array captures the interferometric image resulting from the multiple-slit interference. Hence, a sequence of measurements in the far field can be used, in conjunction with Equation 10.27 (for the one-dimensional case, for example), to establish the dimensions and the number of slits generating the signal. Then, the generalized interference equation can be applied to calculate the interference signals in the near field, where the detector array was unable to provide a measurement.

10.6.6 LASER PRINTING

A multiwavelength laser instrument designed to print a series of lines, at varying intensity levels, was designed, built, and disclosed as a *laser sensitometer* [31]. A schematic of this optical system is shown in Figure 10.14. In essence, this is a laser printer that records a line, on light-sensitive paper, without the need to scan a fast-moving laser beam, with a circular cross section, as is done in alternative optical systems for this type of application [13]. In this instrument, linear polarization is used to vary the intensity of the combined laser beam using a rotating high-extinction coefficient Glan–Thompson polarizer [14,31]. This instrument can be described as a polarizer multiple-prism multiple laser (PMPML) sensitometer or as a PMPML printer.

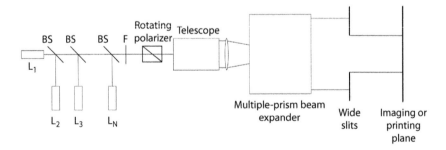

FIGURE 10.14 Schematics of the PMPML printer. A multiple-prism expander in conjunction with a wide aperture produces a nearly constant-intensity laser narrow line in the spatial domain [27]. The narrow line propagates parallel to the plane of propagation. The intensity of this narrow line can be varied continuously by rotating the Glan–Thompson polarizer. Precision movable beam splitters determine whether the exposure is single or multiple wavelength. Various lasers are designated by L_1, L_2, L_3,..., L_N. (Adapted from Duarte, F. J., U.S. Patent 6236461 B1, 2001.)

The collinear laser beams, usually corresponding to a blue, green, and red laser, first encounter a broadband filter to attenuate any excessive intensity. Then, the multiple-wavelength beam propagates through the Glan–Thompson polarizer, where high-precision rotation is used to adjust the intensity of the beam in fine increments [14,31]. The two-dimensional telescope–lens combination yields a tightly focused beam, which is expanded in one dimension by the MPBE. This optical assembly can routinely yield an extremely elongated near-Gaussian beam 30–50 mm wide by a maximum height of 25 μm. As illustrated in [14], deployment of a wide aperture following the MPBE can yield a nearly constant-intensity, or nearly flat, beam in the spatial domain that closely approaches a line. Displacement of a light-sensitive imaging surface, or photographic paper, perpendicular to the plane of propagation renders a series of exposures at different wavelengths and intensity levels. For a detailed description of this instrument, the reader should refer to [31]. An additional laser-printing method using a rotating polygon, in conjunction with a double-mirror arrangement, to produce high-speed displacement of a traditionally highly focused laser beam is described in [32]. This method produces a displacement of the focal point of a combined laser beam to linear speeds of ~4000 m/s.

10.6.7 Wavelength Measurements

One further application of the interferometer described here is its use as a wavelength meter. For instance, the intrinsic dependence of the measurement on wavelength is explicitly illustrated by Equations 10.27 and 10.28, because the interferometric term depends on $2\pi/\lambda$. In this regard, for a given grating and a fixed grating-to-screen distance, the interferogram becomes dependent on the wavelength alone. Hence, changes in wavelength produce changes in the interferogram. Examples on using the NSLI, and the interferometric equations, as a wavelength meter are given in [14]. A natural extension of this approach is to determine *interferometrically* the line-width of the emission source [33,34]. This development follows from the observation that interferograms from narrow-linewidth laser sources yield sharp, well-defined interferograms with a high visibility figure, that is, $V \approx 1.0$. Broadband sources, on the other hand, produce broader, less-defined interferograms with a lower visibility figure ($V \leq 0.8$). Thus, for the same emission wavelength and identical geometrical parameters, the interferogram from the narrow-linewidth laser source is used as a reference, while Equation 10.27 is applied to generate a series of interferograms for different wavelengths departing from the central wavelength. Thus, a graphical representation of the difference of the spatial width, as a function of linewidth, is generated. This graphical representation is then used to estimate the linewidth of the unknown broader source [33,34].

10.6.8 Secure Interferometric Communications in Free Space

The NSLI has also been shown to be applicable as an avenue of secure interferometric communications in free space [35,36], as outlined in Figure 10.15. This class of secure optical communications was originally developed with space-to-space applications in mind, such as satellite-to-satellite communications, as illustrated in Figure 10.16.

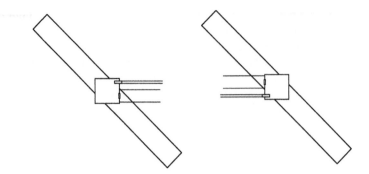

FIGURE 10.15 Secure interferometric satellite-to-satellite communications. This is a pictorial representation of the original idea described by Duarte [35]. An interferometric character is emitted from one satellite 1, or space vehicle 1, to a satellite 2, where it is detected. A reciprocal action can take place from satellite 2 to satellite 1. The interferometric characters are in the form of expanded interferograms to reduce beam divergence. Wider interferometric characters arrive at the intended target. The character is identified by a digital detector, which needs only to detect part of the whole interferogram to identify it via theoretical means.

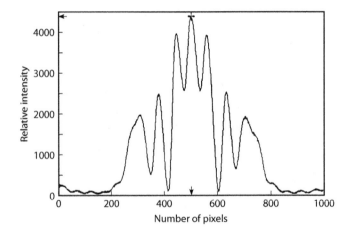

FIGURE 10.16 Interferometric character c generated by the interaction of an expanded TEM_{00} laser beam with four equidistant slits. Each slit is 570 µm wide and $\lambda = 632.82$ nm. The distance from the slits to the digital detector is 723.5 cm, and the small cross indicates the position of the central pixel, each 25 µm wide, in the digital detector. (Reproduced from Duarte, F. J., Secure interferometric communications in free space: Enhanced sensitivity for propagation in the metre range, *J. Opt. A: Pure Appl. Opt.*, 7, 73–75, 2005. With permission from The Institute of Physics.)

The security is provided by the quantum mechanical nature of the interferometric propagation. In other words, any attempt to intercept the intermediate signal to extract information distorts the signal, thus alerting the receiver and subsequently, the emitter. The advantage of this approach over other methods is that it works either in a single-photon mode or with a large population of indistinguishable photons, as provided by a narrow-linewidth laser. So far, this method has been demonstrated in the laboratory over short distances, and it should work well over long distances, via vacuum, in outer space. Nevertheless, preliminary measurements in the laboratory indicate that distortions in the signal due to turbulence induce a different class of distortions than those observed from interception attempts.

For this application, the NSLI is divided in two parts. The laser beam–expander grating assembly of the interferometer comprises the transmitter, while the detector becomes the receiver. Configurationally, in reference to Figures 10.1 and 10.4, all stays the same, albeit the distance between the grating and the detector is allowed to become arbitrarily large.

The concept of secure interferometric communications can be described with the following example, which uses the interferometric character c created by the interaction of an expanded laser beam with four slits in a grating [36]. In Figure 10.16, the initial undisturbed signal being emitted, transmitted, and received is displayed. In Figure 10.17, the effect on the received interferometric signal due to the partial insertion of a thin beam splitter is shown. In Figure 10.18, the effect on the received interferometric signal due to the complete insertion of the thin beam splitter is illustrated. In Figure 10.19, the interferometric signal is displayed as fully restored due to the withdrawal of the thin beam splitter.

The effect of atmospheric turbulence, simulated by the insertion of a thermal source in the path of the interferometric signal, is illustrated in Figure 10.20. As previously mentioned, the pattern of these distortions is different from the violent effect due to the insertion of a thin beam splitter as depicted in Figure 10.18.

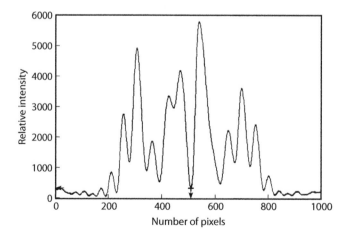

FIGURE 10.17   Severe spatial distortions induced in the interferometric character c by introducing a thin beam splitter at an angle near the Brewster angle relative to the axis of propagation. The laser beam is polarized parallel to the plane of propagation. (Reproduced from Duarte, F. J., Secure interferometric communications in free space: Enhanced sensitivity for propagation in the metre range, *J. Opt. A: Pure Appl. Opt.*, 7, 73–75, 2005. With permission from The Institute of Physics.)

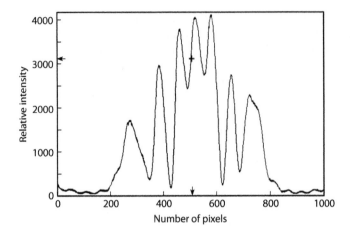

FIGURE 10.18 Spatial distortions in the interferometric character c with the thin beam splitter in place. The intercepted character does not display its original symmetry and is displaced ~300 μm to the right. (Reproduced from Duarte, F. J., Secure interferometric communications in free space: Enhanced sensitivity for propagation in the metre range, *J. Opt. A: Pure Appl. Opt.*, 7, 73–75, 2005. With permission from The Institute of Physics.)

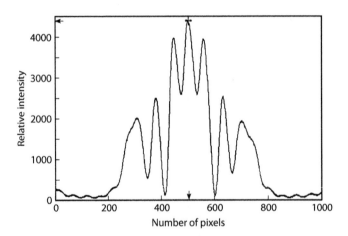

FIGURE 10.19 Removal of the beam splitter restores the original interferometric character c. (Reproduced from Duarte, F. J., Secure interferometric communications in free space: Enhanced sensitivity for propagation in the metre range, *J. Opt. A: Pure Appl. Opt.*, 7, 73–75, 2005. With permission from The Institute of Physics.)

For further details on the generation of interferometric characters, the reader is referred to [37,38]. In a discussion on conceptual countermeasures given in [36], it is underlined that the security of this method of communications is guaranteed by the *principle of interference*. Further, it is mentioned that Feynman [22] considered interference to be a fundamental principle of quantum mechanics. It is also relevant to mention that the principles of N-slit interferometry, as described via Dirac's

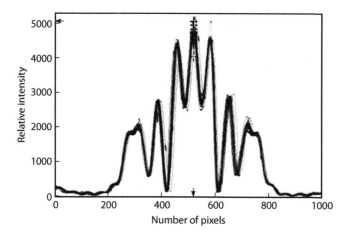

FIGURE 10.20 Cumulative spatial distortions in the interferometric character c caused by turbulence in the propagation air generated by a thermal source.

notation [8], can be used to provide an approximate derivation of Heisenberg's uncertainty principle [14]. Extended N-slit interferometers, with intracavity propagation distances of 35 and 527 m, are discussed by Duarte et al. [37,38].

Going back to space-to-space, or satellite-to-satellite, communications, calculations show that assuming available laser technology, N-slit interferometers emitting via an slit array with a total width of approximately 1 m can propagate an interferogram with a total width of about 4 m at the detection plane for an intra-interferometric distance of $D_{\langle x|j \rangle} = 2 \times 10^6$ m. This might be applicable to a network of satellites including five to six satellites per hemisphere. For space vehicles, or space stations, the intra-interferometric distance might be increased to the $5-10 \times 10^6$ m range [39].

10.6.9 Detection of Clear Air Turbulence

As already seen in Figure 10.20, the interferometric characters are susceptible to variations in the refractive index of the propagation medium as induced by a thermal source that generates turbulence. This phenomenon has been explored further at intra-interferometric propagation distances of $D_{\langle x|j \rangle} = 35$ m [37]. At an ambient temperature of $T \approx 30°C$, a very slight asymmetry is observed in the interferogram for $N=4$, as illustrated in Figure 10.21. A series of interferograms, for $N=4$, under identical conditions reveals a slight wavering pattern in the recorded series of interferograms shown in Figure 10.22. These result illustrate that propagating N-slit interferograms are extremely sensitive to changes in the refractive index of the propagation medium and thus very effective detectors of turbulence in the intra-interferometric path. The use of N-slit interferometers as detectors of clear air turbulence, an aviation hazard, was proposed in [37], and their deployment at thresholds of aviation runways is illustrated in Figure 10.23. The lasers to be used in this application should emit in the eye-safe wavelength range, beyond 1.4 μm, in the near infrared.

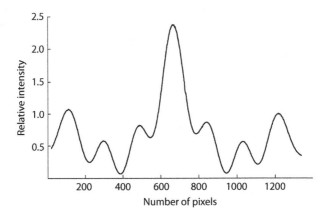

FIGURE 10.21   Interferogram for $N=4$, for $D_{\langle x|j \rangle}=35$ m, at $\lambda=632.8$ nm. The slits are 1000 μm wide separated by 1000 μm. Notice the slight asymmetry induced by very mild atmospheric turbulence. (Reproduced from Duarte, F. J. et al., The N-slit interferometer: An extended configuration, *J. Opt.* 12, 015705, 2010. With permission from The Institute of Physics.)

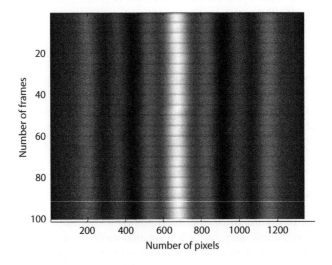

FIGURE 10.22   Series of interferograms for $N=4$, for $D_{\langle x|j \rangle}=35$ m, at $\lambda=632.8$ nm. The slits are 1000 μm wide separated by 1000 μm. Notice the slight wavering pattern induced by very mild atmospheric turbulence. (Reproduced from Duarte, F. J. et al., The N-slit interferometer: An extended configuration, *J. Opt.* 12, 015705, 2010. With permission from The Institute of Physics.)

During the course of experiments on extended intra-interferometric propagation distances [38,40], it was discovered that interception of the propagating interferogram with transparent spider web silk fibers induced subtle and reproducible distortions in the propagating interferograms. In other words, the collapse of the interferogram observed while using classical optical beam splitters could be avoided

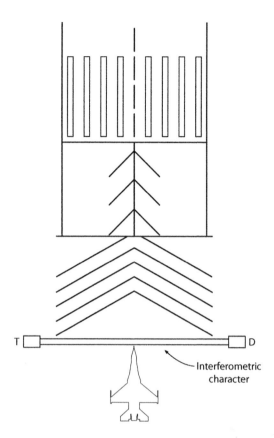

Interferometric
character

FIGURE 10.23 Deployment of *N*-slit interferometer at threshold of aviation runway to alert landing aircraft and pilots of possible clear air turbulence. The transmitter (T) includes the laser, telescope, MPBE, and *N*-slit array. D represents the digital detector. T and D are separated by an appropriate intra-interferometric distance $D_{(x|j)}$, at an adequate height from the ground.

using microscopic soft means of interception via transparent natural fibers. To illustrate this phenomenon, in Figure 10.24, a control interferogram, for $N=3$, is displayed. In Figure 10.25, a measured interferogram is displayed that shows a superimposed diffraction pattern over the propagating interferogram. The measurement is accurately reproduced by the generalized interferometric Equation 10.27, as shown in Figure 10.26. These delicate and predictable interceptions are discussed, via the interferometric equation (Equation 10.27), from a soft measurements perspective by Duarte [27].

10.6.10 INTERFEROMETRY IN TEXTILES

A semi-orderly single-layer textile fabric looks like a grid or a two-dimensional grating, as shown in Figure 10.27 for common cotton. Higher-quality fabrics present a more compact network of finer fibers. From an optics and interferometric

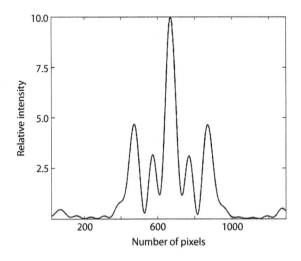

FIGURE 10.24 Control interferogram. (Reproduced from Duarte, F. J., et al., Diffractive patterns superimposed over propagating *N*-slit interferograms, *J. Mod. Opt.* 60, 136–140, 2013. With permission from Taylor & Francis Group.)

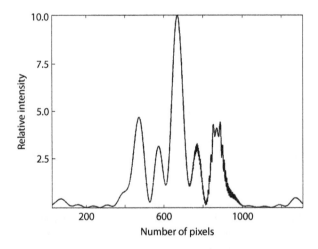

FIGURE 10.25 Measured interferogram showing a superimposed diffraction pattern over the propagating interferogram. (Reproduced from Duarte, F. J., et al., Diffractive patterns superimposed over propagating *N*-slit interferograms, *J. Mod. Opt.* 60, 136–140, 2013. With permission from Taylor & Francis Group.)

perspective, this means that a particular class of single-layered fabric corresponds to a particular grating structure and as such, is applicable to an interferometric classification. An interferogram using the *N*SLI on the type of single-layer cotton fabric mentioned here yields an interferometric signature, as shown in Figure 10.28.

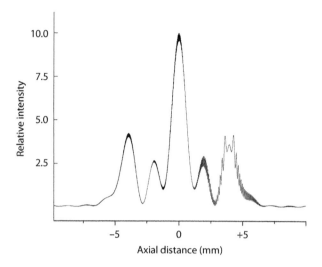

FIGURE 10.26 Theoretical interferogram accurately reproducing the interception phenomenon illustrated in Figure 10.26. (Reproduced from Duarte, F. J., et al., Diffractive patterns superimposed over propagating *N*-slit interferograms, *J. Mod. Opt.* 60, 136–140, 2013. With permission from Taylor & Francis Group.)

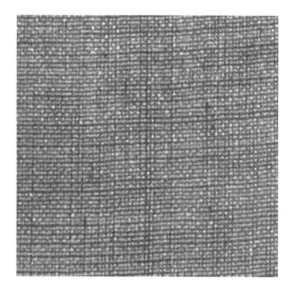

FIGURE 10.27 Single-layered textile 25×25 mm approximately configuring a two-dimensional optical grating.

In the same way as a molecular coating of given characteristics yields a unique interferometric signature, it is not difficult to extrapolate to networks of fibers constituting textile fabrics. This technique could also be used as a forensic tool in the arts to determine the similarity, or differences, between two fabrics. This could be used to establish whether a given fabric came from a particular region or epoch of interest.

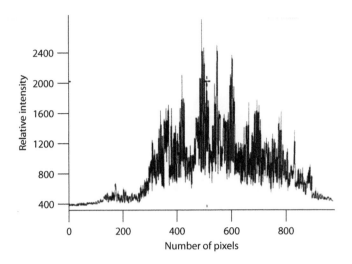

FIGURE 10.28 Interferometric signature of the single-layered textile shown in Figure 13.27.

10.6.11 APPLICATIONS TO BIOMEDICINE

Early detection of certain cancers requires more sensitive and higher-resolution x-ray films. In this regard, microdensitometry is an essential tool applied to determine the granularity of the film. Modulation measurements are also important. As previously discussed, the *N*SLI can be used to quantify both these parameters rapidly and with added sensitivity.

An additional way to think of the *N*SLI is as a laser microscope with a vastly extended field of observation and a vastly extended depth of focus. Microscopy has been used in biomedicine since the seventeenth century, and, as we all know, today it continues to be used in a plethora of biomedical applications (see Chapter 9). The *N*SLI could also be used as a microdensitometer to observe, compare, and study biological samples in the transmission domain. Using a broadly tunable laser greatly enhances its information-gathering capabilities.

The illumination and wide microdetection capabilities of the *N*SLI have been found relevant by researchers and engineers working on instrumentation for structural analysis of organic compounds [41], cytological research [42], and x-ray imaging [43–45].

10.7 CONCLUSIONS

The *N*SLI has been discussed and analyzed. This instrument can be described as a tunable laser microscope with an extensive microillumination capability and a very long depth of focus. Alternatively, the *N*SLI can be thought of as a microdensitometer with wide illumination and extensive depth of focus. Beam propagation through the telescope and multiple-prism expander has been described using ray transfer matrices. This approach enables the prediction of the beam spatial characteristics at the focal plane. For one mode of operation, the optics yields an extremely elongated Gaussian spatial beam ~32 μm high by 35–60 mm wide. An alternative mode of operation is the generation of spatial Gaussian beams ~10 mm high by 35–60 mm wide.

Transmission surfaces can be assessed by positioning the surface of interest in the vertical plane, normal to the plane of propagation, between the multiple-prism expander and the digital detector array. For smooth optical surfaces, the instrument can be used as a classical densitometer. For surfaces with micro and submicron features, such as transmission gratings, the instrument functions as an interferometer. However, in the near field, and for sufficiently wide slits, the instrument measures classical modulation patterns.

The Dirac formalism has been applied to describe the photon propagation from the source to the detection screen via the intermediate grating. The resulting interferometric equations have been successfully applied to predict and quantify the measured interference/diffraction patterns. An important application of this method enables the prediction of interference signals in the near field, where photodiode array detectors are unable to resolve. Thus, the resolution of these detectors can be enhanced.

Other applications include detection of microholes in thin metal films, detection of surface defects in clear transmission surfaces, characterization of grain structure in photographic film, assessment of transmission gratings, and wavelength measurements. The NSLI has also been applied to assess textile fabrics and to demonstrate secure interferometric communications in free space. Various biomedical applications have also been outlined.

The scope of applications is significantly enhanced by the availability of a variety of discretely tunable and broadly tunable laser sources. A requirement for the laser source is emission in a single transverse mode.

ACKNOWLEDGMENTS

The initial part of this work was made possible by the support of the former *Photographic Research Laboratories* of the Eastman Kodak Company, and it was enthusiastically encouraged by J. Merrigan, to whose memory this work is dedicated. Also, the author is grateful to J. C. Kinard and J. P. Terwilliger. For software support, the author is thankful to D. J. Paine, F. J. Duarte Jr., and I. E. Olivares.

REFERENCES

1. Dainty, J. C. and R. Shaw, *Image Science*, Academic, New York, 1974.
2. Duarte, F. J., Static multicolor laser system for microdensitometry: Preliminary report, *Current Awareness Report*, Eastman Kodak Company, Rochester, NY, 1986 (unpublished).
3. Duarte, F. J. and D. J. Paine, Quantum mechanical description of N-slit interference phenomena. In R. C. Sze and F. J. Duarte (Eds), *Proceedings of the International Conference on Lasers '88*, pp. 42–47, STS, McLean, VA, 1989.
4. Duarte, F. J., Dispersive dye lasers. In F. J. Duarte (Ed.), *High Power Dye Lasers*, Chapter 2, Springer, Berlin, 1991.

5. Duarte, F. J., Electro-optical interferometric microdensitometer system, U.S. Patent 5255069, 1993.
6. Duarte, F. J., On a generalized interference equation and interferometric measurements, *Opt. Commun.* 103: 8–14, 1993.
7. Duarte, F. J., Interferometric imaging. In F. J. Duarte (Ed.), *Tunable Laser Applications*, 1st edn, Chapter 5, Marcel-Dekker, New York, 1995.
8. Dirac, P. A. M., *The Principles of Quantum Mechanics*, 4th edn, Oxford University Press, Oxford, 1978.
9. Willett, C. S., *An Introduction to Gas Lasers: Population Inversion Mechanisms*, Pergamon, New York, 1974.
10. Hollberg, L., CW dye laser. In F. J. Duarte and L. W. Hillman (Eds), *Dye Laser Principles*, Chapter 5, Academic, New York, 1990.
11. Johnston, T. F. and F. J. Duarte, Lasers, dye. In R. A. Meyers (Ed.), *Encyclopedia of Physical Science and Technology*, 3rd edn, Volume 8, pp. 315–359, Academic, New York, 2002.
12. Duarte, F. J., Narrow linewidth pulsed dye laser oscillators. In F. J. Duarte and L. W. Hillman (Eds), *Dye Laser Principles*, Chapter 4, Academic, New York, 1990.
13. Duarte, F. J., Multiple-prism grating solid-state dye laser oscillator: Optimized architecture, *Appl. Opt.* 38: 6347–6349, 1999.
14. Duarte, F. J., *Tunable Laser Optics*, Elsevier-Academic, New York, 2003.
15. Olejnicek, J., H. T. Do, Z. Hubicka, R. Hippier, and L. Jastrabik, Blue diode laser absorption spectroscopy of pulse magnetron discharge, *Jpn. J. Appl. Phys.* 45: 8090–8094, 2006.
16. Olivares, I. E., A. E. Duarte, E. A. Saravia, and F. J. Duarte, Lithium isotope separation with tunable diode lasers, *Appl. Opt.* 41: 2973–2977, 2002.
17. Zorabedian, P., Characteristics of a grating-external-cavity semiconductor laser containing intracavity prism beam expanders, *J. Lightwave Technol.* 10: 330–335, 1992.
18. Duarte, F. J., Beam shaping with telescopes and multiple-prism beam expanders, *J. Opt. Soc. Am. A* 4: P30, 1987.
19. Duarte, F. J., Multiple-prism dispersion and 4×4 ray transfer matrices, *Opt. Quant. Electron.* 24: 49–53, 1992.
20. Turunen, J., Astigmatism in laser beam optical systems, *Appl. Opt.* 25: 2908–2911, 1986.
21. Feynman, R. P. and A. R. Hibbs, *Quantum Mechanics and Path Integrals*, McGraw-Hill, New York, 1965.
22. Feynman, R. P., R. B. Leighton, and M. Sands, *The Feynman Lectures on Physics*, Volume III, Addison-Wesley, Reading, MA, 1965.
23. Duarte, F. J., Interference, diffraction, and refraction, via Dirac's notation, *Am. J. Phys.* 65: 637–640, 1997.
24. Kurusingal, J., Law of normal scattering—A comprehensive law for wave propagation at an interface, *J. Opt. Soc. Am. A* 24: 98–108, 2007.
25. Duarte, F. J., Comment on reflection, refraction, and multislit interference, *Eur. J. Phys.* 25: L57–L58, 2004.
26. Lamb, W. E., Quantum measurement theory, *Ann. N. Y. Acad. Sci.* 480: 407–416, 1986.
27. Duarte, F. J., *Quantum Optics for Engineers*, CRC Press, New York, 2014.
28. van Kampen, N. G., Ten theorems about quantum mechanical measurement, *Physica A.* 153: 97–113, 1988.
29. Duarte, F. J., *Tunable Laser Optics*, 2nd edn, CRC Press, New York, 2015.
30. Michelson, A. A., *Studies in Optics*, The University of Chicago, 1927.
31. Duarte, F. J., Laser sensitometer using multiple-prism beam expansion and polarizer, U.S. Patent 6236461 B1, 2001.

32. Duarte, F. J., B. A. Reed, and C. J. Burak, Laser sensitometer, U.S. Patent 6903824 B2, 2005.
33. Duarte, F. J., Coherent electrically-excited organic semiconductors: Visibility of interferograms and emission linewidth, *Opt. Lett.* 32: 412–414, 2007.
34. Duarte, F. J., Coherent electrically-excited organic semiconductors: Coherent or laser emission? *Appl. Phys. B* 90: 101–108, 2008.
35. Duarte, F. J., Secure interferometric communications in free space, *Opt. Commun.* 205: 313–319, 2002.
36. Duarte, F. J., Secure interferometric communications in free space: Enhanced sensitivity for propagation in the metre range, *J. Opt. A: Pure Appl. Opt.* 7: 73–75, 2005.
37. Duarte, F. J., T. S. Taylor, A. B. Clark, and W. E. Davenport, The N-slit interferometer: An extended configuration, *J. Opt.* 12: 015705, 2010.
38. Duarte, F. J., T. S. Taylor, A. B. Black, W. E. Davenport, and P. G. Varmette, N-slit interferometer for secure optical communications: 527 m intra interferometric path length, *J. Opt.* 13: 035710, 2011.
39. Duarte, F. J. and T. S. Taylor, Secure space-to-space interferometric communications, *Laser Focus World* 51: 54–58, 2015.
40. Duarte, F. J., T. S. Taylor, A. M. Black, and I. E. Olivares, Diffractive patterns superimposed over propagating N-slit interferograms, *J. Mod. Optic.* 60: 136–140, 2013.
41. Chrastil, J., Spectrophotometric method for structural analysis of organic compounds, polymers, nucleotides, and peptides, U.S. Patent 5550630, 1996.
42. Ortyn, W. E., L. R. Piloco, and J. W. Hayenga, Cytological system illumination integrity checking apparatus and method, U.S. Patent 6011861, 2000.
43. Sliski, A. P., X-ray phantom apparatus, U.S. Patent 5511107, 1996.
44. Sliski, A. P., CCD X-ray microdensitometer system, U.S. Patent 5623139, 1997.
45. Kwok, C. S., and K. Y. Lee, Microdensitometer system with micrometer resolution for reading radiochromic films, U.S. Patent 6927859, 2005.

11 Tunable Laser Atomic Vapor Laser Isotope Separation

F. J. Duarte

CONTENTS

11.1 INTRODUCTION

According to the open literature, the subject of selective multiple-step laser photoionization and laser isotope separation (LIS) surfaced under the authorship of researchers from the former Soviet Union around 1972 [1–4]. Theoretical interest in the United States was documented in the mid- to late 1970s [5,6], and more explicit interest on this subject was made public in the late 1970s to early 1980s [7–9]. Australian efforts in this research area were disclosed in the open literature in the early 1980s [10–13]. According to the open literature, subsequent LIS efforts can also be documented in France [14], India [15], and Japan [16].

There are two main approaches to LIS: atomic vapor laser isotope separation (AVLIS) and molecular laser isotope separation (MLIS). In this chapter, attention is mainly given to AVLIS and the tunable lasers necessary to achieve AVLIS, while the process of MLIS is only considered from a peripheral perspective. Other commercially based LIS processes are not considered, given the absence of peer-reviewed literature.

Reviews relevant to various aspects of LIS can be found in *Laser Spectroscopy and Its Applications* [17], *Dye Laser Principles* [18], *High Power Dye Lasers* [19], and *Laser Isotope Separation in Atomic Vapor* [20]. Some of these reviews deal with the efficiency and economic advantages of LIS. Technological advances since then have most likely increased these advantages, albeit the topic is beyond the scope of this review. The description provided in this chapter focuses mainly on the tunable laser aspects of LIS.

11.2   ATOMIC VAPOR LASER ISOTOPE SEPARATION

AVLIS applies to numerous elements of the periodic table [17]. In this review chapter, our attention focuses principally on the open literature on isotopic enrichment of atomic uranium, namely, separation of ^{235}U from ^{238}U, and lithium, namely, separation of ^7Li from ^6Li.

11.2.1   GEOMETRY OF EXCITATION

A simplified geometry of excitation of an atomic vapor applicable to LIS is depicted in Figure 11.1. An atomic metal vapor beam is generated using appropriate

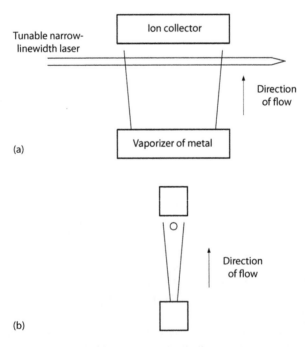

FIGURE 11.1   Simplified schematics of the apparatus used in AVLIS. An electron beam oven vaporizes the atomic species in a vacuum chamber. The atomic beam thus created is excited by a tunable narrow-linewidth laser beam, or a combination of tunable laser beams, causing highly selective excitation of a particular isotope while leaving the unwanted isotope unexcited. Following selective excitation, the excited isotope is ionized and collected by electromagnetic means. (a) Side view. (b) Frontal perspective.

vaporization means, including electron beams. The vaporized atomic species are then selectively and sequentially excited by a high-power tunable narrow-linewidth laser. The narrow-linewidth laser excitation is capable of selectively exciting one isotope of an atomic species while leaving the other isotope in the ground state. Once this sequential selective excitation ionizes the excited isotope, the resulting ions are collected by electromagnetic means.

This type of geometry and excitation configuration is described by Paisner and Solarz [21] as applied to separating ^{235}U from ^{238}U while using narrow-linewidth tunable laser excitation generated by a copper-vapor laser (CVL)-pumped dye laser system.

11.2.2 EXCITATION MECHANISMS

Descriptions of sequential selective excitation toward photoionization can employ the judicious application of population rate equations [5] or quantum-based approaches such as the density matrix technique [6]. According to Eberly, tunable narrow-linewidth laser, or highly coherent, excitation is assumed [5,6].

This subject is treated in detail elsewhere [20,21], and it is only briefly introduced here from an alternative perspective. The Dirac quantum principle [22]

$$\langle \phi \mid \psi \rangle = \sum_{k}^{N} \langle \phi \mid k \rangle \langle k \mid \psi \rangle \tag{11.1}$$

can be expressed as

$$\mid \psi \rangle = \sum_{k}^{N} \mid k \rangle C_k \tag{11.2}$$

and the amplitudes C_k satisfy the linear differential equations

$$i\hbar \frac{dC_j(t)}{dt} = \sum_{k}^{N} H_{jk} C_k(t) \tag{11.3}$$

where H_{jk} is the Hamiltonian.

A multistep selective photon-excitation alternative leading to ionization is shown in Figure 11.2. In this notation, the k index refers to the various successive energy levels existing from the ground state all the way up to the ionization level. Solving Equation 11.3 leads to the probability of the various transitions, which in turn leads to the cross section associated with the various transitions [23]. Once the cross sections are worked out, then the populations at the various energy levels can be predicted.

A detailed density matrix description for sequential selective excitation in lithium was developed by A. E. Duarte and colleagues [24].

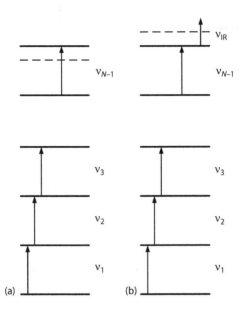

FIGURE 11.2 Selective multiphoton excitation leading to photoionization. (a) Sequential excitation with various similar frequencies leads directly to the ionization of the selected isotope. (b) Sequential excitation with various similar frequencies leaves the atomic isotope near its ionization potential, and the last excitation is performed by a longer wavelength laser.

11.3 MOLECULAR LASER ISOTOPE SEPARATION

MLIS refers to the use of molecular compounds rather than the atomic species. In the case of uranium, uranyl compounds such as UF_6 [25] and UO_2 [11] are used.

The use of molecular compounds such as UF_6 has the advantage of requiring much lower temperatures to achieve a molecular beam to be illuminated by the laser radiation. In fact, it has been reported that a reservoir of UF_6 was maintained at an "ambient temperature" while the population of UF_6 was ~10^9 molecules/cm^2 in the laser-interacting region [25]. The disadvantage, however, is that molecular fluorine is involved.

The isotopic shift between $^{235}UF_6$ and $^{238}UF_6$ is reported to be $(1/\Delta x') \approx 0.7$ cm^{-1} [26], which at a wavelength of $\lambda \approx 16$ μm, translates into $\Delta v \approx 21$ GHz; thus, the excitation laser linewidth has to be below this limit.

The 16 μm coherent excitation source used in these UF_6 uranium isotope enrichment experiments is a p-H_2 Raman cell excited by two pulsed CO_2 lasers. The CO_2 laser transitions used to excite the Raman cell were the $10P(12)$ and $10P(10)$ transitions, and the optimum selectivity (β_h = depletion $^{235}UF_6$/depletion $^{238}UF_6$) reported by these authors was $\beta_h = 1.2 \pm 0.03$ [25]. Although the linewidth of the CO_2 lasers is not mentioned, it is well known that high-power TEA CO_2 laser oscillators can deliver linewidths in the $107 \leq \Delta v \leq 140$ MHz range at $\lambda \approx 10.59$ μm [27,28].

The UO_2 experiments employed a pulsed TEA CO_2 laser and a continuous-wave (CW) CO_2–N_2O laser [9]. The $^{235}U/^{238}U$ enrichment factors measured by these authors were ≤ 1.1[10].

11.4 NARROW-LINEWIDTH TUNABLE LASERS FOR AVLIS

In this section, two of the most widely applied classes of narrow-linewidth tunable lasers are described in the context of isotope enrichment: the tunable organic dye laser and the tunable diode laser. Tunable narrow-linewidth dye laser oscillators lase in the pulse regime at high pulse repetition frequencies (prfs), and they are intrinsically apt to be engineered into high average power oscillator–amplifier systems. Tunable narrow-linewidth diode lasers emit low powers in the CW regime, but they could also be applied to integrate high-power laser systems.

11.4.1 High-Power Tunable Narrow-Linewidth Dye Lasers

The most widely used laser system applied in AVLIS is the CVL-pumped narrow-linewidth tunable dye laser. Early versions of these lasers were disclosed by Pease and Pearson [7] and Hargrove and Kan [29].

High-power narrow-linewidth tunable laser systems for AVLIS applications are mostly composed of oscillator–amplifier systems, in which a crucial component is the oscillator configuration, which enables the generation of low beam divergence, tunable narrow-linewidth emission with a minimum of amplified spontaneous emission (ASE).

An important advancement in the architecture of tunable laser oscillators came with the introduction of multiple-prism Littrow (MPL) grating cavities [30], grazing-incidence (GI) grating cavities [31,32], and hybrid multiple-prism near-grazing incidence (HMPGI) grating cavities [33].

These developments also led to the demonstration of CVL-pumped MPL-grating narrow-linewidth oscillators incorporating intracavity étalons [34], CVL-pumped MPL-grating narrow-linewidth oscillators [13,35], and CVL-pumped HMPGI-grating narrow-linewidth oscillators [13,35]. These high-performance CVL-pumped dispersive laser cavities are illustrated in Figures 11.3 and 11.4.

In the tunable multiple-prism grating laser oscillators depicted in Figures 11.3 and 11.4, the multiple-pass laser linewidth is given by [35,36]

$$\Delta\lambda = \Delta\theta_R \left(MR\nabla_\lambda\Theta_G + R\nabla_\lambda\Phi_P \right)^{-1} \tag{11.4}$$

where:
$\nabla_\lambda\Theta = \partial\Theta/\partial\lambda$
  R is a finite number of intracavity passes
  M is the overall intracavity beam magnification

The multiple return-pass beam divergence $\Delta\theta_R$ is given by [36]

$$\Delta\theta_R = \frac{\lambda}{\pi w}\left(1 + \left(\frac{L_\mathcal{R}}{B_R}\right)^2 + \left(\frac{A_R L_\mathcal{R}}{B_R}\right)^2\right)^{1/2} \tag{11.5}$$

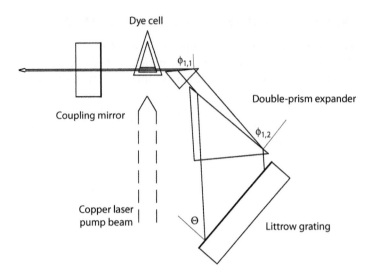

FIGURE 11.3 CVL-pumped tunable narrow-linewidth MPL grating laser oscillator. Its performance is given in Table 11.1. (Reproduced from Duarte, F. J., and J. A. Piper, Narrow-linewidth, high prf copper laser-pumped dye laser oscillators, *Appl. Opt.* 23, 1391–1394, 1988. With permission of Optical Society of America.)

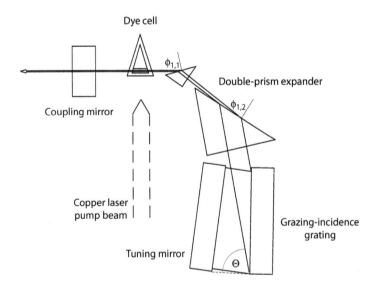

FIGURE 11.4 CVL-pumped tunable narrow-linewidth HMPGI grating laser oscillator. Its performance is given in Table 11.1. (Reproduced from Duarte, F.J., and J. A. Piper, Narrow-linewidth, high prf copper laser-pumped dye laser oscillators, *Appl. Opt.* 23, 1391–1394, 1988. With permission of Optical Society of America.)

where:

$L_R = (\pi w^2 / \lambda)$ is the Rayleigh length

w is the beam waist

A_R and B_R are the corresponding multireturn-pass matrix elements of the $ABCD$ matrix describing the optics of the multiple-prism grating oscillator [36–38]

In a well-designed cavity, the terms in parentheses approach unity, and the beam divergence reduces to its diffraction limit

$$\Delta\theta_R \approx \frac{\lambda}{\pi w}$$

(11.6)

The return-pass multiple-prism dispersion is given by [35,39]

$$\nabla_\lambda \Phi_P = \nabla_\lambda \phi'_{1,m} = \mathcal{H}'_{1,m} \nabla_\lambda n_m + (k'_{1,m} k'_{2,m})\left(\mathcal{H}'_{2,m} \nabla_\lambda n_m \pm \nabla_\lambda \phi'_{1,(m+1)}\right)$$

(11.7)

where

$$k'_{1,m} = \frac{\cos\psi'_{1,m}}{\cos\phi'_{1,m}}$$

(11.8)

$$k'_{2,m} = \frac{\cos\phi'_{2,m}}{\cos\psi'_{2,m}}$$

(11.9)

$$\mathcal{H}'_{1,m} = \frac{\tan\phi'_{2,m}}{n_m}$$

(11.10)

$$\mathcal{H}'_{2,m} = \frac{\tan\phi'_{2,m}}{n_m}$$

(11.11)

In these equations, the prime quantities refer to the return pass where $\phi'_{1,m}$ and $\phi'_{2,m}$ are the exit and incident angles at the mth prism, while $\psi'_{1,m}$ and $\psi'_{2,m}$ are the corresponding refraction angles. For a review on this subject, refer to Chapter 4 of *Dye Laser Principles* [37] or Chapter 4 of *Tunable Laser Optics* [38]. The basic message here is that, as described by Equation 11.4, the main function of a multiple-prism beam expander is to significantly augment the dispersion of the diffraction grating via multiplication by M. This is especially important, since multiple-prism expanders can be designed to yield $\nabla_\lambda \Phi_P \approx 0$, so that the tuning characteristics of the cavity are entirely controlled by the diffraction grating.

Additional CVL-pumped tunable narrow-linewidth oscillators applicable to AVLIS include those of Broyer et al. [14], Singh et al. [15], Maruyama et al. [16], and Bass et al. [40]. In Table 11.1, the performance of these dispersive dye laser oscillators is summarized in chronological order.

TABLE 11.1

Emission Characteristics of CVL-Pumped Tunable Narrow-Linewidth Laser Oscillators

Oscillator	λ Range (nm)	Δθ[a]	Δν (MHz)	η(%)[b]	prf[c] (kHz)	References
MPL	$565 \leq \lambda \leq 605$	×1.1	1400	5	8	[13]
HMPGI	$565 \leq \lambda \leq 603$	×1.1	600[d]	4	8	[13]
MPL[e]	$560 \leq \lambda \leq 650$[f]	—	$50 \leq \Delta \nu \leq 5000$[g]	—	26	[40]
GI	$563 \leq \lambda \leq 607$	—	3000	20	2.5	[14]
HMPGI	$562 \leq \lambda \leq 619$	—	2098	19	6.5	[15]
MPL[e]	—	—	~800[d]	—	6.5	[16]

[a] Times its diffraction-limited value.
[b] Conversion efficiency.
[c] Pulse repetition frequency.
[d] Single-longitudinal-mode emission.
[e] Includes an intracavity étalon.
[f] Uses more than one laser dye.
[g] Single-longitudinal-mode emission at the narrower end of this range.

The type and class of tunable narrow-linewidth oscillators listed in Table 11.1 provide average powers from 80 to 100 mW at a prf of 8 kHz [13] to about 600 mW at a prf of 26 kHz [40]. The total spectrally integrated ASE for the MPL grating cavity delivering a laser linewidth of $\Delta \nu \approx 1.4$ GHz was ~ 1%, while the HMPGI grating cavity, yielding $\Delta \nu \approx 600$ MHz, registered an ASE level of ~ 0.1% [13]. While oscillator ASE figures are not quoted in the Lawrence Livermore publication, it is mentioned that the overall postamplification ASE level was less than 5% [40]. A detailed review on ASE-reducing techniques and measuring protocols is given in [41]. An additional relevant point is that these oscillators can be designed to yield an emission strongly polarized parallel to the plane of propagation [13].

In the Lawrence Livermore experiments, up to four master oscillators (MOs) are used to inject respective power amplifiers (PAs). Each MOPA chain is reported to deliver 1.3–1.5 kW of average power, while the whole system is reported to deliver 2.5–2.8 kW of narrow-linewidth tunable laser radiation [40].

11.4.2 NARROW-LINEWIDTH TUNABLE DIODE LASERS

Tunable narrow-linewidth semiconductor lasers are reviewed in detail in Chapter 5. Further information can be found in *Tunable Laser Optics* [38]. Tunable narrow-linewidth diode lasers used in lithium AVLIS are described by Olivares et al. [42] as using Littrow grating configurations and yielding single-longitudinal-mode laser linewidths of $\Delta \nu \approx 100$ kHz at an approximate tuning range of $659.5 \leq \lambda \leq 684.5$ nm. The beam divergence is diffraction limited, and the CW output power is 9 mW [42].

11.4.2.1 Example

As a means of comparison or reference, here we include the performance of a compact CW semiconductor laser emitting single-longitudinal-mode emission in the red portion of the spectrum. Consider a semiconductor gain waveguide with $2w \approx 2$ µm emitting at $\lambda = 670$ nm. For an MPL grating cavity, as illustrated in Figure 11.5, incorporating a *fully illuminated* 2400 lines/mm grating, the *multiple return-pass* dispersive linewidth becomes

$$\Delta\lambda \approx \Delta\theta \left(RM \frac{\partial\Theta}{\partial\lambda} \right)^{-1}$$

$$(11.12)$$

which in this case is $\Delta\lambda \approx (14 \times 10^{-12}/R)$ m or $\Delta\nu \approx (9.39 \times 10^{9}/R)$ Hz. Previously, for high-power short-pulse multiple-prism oscillators, the multiple return-pass factor has been established as being at least $R \approx 3$ [35–36]. The cavity length of the MPL grating oscillator depicted in Figure 11.5 is about 45 mm, which translates into an intracavity mode spacing of $\delta\nu \approx 3.33 \times 10^{9}$ Hz. This means that for a CW oscillator lasing at $\lambda \approx 670$ nm, single-longitudinal-mode emission should be easily achieved. In this regard, it should be mentioned that Zorabedian reports single-longitudinal-mode oscillation, at $\Delta\nu \approx 100$ kHz, using MPL grating oscillators with cavity lengths in the 50–100 mm range [43–44]. See Chapter 5 for further information on tunable external-cavity diode lasers.

11.5 URANIUM AVLIS

Separation of ^{235}U from ^{238}U has been accomplished in a number of laboratories using high-power CVL-pumped narrow-linewidth tunable dye lasers. The crucial laser parameters of interest are laser wavelength, laser linewidth, linewidth jitter, ASE levels, and beam divergence. Average power, of course, affects yield, but as a

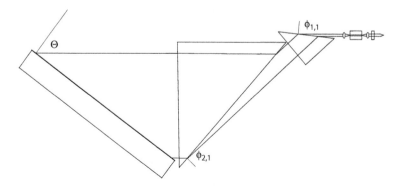

FIGURE 11.5 Tunable CW narrow-linewidth MPL grating external-cavity semiconductor laser. The double-prism expander provides a beam-expansion factor of $M \approx 44$, and the width of the diffraction grating is 25 mm.

parameter it is not as important as the parameters determining the spectral emission and the coherence characteristics of the laser. From a more general perspective, it should be mentioned that an authoritative review of the literature applicable to AVLIS, up to 1990, is given by Akerman [45].

From figures in the open literature [17,40] it is known that the laser wavelengths of interest are in the $550 \leq \lambda \leq 650$ nm range, laser linewidths lie in the $1 \leq \Delta v \leq 3$ GHz range, and frequency jitter should be below ± 30 MHz. Although no specific figures are available for ASE levels, it is known that well-designed tunable narrow-linewidth lasers for this type of application yield very low ASE levels [13,41].

The ionization potential for ^{235}U is quoted at ~6.19 eV [46], which means that three photons of $\lambda \approx 590$ nm are needed for sequential excitation and ionization in a process similar to that outlined in Figure 11.2a. Important additional information relates to the isotopic shift between ^{235}U and ^{238}U, which is known to be at least $\delta v \approx 2$ GHz, a fact already covered in the published laser linewidth requirements.

Using two tunable dye lasers emitting in the $560 \leq \lambda \leq 600$ nm range, Bajaj et al. [45] report on a two-wavelength three-photon scheme to selectively excite and ionize uranium isotopes in an excitation configuration compatible with that illustrated in Figure 11.2a. The wavelengths used by these authors were $\lambda_1 = 589.24$ nm and $\lambda_2 = 592.2$ nm. The first step in the excitation used λ_1, and the two subsequent steps utilized λ_2 [47].

11.6   LITHIUM AVLIS

LIS of ^6Li and ^7Li was achieved by Arizawa et al. [48] using tunable dye lasers as exciters and an Nd:YAG laser as ionizer. LIS of ^6Li and ^7Li using tunable diode lasers was first reported by Olivares et al. [42].

Research in this field requires laser narrow-linewidth radiation tunable in the $670 \leq \lambda \leq 671$ nm range, and the isotopic shift between ^6Li and ^7Li is in the $9 \leq \delta v \leq 11$ GHz range, approximately [42]. Therefore, isotope enrichment in lithium is accessible using either pulsed narrow-linewidth dye lasers or tunable CW narrow-linewidth semiconductor lasers.

Briefly, the approach uses a two-step photoionization process [42] in which one wavelength from the tunable diode laser excites a specific lithium ion to an intermediate level, from which the fourth harmonic from an Nd:YAG laser takes the excited isotope beyond its ionization potential. More specifically, for instance, in the case of ^6Li, the narrow-linewidth diode laser beam tuned at $\lambda_1 = 670.8073$ nm is used to enable the $2s^2S_{1/2} - 2p^2P_{1/2}$ transition. Once excitation to the $2p^2P_{1/2}$ level is accomplished, the ultraviolet laser at $\lambda_2 \approx 266$ nm takes the ^6Li isotope beyond its ionization potential. For excitation of ^7Li, the narrow-linewidth diode laser beam is tuned at $\lambda_1 = 670.7764$ nm.

A simplified apparatus schematics applicable to LIS experiments is shown in Figure 11.6. A lithium beam is illuminated by both lasers, λ_1 and λ_2, and the excited species proceeds toward a Pierce extractor, from where it propagates via a charged particle lens toward a magnetic sector. At the magnetic sector, the beam is separated

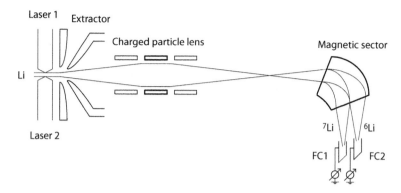

FIGURE 11.6 Simplified apparatus schematics applicable to the lithium isotope separation experiments. The tunable diode radiation (Laser 1) and the UV laser radiation (Laser 2) are focused onto the lithium beam in transit toward a Pierce extractor. Then, the excited species in the beam propagate via an Einzel lens. Next, the excited isotopes are spatially separated at the magnetic sector before entering Faraday cup 1 (FC1) and Faraday cup 2 (FC2). This diagram is derived from the description provided by Saravia and colleagues. (Olivares, I. E., A. E. Duarte, E. A. Saravia, and F. J. Duarte, Lithium isotope separation with tunable diode lasers, *Appl. Opt.* 41, 2973–2977, 2002.)

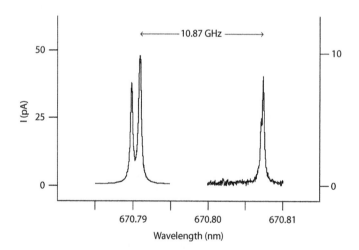

FIGURE 11.7 Composite spectra depicting the D_1 lines of ^{7}Li and ^{6}Li displayed as a function of wavelength. The spectrum of isotope ^{7}Li (left) is recorded at FC1, and the spectrum of ^{6}Li (right) is recorded at FC2. (Reproduced from Olivares, I. E., A. E. Duarte, E. A. Saravia, and F. J. Duarte, Lithium isotope separation with tunable diode lasers, *Appl. Opt.* 41, 2973–2977, 2002. With permission from Optical Society of America.)

into its two isotopic components and collected at their respective Faraday cups (FC1 and FC2) [42].

In Figure 11.7, the D_1 lines due to ^{7}Li and ^{6}Li are displayed as a function of wavelength. The ^{7}Li spectrum is recorded at FC1, and the ^{6}Li spectrum is recorded at FC2.

11.7 HISTORICAL NOTE

A. W. Pryor provides a revealing account of LIS efforts in Australia [49]. In this account, he refers to MLIS, AVLIS, and a secretive approach based on a phase transition transformation of UF_6 known only as the Ward process [49], named after the well-known quantum and particle physicist J. C. Ward. A second corroborative article, focused on AVLIS, was published by Duarte [50], who also describes a contemporaneous, and yet parallel, effort to continue and extend AVLIS development in Australia.

REFERENCES

1. Ambartzumian, R. V., and V. S. Letokhov, Selective two-step (STS) photoionization of atoms and photodissociation of molecules by laser radiation, *Appl. Opt.* 11: 354–358, 1972.
2. Karlov, N. V. and A. M. Prokhorov, Laser isotope separation, *Sov. Phys. Usp.* 19: 285–300, 1976.
3. Basov, N. G., E. M. Belenov, V. A. Isakov, E. P. Markin, A. N. Oraevskii, and V. I. Romanenko, New methods of isotope separation, *Sov. Phys. Usp.* 20: 209–225, 1977.
4. Letokhov, V. S., Laser selective photophysics and photochemistry, *Prog. Optics* 16: 1–69, 1978.
5. Ackerhalt, J. R. and J. H. Eberly, Coherence versus incoherence in stepwise laser excitation of atoms and molecules, *Phys. Rev. A* 14: 1705–1710, 1976.
6. Eberly, J. H. and S.V. O'Neil, Coherence versus incoherence: Time-independent rates for resonant two-photon ionization, *Phys. Rev. A* 19: 1161–1168, 1979.
7. Pease, A. A. and W. M. Pearson, Axial mode structure of a copper vapor pumped dye laser, *Appl. Opt.* 16: 57–60, 1977.
8. Davis, J. I., J. Z. Holtz, and M. L. Spaeth, Status and prospects for lasers in isotope separation, *Laser Focus* 18(9): 49–54, 1982.
9. Emmett, J. L, W. F. Krupke, and J. I. Davis, Laser R & D at the Lawrence Livermore National Laboratory for fusion and isotope separation applications, *IEEE J. Quantum Elect.* QE-20: 591–602, 1984.
10. Eberhardt, J. E., R. B. Knott, and A. W. Pryor, Master equation description of the multiphoton decomposition of ethyl acetate, *Chem. Phys.* 69: 45–59, 1982.
11. Eberhardt, J. E., R. B. Knott, and A. W. Pryor, Multiphoton dissociation of some volatile uranyl complexes. II. Frequency and isotopic effects, *Chem. Phys.*72: 51–59, 1982.
12. Duarte, F. J. and J. A. Piper, Comparison of prism-expander and grazing-incidence grating cavities for copper laser pumped dye lasers, *Appl. Opt.* 21: 2782–2786, 1982.
13. Duarte, F. J. and J. A. Piper, Narrow-linewidth, high prf copper laser-pumped dye laser oscillators, *Appl. Opt.* 23: 1391–1394, 1984.
14. Broyer, M., J. Chevaleyre, G. Delacretaz, and L. Woste, CVL-pumped dye laser for spectroscopic application, *Appl. Phys. B* 35: 31–36, 1984.
15. Singh, S., K. Dasgupta, S. Kumar, K. G. Manohar, L. G. Nair, and U. K. Chatterjee, High-power high-repetition-rate copper-vapor-pumped dye laser, *Opt. Eng.* 33: 1894–1904, 1994.
16. Sugiyama, A., T. Nakayama, M. Kato, Y. Maruyama, and T. Arisawa, Characteristics of a pressure-tuned single-mode dye laser pumped by a copper vapor laser, *Opt. Eng.* 35: 1093–1097, 1996.
17. Radziemski, L. J., R. W. Solarz, and J. A. Paisner (Eds), *Laser Spectroscopy and Its Applications*, Marcel Dekker, New York, 1987.
18. Duarte, F. J. and L. W. Hillman (Eds), *Dye Laser Principles*, Academic, New York, 1990.
19. Duarte, F. J. (Ed.), *High Power Dye Lasers*, Springer, Berlin, 1991.

20. Bokhan, P. A., V. Buchanov, N. V. Fateev, M. M. Kalugin, M. A. Kazaryan, A. M. Prokhorov, and D. E. Zakrevskii, *Laser Isotope Separation in Atomic Vapor*, Wiley-VCH, Weinheim, 2006.

21. Paisner, J. A. and R. W. Solarz, Resonance photoionization spectroscopy. In L. J. Radziemski, R. W. Solarz, and J. A. Paisner (Eds), *Laser Spectroscopy and Its Applications*, Chapter 3, Marcel Dekker, New York, 1987.

22. Dirac, P. A. M., *The Principles of Quantum Mechanics*, 4th edn, Oxford University, Oxford, 1978.

23. Duarte, F. J., *Quantum Optics for Engineers*, CRC Press, New York, 2014.

24. Olivares, I. E., A. E. Duarte, T. Lokajczyk, A. Dinklage, and F. J. Duarte, Doppler-free spectroscopy and collisional studies with tunable diode lasers of lithium isotopes in a heat-pipe oven, *J. Opt. Soc. Am. B* 15: 1932–1939, 1998.

25. Rabinowitz, P., A. Kaldor, A. Gnauck, R. L. Woodin, and J. S. Gethner, Two-color infrared isotopically selective decomposition of UF_6, *Opt. Lett.* 7: 212–214, 1982.

26. Cox, D. M. and J. Elliott, IR spectroscopy of UF_6, *Spectrosc. Lett.* 12: 275–280, 1979.

27. Duarte, F. J., Variable linewidth high-power TEA CO_2 laser, *Appl. Opt.* 24: 34–37, 1985.

28. Duarte, F. J., Multiple-prism Littrow and grazing-incidence pulsed CO_2 lasers, *Appl. Opt.* 24: 1244–1245, 1985.

29. Hargrove, R. S. and T. Kan, High-power efficient dye amplifier pumped by copper vapor lasers, *IEEE J. Quantum Elect.* QE-16: 1108–1113, 1980.

30. Duarte, F. J. and J. A. Piper, A double-prism beam expander for pulsed dye lasers, *Opt. Commun.* 35: 100–104, 1980.

31. Shoshan, I., N. N. Danon, and U. P. Oppenheim, Narrowband operation of a pulsed dye laser without intracavity beam expansion, *J. Appl. Phys.* 48: 4495–4497, 1977.

32. Littman, M. G. and H. J. Metcalf, Spectrally narrow pulsed dye laser without beam expander, *Appl. Opt.* 17: 2224–2227, 1978.

33. Duarte, F. J. and J. A. Piper, Prism preexpanded grazing-incidence grating cavity for pulsed dye lasers, *Appl. Opt.* 20: 2113–2116, 1981.

34. Bernhardt, A. F. and Rasmussen, P., Design criteria and operating characteristics of a single-mode pulsed dye laser, *Appl. Phys. B* 26: 141–146, 1981.

35. Duarte, F. J. and J. A. Piper, Multi-pass dispersion theory of prismatic pulsed dye lasers, *Opt. Acta* 31: 331–335, 1984.

36. Duarte, F. J., Multiple-return-pass beam divergence and the linewidth equation, *Appl. Opt.* 40: 3038–3041, 2001.

37. Duarte, F. J., Narrow-linewidth pulsed dye laser oscillators. In F. J. Duarte and L. W. Hillman (Eds), *Dye Laser Principles*, Chapter 6, Academic, New York, 1990.

38. Duarte, F. J., *Tunable Laser Optics*, 2nd edn, CRC Press, New York, 2015.

39. Duarte, F. J. and J. A. Piper, Dispersion theory of multiple-prism beam expander for pulsed dye lasers, *Opt. Commun.* 43: 303–307, 1982.

40. Bass, I. L., R. E. Bonanno, R. P. Hackel, and P. R. Hammond, High-average-power dye-laser at Lawrence Livermore National Laboratory, *Appl. Opt.* 31: 6993–7006, 1992.

41. Duarte, F. J., Technology of pulsed dye lasers. In F. J. Duarte and L. W. Hillman (Eds), *Dye Laser Principles*, Chapter 6, Academic, New York, 1990.

42. Olivares, I. E., A. E. Duarte, E. A. Saravia, and F. J. Duarte, Lithium isotope separation with tunable diode lasers, *Appl. Opt.* 41: 2973–2977, 2002.

43. Zorabedian, P., Characteristics of grating-external-cavity semiconductor laser containing intracavity prism beam expanders, *J. Lightwave Technol.* 10: 330–335, 1992.

44. Zorabedian, P., Tunable external cavity semiconductor lasers. In F. J. Duarte (Ed.), *Tunable Lasers Handbook*, Chapter 8, Academic, New York, 1995.

45. Akerman, M. A., Dye-laser isotope separation. In F. J. Duarte and L. W. Hillman (Eds), *Dye Laser Principles*, Chapter 9, Academic, New York, 1990.

46. Paisner, J. A., Atomic vapor laser isotope separation, *Appl. Phys. B* 46: 253–260, 1988.
47. Bajaj, P. N., K. G. Manohar, B. M. Suri, K. Dasgupta, R. Talukdar, P. K. Chakraborti, and P. R. K. Rao, Two colour multiphoton ionization spectroscopy of uranium from a metastable state, *Appl. Phys. B* 47: 55–59, 1988.
48. Arizawa, Y., Y. Maruyama, Y. Suzuki, and K. Shiba, Lithium isotope separation by laser, *Appl. Phys. B* 28: 73–76, 1982.
49. Pryor, A. W., Personal memories of two advanced uranium enrichment projects at Lucas Heights in the years 1972–1980, *Aust. N Z Phys.* 33(3–4): 53–58, 1997.
50. Duarte, F. J., Tunable lasers for atomic vapor laser isotope separation: The Australian contribution, *Aust. Phys.* 47(2): 38–40, 2010.

12 Coherent Electrically Excited Organic Semiconductors

F. J. Duarte

CONTENTS

12.1 INTRODUCTION

Since the early days of organic tunable lasers, there has been interest in solid-state tunable organic dye lasers [1,2]. Early interest in the electrical excitation of these molecular species has also been documented in the literature [3,4].

For many years, interest in solid-state tunable organic dye lasers was sporadic, until in the early 1990s, when advances in solid-state organic dye gain media reenergized activity in the field. For a generalized perspective on solid-state organic dye lasers, the reader can consult Chapters 3 and 4.

Despite the enormous success of broadly tunable optically pumped lasers, as evidenced in the various chapters on the subject included in this book, the issue of *direct electrical excitation* for organic gain media continues to evoke interest among scientists and researchers. Indeed, the possibility of direct electrical excitation has been considered in various recent reviews [5–7]. These review papers also describe the work on optically pumped organic semiconductor gain media [8].

In this chapter, a succinct review of recent experiments [9–11] designed to produce coherent emission from direct electrical excitation of organic semiconductors is provided. The relevant background necessary to the discussion is presented in the next few sections. Potential applications are also mentioned.

12.2 AMPLIFIED SPONTANEOUS EMISSION (ASE) IN ORGANIC LASERS

Understanding, controlling, and reducing the level of ASE in high-gain organic lasers has been central to the successful development of narrow-linewidth tunable organic dye lasers [12]. ASE in the context of organic semiconductor lasers has been reviewed in detail by Duarte [13]. Here, the salient aspects of this topic are highlighted.

ASE in high-gain organic lasers is characterized by highly divergent broadband emission. More specifically, the word *broadband* in ASE means emission with a spectral width in the 50–60 nm range [14–17]. *Broadband laser emission* in high-gain organic dye lasers is different from ASE, and is characterized by lower beam divergence and spectral widths in the $4.5 \leq \Delta\lambda \leq 10$ nm range [18–20].

In well-designed, narrow-linewidth tunable organic dye lasers, a great deal of effort is devoted to suppressing the ASE level. Explicitly, in tunable narrow-linewidth flashlamp-pumped multiple-prism grating dye laser oscillators, researchers have measured the total spectrally integrated ASE, in terms of energy spectral density, to be

$$\frac{\rho_{ASE}}{\rho_{laser}} \approx \frac{(\Delta\Lambda)^{-1} \int_{\Lambda_1}^{\Lambda_2} W(\Lambda)d\Lambda}{(\Delta\lambda)^{-1} \int_{\lambda_1}^{\lambda_2} E(\lambda)d\lambda} \approx 10^{-9} \qquad (12.1)$$

for an oscillator yielding a laser linewidth of $\Delta\nu \approx 360$ MHz at $\lambda \approx 590$ nm (or $\Delta\lambda \approx 0.00042$ nm) [21]. In the aforementioned definition, $\Delta\Lambda$ is the total bandwidth of the broadband ASE and $\Delta\lambda$ is the laser linewidth at full width.

This introduction to ASE is given here to articulate explicitly that the differences between broadband lasing and ASE are clearly specified in the published literature [12–21]. More specifically, this brief review of basic ASE characteristics, and their differences from broadband laser emission in high-gain pulsed organic lasers, is necessary, given the ambiguities and confusion evident in some of the published literature.

12.3 TUNABLE NARROW-LINEWIDTH SOLID-STATE ORGANIC LASERS

As discussed in Chapter 4, the availability of highly homogeneous dye-doped polymer gain media [22] led to the demonstration of broadly tunable narrow-linewidth emission in the yellow-red portion of the spectrum [23–27]. One particular optimized tunable solid-state dye laser oscillator yielded single-longitudinal-mode lasing in the $550 \leq \lambda \leq 603$ nm portion of the spectrum with a laser linewidth of $\Delta v \approx 350$ MHz (or $\Delta \lambda \approx 0.0004$ nm at $\lambda \approx 590$ nm) [27]. This emission was provided at ~5% conversion efficiency with extremely low levels of ASE, measured to be $\sim 10^{-6}$. The beam divergence of the single-transverse-mode emission was measured to be ~1.5 times the diffraction limit.

It should be mentioned that while using broadband emission cavity configurations, these dye-doped polymer lasers have been *conservatively* reported to demonstrate conversion efficiencies in the 40%–63% range [22,23,28].

As explained previously [27,29], highly coherent emission from this class of oscillator is determined first of all by the emission of a single-transverse-mode in the spatial domain, a smooth near-Gaussian profile in the temporal domain, and a single-longitudinal-mode in the frequency domain. For the optimized multiple-prism grating solid-state dye laser depicted in Figure 12.1, the near-Gaussian temporal profile of the emission is shown in Figure 12.2, and the Fabry–Perot interferogram recording single-longitudinal-mode emission is shown in Figure 12.3.

As already mentioned in Chapter 4, the measured laser linewidth ($\Delta v \approx 350$ MHz) from this optimized multiple-prism Littrow (MPL) grating laser oscillator appears to be approximately limited by the length of the temporal emission ($\Delta t \approx 3$ ns) according to

$$\Delta v \Delta t \approx 1 \tag{12.2}$$

which, as explained in [29], is a direct consequence of Heisenberg's uncertainty principle [30]:

$$\Delta p \Delta x \approx h \tag{12.3}$$

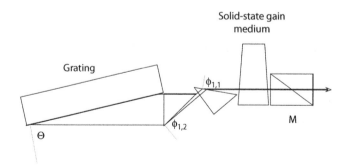

FIGURE 12.1 Optimized multiple-prism grating tunable laser oscillator incorporating an organic dye-doped polymer gain medium. This oscillator is of the MPL grating class, with the added feature of a fully illuminated Littrow grating deployed at a relatively high angle of incidence. The excitation of this laser is accomplished in a longitudinal configuration. (Reproduced from Duarte, F. J., Multiple-prism grating solid-state dye laser oscillator: Optimized architecture, *Appl. Optics* 38, 6347–6349, 1999. With permission of Optical Society of America.)

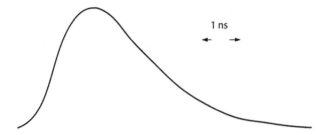

FIGURE 12.2 Smooth near-Gaussian temporal profile of the single-longitudinal-mode emission. Each division corresponds to 1 ns. (Reproduced from Duarte, F. J., Multiple-prism grating solid-state dye laser oscillator: Optimized architecture, *Appl. Optics* 6347–6349, 1999. With permission of Optical Society of America.)

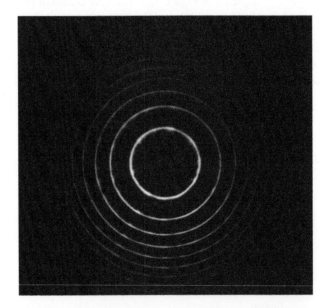

FIGURE 12.3 Silver-halide photograph of a Fabry–Perot interferogram showing single-longitudinal-mode emission at a laser linewidth of $\Delta v \approx 350$ MHz. (Reproduced from Duarte, F. J., Multiple-prism grating solid-state dye laser oscillator: Optimized architecture, *Appl. Optics* 6347–6349, 1999. With permission of Optical Society of America.)

Hence, following [11], a description of the linewidth-narrowing process is provided here.

Multiple-prism grating oscillators benefit from an extraordinarily large intracavity dispersion, which is illustrated by the dispersive linewidth equation [29]:

$$\Delta\lambda \approx \Delta\theta_R \left(MR\nabla_\lambda\Theta_G \right)^{-1} \tag{12.4}$$

where:

    M is the intracavity beam expansion

    R is the number of return cavity passes necessary to achieve laser threshold

    $\nabla_\lambda \Theta_G$ is the dispersion of the grating deployed in either Littrow or near grazing-incidence configuration

The multiple-pass beam divergence is given by [29,31]

$$\Delta\theta_R \approx \frac{\lambda}{\pi w}\left[1+\left(\frac{L_\mathcal{R}}{B_R}\right)^2+\left(\frac{L_\mathcal{R}A_R}{B_R}\right)^2\right]^{1/2} \tag{12.5}$$

where:

    w is the beam waist

    $L_R = (\pi w^2/\lambda)$ is known as the Rayleigh length

    A_R and B_R are the corresponding multiple-return pass propagation matrix elements [29,31]

In an optimized cavity configuration, using a liquid gain medium, it is often possible to reduce the terms in parentheses toward unity, so that

$$\Delta\theta_R \approx \frac{\lambda}{\pi w} \tag{12.6}$$

is achieved, which is the diffraction-limited divergence allowed by Heisenberg's uncertainty principle [29]. For the solid-state gain matrices used in these oscillators, thermal lensing effects limit the reduction in beam divergence to

$$\Delta\theta_R \approx \frac{3}{2}\left(\frac{\lambda}{\pi w}\right) \tag{12.7}$$

In these highly dispersive oscillators, as the ASE photons leave the gain medium, they encounter the entrance of the multiple-prism beam expander, which acts as the entrance to a highly discriminatory frequency filter. Only photons highly resonant with the multiple-prism grating frequency band pass return to the gain medium for further amplification [11].

12.4 SPATIAL AND SPECTRAL COHERENCE

This topic is discussed in detail in [11], and some of the basics are presented here. The link between spatial coherence, that is, low beam divergence, and laser emission is intimately entangled with the history of the laser. In fact, Siegman in his book *Lasers* reminds us of the "beam of heat" [32]. This link is justified, since the first explicit observation of high-intensity emission in low-divergence beams was made by Maiman et al. [33]. More recently, Wolf and Carter [34] have stated: "a source with a high degree of spatial coherence, such as a laser, generates light that is highly directional."

In the spectral domain, the highest form of coherence can be described using the Dirac definition of interference [30] as a single-photon phenomenon. In practice, the experimentalists observe that the sharpest interferograms are generated by sources of indistinguishable photons or narrow-linewidth lasers.

In [11], it was observed that a more accurate description of diffraction-limited beam divergence is given by

$$\Delta\theta \approx \frac{(\lambda \pm \Delta\lambda)}{\pi w} \qquad (12.8)$$

which illustrates how spectral coherence influences spatial coherence. A broadband detector, such as a photographic plate, registers the larger value:

$$\Delta\theta \approx \frac{(\lambda + \Delta\lambda)}{\pi w} \qquad (12.9)$$

For narrow-linewidth, or spectrally coherent, emission, which can exhibit $\Delta\lambda \approx 0.0004$ nm at $\lambda \approx 590$ nm [27], this effect is negligible. However, in the case of broadband radiation, the red end of the spectrum should originate some augmentation of the measurable beam divergence [11]. Thus, in principle, narrow-linewidth emission should be more likely to yield beams with a divergence close to the diffraction limit.

12.5 ELECTRICALLY EXCITED INTERFEROMETRIC EMITTER

Using an electrically excited organic semiconductor comprising a double emitting region, in series, also described as a tandem organic light-emitting diode (OLED), an interferometric emitter was built [9–11]. The active medium in both regions is a coumarin 545 tetramethyl (C 545 T) dye-doped Alq_3 matrix used in the engineering of high-brightness organic semiconductors [35,36]. In addition, the C 545 T dye (see Figure 12.4) was shown to oscillate as an efficient broadly tunable laser [37]. The cavity used in these experiments is shown in Figure 12.5, and the tuning curve for this laser, showing a useful tuning range of $501 \leq \lambda \leq 574$ nm, is shown in Figure 12.6. The emission linewidth of this laser was measured to be $\Delta\lambda \approx 3$ nm (full width half-maximum [FWHM]) at $\lambda \approx 540$ nm [37].

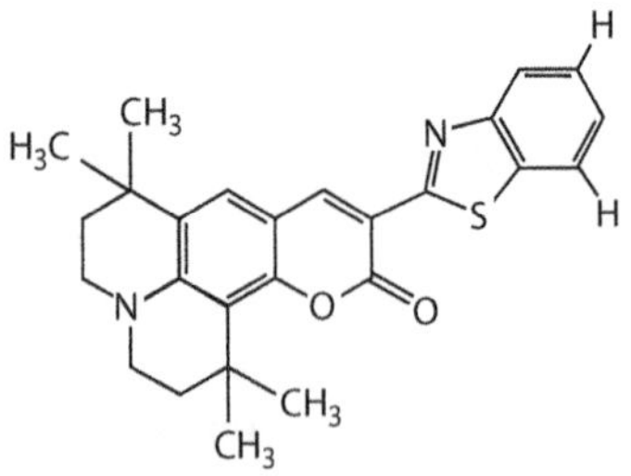

FIGURE 12.4 Molecular structure for the coumarin 545 tetramethyl (C 545 T) dye. (Reproduced from Duarte, F. J., L. S. Liao, K. M. Vaeth, and A. M. Miller, Widely tunable green laser emission using the coumarin 545 tetramethyl dye as the gain medium, *J. Opt. A: Pure Appl. Op.* 8, 172–174, 2008. With permission from the Institute of Physics.)

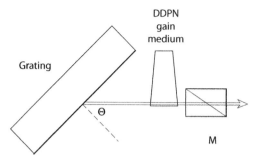

FIGURE 12.5 Transversely excited C 545 T dye laser. The output coupler is a Glan–Thompson polarizer with ~20% reflectivity at its external surface. The tuning element is a 3000 lines/mm diffraction grating deployed in Littrow configuration. The excitation laser is a nitrogen laser emitting at $\lambda \approx 337$ nm. (Reproduced from Duarte, F. J., L. S. Liao, K. M. Vaeth, and A. M. Miller, Widely tunable green laser emission using the coumarin 545 tetramethyl dye as the gain medium, *J. Opt. A: Pure Appl. Op.* 8, 172–174, 2008. With permission from the Institute of Physics.)

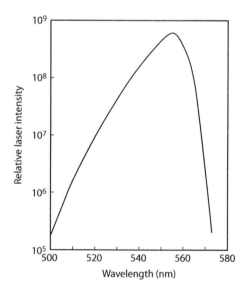

FIGURE 12.6 Laser tuning curve of the C 545 T laser at a concentration of 2 mM in ethanol. (Reproduced from Duarte, F. J., L. S. Liao, K. M. Vaeth, and A. M. Miller, Widely tunable green laser emission using the coumarin 545 tetramethyl dye as the gain medium, *J. Opt. A: Pure Appl. Op.* 8, 172–174, 2008. With permission from the Institute of Physics.)

The tandem dye-doped organic semiconductor was excited in the pulsed domain using nanosecond rise-time pulses up to ~100 V high [9]. The interferometric emitter is shown in Figure 12.7. A cavity, with a length of $l \approx 300$ nm, is configured with a high-reflectivity back mirror ($R_1 \approx 0.9$), which is also the cathode, and an output-coupler mirror ($R_2 \approx 0.08$), which is also the anode. The output-coupler mirror has a layer of indium tin oxide (ITO) and a glass interface. The external surface of

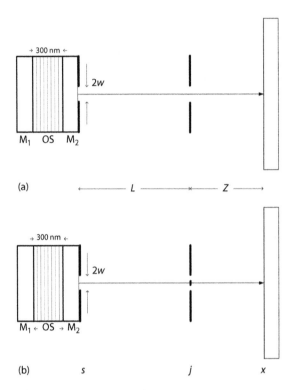

FIGURE 12.7 Schematics of the electrically excited DICOS emitter powered by a submicron cavity with a length of $l \approx 300$ nm. In this integrated device, the backreflector (M_1) is also the cathode, and the output-coupler mirror (M_2) is also the anode. The active region is labeled *organic semiconductor* (OS). (a) In its primary form, the interferometric emitter is comprised of two sequential slits of width $2w$ separated by a distance L. (b) In its analytical version, the secondary slit is replaced by a multiple-slit arrangement ($N=2$, in these experiments) to perform interferometry of the emitted radiation. Detection occurs at position x using either a photographic silver halide film or a digital detector. Drawing not to scale. (Adapted from Duarte, F. J., Coherent electrically excited organic semiconductors: Visibility of interferograms and emission linewidth, *Opt. Lett.* 32, 412–414, 2007. With permission of Optical Society of America.)

the output coupler is antireflection coated with MgF_2 to suppress possible intraglass interference. This integrated interferometric emitter (IIE) can be described as a doubly interferometrically confined organic semiconductor (DICOS) emitter in which the emission medium is a laser dye-doped Alq_3 matrix [9–11]. Here, the terms *interferometric emitter* and *DICOS emitter* are used as synonyms.

Excitation was also performed with the transmission line of a gas laser, which yielded nanosecond pulses at a voltage approaching 10 kV at the semiconductor load [11]. The principle of operation of this interferometric emitter is as follows. The first aperture of width $2w$ induces divergence in the emission radiation. The second aperture, also of width $2w$, and positioned along the optical axis at a distance L from the first aperture, serves as the second spatial discriminator. This double-aperture arrangement ensures that only the emission precisely along the optical axis is allowed transmission by the second aperture. Since both these apertures can be physically represented as an array of a large number of subapertures, they can be considered as interferometric arrays. Subsequently, interferometry of the emission is performed by replacing the second aperture with a double-slit arrangement, also known as a Young-slit configuration [38]. In the present experiment, $2w = 150$ µm, $L \approx 130$ mm, and the width of the slits of the interferometer (Figure 12.7b) is 50 µm separated by 50 µm.

12.6 MEASURED BEAM DIVERGENCE AND INTERFEROGRAMS

The emission beam profile was measured both digitally and using archival black-and-white silver halide film. Digitally, it was verified that the emission beam profile was near Gaussian [9]. A beam profile, at a distance of $z \approx 340$ mm, is shown in Figure 12.8. The beam profile measured while under the excitation of nanosecond pulses at voltages approaching 10 kV was also recorded photographically [11].

Using the experimental arrangement depicted in Figure 12.7b, high-visibility interferograms were recorded, as shown in Figure 12.9 for $z \approx 50$ mm. An interferometric comparison, using the same two-slit interferometer and emission from a beam-expanded He–Ne laser emitting from its $3s_2 - 2p_{10}$ transition at $\lambda \approx 543.3$ nm, is shown in Figure 14.10. A further interferometric comparison, this time with the emission from the C 545 T high-power pulsed dye laser, is shown in Figure 12.11.

The emission was determined to be in the nanowatt regime [9,10], and the measurements caused irreversible damage to the organic semiconductor. Damage was noticed as the emission intensity decreased with each voltage sweep up to 100 V. The experiments at ~10 kV caused visible irreversible damage after a few pulses, as evidenced by the emission of red sparks from the semiconductor. Thus, after many attempts, only a few beam profiles could be recorded, and no interferometry could be performed at this excitation level.

12.7 ENERGETICS

For a discussion on energetic aspects of these experiments, please refer to [9–11]. Some points worth highlighting here include the fact that C 545 T under optical excitation offers tunable laser emission over a range of 60 nm, and its intensity dynamic range spans nearly four orders of magnitude [37] (see Figure 12.6). The quoted laser efficiency in the diffraction grating tuned cavity, under UV laser excitation, is ~14% [37]. This is consistent with previously published laser efficiencies for other coumarin tetramethyl dyes [38]. At this stage, there is no published data that would enable a formal excitation analysis of the emission, as has been done with other better-known laser dyes. Also, the relevant information to perform an analysis under electrical excitation in a semiconductor matrix is not available.

The main issue that will be highlighted here is the observed behavior of the output power as a function of excitation current density, which is associated with an observed change in gradient. This change in gradient as the excitation current density is increased is characterized by a ratio of gradients of $(\eta_2/\eta_1) \approx 2.33$. Comparison

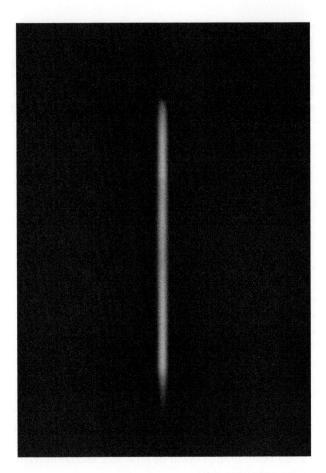

FIGURE 12.8 Beam profile recorded using black-and-white photographic film at a distance of $z \approx 340$ mm. The excitation voltage was ~100 V. The longitudinal profile is perpendicular to the plane of propagation. (Reproduced from Duarte, F. J., L. S. Liao, and K. M. Vaeth, Coherence characteristics of electrically excited tandem organic light-emitting diodes, *Opt. Lett.* 30: 3072–3074, 2005. With permission of Optical Society of America.)

of this ratio with existing laser data indicates that this ratio is at least compatible with soft threshold behavior observed in semiconductor lasers with asymmetrical cavities and some optically excited semiconductor lasers [11].

However, as indicated in [13], the situation becomes far more interesting when it is considered that experiments published on optically pumped liquid dye lasers with a cavity length $l \leq \lambda$ indicate that a near "zero-threshold-laser" emission is observed for $l \approx \lambda/2$ [39]. The relevant fact here is that De Martini et al. [39] did observe a near "zero-threshold-laser" emission under multiple-transverse-mode conditions. These experiments provide very persuasive evidence in support of threshold behavior at very low excitation densities. In other words, the experiments reported in [39] strongly suggest that with a suitable gain medium and microcavity configurations, high threshold energy densities are not required. In other words, low threshold

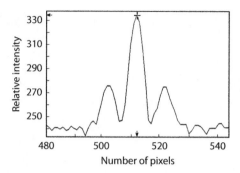

FIGURE 12.9 Interferogram of the emission from the DICOS emitter, at $\lambda \approx 540$ nm, for $z \approx 50$ mm. (Reproduced from Duarte, F. J., L. S. Liao, and K. M. Vaeth, Coherence characteristics of electrically excited tandem organic light-emitting diodes, *Opt. Lett.* 30: 3072–3074, 2005. With permission of Optical Society of America.)

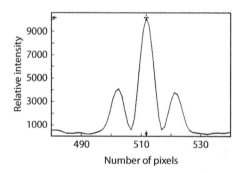

FIGURE 12.10 Interferogram using the identical interferometer of radiation from a He–Ne laser, at $\lambda \approx 543.3$ nm, for $z \approx 50$ mm. (Reproduced from Duarte, F. J., L. S. Liao, and K. M. Vaeth, Coherence characteristics of electrically excited tandem organic light-emitting diodes, *Opt Lett.* 30: 3072–3074, 2005. With permission of Optical Society of America.)

behavior at $0.8 \leq \rho \leq 0.9$ A/cm^2 [9,10] is consistent with what would be expected in a submicrometer cavity where the condition $l \leq \lambda$ applies [13].

An additional point of interest is that the excitation experiments at high-pulsed voltages indicate that it only takes a few excitation pulses in the nanosecond regime to obliterate the organic semiconductor at ~10 kV. It is estimated that this excitation took place at current densities of $\rho \approx 190$ A/cm^2 [11].

12.8 PHYSICAL INTERPRETATION OF THE MEASUREMENTS

The pulsed electrically pumped organic semiconductor integrated device illustrated in Figure 12.7 emits in a low-divergence directional beam, and its spectral emission is characterized by high-visibility interferograms. In this section, these characteristics are analyzed further.

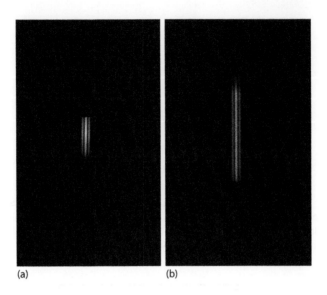

(a)   (b)

FIGURE 12.11 Interferometric comparison of the emission from the high-power C 545 T dye laser (a) and the emission from the DICOS emitter (b). Both measurements were performed at $z \approx 50$ mm. The recording medium was black-and-white silver halide film. (Reproduced from Duarte, F. J., L. S. Liao, and K. M. Vaeth, Coherence characteristics of electrically excited tandem organic light-emitting diodes, *Opt. Lett.* 30: 3072–3074, 2005. With permission of Optical Society of America.)

12.8.1 BEAM DIVERGENCE

As seen previously, the beam divergence is given by

$$\Delta\theta_R \approx \frac{\lambda}{\pi w}\left(1+\left(\frac{L_R}{B_R}\right)^2+\left(\frac{L_R A_R}{B_R}\right)^2\right)^{1/2}$$

where $L_R = (\pi w^2/\lambda)$. For a simple mirror–mirror microcavity, assuming a single-return pass $(R=1)$, and in the absence of intracavity beam expansion, $A \approx 1$ and $B \approx 2l$, so that [13]

$$\Delta\theta \approx \frac{\lambda}{\pi w}\left(1+2\left(\frac{L_R}{2l}\right)^2\right)^{1/2} \qquad (12.10)$$

In a microcavity, the condition $l \leq \lambda$ applies. Assuming just $l \approx \lambda$,

$$\Delta\theta \approx \frac{\lambda}{\pi w}\left(1+2\left(\frac{\pi w^2}{2\lambda^2}\right)^2\right)^{1/2} \qquad (12.11)$$

and assuming $l \approx (\lambda/2)$,

$$\Delta\theta \approx \frac{\lambda}{\pi w}\left(1+2\left(\frac{\pi w^2}{\lambda^2}\right)^2\right)^{1/2} \tag{12.12}$$

In either case,

$$\Delta\theta \gg \frac{\lambda}{\pi w} \tag{12.13}$$

Now, for an integrated device such as the interferometric emitter depicted in Figure 12.7, l is replaced by L, $l \approx 300$ nm, $L \approx 130$ mm, so that $L \gg l$. Under those circumstances, for $A \approx 1$ and $B \approx 2L$:

$$\Delta\theta \approx \frac{\lambda}{\pi w}\left(1+2\left(\frac{L_R}{2L}\right)^2\right)^{1/2} \tag{12.14}$$

For $2w \approx 150$ μm, $L_R \approx 32.43$ mm, and $L \approx 130$ mm, this equation reduces to

$$\Delta\theta \approx 1.015\frac{\lambda}{\pi w} \tag{12.15}$$

Experimentally, the divergence of the beam shown in Figure 12.8 was measured to be $\Delta\theta = 2.53 \pm 0.13$ mrad, which, for $2w \approx 150$ μm, is ~1.09 times the diffraction limit, or $\Delta\theta_R \approx 1.1 \times (\lambda/\pi w)$. Thus, considering the experimental error, the single-return pass beam divergence is close to the measured multiple-return pass beam divergence, or $\Delta\theta \approx \Delta\theta_R$. This implies that spatial coherence is reached within $R \approx 1$, which is compatible with a near "zero-threshold-laser" hypothesis advanced for microcavity laser emission [39].

Also, the near-Gaussian profile of this beam [9] allows us to conclude that the emission is equivalent to what we know in laser development as *single transverse mode*. This means that the on-axis emission from the electrically pumped organic semiconductor interferometric emitter has a high degree of spatial coherence.

12.8.2 INTERFEROMETRIC LINEWIDTH ESTIMATE

Using the visibility definition introduced by Michelson [40]:

$$\mathcal{V} = \frac{I_1 - I_2}{I_1 + I_2} \tag{12.16}$$

it can be estimated that for the DICOS emitter, $\mathcal{V} = 0.901 \pm 0.088$, while the visibility for the He–Ne laser emitting at $\lambda \approx 543.3$ nm is $\mathcal{V} = 0.952 \pm 0.031$ [10].

Results in the published literature indicate that the visibility measurements for partially coherent emission, ASE, and emission from organic semiconductors are in the range of $0.40 \leq V \leq 0.65$, corresponding to emission linewidths in the $17 \leq \Delta\lambda \leq 100$ nm range [41–43]. In this set of results, the narrower linewidth corresponds to the ASE from a laser dye exhibiting a visibility of $V \approx 0.65$ [42]. These results indicate that the visibility of the interferograms recorded with the radiation from the DICOS emitter is higher than the visibility associated with ASE sources and approaches the visibility values associated with laser emission, as is evident by comparing the interferograms shown in Figures 12.9 and 12.10 and by observing the interferograms displayed in Figure 12.11.

Strong evidence of highly spatially coherent emission plus interferograms showing high visibility might be sufficient to draw some conclusions on the nature of the emission being observed. More specifically, this emission is narrower than ASE (see Section 12.2). Thus, the question confronted in [10] was how to use the available interferometric data and extract information about the *linewidth* of the emission. Given the low-intensity nature of the emission, the possible use of conventional methods to perform this measurement had to be abandoned [11].

To elucidate this issue, it must be realized that the generalized interferometric equation [29,44]:

$$\left| \langle x | s \rangle \right|^2 = \sum_{j=1}^{N} \Psi(r_j)^2 + 2 \sum_{j=1}^{N} \Psi(r_j) \left(\sum_{m=j+1}^{N} \Psi(r_m) \cos(\Omega_m - \Omega_j) \right) \quad (12.17)$$

can be used, in conjunction with measured interferograms, to determine the wavelength of the emission under observation [29]. That is because, as explained in Chapter 10, the interferometric term (in parentheses) in Equation 12.17 depends on the exact geometry of the interferometer and the wavelength of the emission under observation. Thus, if the emission of different laser wavelengths is observed, under identical geometrical conditions, in an N-slit interferometer, the interferograms thus recorded will be uniquely a function of emission wavelength [29]. It follows that if this interferometric method can yield information about the wavelength λ, it should also yield information about the linewidth of the emission $\Delta\lambda$.

For completeness, it should be mentioned that, in Equation 12.17, $\Psi(r_j)$ are wave functions of "ordinary wave optics" [30], and the j index refers to the jth slit of the N-slit interferometer. Also, the application of quantum techniques [30,45] to a situation related to populations of indistinguishable photons is compatible with the approach of van Kampen to quantum mechanics [46].

Experimentally, it is observed that narrow-linewidth lasers yield sharp, well-defined N-slit interferograms, while broadband sources yield broad, less-defined interferograms [9,29]. This observation can be explained following the Dirac description of interference, as a single-photon phenomenon, or as a phenomenon that takes place between indistinguishable photons.

Thus, the sharpest and purest interferogram is provided by a single photon whose probability amplitudes, within the N-slit interferometer, are handled according to the mechanics described by Equation 12.17. As described in [10,11], interference for broadband emission takes place in the same manner, but now a multitude of interferograms are integrated at the detector, which is either a silver halide photographic plate or a digital detector. Both methods of detection provide an integrated view of the interferometric event [10,11,47].

This description of interference is compatible with the link between sharp, well-defined interferograms with narrow-linewidth laser emission and the emission of populations of indistinguishable photons. It also allows the link between broad, less-defined interferograms and the emission of broadband radiation. Thus, for radiation at the same wavelength and observation at the same N-slit interferometer, it is possible to use narrow-linewidth laser emission as a reference to estimate the bandwidth of broader emission.

The approximate spatial-graphical technique for estimating $\Delta\lambda$ has been covered in [10,11], and it is described briefly here. First, either the full width, or half-width, of the interferogram under examination is defined. Once this definition is done, then the width of the narrow reference interferogram (W_r) and the width of the broader interferogram (W_m) are measured. Then, the broadening factor Δb can be defined as

$$\Delta b = \frac{W_m - W_r}{W_r} \tag{12.18}$$

Using this definition, the broadening factor of the interferogram of the DICOS emitter (Figure 12.10), relative to the interferogram generated with the $3s_2 - 2p_{10}$ transition of the He–Ne laser (Figure 12.10), was determined to be $\Delta b \approx 0.04$.

The second part of the method consists in generating a calculated interferogram at the reference wavelength, followed by a series of calculations at various wavelength increments above and below the reference wavelength. This approximate technique then uses graphical methods to relate the broadening factor Δb to $\Delta\lambda$. As reported in [10,11], for the case at hand, the linewidth related to $\Delta b \approx 0.04$ was $\Delta\lambda \approx 11$ nm.

Certainly, the accuracy of this graphical approach is limited, and it would be useful to extend the scope of the theory to provide equations that would make this task faster and improve accuracy.

Going back to Section 12.2, it can be concluded that a linewidth of $\Delta\lambda \approx 11$ nm is narrower than should be expected for ASE generated by organic gain media, and it is compatible with broadband dye laser emission. Thus, the conclusion is that on-axis emission from the electrically pumped organic semiconductor interferometric emitter shows a linewidth compatible with the linewidth observed from broadband dye lasers.

12.9 COHERENT EMISSION AND LASER EMISSION

Following the previous exposition, the set of variables related to the radiation from the interferometric emitter, or DICOS emitter, are

$$\Delta\theta_R \approx 1.1\left(\frac{\lambda}{\pi w}\right)$$

$$\mathcal{V} \approx 0.9$$

$$\Delta\lambda \approx 11 \text{ nm}$$

All these parameters reaffirm the coherent nature of the emission.

12.9.1 INTERFEROMETRIC VISIBILITY OF THE INTERFEROMETRIC EMITTER

At this stage, it is important to reiterate that visibility measurements for partially coherent emission, ASE, and emission from organic semiconductors is in the range of $0.40 \leq \mathcal{V} \leq 0.65$, corresponding to emission linewidths in the $17 \leq \Delta\lambda \leq 100$ nm range [41–43]. The narrower linewidth corresponds to the ASE from a laser dye exhibiting a visibility of $\mathcal{V} \approx 0.65$ [42]. Furthermore, Newton's ring interferometry has been used on standard C 545 T dye-doped OLED devices yielding measured linewidths in the $40 \leq \Delta\lambda \leq 110$ nm range, with the authors attributing the narrower linewidth ($\Delta\lambda \approx 40$ nm) to "microcavity effects" [48]. In addition, it is well known that true ASE in dye lasers is characterized by bandwidths in the $50 \leq \Delta\lambda \leq 60$ nm range [14–15].

In the light of previous data [14–15,41–43,48], it is reasonable to deduce that emission characterized with a measured visibility of $\mathcal{V} \approx 0.9$ for the interferometric emitter, which is related to a linewidth of $\Delta\lambda \approx 11$ nm, exhibits significantly higher coherence than ASE.

12.9.2 INTERFEROMETRIC VISIBILITY AND LASER EMISSION

The use of double-slit interference techniques to characterize the coherence of laser emission is a standard and accepted practice, well documented in the laser literature since the dawn of the laser age [49], and in particular in the x-ray laser literature [50–53]. In this regard, laser emission is associated with visibilities in the approximate $0.85 \leq \mathcal{V} \leq 1.00$ range [51,53].

In the experiments considered here, a visibility of $\mathcal{V} \approx 0.95$ was measured using the He–Ne laser transition $3s_2 - 2p_{10}$, with a laser linewidth of $\Delta v \approx 1$ GHz at $\lambda \approx 543.3$ nm, in the interferometric configuration depicted in Figure 12.7b [9–11]. Using an identical interferometric configuration, with the pulsed electrically excited organic semiconductor as source, the measured interferometric visibility is $\mathcal{V} \approx 0.9$ [9–11]. This visibility is perfectly within the $0.85 \leq \mathcal{V} \leq 1.00$ range accepted as *laser-class visibility* [51,53].

From the experimental results presented in Figure 12.11, it is evident that the interferogram produced with radiation from the DICOS emitter is almost identical to the interferogram recorded, in the same interferometer, with radiation from the high-power C 545 T dye laser tuned at $\lambda \approx 540$ nm. In other words, the interferogram produced with radiation from the electrically excited organic interferometric emitter, doped with C 545 T, is nearly indistinguishable, in its spatial features, from the interferogram recorded with radiation from the high-power C 545 T dye laser.

Independently of the literature information presented thus far, the interferometric analysis described in Section 12.7 indicates that the emission linewidth of the

DICOS emitter is $\Delta\lambda \approx 11$ nm [10,11], which is comparable to the linewidth reported for a broadband dye laser by Schäfer et al. [18]. Albeit at first glance this linewidth is comparable with multimode broadband laser emission [18], a more careful analysis using

$$\delta\lambda \approx \frac{\lambda^2}{2l}$$

(12.19)

reveals that the longitudinal mode separation, also known as the free spectral range of the microcavity, is $\delta\lambda \approx 486$ nm, which implies that emission at a linewidth of $\Delta\lambda \approx 11$ nm corresponds to single-longitudinal-mode emission [11,13]. This observation helps to explain how the interferometric emitter might work as an integrated device: in reference to Figure 14.7, the apertures positioned at s and j provide a high-selectivity spatial filter that allows passage of emission along the optical axis only. It is this on-axis emission that is both spatially and spectrally coherent.

12.10 CONCLUSION

The results presented here indicate that this electrically powered pulsed organic interferometric emitter yields a nearly diffraction-limited beam, with a Gaussian profile, compatible with single-transverse-mode emission and low beam divergence, with $\Delta\theta_R \approx 1.1 \times (\lambda/\pi w)$. Also, given the extremely short length of the active region ($l \approx 300$ nm), the emission linewidth of $\Delta\lambda \approx 11$ nm is compatible with single-longitudinal-mode emission. Furthermore, the high visibility of the measured interferogram $\mathcal{V} \approx 0.9$ is within the range of the visibility of interferograms, $0.85 \leq \mathcal{V} \leq 1.00$, associated with laser emission [51,53].

Albeit no mirror-alignment dependence of the emission has been demonstrated, thus leading to no claim of traditional laser emission [9–11], the evidence for spatially and spectrally coherent emission is overwhelming. In other words, an integrated interferometric emitter powered by a pulsed electrically pumped organic semiconductor has been shown to emit coherent emission. Avenues to miniaturize this integrated coherent emitter have been discussed previously [11].

In summary, the interpretation of Duarte et al. [9] and Duarte [10,11] that the emission observed from the electrically excited doubly interferometrically confined organic semiconductor emitter is, coherently speaking, *indistinguishable from broadband dye laser emission* [13] is reiterated.

Electrically driven miniature tunable coherent integrated organic semiconductor devices yielding spatially well-defined low-divergence emission beams could find a number of applications in spectroscopy, interferometry, medicine, and still other unimagined uses.

REFERENCES

1. Soffer, B. H., and B. B. McFarland, Continuously tunable narrow-band organic dye lasers, *Appl. Phys. Lett.* 10: 266–267, 1967.
2. Peterson, O. G. and B. B. Snavely, Stimulated emission from flashlamp-excited organic dyes in polymethyl methacrylate, *Appl. Phys. Lett.* 12: 238–240, 1968.

3. Steyer, B. and F. P. Schäfer, A vapor phase dye laser, *Opt. Commun.* 10: 219–220, 1974.

4. Marowsky, G., F. P. Schäfer, J. W. Keto, and F. K. Tittel, Fluorescence studies of electron beam pumped POPOP dye vapor, *Appl. Phys.* 9: 143–146, 1976.

5. Kranzelbinder, G. and G. Leising, Organic solid-state lasers, *Rep. Prog. Phys.* 63: 729–762, 2000.

6. Baldo, M. A., R. J. Holmes, and S. R. Forrest, Prospects for electrically pumped organic lasers, *Phys. Rev. B* 66: 035321, 2002.

7. Samuel, I. D. W. and G. A. Turnbull, Organic semiconductor lasers, *Chem. Rev.* 107: 1272–1295, 2007.

8. Holzer, W., A. Penzkofer, T. Pertsch, N. Danz, A. Abräuer, E. B. Kley, H. Tillmann, et al., Corrugated neat thin-film conjugated polymer distributed-feedback lasers, *Appl. Phys. B* 74, 333–342, 2002.

9. Duarte, F. J., L. S. Liao, and K. M. Vaeth, Coherence characteristics of electrically excited tandem organic light-emitting diodes, *Opt. Lett.* 30: 3072–3074, 2005.

10. Duarte, F. J., Coherent electrically excited organic semiconductors: Visibility of interferograms and emission linewidth, *Opt. Lett.* 32: 412–414, 2007.

11. Duarte, F. J., Coherent electrically-excited organic semiconductors: Coherent or laser emission? *Appl. Phys. B* 90: 101–108, 2008.

12. Duarte, F. J., Narrow-linewidth pulsed dye laser oscillators. In F. J. Duarte (Ed.), *Dye Laser Principles*, Chapter 4, Academic, New York, 1990.

13. Duarte, F. J., Electrically-pumped organic semiconductor coherent emission: A review. In F. J. Duarte (Ed.), *Coherence and Ultrashort Pulsed Laser Emission*, Chapter 1, InTech, Rijeka, 2010.

14. Dujardin, G. and P. Flamant, Amplified spontaneous emission and spatial dependence of gain in dye amplifiers, *Opt. Commun.* 24: 243–247, 1978.

15. Duarte, F. J. and J. A. Piper, A double-prism beam expander for pulsed dye lasers, *Opt. Commun.* 35: 100–104, 1980.

16. Bor, Z. (1981). Amplified spontaneous emission from N_2 laser pumped dye lasers, *Opt. Commun.* 39: 383–386, 1981.

17. McKee, T. J., J. Lobin, and W. A. Young, Dye laser spectral purity, *Appl. Opt.* 21: 725–728, 1982.

18. Schäfer, F. P., W. Schmidt, and J. Volze, Organic dye solution laser, *Appl. Phys. Lett.* 9: 306–309, 1966.

19. Spaeth, M. L. and D. P. Bortfeld, Stimulated emission from polymetine dyes, *Appl. Phys. Lett.* 9: 179–181, 1966.

20. Baltakov, F. N., B. A. Barikhin, V. G. Kornilov, S. A. Mikhnov, A. N. Rubinov, and L. V. Sukhanov, 110-J pulsed laser using a solution of rhodamine 6G in ethyl alcohol, *Sov. Phys. Tech. Phys.* 17: 1161–1163, 1973.

21. Duarte, F. J., J. J. Ehrlich, W. E. Davenport, and T. S. Taylor, Flashlamp pumped narrow-linewidth dispersive dye laser oscillators: Very low amplified spontaneous emission levels and reduction of linewidth instabilities, *Appl. Opt.* 29: 3176–3179, 1990.

22. Maslyukov, A., S. Solokov, M. Kaivola, K. Nyholm, and S. Popov, Solid-state dye laser with modified poly(methyl methacrylate)-doped active elements, *Appl. Opt.* 34: 1516–1518, 1995.

23. Duarte, F. J., Solid-state multiple-prism grating dye-laser oscillators, *Appl. Opt.* 33: 3857–3860, 1994.

24. Duarte, F. J., Solid-state dispersive dye laser oscillator: Very compact cavity, *Opt. Commun.* 117: 480–484, 1995.

25. Duarte, F. J., Multiple-prism near-grazing-incidence grating solid-state dye laser oscillator, *Opt. Laser Technol.* 29: 513–516, 1997.

26. Duarte, F. J., T. S. Taylor, A. Costela, I. García-Moreno, and R. Sastre, Long-pulse narrow-linewidth dispersive solid-state dye laser oscillator, *Appl. Opt.* 37: 3987–3989, 1998.

27. Duarte, F. J., Multiple-prism grating solid-state dye laser oscillator: Optimized architecture, *Appl. Opt.* 38: 6347–6349, 1999.

28. Duarte, F. J. and R. O. James, Tunable solid-state lasers incorporating dye-doped polymer-nanoparticle gain media, *Opt. Lett.* 28: 2088–2090, 2003.

29. Duarte, F. J., *Tunable Laser Optics*, Elsevier Academic, New York, 2003.

30. Dirac, P. A. M., *The Principles of Quantum Mechanics*, 4th edn, Oxford, London, 1978.

31. Duarte, F. J., Multiple-return-pass beam divergence and the linewidth equation, *Appl. Opt.* 40: 3038–3041, 2001.

32. Siegman, A. E., *Lasers*, Chapter 1, University Science, Mill Valley, 1986.

33. Maiman, T. H., R. H. Hoskins, I. J. D'Haenens, C. K. Asawa, and V. Evtuhov, Stimulated optical emission in fluorescent solids II: Spectroscopy and stimulated emission in ruby, *Phys. Rev.* 123: 1151–1157, 1961.

34. Wolf, E. and W. H. Carter, Angular distribution of radiant intensity from sources of different degrees of spatial coherence, *Opt. Commun.* 13: 205–209, 1975.

35. Liao, L. S., K. P. Klubek, and C. W. Tang, High-efficiency tandem organic light-emitting diodes, *Appl. Phys. Lett.* 84: 167–169, 2004.

36. Chang, C-C., S. W. Hwang, C. H. Chen, and J-F. Chen, High-efficiency organic electroluminescent device with multiple-emitting units, *Jpn. J. Appl. Phys.* 43: 6418–6422, 2004.

37. Duarte, F. J., L. S. Liao, K. M. Vaeth, and A. M. Miller, Widely tunable green laser emission using the coumarin 545 tetramethyl dye as the gain medium, *J. Opt. A: Pure Appl. Op.* 8: 172–174, 2008.

38. Chen, C. H., J. L. Fox, F. J. Duarte, and J. J. Ehrlich, Lasing characteristics of new coumarin-analog dyes: Broadband and narrow-linewidth performance, *Appl. Opt.* 27: 443–445, 1988.

39. De Martini, F. and J. R. Jakobovitz, Anomalous spontaneous-emission-decay phase transition and zero-threshold laser action in a microscopic cavity, *Phys. Rev. Lett.* 60: 1711–1714, 1988.

40. Michelson, A. A., *Studies in Optics*, The University of Chicago, Chicago, 1927.

41. Thompson, B. J. and E. Wolf, Two beam interference with partially coherent light, *J. Opt. Soc. Am.* 47: 895–902, 1957.

42. Saxena, K., D. S. Mehta, R. Srivastava, and M. N. Kamalasanan, Spatial coherence properties of electroluminescence from Alq_3-based organic light emitting diodes, *Appl. Phys. Lett.* 89: 061124, 2006.

43. Dharmadhikari, J. A., A. K. Dharmadhikari, and G. R. Kumar, High-contrast interference pattern of amplified spontaneous emission from dyes under transient grating excitation, *Opt. Lett.* 30: 765–767, 2005.

44. Duarte, F. J., On a generalized interference equation and interferometric measurements, *Opt. Commun.* 103: 8–14, 1993.

45. Feynman, R. P., R. B. Leighton, and M. Sands, *The Feynman Lectures on Physics*, Volume III, Addison-Wesley, Reading, 1965.

46. van Kampen, N. G., Ten theorems about quantum mechanical measurement, *Physica A* 153: 97–113, 1988.

47. Duarte, F. J., Comment on "Reflection, refraction, and multislit interference", *Eur. J. Phys.* 25: L57–L58, 2004.

48. Tsai, C-H., K-C. Tien, M-C. Chen, K-M. Chang, M-S. Lin, H-C. Cheng, Y-H. Lin, et al. Characterizing coherence lengths of organic light-emitting devices using Newton's rings apparatus, *Org. Electron.* 11: 439–444, 2009.

49. Nelson, D. F. and R. J. Collins, Spatial coherence in the output of an optical maser, *J. Appl. Phys.* 32: 739–740, 1961.
50. Shimkaveg, G. M., M. R. Carter, R. S. Walling, J. M. Ticehurst, J. A. Koch, S. Mrowka, J. E. Trebes, et al. X-ray laser coherence experiments in neon-like yttrium. In F. J. Duarte and D. G. Harris (Eds), *Proceedings of The International Conference on Lasers'91*, pp. 84–92, STS, Mc Lean, VA, 1992.
51. Trebes, J. E., K. A. Nugent, S. Mrowka, R. A. London, T. W. Barbee, M. R. Carter, J. A. Koch, et al. Measurements of spatial coherence of a soft x-ray laser, *Phys. Rev. Lett.* 68: 588–591, 1992.
52. Ditmire, T., E. T. Gumbrell, R. A. Smith, J. W. G. Tisch, D. D. Meyerhofer, and M. H. R. Hutchison, Spatial coherence measurements of soft x-ray radiation produced by high-order harmonic generation, *Phys. Rev. Lett.* 77: 4756–4759, 1996.
53. Lucianetti, A., K. A. Janulewicz, R. Kroemer, G. Priebe, J. Tümmler, W. Sandner, P. V. Nickless, et al., Transverse spatial coherence of a transient nickellike silver soft-x-ray laser pumped by a single picosecond laser pulse, *Opt. Lett.* 29: 881–883, 2004.

13 Multiple-Prism Arrays and Multiple-Prism Beam Expanders
Laser Optics and Scientific Applications

F. J. Duarte

CONTENTS

13.1 INTRODUCTION

Multiple-prism arrays were introduced by Newton in his book entitled *Opticks* in 1704 [1]. In addition to the introduction of the reflection telescope and a detailed qualitative description of multiple-prism arrays, the use of the prism as a beam expander was also suggested in that prophetic book [2]. A subsequent significant contribution was made by Brewster, who introduced prism pairs as beam expanders in 1813 [3].

13.2 DISPERSION THEORY OF MULTIPLE-PRISM ARRAYS

Multiple-prism wavelength tuners were introduced by Strome and Webb [4] in 1971. The introduction of a prism as an intracavity beam-expansion element in tunable lasers by Hanna et al. [5] was followed by the introduction of multiple-prism beam expanders to achieve efficient illumination of the diffraction grating in narrow-linewidth tunable laser oscillators [6–8]. Prismatic and multiple-prism intracavity beam expansion in oscillators using near grazing-incidence grating configurations was demonstrated shortly thereafter [9–11]. Comprehensive reviews on this subject are given in [12,13].

The emission linewidth in a pulsed tunable laser oscillator is given by [4,12–16]

$$\Delta\lambda \approx \Delta\theta\left(\nabla_\lambda\Theta\right)^{-1} \tag{13.1}$$

where

$$\nabla_\lambda\Theta = \frac{\partial\Theta}{\partial\lambda} \tag{13.2}$$

is the overall intracavity dispersion (see Chapter 4 for further details). This cavity linewidth equation was originally introduced from a classical perspective [4,15] and was subsequently shown to be compatible with interferometric principles derived using Dirac's notation [13,16].

Soon after the introduction of intracavity multiple-prism beam expanders, it became necessary to develop a generalized multiple-prism dispersion theory. That was provided in 1982 by Duarte and Piper [17,18]. For a generalized array of m prisms, as depicted in Figure 13.1, the cumulative dispersion at the mth prism is given by [17,18]

$$\nabla_\lambda\phi_{2,m} = \mathcal{H}_{2,m}\nabla_\lambda n_m + \left(k_{1,m}k_{2,m}\right)^{-1}\left(\mathcal{H}_{1,m}\nabla_\lambda n_m \pm \nabla_\lambda\phi_{2,(m-1)}\right) \tag{13.3}$$

where

$$\mathcal{H}_{1,m} = \frac{\tan\phi_{1,m}}{n_m} \tag{13.4}$$

$$\mathcal{H}_{2,m} = \frac{\tan\phi_{2,m}}{n_m} \tag{13.5}$$

are geometrical coefficients while

$$k_{1,m} = \frac{\cos\psi_{1,m}}{\cos\phi_{1,m}} \tag{13.6}$$

is the beam expansion experienced by the beam at the incidence surface of the mth prism and

$$k_{2,m} = \frac{\cos\phi_{2,m}}{\cos\psi_{2,m}} \tag{13.7}$$

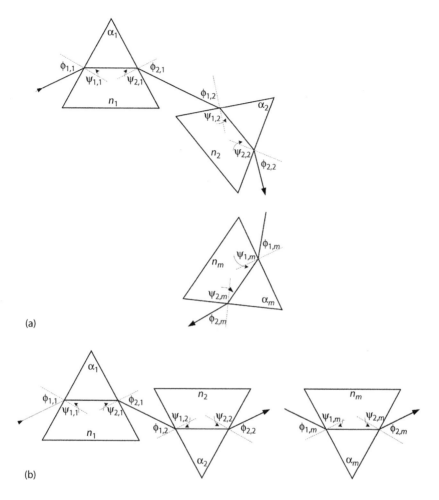

(a)

(b)

FIGURE 13.1 Generalized multiple-prism array deployed in (a) an additive configuration and (b) a compensating configuration. (Adapted with permission from Duarte, F. J. and J. A. Piper, Generalized prism dispersion theory, *Am. J. Phys.* 51: 1132–1134, 1983. Copyright 1983, American Association of Physics Teachers.)

is the corresponding term at the exit surface of the mth prism, where $\phi_{1,m}$ and $\phi_{2,m}$ are the incidence and exit angles, respectively, at each individual prism, while $\psi_{1,m}$ and $\psi_{2,m}$ are the corresponding angles of refraction as determined by Snell's law. In Equation 13.3, the term $\nabla\lambda\phi_{2,(m-1)}$ refers to the cumulative dispersion up to the $(m-1)$ prism. Equations for the generalized double-pass dispersion are given in [12,13,17,18]. In [12,13], these double-pass equations are also expressed in explicit notation directly applicable to designs and calculations. Using explicit notation, Equation 13.3 can be expressed as [12–14]

$$\nabla_\lambda \phi_{2,r} = \sum_{m=1}^{r} (\pm 1) \mathcal{H}_{1,m} \left(\prod_{j=m}^{r} k_{1,j} \prod_{j=m}^{r} k_{2,j} \right)^{-1} \nabla_\lambda n_m$$

$$+ (M_1 M_2)^{-1} \sum_{m=1}^{r} (\pm 1) \mathcal{H}_{2,m} \left(\prod_{j=1}^{m} k_{1,j} \prod_{j=1}^{m} k_{2,j} \right) \nabla_\lambda n_m \qquad (13.8)$$

where

$$M_1 = \prod_{j=1}^{r} k_{1,j} \qquad (13.9)$$

$$M_2 = \prod_{j=1}^{r} k_{2,j} \qquad (13.10)$$

For the important practical case of an array of r right-angle prisms designed for orthogonal beam exit (i.e., $\phi_{2,m} = \psi_{2,m} = 0$), Equation 13.8 reduces to [13]

$$\nabla_\lambda \phi_{2,r} = \sum_{m=1}^{r} (\pm 1) \mathcal{H}_{1,m} \left(\prod_{j=m}^{r} k_{1,j} \right)^{-1} \nabla_\lambda n_m \qquad (13.11)$$

Furthermore, if the prisms in the array have an identical apex angle $(\alpha_1 = \alpha_2 = \alpha_3 = \cdots = \alpha_m)$ and are configured to have the same angle of incidence $(\phi_{1,1} = \phi_{1,2} = \phi_{1,3} = \cdots = \phi_{1,m})$, then Equation 13.11 reduces to [12–14]

$$\nabla_\lambda \phi_{2,r} = \tan \psi_{1,1} \sum_{m=1}^{r} (\pm 1) \left(\frac{1}{k_{1,m}} \right)^{m-1} \nabla_\lambda n_m \qquad (13.12)$$

This class of multiple-prism beam expander, for $r = 3$, is illustrated in Figure 13.2 for additive and compensating dispersion configurations.

For an array of r right-angle prisms, with identical apex angle $(\alpha_1 = \alpha_2 = \cdots = \alpha_m)$, deployed at the Brewster angle of incidence and designed for orthogonal beam exit, Equation 15.8 assumes the rather elegant form of [12,13]

$$\nabla_\lambda \phi_{2,r} = \sum_{m=1}^{r} (\pm 1) \left(\frac{1}{n_m} \right)^{m} \nabla_\lambda n_m \qquad (13.13)$$

In this power series, n_m is the refractive index of the mth prism. Under these special circumstances, the overall beam expansion is given by [12]

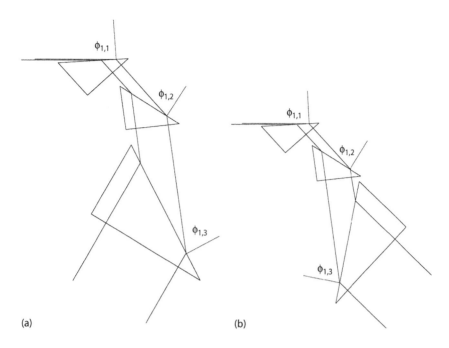

(a)   (b)

FIGURE 13.2 Multiple-prism expander, $r=3$, designed for orthogonal beam exit. (a) Deployment in an additive configuration. (b) Deployment in a compensating configuration yielding $\nabla\lambda\phi_{2,3}\approx0$. This particular depiction approximates a calculation suggested as a problem in using crown glass at $\lambda=590$ nm ($n\approx1.5167$). (Duarte, F. J., *Tunable Laser Optics*, Elsevier-Academic, New York, 2003.)

$$M = n^r \qquad (13.14)$$

One further case of practical significance is that of an array of r identical isosceles prisms, deployed symmetrically in additive configuration, so that $\phi_{1,m}=\phi_{2,m}$; then, Equation 13.3 reduces to [12,13]

$$\nabla_\lambda\phi_{2,r} = r\nabla_\lambda\phi_{2,1} \qquad (13.15)$$

The use of the generalized dispersion equations to design multiple-prism beam expanders with zero dispersion at a given wavelength, that is,

$$\nabla_\lambda\phi_{2,m} \approx 0 \qquad (13.16)$$

is described and discussed in [12,13,19]. Equations describing multiple-pass intracavity dispersion are given by Duarte and Piper [20] and also in [12,13,21].

13.2.1 MULTIPLE-PRISM DISPERSION THEORY OF LASER PULSE COMPRESSION

The generalized multiple-prism dispersion theory for laser pulse compression was introduced in 1982 [18]; in 1987, the second derivative of the refraction angle,

$\nabla_\lambda^2 \phi_{2,m}$, was exactly quantified [22]; and more recently, the theory has been extended to higher-phase derivatives [23,24]. For pulse compression, it is necessary to use the identity:

$$\nabla_n \phi_{2,m} = \nabla_\lambda \phi_{2,m} \left(\nabla_\lambda n_m \right)^{-1} \tag{13.17}$$

which allows Equation 13.3 to be reexpressed as [22]

$$\nabla_n \phi_{2,m} = \mathcal{H}_{2,m} + \left(\mathcal{M} \right)^{-1} \left(\mathcal{H}_{1,m} \pm \nabla_n \phi_{2,(m-1)} \right) \tag{13.18}$$

where

$$k_{1,m}^{-1} k_{2,m}^{-1} = \left(\mathcal{M}^{-1} \right) \tag{13.19}$$

Observing the progression of the higher derivatives, a generalized expression can be found to be [23,24]

$$\nabla_n^r \phi_{2,m} = \nabla_n^{r-1} \mathcal{H}_{2,m} + \left(\mathcal{M} \right)^{-1} \left(\nabla_n + \zeta \right)^{r-1} \tag{13.20}$$

where

$$\zeta^s = \nabla_n^s \mathcal{H}_{1,m} \pm \nabla_n^{s+1} \phi_{2,(m-1)} \tag{13.21}$$

$$\zeta^0 = 1 = \mathcal{H}_{1,m} \pm \nabla_n \phi_{2,(m-1)} \tag{13.22}$$

Here, it is very important that when writing the expansion in r in Equation 13.21, the term $\zeta^0 = 1$ be included as defined in Equation 13.22. Also, in Equation 13.21, the maximum value of the s exponent is $s = (r - 1)$. More specifically,

$$\nabla_n^1 \phi_{2,m} = \nabla_n^0 \mathcal{H}_{2,m} + \left(\mathcal{M} \right)^{-1} \left(\nabla_n + \zeta \right)^0 \tag{13.23}$$

$$\nabla_n^1 \phi_{2,m} = \nabla_n^0 \mathcal{H}_{2,m} + \left(\mathcal{M} \right)^{-1} 1 \tag{13.24}$$

$$\nabla_n \phi_{2,m} = \mathcal{H}_{2,m} + \left(\mathcal{M} \right)^{-1} \left(\mathcal{H}_{1,m} \pm \nabla_n \phi_{2,(m-1)} \right) \tag{13.25}$$

$$\begin{aligned} \nabla_n^2 \phi_{2,m} = \ &\nabla_n \mathcal{H}_{2,m} \\ &+ \left(\nabla_n \mathcal{M}^{-1} \right) \left(\mathcal{H}_{1,m} \pm \nabla_n \phi_{2,(m-1)} \right) \\ &+ \left(\mathcal{M}^{-1} \right) \left(\nabla_n \mathcal{H}_{1,m} \pm \nabla_n^2 \phi_{2,(m-1)} \right) \end{aligned} \tag{13.26}$$

$$\nabla_n^3 \phi_{2,m} = \nabla_n^2 \mathcal{H}_{2,m}$$

$$+\left(\nabla_n^2 \mathcal{M}^{-1}\right)\left(\mathcal{H}_{1,m} \pm \nabla_n \phi_{2,(m-1)}\right)$$

$$+2\left(\nabla_n \mathcal{M}^{-1}\right)\left(\nabla_n \mathcal{H}_{1,m} \pm \nabla_n^2 \phi_{2,(m-1)}\right) \tag{13.27}$$

$$+\left(\mathcal{M}^{-1}\right)\left(\nabla_n^2 \mathcal{H}_{1,m} \pm \nabla_n^3 \phi_{2,(m-1)}\right)$$

Higher-phase derivatives are given explicitly by Duarte [23–25], for instance,

$$\nabla_n^7 \phi_{2,m} = \nabla_n^6 \mathcal{H}_{2,m}$$

$$+\left(\nabla_n^6 \mathcal{M}^{-1}\right)\left(\mathcal{H}_{1,m} \pm \nabla_n \phi_{2,(m-1)}\right)$$

$$+6\left(\nabla_n^5 \mathcal{M}^{-1}\right)\left(\nabla_n \mathcal{H}_{1,m} \pm \nabla_n^2 \phi_{2,(m-1)}\right)$$

$$+15\left(\nabla_n^4 \mathcal{M}^{-1}\right)\left(\nabla_n^2 \mathcal{H}_{1,m} \pm \nabla_n^3 \phi_{2,(m-1)}\right)$$

$$+20\left(\nabla_n^3 \mathcal{M}^{-1}\right)\left(\nabla_n^3 \mathcal{H}_{1,m} \pm \nabla_n^4 \phi_{2,(m-1)}\right)$$

$$+15\left(\nabla_n^2 \mathcal{M}^{-1}\right)\left(\nabla_n^4 \mathcal{H}_{1,m} \pm \nabla_n^5 \phi_{2,(m-1)}\right)$$

$$+6\left(\nabla_n \mathcal{M}^{-1}\right)\left(\nabla_n^5 \mathcal{H}_{1,m} \pm \nabla_n^6 \phi_{2,(m-1)}\right)$$

$$+\left(\mathcal{M}^{-1}\right)\left(\nabla_n^6 \mathcal{H}_{1,m} \pm \nabla_n^7 \phi_{2,(m-1)}\right) \tag{13.28}$$

For the special case of four isosceles prisms [26], at minimum deviation, and deployed at the Brewster angle of incidence, the dispersion and its derivative become [13,22]

$$\nabla_n \phi_{2,1} = \nabla_n \phi_{2,3} = 2 \tag{13.29}$$

$$\nabla_n \phi_{2,2} = \nabla_n \phi_{2,4} = 0 \tag{13.40}$$

$$\nabla_n^2 \phi_{2,1} = \nabla_n^2 \phi_{2,3} = 4n - \left(2/n^3\right) \tag{13.41}$$

$$\nabla_n^2 \phi_{2,2} = \nabla_n^2 \phi_{2,4} = 0 \tag{13.42}$$

A basic four-prism pulse compressor indicating the various incident and exit angles is depicted in Figure 13.3.

13.2.2 THE INTERFEROMETRIC ORIGIN OF ANGULAR DISPERSION

In a paper published in 1997, a succinct derivation of refraction was given, which established the following hierarchic description of optics: interference, diffraction, and refraction [27]. The next reductive step following refraction, namely, reflection, was added in 2003 [13]. Apart from succinctness, the beauty of this interferometric

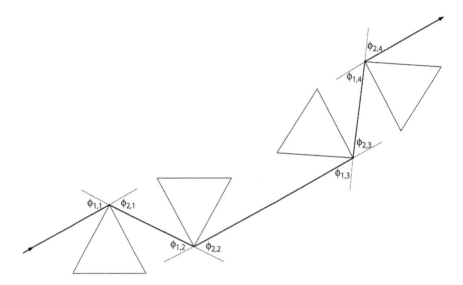

FIGURE 13.3 Four-prism pulse compressor configured from two basic two-prism components unfolded at the symmetry axis.

approach, via Dirac's notation, is that it naturally opens further refractive avenues. A brief description of this approach is provided here from a slightly different perspective from that published in the recent literature [28].

Following the convention introduced in [28], and in reference to Figure 13.4, for incidence above the normal, the sign of the angle is defined as positive (+). For diffraction below the normal, the diffraction angle is defined as negative (−). In reference to Figure 13.5, for incidence below the normal, the sign of the angle is defined as negative (−). For diffraction below the normal, the diffraction angle is also defined as negative (−). Alternative cases of incidence and diffraction are illustrated in [28], and it is clear that there is a ± alternative associated with diffraction. The traditional description associated with incidence below the normal (−) and diffraction above the normal (+) is described in [28].

Interference associated with ± incidence or ± diffraction, as it occurs in nature, is accurately described by the generalized interferometric equation introduced in Chapter 10 [13,29–31]:

$$|\langle x \mid s \rangle|^2 = \sum_{j=1}^{N} \Psi(r_j)^2 + 2 \sum_{j=1}^{N} \Psi(r_j) \left(\sum_{m=j+1}^{N} \Psi(r_m) \cos(\Omega_m - \Omega_j) \right) \quad (13.43)$$

The interferometric term of this equation, given in the inner parentheses, in conjunction with the detailed geometrical terms [13,31], leads to the following diffraction equation allowing all the incidence and diffraction alternatives:

$$d_m \left(\pm n_1 \sin \Theta_m \pm n_2 \sin \Phi_m \right) \left(\frac{2\pi}{\lambda_v} \right) = L\pi \quad (13.44)$$

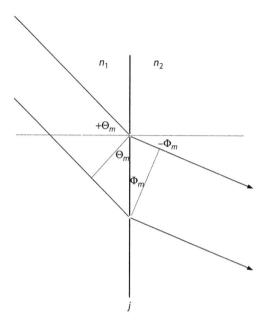

FIGURE 13.4 The plane of the slits (j) illustrating incidence above the normal $+\Theta_m$ and diffraction below the normal $-\Phi_m$. This diffraction alternative eventually leads to the equation for positive refraction known as Snell's law (see Equation 13.47).

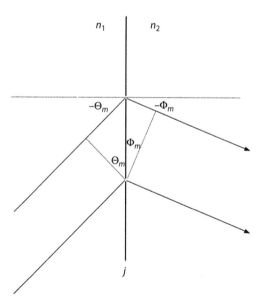

FIGURE 13.5 The plane of the slits (j) illustrating incidence below the normal $-\Theta_m$ and diffraction below the normal $-\Phi_m$ (see text). This diffraction alternative eventually leads to the equation for negative refraction given by Equation 13.50.

This is a generalized form of the diffraction grating equation, in which, in reference to Figures 13.4 and 13.5, n_1 and n_2 represent the refractive indices of two adjacent regions separated by the slit array comprising the diffraction grating, Θ_m is the angle of incidence, Φ_m is the angle of refraction, d_m is the sum of the dimensions of the mth slit plus the corresponding isle, and $L = 0, 2, 4, \ldots$. Also, in this equation, $2\pi/\lambda_v$ is related to the wavenumbers associated with the two refractive index regions [31].

For incidence above the normal and diffraction below the normal (see Figure 13.4), Equation 13.44 becomes

$$d_m \left(+n_1 \sin \Theta_m - n_2 \sin \Phi_m \right) \left(\frac{2\pi}{\lambda_v} \right) = L\pi \qquad (13.45)$$

As explained in [13,27], for the condition $d_m \ll \lambda$, diffraction ceases to occur, and the equation can only be solved for $L = 0$, so that

$$\left(+n_1 \sin \Theta_m - n_2 \sin \Phi_m \right) = 0 \qquad (13.46)$$

which leads directly to the well-known law of refraction also known as Snell's law:

$$n_1 \sin \Theta_m = n_2 \sin \Phi_m \qquad (13.47)$$

For incidence below the normal and diffraction below the normal (see Figure 13.5), Equation 13.44 becomes

$$d_m \left(-n_1 \sin \Theta_m - n_2 \sin \Phi_m \right) \left(\frac{2\pi}{\lambda_v} \right) = L\pi \qquad (13.48)$$

which again, for the condition $d_m \ll \lambda$, can only be solved for $L = 0$, so that

$$\left(-n_1 \sin \Theta_m - n_2 \sin \Phi_m \right) = 0 \qquad (13.49)$$

leading directly to the equation for negative refraction:

$$-n_1 \sin \Theta_m = n_2 \sin \Phi_m \qquad (13.50)$$

Using these results and the two alternative cases discussed in [28], a more general refraction equation emerges:

$$\pm n_1 \sin \Theta_m \pm n_2 \sin \Phi_m = 0 \qquad (13.51)$$

Thus, the equations describing propagation via a generalized hypothetical prism, exhibiting both positive and negative refraction, become [28]

$$\phi_{1,m} + \phi_{2,m} = \varepsilon_m \pm \alpha_m \qquad (13.52)$$

$$\psi_{1,m} + \psi_{2,m} = \alpha_m \tag{13.53}$$

$$\sin\phi_{1,m} = \pm n_m \sin\psi_{1,m} \tag{13.54}$$

$$\sin\phi_{2,m} = \pm n_m \sin\psi_{2,m} \tag{13.55}$$

and the generalized single-pass multiple-prism dispersion equation is modified to [28]

$$\nabla_\lambda\phi_{2,m} = \pm\mathcal{H}_{2,m}\nabla_\lambda n_m \pm \left(k_{1,m}k_{2,m}\right)^{-1}\left(\mathcal{H}_{1,m}\nabla_\lambda n_m \left(\pm\right)\nabla_\lambda\phi_{2,(m-1)}\right) \tag{13.56}$$

where the signs in parentheses refer to deployment at either a positive (+) or a compensating (−) configuration, while the simple ± is indicative of either positive or negative refraction. Thus, the interferometric foundations for either positive or negative refraction have been established [28]. As discussed in this chapter, the geometrical implications of negative refraction, for a double-prism beam expansion alone, signify a potential increase of ×4 in the number of possible geometrical permutations [28]. This chapter also discussed the use of a multiple-prism beam expander "in reverse," thus performing the function of a geometrical beam compressor. Relative to Figure 13.2, propagation toward the right results in spatial expansion, while propagation toward the left results in spatial compression (see Section 13.3.1).

13.3 DUAL MULTIPLE-PRISM BEAM EXPANDERS

The multiple-prism beam expanders illustrated in Figure 13.2 expand in one plane only. Thus, they are sometimes referred to as *one-dimensional beam expanders*. The expansion occurs parallel to the plane of incidence, which is perpendicular to the direction of propagation, as illustrated in Figure 13.2 for a double-prism beam expander. Obviously, if an identical second multiple-prism beam expander is deployed following a first multiple-prism beam expander, providing a beam expansion M but at an angle of $\pi/2$, while also providing a beam-expansion factor of $M_{\pi/2}=M$, then the resulting beam has a circular cross section, as illustrated in Figure 13.6.

The single double-prism beam expander is discussed in detail by Duarte [25] and consists of two prisms made of fused silica, with $n=1.4583$ at $\lambda\approx590$ nm and an apex angle of 42.7098°. Both prisms are deployed to yield identical magnifications and for orthogonal beam exit, so that

$$\phi_{1,1} = \phi_{1,2} = 81.55° \quad \psi_{1,1} = \psi_{1,2} = 42.7098° \quad \phi_{2,1} = \phi_{2,2} = 0° \quad \psi_{2,1} = \psi_{2,2} = 0°$$

$$\psi_{2,1} = \psi_{2,2} = 0°$$

and

$$M = k_{1,1}\,k_{1,2} = 25.0045$$

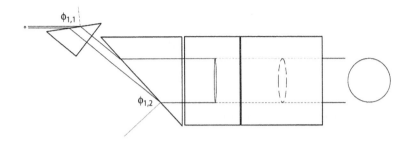

FIGURE 13.6 Dual multiple-prism beam expander producing circular beam expansion. The first double-prism beam expander, viewed from the top, expands the input beam by a factor of $M_1 \approx 25$ parallel to the plane of incidence. The second identical double-prism beam expander, rotated by $\pi/2$ relative to the first array and viewed from the side, also expands the beam by a factor of 25, but in a direction perpendicular to the plane of incidence. Thus, the resulting beam is not an extremely elongated Gaussian beam, but a Gaussian beam with a *circular cross section*, with a total beam expansion of 25.

This alternative might be attractive relative to traditional telescopic beam expansion if a nonfocusing beam expansion is needed or if a given circular beam expansion is required in applications demanding a reduced, or tight, longitudinal space.

13.3.1 MULTIPLE-PRISM ARRAYS FOR BEAM GEOMETRICAL COMPRESSION

Duarte [28] also discussed the use of a multiple-prism beam expander "in reverse," thus performing the function of a geometrical beam compressor. Relative to Figure 13.2, propagation toward the right results in spatial, or geometrical, beam expansion, while propagation toward the left results in geometrical beam compression. More specifically, using the double-prism expander example discussed previously, geometrical beam compression is illustrated in Figure 13.7. Thus, an extremely elongated Gaussian beam is compressed into a small circular Gaussian beam. Obviously, the principle is also applicable to compression from a large circular

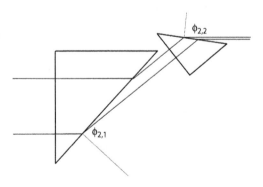

FIGURE 13.7 Multiple-prism beam compressor compressing the incidence beam by a factor of $C \approx 25$ parallel to the plane of incidence.

Gaussian beam to a small cross section circular Gaussian beam, as illustrated in the right-to-left propagation of Figure 13.5.

13.4   APPLICATIONS TO LASER OPTICS

The application of multiple-prism beam expanders as intracavity elements in narrow-linewidth tunable lasers has been well documented in various reviews [2,12,13,32]. Beam-expansion factors provided by these prismatic expanders are approximately in the $25 \leq M \leq 100$ range [12], depending on the type of cavity configuration, although higher magnifications can be easily provided. Multiple-prism expanders in multiple-prism Littrow grating oscillators and hybrid multiple-prism grazing-incidence grating oscillators are depicted in Chapters 4 and 5.

In addition to the initial application of multiple-prism assemblies, in multiple-prism grating configurations for dye lasers [8–12], these prismatic beam expanders have also been applied to gas lasers [33–35] and semiconductor lasers [36,37]. For the case of gas lasers, single-longitudinal-mode oscillation has been reported for cavity lengths of approximately 107 cm at $\Delta v \approx 140$ MHz [34]. This result is particularly relevant to contemporary fiber lasers, in which well-designed multiple-prism grating configurations should yield tunable single-longitudinal-mode lasing. A multiple-prism grating configuration for tunable fiber lasers is described in Chapter 6.

The use of prism pairs, as first outlined by Brewster [3], as extracavity components to correct the beam profile of semiconductor or diode lasers is also a well-known application [38].

13.5   APPLICATIONS TO LASER SPECTROSCOPY AND LASER ISOTOPE SEPARATION

One of the first applications of tunable lasers, incorporating intracavity multiple-prism beam expansion to illuminate the whole width of the tuning grating, was laser spectroscopy [39–41]. In particular, double-resonance spectroscopy, where one of the lasers was a tunable narrow-linewidth ultraviolet dye laser incorporating a multiple-prism beam expander and a 3600 line/mm holographic grating [39,40]. Recent interesting experiments performed with multiple-prism grating tunable lasers have studied time-resolved atomic spectroscopy in beryllium [42] and ionized iron [43].

An additional application for narrow-linewidth multiple-prism grating tunable lasers is the sequential excitation of atomic species and atomic vapor laser isotope separation [10,11,44–48], as discussed in Chapter 11. Further references on this topic are given in Chapter 1.

13.6   APPLICATIONS TO GUIDE STARS AND ASTRONOMY

Copper-vapor laser (CVL)-pumped narrow-linewidth dye lasers, incorporating multiple-prism grating cavity configurations, emit in the $565 \leq \lambda \leq 605$ nm range [11]. A high average power CVL-pumped dye laser system, using multiple-prism beam expansion in its oscillator, was used in early experiments for *guide star* applications [46]. The guide star concept is used to correct for atmospheric turbulence, in conjunction with adaptive optics, at large terrestrial telescopes. This laser beacon principle [49] uses the sodium layer in the mesosphere, which is at an altitude of 80–100 km. Fugate [49] discusses pulse energy requirements and provides a historical introduction to the subject. The sodium transition used is the D_2 line, at $\lambda = 588.9963$ nm, which has an absorption linewidth of ~3 GHz. These requirements make high-power narrow-linewidth dye lasers, yielding laser linewidths in the $350 \leq \Delta v \leq 700$ MHz range, ideally suited for this application. The use of continuous-wave dye laser systems for this application is discussed in [50].

Multiple-prism beam expanders have also been found useful by researchers working in imaging systems for astronomy, in particular in the subfield of astrometry [51]. The imaging application discussed by these authors is related to the precise cataloguing of large numbers of stars [51].

Multiple-prism arrays, in compensating configurations, with prisms right next to each other, as illustrated in Figure 13.8, are known as Amici prisms, compound prisms, or direct vision prisms. These prism arrays are used in astronomy [52] to correct for atmospheric refraction while yielding a direct line of sight. Recently, Duarte [24,25], calculated the overall dispersion of Amici prisms composed of three prisms via Equation 13.3. For a single prism, the beam is deviated while yielding a dispersion of [25]

$$\nabla_\lambda \phi_{2,1} \approx -0.0386$$

while for a three-prism Amici configuration, the beam is straight while yielding an overall dispersion of [25]

$$\nabla_\lambda \phi_{2,3} \approx +0.0720$$

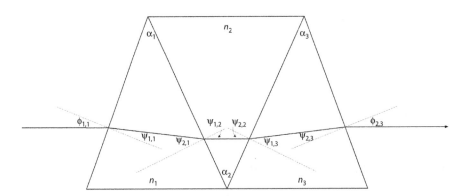

FIGURE 13.8 Amici prism composed of three prisms. The first and third prisms are made of fused silica, while the complementary prism at the center is made of a higher refractive index SF10 prism. Drawing not to scale. (Reproduced from Duarte, F. J., *Tunable Laser Optics*, 2nd edn, CRC Press, New York, 2015. With permission from Taylor & Francis Group.)

13.7 APPLICATIONS TO PULSE COMPRESSION IN ULTRASHORT PULSE LASERS

The dispersive laser linewidth equation:

$$\Delta\lambda = \Delta\theta(\nabla_\lambda\Theta)^{-1}$$

directly links the laser linewidth to intracavity dispersion. This equation immediately suggests that minimizing intracavity dispersion leads to broadband laser emission: that is, very large $\Delta\lambda$, and hence very large Δv. Heisenberg's uncertainty principle [53]:

$$\Delta p\Delta x \approx h \tag{13.57}$$

leads directly to [13]

$$\Delta v\Delta t \approx 1 \tag{13.58}$$

Thus, for minimal intracavity dispersion, broad bandwidth emission is possible, which allows ultrashort pulse emission. As discussed in Section 13.2.1, detailed and exact multiple-prism dispersion equations to evaluate the various derivatives applicable to laser pulse compression are available.

Prismatic pulse compression was first demonstrated by Dietel et al. [54]. Multiple-prism arrays in the form of double prisms [55], four prisms [23], double-prism pairs [56], and six prisms [57] have become widely used as pulse compressors in lasers yielding ultrashort pulses in the femtosecond domain.

The effect of minute beam deviations on the overall multiple-prism dispersion $\nabla_n\phi_{2,m}$ and its derivative $\nabla_n^2\phi_{2,m}$ was calculated by Duarte [58]. In a series of experiments, Osvay et al. [59–61] investigated the fine-tuning of intracavity dispersions in femtosecond lasers, obtaining excellent agreement between theory [22,58] and experiment in an 18 fs laser incorporating a prism-pair pulse compressor [61].

An extensive review on prismatic pulse compression is given by Diels and Rudolph [62], and a recent study on pulse compression with prism pairs was reported in [63].

13.8 APPLICATIONS TO MICROSCOPY AND ULTRAFAST SPECTROSCOPY

Ultrashort pulse lasers emitting in the femtosecond region have generated a renaissance in the field of microscopy. An introduction to this subject is given by Diels and Rudolph [62], and it is treated in detail by Rudolph and Thomas [64] in reference to biology. Microscopy in reference to the field of imaging is discussed in detail in Chapter 9.

Using a double-prism dispersion compensator, Nachay et al. [65] developed a femtosecond microscope with ~150 nm lateral resolution and ~250 fs temporal resolution. These authors applied their microscope to produce two-dimensional scans of GaAs/AlGaAs semiconductor structures [65]. The application of this type of instrument to characterize nanostructured materials, including single semiconductor quantum wires, with remarkable temporal and spatial resolution was reported by Siegner et al. [66].

Ultrafast dynamic studies of halogens in rare gas solids, using a laser system including prismatic compressors, have been performed by Gürh et al. [67]. The use of multiple-prism beam expanders in microscopes illuminated by tunable laser radiation is described in Chapter 9.

13.9 APPLICATIONS TO INTERFEROMETRY AND OPTICAL METROLOGY

Multiple-prism beam expanders have become integral components of various improved, and some unique optical instruments, including

Densitometers
Digital microscopes
Nanoscopes
Interferometric wavelength meters
Laser printers
Microdensitometers
N-slit interferometers
Spectrometers

These optical instruments are described in detail in the second edition of *Tunable Laser Optics* [25] and described in part in Chapter 10.

REFERENCES

1. Newton, I., *Opticks*, Royal Society, London, 1704.
2. Duarte, F. J., Newton, prisms, and the *opticks* of tunable lasers, *Opt. Photonics News* 11(5): 24–28, 2000.
3. Brewster, D., *A Treatise on New Philosophical Instruments for Various Purposes in the Arts and Sciences with Experiments on Light and Colours*, Murray and Blackwood, Edinburgh, 1813.
4. Strome, F. C. and J. P. Webb, Flashtube-pumped dye laser with multiple-prism tuning, *Appl. Opt.* 10: 1348–1353, 1971.
5. Hanna, D. C., P. A. Kärkkäinen, and R. Wyatt, A simple beam expander for frequency narrowing of dye lasers, *Opt. Quantum Elect.* 7: 115–119, 1975.
6. Klauminzer, G. K., Optical beam expander for dye laser, U.S. Patent 4127828, 1978.
7. Kasuya, T., T. Suzuki, and K. Shimoda, A prism anamorphic system for Gaussian beam expander, *Appl. Phys.* 17: 131–136, 1978.
8. Duarte, F. J. and J. A. Piper, A double-prism beam expander for pulsed dye lasers, *Opt. Commun.* 35: 100–104, 1980.
9. Duarte, F. J. and J. A. Piper, Prism preexpanded grazing-incidence grating cavity for pulsed dye lasers, *Appl. Opt.* 20: 2113–2116, 1981.
10. Duarte, F. J. and J. A. Piper, Comparison of prism-expander and grazing-incidence grating cavities for copper laser pumped dye lasers, *Appl. Opt.* 21: 2782–2786, 1982.
11. Duarte, F. J. and J. A. Piper, Narrow-linewidth, high-prf copper laser-pumped dye-laser oscillators, *Appl. Opt.* 23: 1391–1394, 1984.

12. Duarte, F. J., Narrow linewidth pulsed dye laser oscillators. In F. J. Duarte and L. W. Hillman (Eds), *Dye Laser Principles*, 1990, Chapter 4, Academic, New York.

13. Duarte, F. J., *Tunable Laser Optics*, Elsevier-Academic, New York, 2003.

14. Duarte, F. J., Transmission efficiency in achromatic nonorthogonal multiple-prism laser beam expanders, *Opt. Commun.* 71: 1–5, 1989.

15. Hänsch, T. W., Repetitively pulsed tunable dye laser for high resolution spectroscopy, *Appl. Opt.* 11: 895–898, 1972.

16. Duarte, F. J., Cavity dispersion equation $\Delta\lambda \approx \Delta\theta(\partial\theta/\partial\lambda)^{-1}$: A note on its origin, *Appl. Opt.* 31: 6979–6982, 1992.

17. Duarte, F. J. and J. A. Piper, Dispersion theory of multiple-prism beam expander for pulsed dye lasers, *Opt. Commun.* 43: 303–307, 1982.

18. Duarte, F. J. and J. A. Piper, Generalized prism dispersion theory, *Am. J. Phys.* 51: 1132–1134, 1983.

19. Duarte, F. J., Note on achromatic multiple-prism beam expanders, *Opt. Commun.* 53: 259–262, 1985.

20. Duarte, F. J. and J. A. Piper, Multi-pass dispersion theory of prismatic pulsed dye lasers, *Opt. Acta* 31: 331–335, 1984.

21. Duarte, F. J., Multiple-return-pass beam divergence and the linewidth equation, *Appl. Opt.* 40: 3038–3041, 2001.

22. Duarte, F. J., Generalized multiple-prism dispersion theory for pulse compression in ultrafast dye lasers, *Opt. Quantum Elect.* 19: 223–229, 1987.

23. Duarte, F. J., Generalized multiple-prism dispersion theory for laser pulse compression: Higher order phase derivatives, *Appl. Phys. B* 96: 809–814, 2009.

24. Duarte, F. J., Tunable laser optics: Applications to optics and quantum optics, *Prog. Quantum Elect.* 37: 326–347, 2013.

25. Duarte, F. J., *Tunable Laser Optics*, 2nd edn, CRC Press, New York, 2015.

26. Fork, R. L., O. E. Martínez, and J. P. Gordon, Negative dispersion using pairs of prisms, *Opt. Lett.* 9: 150–152, 1984.

27. Duarte, F. J., Interference, diffraction, and refraction, via Dirac's notation, *Am. J. Phys.* 65: 637–640, 1997.

28. Duarte, F. J., Multiple-prism dispersion equations for positive and negative refraction, *Appl. Phys. B* 82: 35–38, 2006.

29. Duarte, F. J. and D. J. Paine, Quantum mechanical description of N-slit interference phenomena. In R. C. Sze and F. J. Duarte (Eds), *Proceedings of the International Conference on Lasers '88*, pp. 42–27, STS, McLean, VA, 1989.

30. Duarte, F. J., Dispersive dye lasers. In F. J. Duarte (Ed.), *High Power Dye Lasers*, Chapter 2, Springer, Berlin, 1991.

31. Duarte, F. J., On a generalized interference equation and interferometric measurements, *Opt. Commun.* 103: 8–14, 1993.

32. Duarte, F. J., Multiple-prism arrays in laser optics, *Am. J. Phys.* 68: 162–166, 2000.

33. Duarte, F. J., Variable linewidth high-power TEA CO_2 laser, *Appl. Opt.* 24: 34–37, 1985.

34. Duarte, F. J., Multiple-prism Littrow and grazing-incidence pulsed CO_2 lasers, *Appl. Opt.* 24: 1244–1245, 1985.

35. Sze, R. C. and D. G. Harris, Tunable excimer lasers. In F. J. Duarte (Ed.), *Tunable Lasers Handbook*, Chapter 3, Academic, New York, 1995.

36. Duarte, F. J., Dispersive external-cavity semiconductor lasers. In F. J. Duarte (Ed.), *Tunable Laser Applications*, 1st edn, Chapter 3, Marcel-Dekker, New York, 1995.

37. Zorabedian, P., Tunable external-cavity semiconductor lasers. In F. J. Duarte (Ed.), *Tunable Lasers Handbook*, Chapter 8, Academic, New York, 1995.

38. Hughes, D. W. and J. R. M. Barr, Laser diode pumped solid state lasers, *J. Phys. D: Appl. Phys.* 25: 563–586, 1992.

39. Duval, A. B., D. A. King, R. Haines, N. R. Isenor, and B. J. Orr, Fluorescence-detected Raman-optical double-resonance spectroscopy of glyoxal vapor, *J. Opt. Soc. Am. B* 2: 1570–1581, 1985.

40. Duarte, F. J., Technology of pulsed dye lasers. In F. J. Duarte and L. W. Hillman (Eds), *Dye Laser Principles*, Chapter 6, Academic, New York, 1990.

41. Murray, J. R., Lasers for spectroscopy. In L. J. Radziemski, R. W. Solarz, and J. A. Paisner (Eds), *Laser Spectroscopy and its Applications*, Chapter 2, Marcel Dekker, New York, 1987.

42. Schnabel, R. and M. Kock, *f*-value measurements of the Be I resonance line using a nonlinear time-resolved laser-induced-fluorescence technique, *Phys. Rev. A* 61: 062506, 2000.

43. Schnabel, R. and M. Kock, Time-resolved nonlinear laser-induced fluorescence technique for a combined lifetime and branching-fraction measurement, *Phys. Rev. A* 63: 012519, 2000.

44. Broyer, M. and J. Chevaleyre, CVL-pumped dye laser for spectroscopic applications, *Appl. Phys. B* 35: 31–36, 1984.

45. Webb, C. E., High-power dye lasers pumped by copper-vapor lasers. In F. J. Duarte (Ed.), *High Power Dye Lasers*, Chapter 5, Springer, Berlin, 1991.

46. Bass, I. L., R. E. Bonanno, R. P. Hackel, and P. R. Hammond, High-average-power dye laser at Lawrence Livermore National Laboratory, *Appl. Opt.* 31: 6993–7006, 1992.

47. Singh, S., K. Dasgupta, S. Kumar, K. G. Manohar, L. G. Nair, and U. K. Chatterjee, High-power high-repetition-rate copper-vapor-pumped dye laser, *Opt. Eng.* 33: 1894–1904, 1994.

48. Sugiyama, A., T. Nakayama, M. Kato, Y. Maruyama, and T. Arisawa, Characteristics of a pressure-tuned single-mode dye laser oscillator pumped by a copper vapor laser, *Opt. Eng.* 35: 1093–1097, 1996.

49. Fugate, R. Q., Laser beacon adaptive optics, *Opt. Photon. News.* 4(6): 14–19, 1993.

50. Pique, J.-P. and S. Farinotti, Efficient modeless laser for mesospheric sodium laser guide star, *J. Opt. Soc. Am. B* 20: 2093–2101, 2003.

51. Sirat, G. Y., K. Wilner, and D. Neuhauser, Uniaxial crystal interferometer: Principles and forecasted applications to imaging astrometry, *Opt. Express.* 13: 6310–6322, 2005.

52. Wynne, C. G., Atmospheric dispersion in very large telescopes with adaptive optics, *MNRAS* 285: 130–134, 1997.

53. Dirac, P. A. M., *The Principles of Quantum Mechanics*, 4th edn, Oxford University, London, 1978.

54. Dietel, W., J. J. Fontaine, and J.-C. Diels, Intracavity pulse compression, with glass: A new method of generating pulses shorter than 60 fsec, *Opt. Lett.* 8: 4–6, 1983.

55. Kafka, J. D. and T. Baer, Prism-pair delay lines in optical pulse compression, *Opt. Lett.* 12: 401–403, 1987.

56. Chou, Y-F., C-H. Lee, and J. Wang, Characteristics of a femtosecond transform-limited Kerr-lens mode-locked dye laser, *Opt. Lett.* 19: 975–977, 1994.

57. Pang, L. Y., J. G. Fujimoto, and E. S. Kintzer, Ultrashort-pulse generation from high-power diode arrays by using intracavity optical nonlinearities, *Opt. Lett.* 17: 1599–1601, 1992.

58. Duarte, F. J., Prismatic pulse compression: Beam deviations and geometrical perturbations, *Opt. Quantum Elect.* 22: 467–471, 1990.

59. Osvay, K., P. Dombi, A. P. Kovács, and Z. Bor, Fine tuning of the higher-order dispersion of a prismatic pulse compressor, *Appl. Phys. B.* 75: 649–654, 2002.

60. Osvay, K., A. P. Kovács, Z. Heiner, G. Kurdi, J. Klebniczki, and M. Csatári, Angular dispersion and temporal change of femtosecond pulses from misaligned pulse compressors, *IEEE. J. Sel. Top. Quant.* 10: 213–220, 2004.

61. Osvay, K., A. P. Kovács, G. Kurdi, Z. Heiner, M. Divall, J. Klebniczki, and I. E. Ferincz, Measurement of non-compensated angular dispersion and the subsequent temporal lengthening of femtosecond pulses in a CPA laser, *Opt. Commun.* 248: 201–209, 2005.
62. Diels, J.-C. and W. Rudolph, *Ultrashort Laser Pulse Phenomena*, 2nd edn, Academic, New York, 2006.
63. Arissian, L. and J.-C. Diels, Carrier to envelope and dispersion control in a cavity with prism pairs, *Phys. Rev. A* 75: 013814, 2007.
64. Thomas, J. L. and W. Rudolph, Biological microscopy with ultrashort laser pulses. In F. J. Duarte (Ed.), *Tunable Laser Applications*, Chapter 9, 2nd edn, CRC Press, New York, 2009.
65. Nechay, B. A., U. Siegner, M. Achermann, H. Bielefeldt, and U. Keller, Femtosecond pump-probe near-field optical microscopy, *Rev. Sci. Instrum.* 70: 2758–2764, 1999.
66. Siegner, U., M. Achermann, and U. Keller, Spatially resolved femtosecond spectroscopy beyond the diffraction limit, *Meas. Sci. Technol.* 12: 1847–1857, 2001.
67. Gühr, M., M. Bargheer, M. Fushitani, T. Kiljunen, and N. Schwentner, Ultrafast dynamics of halogens in rare-gas solids, *Phys. Chem. Chem. Phys.* 9: 779–801, 2007.

14 Optical Quantities and Conversions of Units

F. J. Duarte

CONTENTS

14.1   INTRODUCTION

In this book, electromagnetic radiation is described in both frequency and wavelength units. For the sake of completeness, a brief description of the identities relating these units is provided here, in addition to relevant physical constants commonly used throughout the book.

The basic relation between wavelength, λ, and frequency, ν, is given by

$$\lambda = \frac{c}{\nu}$$

(14.1)

where:
  c is the speed of light
  c is given in meters per second
  λ is in meters
  ν is in Hz

Standard physical constants, such as c, are given in Table 14.1. The values of these constants are those listed by the National Institute of Science and Technology (NIST) available at the time of publication.

The Planck quantum energy is given by

$$E = h\nu$$

(14.2)

and the wavenumber, k, is defined as

$$k = \frac{2\pi}{\lambda}$$

(14.3)

TABLE 14.1
Physical Constants

Name	Symbol	Value	Units
Elementary charge	e	$1.602176487 \times 10^{-19}$	C
Permeability of vacuum[a]	μ_0	$4\pi \times 10^{-7}$	N/A^2
Permittivity of vacuum	ε_0	$8.854187817 \times 10^{-12}$	F/m
Planck constant	h	$6.62606896 \times 10^{-34}$	Js
Speed of light in vacuum	c	2.99792458×10^{8}	m/s

[a] $\pi \approx 3.141592654 \ldots$

14.2 LINEWIDTH EQUIVALENCE

For laser emission at any particular wavelength, λ, it is important to estimate the purity, or bandwidth, of this radiation. This is quantified by the width of the laser line, or linewidth, $\Delta\lambda$. As explained in [1], starting from Heisenberg's uncertainty principle [2]:

$$\Delta p \Delta x \approx h \tag{14.4}$$

one can write

$$\Delta\lambda \approx \frac{\lambda^2}{\Delta x} \tag{14.5}$$

which is an expression for linewidth in units of meters. Its equivalent expression in the frequency domain is

$$\Delta v \approx \frac{c}{\Delta x} \tag{14.6}$$

which provides the linewidth in Hz. It should also be mentioned that in spectroscopy, the *reciprocal centimeter* (cm⁻¹) is widely used as a unit of linewidth (see Chapter 2). This spectroscopist's linewidth can be obtained from Equation 14.6 in the form of

$$\frac{\Delta v}{c} \approx \frac{1}{\Delta x} \tag{14.7}$$

in units of 1/m. Conversion to units of reciprocal centimeters requires multiplication of Δx by 100, so that the spectroscopist's linewidth is calculated according to

$$\frac{1}{\Delta x'} \approx \frac{1}{100\Delta x} \tag{14.8}$$

TABLE 14.2

Linewidth Equivalence for $\Delta\lambda \approx 0.000406$ nm at $\lambda \approx 590$ nm

Linewidth Domain	Value
Wavelength	$\Delta\lambda \approx 0.0004064$ nm at $\lambda \approx 590$ nm
Frequency	$\Delta\nu \approx 350$ MHz
Spatial	$(1/\Delta x') \approx 0.0116747$ cm^{-1}

Thus, for a linewidth of $\Delta\nu \approx 30$ GHz, we get $(1/\Delta x') \approx 1$ cm^{-1}. To illustrate these conversions further, consider the laser linewidth of $\Delta\lambda \approx 0.0004064$ nm at $\lambda \approx 590$ nm, given in its three versions in Table 14.2.

By definition, according to Equation 14.5, when a linewidth is quoted as $\Delta\lambda$, the wavelength at which it was measured, or calculated, must also be quoted. Linewidths in the frequency or spatial domain are not a function of wavelength. For an introduction to reciprocal centimeter units, the reader is referred to Herzberg [3].

14.3 PHOTON-ENERGY WAVELENGTH EQUIVALENCE

In the x-ray field, as well as in spectroscopy [3] and semiconductor physics [4,5], the absorption and emission spectra can be characterized in units of electronvolts. The equivalence between energy and frequency is established in Planck's quantum energy equation. Thus, using Equations 14.1 and 14.2,

$$\lambda = \frac{hc}{E} \tag{14.9}$$

the equivalence is also made explicit for the wavelength domain. In Table 14.3, the equivalence of photon energy in electronvolts and wavelength is given for a few spectral values of interest. A graphical equivalence between the two domains is given in [6].

TABLE 14.3

Photon-Energy Wavelength Equivalence

Photon Energy	Wavelength (nm)[a]
1 eV	~ 1239.842
10 eV	~ 123.9842
100 eV	~ 12.39842
1 keV	~ 1.239842
10 keV	~ 0.123984

[a] Using 1 eV $= 1.602176487 \times 10^{-19}$ J.

REFERENCES

1. Duarte, F. J., *Tunable Laser Optics*, Elsevier-Academic, New York, 2003.
2. Dirac, P. A. M., *The Principles of Quantum Mechanics*, 4th edn, Oxford University, London, 1978.
3. Herzberg, G., *Spectra of Diatomic Molecules*, 2nd edn, Van Nostrand Reinhold, New York, 1950.
4. Kittel, C., *Introduction to Solid State Physics*, 4th edn, Wiley, New York, 1971.
5. Yariv, A., *Optical Electronics*, 3rd edn, Holt Rinehart and Winston, New York, 1985.
6. Carroll, F. and C. A. Brau, Medical applications of the free electron laser. In F. J. Duarte (Ed.), *Tunable Laser Applications*, Chapter 6, 1st edn, Marcel-Dekker, New York.

Index

Printed and bound by CPI Group (UK) Ltd, Croydon, CR0 4YY

01/11/2024

01782619-0017